T0314281

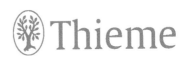

Medical Biochemistry

An Essential Textbook

Second Edition

Sankhavaram R. Panini, PhD
Associate Chair of Basic Biomedical Sciences
Professor and Course Director of Medical Biochemistry and Medical Genetics
Department of Basic Biomedical Sciences
Touro College of Osteopathic Medicine
Middletown, New York, USA

388 illustrations

Thieme
New York • Stuttgart • Delhi • Rio de Janeiro

Library of Congress Cataloging-in-Publication Data
is available from the publisher.

Important note: Medicine is an ever-changing science undergoing continual development. Research and clinical experience are continually expanding our knowledge, in particular our knowledge of proper treatment and drug therapy. Insofar as this book mentions any dosage or application, readers may rest assured that the authors, editors, and publishers have made every effort to ensure that such references are in accordance with **the state of knowledge at the time of production of the book.**

Nevertheless, this does not involve, imply, or express any guarantee or responsibility on the part of the publishers in respect to any dosage instructions and forms of applications stated in the book. **Every user is requested to examine carefully** the manufacturers' leaflets accompanying each drug and to check, if necessary in consultation with a physician or specialist, whether the dosage schedules mentioned therein or the contraindications stated by the manufacturers differ from the statements made in the present book. Such examination is particularly important with drugs that are either rarely used or have been newly released on the market. Every dosage schedule or every form of application used is entirely at the user's own risk and responsibility. The authors and publishers request every user to report to the publishers any discrepancies or inaccuracies noticed. If errors in this work are found after publication, errata will be posted at www.thieme.com on the product description page.

Some of the product names, patents, and registered designs referred to in this book are in fact registered trademarks or proprietary names even though specific reference to this fact is not always made in the text. Therefore, the appearance of a name without designation as proprietary is not to be construed as a representation by the publisher that it is in the public domain.

© 2021. Thieme. All rights reserved.

Thieme Medical Publishers, Inc.
333 Seventh Avenue, 18th Floor
New York, NY 10001, USA
www.thieme.com
+1 800 782 3488, customerservice@thieme.com

Cover design: Thieme Publishing Group
Cover illustrations:
DNA illustration © Sergey Nivens/stock.adobe.com
Human check © vegefox.com/stock.adobe.com
Typesetting by DiTech Process Solutions, India

Printed in the USA by King Printing Co., Inc.   5 4 3 2 1

ISBN 978-1-62623-744-5

Also available as an e-book:
eISBN 978-1-62623-745-2

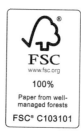

FSC
www.fsc.org
100%
Paper from well-managed forests
FSC® C103101

This book, including all parts thereof, is legally protected by copyright. Any use, exploitation, or commercialization outside the narrow limits set by copyright legislation, without the publisher's consent, is illegal and liable to prosecution. This applies in particular to photostat reproduction, copying, mimeographing, preparation of microfilms, and electronic data processing and storage.

This book is dedicated to my precious granddaughters:

Camila Panini Diez de Bonilla
Frida Panini Diez de Bonilla
Maya Grace Panini
Elina Jolie Panini

Key to *Medical Biochemistry: An Essential Textbook, Second Edition*

Color-Coded integration boxes

Therapeutics

Provides a clinical context and may include topics pertaining to disease and treatment.

Normal

Provides insights into normal functioning and may include biomechanics, physiology, hormone levels, etc.

Foundations

Provides fundamental information and links to the basic sciences.

Symbols

Shows clinical correlations at a glance

Inhibitors/negative regulators

⊖   —⊙⊣

Activators/stimulators/positive regulators

⊕   —⊙▶

Contents

Contents

Preface to the First Edition

In the past decade, the graduate medical curriculum, particularly in the first two years of medical school, has undergone innovative transformation. A major thrust of this transformation has been to present the core knowledge of basic and clinical sciences, spanning a number of disciplines, in a single integrated "Foundations" course. The goal is to train a competent physician who demonstrates knowledge of health problems and their prevention, based on current scientific thinking. It is my belief that while knowledge of the "who, what, where, and when" of health problems can be acquired from the study of many disciplines, it is biochemistry that provides the foundation for a thorough understanding of "why" such problems arise and "how" they can be effectively managed. The traditional, large textbooks were best-suited for use in the stand-alone biochemistry courses of the past, but with the advent of curricular reform, the need and demand for concise texts that emphasize the clinical relevance of basic biochemical knowledge and allow for quick review and self-directed learning has grown. *Medical Biochemistry – An Illustrated Review* was created to fulfill this need.

The biochemical principles in *Medical Biochemistry – An Illustrated Review* are structured and presented in a manner that allows for easy learning/review of key concepts and clear understanding of their connections to clinical conditions and other basic science subjects (e.g., physiology, pathology, and pharmacology). The more than 200 full-color illustrations of biochemical pathways/systems were designed specifically to meet the high-yield learning needs of medical students. Key features of these illustrations include the use of easily identifiable color-coded symbols that, for critical enzymes, highlight their modes of regulation, sensitivities to pharmacological agents, and associated clinical disorders. The more than 400 color-coded correlation boxes serve to connect key biochemical concepts with the other basic sciences and clinical conditions. The collection of 400 factual and USMLE style questions (with full explanatory answers) available on our companion website (200 of which are included in the book) are important tools for students to test their knowledge of the basic biochemical concepts and their ability to apply this knowledge in identifying and solving clinical problems.

In this book, I have used art from the Thieme Flexibook series to support and enhance the text and summarize many of the key points in a way that reinforces learning. I am particularly grateful to the illustrator Jürgen Wirth and the authors Professors Jan Koolmon and Klaus-Heinrich Roehm of *Color Atlas of Biochemistry*, second edition, revised and enlarged, from which a significant portion was adapted.

I am indebted to so many colleagues without whose contributions, generosity, and expertise, this project could not come to fruition. First of all, I am grateful to Anne Vinnicombe who oversaw the development and production aspects of the publication of the book and provided the needed guidance. She made sure that the wheels of this project kept turning despite various obstacles. My special thanks to Avalon Garcia, the developmental editor and a biochemist by training, who worked patiently and tirelessly with me not only in developing the content of many chapters but also in adapting and creating a majority of the illustrations and in developing questions. Renee Schwartz, Megan Conway, and Thieme's production team provided able editorial and production assistance. Julie O'Meara edited and wrote many of the boxes in Units IV (Metabolism) and V (Genetics and Cell Cycle). I particularly thank David Watt (University of Kentucky College of Medicine) for drafting the content in Chapter 16, Nucleotide and Heme Metabolism. I am thankful to several of my colleagues at Emory University School of Medicine who provided the inspiration for the content of many of the chapters in this book. The contributions of Engelbert Buxbaum (Ross University), Joseph D. Fontes (University of Kansas Medical Center), Karla Rodgers (University of Oklahoma Health Sciences Center) and J. David Warren (Weil Cornell Medical College) to the problem sets and to the review of the content are gratefully acknowledged. My thanks also to all of the reviewers of the manuscript for their many helpful suggestions.

All of the individuals involved in the publication of *Medical Biochemistry – An Illustrated Review* were united by a common goal which was to make concepts in biochemistry unintimidating, clinically relevant, and interesting. I hope we have accomplished this goal and welcome suggestions for improvements for future editions.

Sankhavaram R. Panini, PhD

Acknowledgments

I wish to express my gratitude to my colleagues at the Touro College of Osteopathic Medicine, New York for their generous help in reviewing several chapters of *Medical Biochemistry: An Essential Textbook, Second Edition*. Drs. Judith Binstock, Mariluz Henshaw, and Vasudeva Kamath provided invaluable suggestions for improvement of the content.

I sincerely thank Dr. Shilpika Bagh of Medical University of the Americas (Nevis, West Indies) for revising many of the problem sets at the end of each unit as well as writing several new questions.

I acknowledge the Thieme editorial and production teams for making the second edition possible. In particular, I thank Delia DeTurris, Sarah Landis, Brenda Bunch, Mary Wilson, Torsten Scheihagen, and Jyothi Sriram for their patience and perseverance.

I thank all the reviewers for their critical reading of the manuscript.

Sankhavaram R. Panini, PhD

Part I

Nutrition and Biomolecules

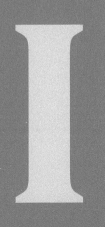

1 Nutrition and Digestion

1.1 Nutrition and Energy Requirements

1.1.1 Nutrients

Nutrients are organic and inorganic molecules that support the growth and survival of a living organism. Those utilized by humans can be divided into six major classes: carbohydrates, lipids, proteins, vitamins, water, and minerals. Nutrients are used for three major purposes:
1. To supply the energy needed for the body to perform work
2. To provide the building blocks for the synthesis of other important molecules
3. To support the function of metabolic pathways

Energy content of nutrients

The energy content of nutrients is an expression of the amount of heat released upon burning 1 g of a nutrient. This energy is measured in kilocalories (kcal); however, it is conventionally expressed as "calories" on the Nutrition Facts labels of foods. The energy content for the major energy nutrients are as follows:
- Carbohydrates: 4.1 kcal/g
- Proteins: 4.1 kcal/g
- Lipids: 9.3 kcal/g

> **Foundations**
> **Caloric content of alcohol**
> Ethanol (alcohol) can serve as a source of energy because its energy content is 7 kcal/g, which is higher than that of carbohydrates and proteins.

1.1.2 Diet

The daily energy requirements are met through the consumption of food. The Food and Nutrition Board (Institute of Medicine, National Academies) has defined the following terms as part of the Dietary Reference Intake (DRI) values for the six major groups of nutrients (▶ Fig. 1.1):

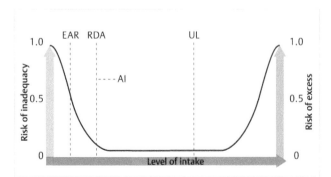

Fig. 1.1 Measures of nutrient intake. The risk of adverse effects (due to inadequate or excessive amounts of a specific nutrient) increases when nutrient intake is below the recommended dietary allowance (RDA) or above the upper level intake (UL). AI, adequate intake; EAR, estimated average requirement.

- **Adequate intake (AI)** is a recommended average daily nutrient intake level assumed to be adequate based on observed or experimentally determined estimates of daily nutrient intake by a group (or groups) of healthy people. AI is used when an RDA cannot be determined (e.g., for certain minerals).
- **Tolerable upper intake level (UL)** is the highest average daily nutrient intake level likely to pose no risk of adverse health effects to almost all individuals in a particular life stage and gender group. As intake increases above the UL, the potential risk of adverse health effects increases (see Section "Lipid-soluble Vitamins).
- **Estimated average requirement (EAR)** is the average daily nutrient intake level estimated to meet the requirement of 50% of the healthy individuals in a particular life stage and gender group.
- **Recommended dietary allowance (RDA)** is a value that represents the amount of a nutrient that, if consumed by every member of a population, will keep 98% of individuals (of a particular life stage and gender group) in good health.
  - The respective RDA for carbohydrates, lipids, and proteins is 60%, 30%, and 10% of an individual's daily caloric intake, which is further described in ▶ Table 1.1.
  - Consumption of a diet that is high in carbohydrates but deficient in protein causes a type of malnutrition called kwashiorkor; consumption of a diet that is deficient in both carbohydrates and proteins leads to another type of malnutrition called marasmus.

> **Therapeutics**
> **Kwashiorkor**
> Kwashiorkor is a form of malnutrition caused by consumption of a diet that lacks sufficient protein but is high in carbohydrates. In such cases, the total caloric intake is adequate, but not enough of it comes from protein. Individuals with this condition appear emaciated and irritable. They present with edema of the feet and hands, a swollen "moon" face, a distended abdomen, skin discolorations and lesions, and an enlarged fatty liver. Kwashiorkor is prevalent in weaning children from developing countries in which the food supply is limited.

> **Therapeutics**
> **Marasmus**
> Marasmus is a form of malnutrition caused by consumption of a calorie-deficient diet that lacks adequate amounts of carbohydrates and proteins. Patients with this condition appear emaciated with decreased subcutaneous fat. Unlike kwashiorkor, individuals with marasmus do not present with a distended abdomen.

Table 1.1 Nutrients' recommended dietary allowance (RDA)

Nutrient	% of Kcal	Kcal Based on a 2,000 kcal/d Diet (130–150 lb person)
Carbohydrates	60	1,200
Lipids	30	600
Proteins	10	200

Table 1.2 Factors that influence basal metabolic rate and its use in calculating the total energy expenditure

Factor	Effects on basal metabolic rate (BMR)
Gender	Male > female
Age	Child > adult
Health	• Elevated by fever • Elevated in individuals with hyperthyroidism (e.g., Graves disease) • Low in individuals with hypothyroidism (e.g., Hashimoto thyroiditis)
Hormones	• Elevated by high levels of thyroid hormones (e.g., thyroxine), growth hormones, sex hormones, epinephrine, and cortisol

Calculating BMR and total energy expenditure:
Men: BMR = 66 + (6.23 × weight in lb) + (12.7 × height in in.) – (6.8 × age in years)
Women: BMR = 655 + (4.35 × weight in lb) + (4.7 × height in in.) – (4.7 × age in years)
Total energy expenditure = BMR × physical activity level (PAL)

1.1.3 Total Energy Expenditure

Total energy expenditure is the amount of calories needed to meet the body's energy demands. It is dependent on age, weight, gender, diet, physical activity, and overall health, which are expressed in the following terms:

- **Basal metabolic rate (BMR)** is the amount of calories required to maintain normal physiological functions when the body is at rest and accounts for 60 to 70% of total energy expenditure. BMR varies with gender, age, health, and hormone levels (▶ Table 1.2) and is estimated using a formula that takes these factors into account.
- **Thermic effect of food (TEF)** represents the amount of calories expended during the digestion, absorption, and metabolism of nutrients. It accounts for ~10% of total energy expenditure.
- **Physical activity level (PAL)** accounts for the amount of calories required to support certain levels of physical exertion. It is expressed in values that range from 1.2 to 2.4. The lowest value represents the PAL of individuals engaged in no physical activity (e.g., bedridden persons); the highest value represents that of individuals engaged in strenuous forms of physical activity (e.g., performance athletes).

Therapeutics
Hashimoto thyroiditis
Another type of autoimmune disease that affects the thyroid is Hashimoto thyroiditis. In this case, the antibodies attack the thyroid gland and destroy its ability to synthesize thyroid hormones. This results in hypothyroidism, which is marked by fatigue, depression, constipation, abnormal sensitivity to cold, and modest weight gain. Treatment involves the administration of thyroid hormone.

Therapeutics
Graves disease
Graves disease is an autoimmune disorder in which antibodies bind to the thyroid-stimulating hormone (TSH) receptor on the surface of the thyroid gland and mimic the actions of TSH. This results in the production of excessive levels of thyroid hormones and hyperthyroidism, which is marked by goiter (enlarged thyroid gland), fatigue, restlessness, increased bowel movement, increased perspiration and heat intolerance, and weight loss. Treatment includes surgical resection of the thyroid gland, radioactive iodine to decrease the thyroid mass, or pharmacological intervention with antithyroid drugs such as propylthiouracil and methimazole.

Calculating total energy expenditure

Total energy expenditure is calculated by multiplying BMR and PAL. Weight gain occurs when caloric intake exceeds that of total energy expenditure. Likewise, weight loss occurs when caloric intake is less than that of total energy expenditure.

- For instance, because 1 lb of fat is equivalent to 3,500 kcal, individuals ingesting 3,500 kcal more than their total energy expenditure will gain 1 lb, or they will lose 1 lb if they ingest 3,500 kcal less than their total energy expenditure, over a certain period of time.

1.1.4 Body Mass Index

Body mass index (BMI) is an indirect method of determining "fatness" based on a person's weight and height. BMI is obtained by calculating the ratio of a person's weight to the square of his or her height, as seen in the following equation.

$$BMI = \frac{Weight(kg)}{Height(m)^2}$$

BMI is a useful tool for gauging an individual's risk for developing health problems based on the person's age-dependent category. The BMI ranges for the four categories (underweight, healthy, overweight, and obese) of those ages 19 to 34 are described in ▶ Fig. 1.2.

1.2 Digestion and Absorption

The energy nutrients—carbohydrates, lipids, and proteins—undergo enzymatic hydrolysis into their constituent parts

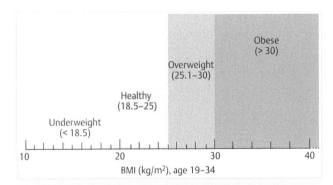

Fig. 1.2 Body mass index (BMI) of adults ages 19 to 34. The BMI of underweight individuals is less than 18.5 kg/m², and that of healthy individuals is between 18.5 and 25 kg/m². At a BMI of between 25.1 and 30 kg/m², a person may be classified as overweight; a BMI higher than 30 kg/m² identifies an individual as obese.

during digestion. These cleavage products, along with ingested vitamins and minerals, are absorbed by cells (enterocytes) of the gastrointestinal tract and delivered to the liver or the bloodstream. The segments of the gastrointestinal tract are the mouth, stomach, small intestine (duodenum, jejunum, ileum), large intestine, rectum, and anus. They work cooperatively with several glands and organs to ensure proper digestion, absorption, and excretion of nutrients and their degradation products, as follows (▶ Fig. 1.3):

- **Mouth:** It contains salivary glands that produce and secrete saliva, as well as salivary a-amylase and salivary lipase enzymes that respectively digest carbohydrates and lipids in the oral cavity.
- **Stomach:** It provides an acidic environment (pH < 2) that supports the function of gastric lipases and pepsin enzymes that respectively hydrolyze short- or medium-chain fatty acids and proteins.
- **Small intestine:** The first part, the duodenum, specifically provides an environment that supports further digestion of carbohydrates, lipids, and proteins with the aid of enzymes secreted by intestinal cells (for the hydrolysis of carbohydrates) and the pancreas (for the hydrolysis of carbohydrates, proteins, and lipids). The products of carbohydrate, protein, and lipid hydrolysis, as well as water, vitamins, and minerals, are absorbed from the lumen of the intestines via intestinal epithelial cells called enterocytes.
  - Disorders such as Crohn disease and celiac disease (nontropical sprue) are attributed to defects that disrupt the proper functioning of the small intestine.

- **Pancreas:** It functions as an exocrine gland that produces digestive enzymes, which are secreted into the duodenum, where they break down carbohydrates, lipids, and proteins. The pancreas also functions as an endocrine gland because its α- and β-cells respectively produce and secrete glucagon and insulin (glucagon when blood glucose levels are low and insulin when blood glucose is high). These hormones regulate nutrient uptake and metabolism.
  - Disorders such as cystic fibrosis and diabetes mellitus are marked by defects in the exocrine and endocrine functions of the pancreas, respectively.
- **Liver:** It synthesizes lipid-emulsifying molecules called bile salts, which are sent to the gallbladder for storage in bile. The products of nutrient digestion are sent to the liver for storage and metabolism.
- **Gallbladder:** It stores bile, a solution that contains lipid-emulsifying molecules such as conjugated bile salts. Bile is sent to the duodenum to aid in the digestion of lipids.
- **Kidneys:** They filter blood so that nutrients, minerals, and water are reabsorbed into the bloodstream, and metabolic waste products are excreted in urine.
- **Large intestine:** It is the site where most of the remaining water is absorbed, which contributes to the production of a solid stool. The latter is then stored in the rectum and excreted through the anus.

Therapeutics
Crohn disease

Crohn disease is an autoimmune disease that causes chronic inflammation and damage of bowel mucosa. The distal ileum is the most frequently involved site, and the disease often manifests as segments of diseased bowel separated by intervening sequences of normal bowel. In addition to nutritional deficiencies caused by malabsorption in the affected areas, abdominal pain, diarrhea, flatulence, bloating, anal itching, and skin lesions are common symptoms. Treatment includes surgical resection of the diseased segments of the intestine, pharmacological therapy consisting of antiinflammatory and immunosuppressive agents, and nutritional supplements.

Normal
Cystic fibrosis versus diabetes mellitus

As an endocrine gland, the pancreas synthesizes and secretes insulin and glucagon. As an exocrine gland, it secretes enzymes (e.g., α-amylase and lipase), in an alkaline fluid, directly into the duodenum to aid in digestion. When damage or inflammation of the pancreas (pancreatitis) is suspected, serum amylase and lipase levels are measured to confirm the diagnosis. Cystic fibrosis affects the function of the pancreas by forming mucous plugs that block the pancreatic ducts. This causes dilation of the ducts and atrophic fibrosis of the secretory cells. As a result, both exocrine and endocrine functions of pancreas are affected, leading to nutrient malabsorption and cystic fibrosis-related diabetes mellitus. Type 1 diabetes mellitus, on the other hand, affects the endocrine function of the pancreas but does not affect its exocrine function.

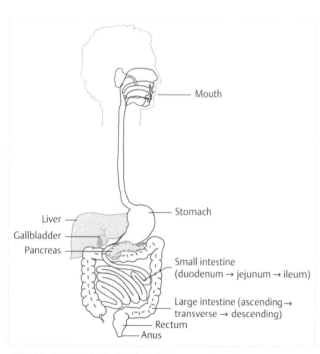

Fig. 1.3 Gastrointestinal tract and supportive organs. The gastrointestinal tract consists of the mouth, stomach, small intestine (duodenum, jejunum, ileum), large intestine (ascending, transverse, descending), rectum, and anus. The digestion/absorption-supportive organs include the pancreas, gall bladder, liver, and kidneys. Together they work in a cooperative manner to ensure the proper digestion, absorption, and excretion of nutrients and their degradation products.

1.3 Energy Nutrients: Carbohydrates, Lipids, and Proteins

1.3.1 Carbohydrates

Carbohydrates are the most plentiful energy source in the human diet and are available in the following forms (▶ Fig. 1.4):

- **Monosaccharides:** These simple sugars, such as glucose and fructose, are found in fruits and honey.
- **Disaccharides:** These carbohydrates, such as sucrose, lactose, and maltose, are composed of two monosaccharide units linked via a glycosidic bond. Sucrose is found in table sugar and fruits, lactose is found in milk, and maltose is found in malt sugar.
- **Oligosaccharides:** These carbohydrates are composed of from 3 to 10 monosaccharide units and are found in vegetables. Oligosaccharides are also found attached to proteins and lipids (e.g., glycoproteins and glycolipids, respectively) on the outer surface of cellular membranes in animals.
- **Polysaccharides:** These carbohydrates are composed of more than 10 monosaccharide units and are exemplified by glycogen (from animal products) and starch (from plant products).

Digestion and absorption

Various enzymes that contribute to the digestion and absorption of carbohydrates as they pass from the mouth to the intestines are as follows:

- α-Amylase: The breakdown of polysaccharides into oligosaccharides and disaccharides is catalyzed by salivary a-amylase (in the oral cavity) and pancreatic a-amylase (in the duodenum).
- Lactase, sucrase, maltase: Oligosaccharides and disaccharides are hydrolyzed into monosaccharides by the enzymes lactase (which targets lactose), sucrase (which targets sucrose), and maltase (which targets maltose). These enzymes are produced and secreted by intestinal cells. The resulting monosaccharides (e.g., glucose, galactose, and fructose) are absorbed by epithelial cells of the intestinal mucosa and transported by the portal circulation to target tissues.

Function

Glucose, the most important molecule for energy, is stored in the liver and muscle as glycogen, which can be degraded when energy is needed. Carbohydrates are also important components of cellular membranes (as components of glycolipids and glycoproteins), tissues (as components of bones and cartilage), and genetic material (as the sugar molecules in nucleic acids).

The metabolic pathways that harness the energy from carbohydrates and those that incorporate carbohydrates into macromolecules are described in Chapters 9 and 12.

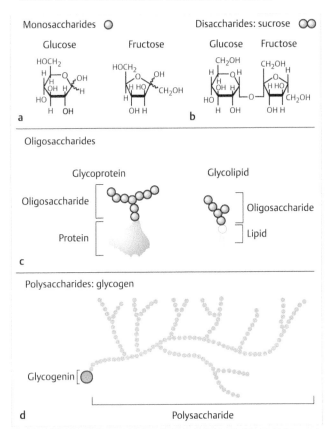

Fig. 1.4 Carbohydrates. Sugars may be classified as mono-, di-, oligo-, or polysaccharides. (**a**) Monosaccharides contain a single sugar molecule (e.g., glucose, fructose, and galactose). (**b**) Disaccharides contain two monosaccharides, which may be the same or different. In the example shown here, the disaccharide sucrose is made up of one glucose and one fructose. (**c**) Oligosaccharides are composed of 3 to 10 monosaccharide units. They are usually found attached to glycoproteins or glycolipids. (**d**) Polysaccharides (also called glycans) are linear or branched polymers of multiple monosaccharide units and can be quite large. One such example is glycogen, a branched polymer of glucose molecules.

Foundations

Hepatic portal system

The hepatic portal system consists of the portal vein and its associated blood vessels (splenic, superior mesenteric, and inferior mesenteric veins). It connects the gastrointestinal tract to the liver and mediates the transport of absorbed nutrients and drugs to the liver first. Many orally administered prodrugs are thus converted to their active forms in the liver (e.g., the cough suppressant dextromethorphan). Portal hypertension can often be caused by pre-, intra-, or posthepatic causes. Prehepatic causes include portal vein thrombosis. Intrahepatic causes include liver cirrhosis and fibrosis due to disorders such as hemochromatosis and Wilson disease. Posthepatic causes include thrombosis in the hepatic vein and the inferior vena cava. High blood pressure in the portal system forces blood into the systemic venous system leading to ascites, splenomegaly, and hepatic encephalopathy.

Foundations

Glucose transporters

The absorption of the monosaccharides glucose, galactose, and fructose by the epithelial cells that line the walls of the small intestine is mediated by glucose transporters (GLUTs). GLUTs bind to their target monosaccharide on one side of the cell membrane and undergo a conformational change to release it to the other side. For instance, sodium-glucose transporter 1 (SGLT1) cotransports one molecule of glucose or galactose along with two Na^+ molecules from the intestinal lumen to the cytosol of enterocytes. SGLT1 is unique among GLUTs in that it has two binding sites instead of one and can function even against a concentration gradient. Another example is GLUT5, a transporter that allows cells to take up or expel fructose via facilitated diffusion. The uptake of monosaccharides by cells of other tissues is facilitated by additional members of the GLUT family of transporters (see Chapter 12, box "GLUT2 in glucose sensing").

Normal

Type 1 diabetes mellitus

Diabetes mellitus (DM) is diagnosed when fasting plasma glucose is ≥ 126 mg/dL and/or when it is > 199 mg/dL 2 h after an oral dose of 75 g of glucose. It affects ~10% of the general population. A small fraction of the affected individuals (10%) are classified as type 1 or insulin-dependent DM. Type 1 DM results from a loss of pancreatic β cells in the islets of Langerhans (which secrete insulin), usually due to an autoimmune disorder. Symptoms of type 1 DM include polyuria, polydipsia, polyphagia, fatigue, and weight loss. An acute complication of type 1 DM is diabetic ketoacidosis. Treatment involves intramuscular administration of exogenous insulin (e.g., recombinant human insulin) to maintain fasting glucose levels < 100 mg/dL and postprandial glucose levels < 140 mg/dL.

1.3.2 Lipids

Ingested lipids consist of a heterogeneous mixture of hydrophobic molecules (▶ Fig. 1.5) that includes the following:
- Fatty acids: These monocarboxylic acids, which contain hydrocarbon chains, are either saturated (zero double bonds), monounsaturated (one double bond), or polyunsaturated (two or more double bonds).
- Triacylglycerols: These lipids are composed of three fatty acids attached to a glycerol backbone. They are stored in adipose tissue as fat.
- Cholesterol and cholesterol esters: These hydrophobic molecules respectively consist of free cholesterol and a cholesterol molecule esterified to a fatty acid.
- Membrane lipids: Phospholipids are found in cellular membranes and are composed of fatty acids attached to a glycerol backbone (glycerophospholipids) or a sphingosine backbone (sphingophospholipids). A phosphate group is esterified to the glycerol and sphingosine backbones. Other membrane lipids, called glycolipids, include those that

contain a fatty acid chain attached to a sphingosine backbone, which is in turn attached to carbohydrate residues.
- Lipid-soluble vitamins: These include vitamins A, D, E, and K.

Digestion and absorption

The digestion of lipids (▶ Fig. 1.6) is catalyzed by lipases (enzymes that hydrolyze ester bonds) and is aided by the lipid-emulsifying molecules in bile.
- Salivary (lingual) lipase and gastric lipases hydrolyze only short-chain and medium-chain fatty acids. Short-chain fatty acids then diffuse through the stomach to enter the circulatory system.
- Bile acids/salts are amphipathic molecules that emulsify dietary lipids in the duodenum, making it easier for digestive enzymes (released by the pancreas and cells lining the intestines) to hydrolyze them. Hydrolysis of ester bonds in triacylglycerols, cholesterol esters, and phospholipids are catalyzed by lipases, cholesterol esterases, and phospholipases, respectively.

The lipid-soluble vitamins, as well as the products of lipid digestion—free fatty acids, 2-monoacylglycerols, and cholesterol—are assembled into spherical particles called micelles. Monomeric lipids are absorbed from the micelles by the villi of the intestinal mucosa. In these cells, the fatty acids are reassembled into triacylglycerols, phospholipids, and cholesterol esters. The reassembled lipids are then incorporated into large spherical lipoproteins called chylomicrons for delivery to the lymphatic system.
- The mechanisms involved in the transport, metabolism, and storage of lipids are described in Chapters 13 and 14.

Therapeutics

Steatorrhea

Steatorrhea is the presence of excess fat in stool and may be associated with fecal incontinence. Steatorrhea may occur due to malabsorption or maldigestion of fat. Malabsorption could result from inflammatory bowel disease, celiac disease, or abetalipoproteinemia. A problem with digestion of fat could be due to decreased lipase activity caused by diminished pancreatic function, problems with bile secretion/production, or obstruction of the bile duct. Pancreatic insufficiency can occur due to cancer or cystic fibrosis. Lipaseblocker drugs such as orlistat or indigestible fats such as olestra can also cause steatorrhea. Malabsorption of lipid-soluble vitamins A, D, E, and K is a concern in cases of steatorrhea.

Function

Lipids are important long-term energy providers, yielding 9 kcal/g. They are also the major structural components of cell membranes (e.g., phospholipids, glycolipids, and cholesterol). Lipids are used to generate lipophilic molecules, such as steroid hormones, bile acids, eicosanoids, and the lipid-soluble vitamins, A, D, E, and K. Several enzymes require lipids for their activity.

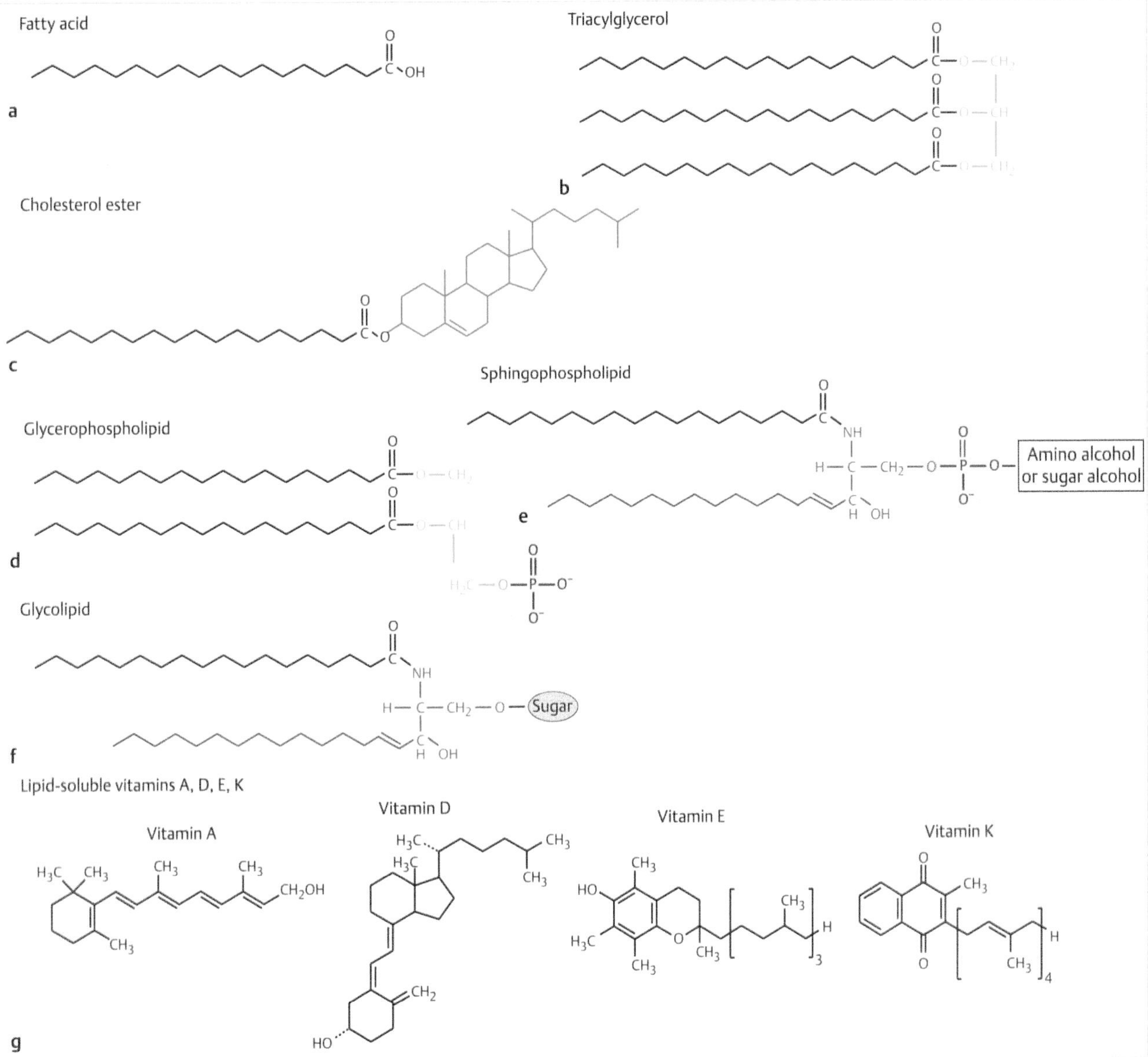

Fig. 1.5 Dietary lipids. (a) Fatty acids are monocarboxylic acids with hydrocarbon chains that are either saturated (zero double bonds), monounsaturated (one double bond), or polyunsaturated (two or more double bonds). Other lipids are composed of fatty acids attached to various molecules. For instance, **(b)** triacylglycerols (fats) are composed of three fatty acids attached to a glycerol molecule. **(c)** Cholesterol esters are composed of a fatty acid esterified to the OH group of cholesterol. **(d)** Phospholipids composed of two fatty acids attached to a glycerol backbone, which is also esterified to a phosphate group, are referred to as glycerophospholipids. **(e)** Phospholipids composed of one fatty acid chain attached to a sphingosine backbone, which is esterified to a phosphate, are referred to as sphingophospholipids. **(f)** Glycolipids are those membrane lipids that contain a fatty acid chain attached to a sphingosine backbone, which is also attached to sugar residues. **(g)** Lipid-soluble vitamins A, D, E, and K.

Therapeutics

Lipoproteins and atherosclerosis

Lipids are packaged into lipoproteins (spherical particles composed of lipids and proteins) for transport in the bloodstream. In order from largest and least dense to smallest and most dense, these lipoproteins are chylomicrons, very low-density lipoproteins (VLDL), intermediate-density lipoproteins (IDL), low-density lipoproteins (LDL), and high-density lipoproteins (HDL). Chylomicrons are made by the intestinal cells, whereas VLDL

are synthesized in the liver. IDL and LDL are formed from VLDL due to its metabolism in circulation. HDL are also assembled in circulation using protein components from the liver and intestine and lipid components from peripheral cells and other lipoproteins. About 70% of total cholesterol in human plasma is carried on LDL. LDL cholesterol levels > 100 mg/ dL are known to be associated with atherosclerosis. On the other hand, HDL cholesterol levels > 40 mg/ dL are protective against atherosclerosis.

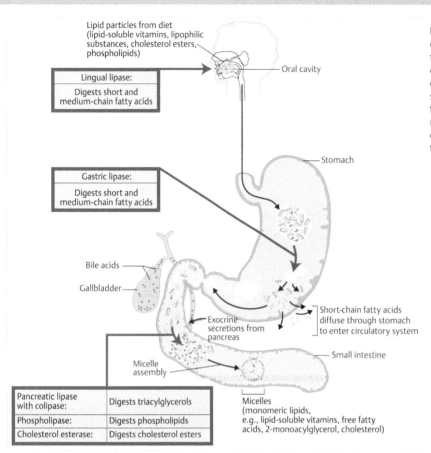

Lipid particles from diet
(lipid-soluble vitamins, lipophilic
substances, cholesterol esters,
phospholipids)

| Lingual lipase: |
| Digests short and medium-chain fatty acids |

| Gastric lipase: |
| Digests short and medium-chain fatty acids |

Oral cavity

Stomach

Bile acids

Gallbladder

Exocrine secretions from pancreas

Short-chain fatty acids diffuse through stomach to enter circulatory system

Small intestine

Micelle assembly

Pancreatic lipase with colipase:	Digests triacylglycerols
Phospholipase:	Digests phospholipids
Cholesterol esterase:	Digests cholesterol esters

Micelles
(monomeric lipids,
e.g., lipid-soluble vitamins, free fatty
acids, 2-monoacylglycerol, cholesterol)

Fig. 1.6 Lipid digestion. Ingested fat particles contain many lipid-soluble substances. Lipases in the saliva and stomach do not significantly break down the emulsified lipids. Significant hydrolysis occurs in the duodenum. Lipid-soluble substances aggregate spontaneously in water, forming mixed micelles in the small intestine. The mixed micelles are 100 times smaller than the fat emulsions; their increased surface area increases the efficiency of absorption (by the intestines).

1.3.3 Proteins

Proteins are created from linear polymers of amino acids linked to each other via peptide bonds.
- Oligopeptides: small peptide polymers containing between 2 and 50 amino acids
- Polypeptides: large peptide polymers containing more than 50 amino acids

Although 20 amino acids are used to construct proteins, 10 of them are considered essential (including arginine, which is essential in growing children), because they cannot be synthesized de novo and therefore must be obtained from the diet. They can be remembered with the mnemonic PVT TIM HALL, which refers to

Phenylalanine	Threonine	Histidine
Valine	Isoleucine	Arginine
Tryptophan	Methionine	Leucine
		Lysine

Proteins from animal sources contain all 10 essential amino acids and are therefore considered high quality. Proteins from plant sources, however, contain some but not all essential amino acids. A judicious combination of different plant sources can provide a balanced supply of high-quality protein.

Digestion and absorption

The acidic pH (< 2) of the stomach denatures proteins and thus makes their polypeptide chains more susceptible to enzymatic degradation by peptidases, as follows:

- Pepsin: Proteins are initially digested in the stomach by the gastric enzyme pepsin. It is most effective at low pH and is inactive at a higher pH such as that observed in the duodenum (pH > 7).
- Pancreatic peptidases: The short polypeptides generated from the action of pepsin are further cleaved in the duodenum by pancreatic peptidases. Cleavage by these peptidases releases amino acids, which are absorbed by intestinal cells.

Function

Proteins are a major source of fuel, enzymatic activity, and structural support (e.g., keratin, collagen). Their degradation into amino acids provides the building blocks for the synthesis of other important molecules (e.g., heme molecules and nucleotides).
- The pathways that describe the metabolism of proteins and amino acids are found in Chapters 15 and 19.

Therapeutics
Celiac disease
Celiac disease, or nontropical sprue, is an immune disorder of the intestine in which there is hypersensitivity to gluten proteins of wheat, barley, and rye. It is associated with cramping, diarrhea, and growth defects in infants. The immune reaction causes villus atrophy, which interferes with absorption of macronutrients, minerals, and lipid-soluble vitamins.

1.4 Vitamins

Vitamins are a heterogeneous class of organic materials that do not provide energy but are essential for normal function. They include the lipid-soluble and water-soluble vitamins.

1.4.1 Lipid-soluble Vitamins (A, D, E, K)

The lipid-soluble vitamins include vitamins A, D, E, and K. They are either synthesized de novo or obtained from the diet. In the latter case, these vitamins are packaged into micelles with other diet-derived lipids for absorption by the enterocytes (villus cells) of the intestinal mucosa. They are transported on plasma lipoproteins (e.g., chylomicrons) and stored in both the liver and adipose tissue. Because they are not excreted, lipid-soluble vitamins may reach toxic levels in the liver. The dietary sources of these vitamins are summarized in ▶ Table 1.3.

Function

Vitamin A

The effects of vitamin A are attributed to its provitamin form β-carotene and its various derivatives, which include retinol (alcohol form), retinal (aldehyde form), retinoic acid (carboxylic acid form), and synthetic forms (drugs). Their functions are as follows:

- β-Carotene functions as an antioxidant.
- Retinal is used to produce the visual pigment rhodopsin.
- Retinoic acid is a nuclear hormone that binds to intracellular DNA-binding receptors known as transcription factors to influence the transcription of specific genes. As a result, retinoic acid contributes to the proper differentiation of epithelial cells.

Table 1.3 Lipid-soluble vitamins: Sources

Vitamin	Source
A	• The vitamin A precursor, β-carotene, is found in spinach, carrots, dark green leafy vegetables, and yellow vegetables • The vitamin A derivative retinol is found in liver, cod liver oil, dairy products, and eggs • Synthetic derivatives of vitamin A include the drugs tretinoin and isotretinoin
D	• Vitamin D_2 (ergocalciferol) and vitamin D_3 (cholecalcif-erol) are found in liver, eggs, fish, plants, and vitamin D–fortifed foods such as milk and cereal • Vitamin D_3 (cholecalciferol) is also produced in the skin via a mechanism that requires exposure to sunlight • Calcitriol, the bioactive form of vitamin D, is derived from vitamins D_2 and D_3
E	• Tocopherols, which are members of the vitamin E family, are found in vegetable oils, seeds, nuts, and green leafy vegetables
K	• Vitamin K_1 is obtained from green leafy vegetables • Vitamin K_2 is synthesized by bacteria in the large intestine and colon

- Topical tretinoin is used to treat acne and wrinkles, and oral tretinoin (all-*trans*-retinoic acid) is used in the treatment of acute promyelocytic leukemia (APL). Oral isotretinoin is used to treat severe acne, but it is teratogenic; it can disrupt the development of an embryo or fetus if the individual being treated is pregnant.

Therapeutics
Disorders associated with vitamin A

Malnutrition (due to inadequate intake or absorption) causes deficiencies in vitamin A that manifest as night blindness, visual impairment, xerophthalmia (dry eye syndrome), and Bitot's spots (due to keratin debris in the conjunctiva). Additional presentations of vitamin A deficiency include growth impediment, failure of wounds to heal well, dry skin, follicular hyperkeratosis, alopecia, and lung conditions such as bronchitis and pneumonia. Intake of copious amounts of vitamin A supplements causes an excess of vitamin A, which leads to liver toxicity and joint pain. Infants exposed to isotretinoin in the womb may have birth defects such as cleft palates and heart abnormalities.

Therapeutics
Acute promyelocytic leukemia

Acute promyelocytic leukemia (APL) is a cancer of the blood and bone marrow marked by the buildup of immature white blood cells (promyelocytes). It is linked to the presence of PML-RARα, the product of a fusion between the promyelocytic leukemia (PML) gene and the retinoic acid receptor-α (RARα) gene. PML-RARα acts to repress the transcription of certain genes and thus prevent cell differentiation. This results in the accumulation of immature promyelocytes. Treatment with all-*trans*-retinoic acid relieves PML-RARα's repression of transcription and thus stimulates the differentiation and maturation of promyelocytes and contributes to APL remission.

Vitamin D

The effects of vitamin D are attributed to its active form, calcitriol, which has three OH groups. It is created when cholecalciferol (D_3, the inactive form of vitamin D produced in intestinal cells and by UV irradiation of the skin) is first hydroxylated in the liver and then hydroxylated a second time in the kidneys (▶ Fig. 1.7).

- The first hydroxylation is catalyzed by a liver hydroxylase (25-hydroxylase), and the second is catalyzed by a kidney hydroxylase (1-α-hydroxylase).
- Calcitriol binds to intracellular receptors (transcription factors) that influence the transcription of specific genes that stimulate the absorption of Ca^{2+} and PO_4^{3-} from the intestines, increase the reabsorption of Ca^{2+} by the kidneys, and promote resorption of Ca^{2+} from bone. The resulting effect of calcitriol is an elevation in blood Ca^{2+} and PO_4^{3-} levels for the maintenance of proper bone mineralization or bone density.

I

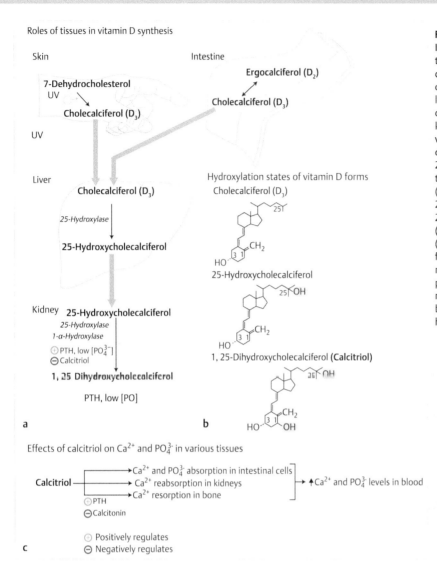

Roles of tissues in vitamin D synthesis

Skin

7-Dehydrocholesterol
UV
Cholecalciferol (D$_3$)

UV

Intestine

Ergocalciferol (D$_2$)

Cholecalciferol (D$_3$)

Liver

Cholecalciferol (D$_3$)

25-Hydroxylase

25-Hydroxycholecalciferol

Kidney 25-Hydroxycholecalciferol
25-Hydroxylase
1-α-Hydroxylase
⊕ PTH, low [PO$_4^{3-}$]
⊖ Calcitriol

1, 25 Dihydroxycholecalciferol

PTH, low [PO]

a

Hydroxylation states of vitamin D forms
Cholecalciferol (D$_3$)

25-Hydroxycholecalciferol

1, 25-Dihydroxycholecalciferol (**Calcitriol**)

b

Effects of calcitriol on Ca^{2+} and PO$_4^{3-}$ in various tissues

Calcitriol
→ Ca^{2+} and PO$_4^{3-}$ absorption in intestinal cells
→ Ca^{2+} reabsorption in kidneys
→ Ca^{2+} resorption in bone
⊕PTH
⊖Calcitonin

→ ↑Ca^{2+} and PO$_4^{3-}$ levels in blood

⊕ Positively regulates
⊖ Negatively regulates

c

Fig. 1.7 Vitamin D synthesis and signaling. (a) In intestinal cells, ergocalciferol (D$_2$) is converted to cholecalciferol (D$_3$). In the skin, 7-dehydrocholesterol is converted to cholecalciferol D$_3$ with the aid of ultraviolet (UV) light. Two subsequent hydroxylations of cholecalciferol (first in the liver and then in the kidneys) generate calcitriol, the active form of vitamin D. The first hydroxylation of cholecalciferol is catalyzed by the liver enzyme 25-hydroxylase, and the second is catalyzed by the kidney enzyme 1-a-hydroxylase. (Note that the full structures of cholecalciferol, 25-hydroxycholecalciferol, and 1, 25-dihydroxycholecalciferol are shown in (b).) (c) Calcitriol stimulates intestinal cells to absorb (or increase the absorption of) Ca^{2+} and PO4 from the intestinal lumen, increase the reabsorption of Ca^{2+} by the kidneys, and promote resorption of Ca^{2+} from bone. The resulting effect of calcitriol is an elevation in blood Ca^{2+} and PO$_4$~ levels. PTH, parathyroid hormone.

Therapeutics

Disorders associated with vitamin D

Normal blood Ca^{2+} levels are 8.4 to 10.2 mg/dL. Deficiencies in vitamin D occur due to (1) inadequate dietary intake, (2) conditions that disrupt the absorption of lipids, (3) poor functioning of the liver and kidneys, (4) hypoparathyroidism, and (5) lack of exposure to sunlight (e.g., winter days in northern latitudes or excessive use of sunscreen). Vitamin D deficiency manifests as brittle bones observed as rickets in children (marked by growth deficiency and skeletal deformities), osteomalacia in adults (marked by "pathological fractures"), and hypocalcemic tetany (involuntary muscle contractions due to low blood Ca^{2+}). Intake of too many vitamin D supplements causes an excess of vitamin D, which results in elevated levels of Ca^{2+} in blood (hypercalcemia) and urine (hypercalciuria). Patients with this condition appear dazed, have a loss of appetite, and may present with sarcoidosis. The latter is an inflammation of tissues marked by the presence of clusters of immune cells (granulomas) in various tissues, such as the lungs, skin, and lymph nodes.

Vitamin E

Compounds that are members of the vitamin E family include γ-tocopherol and α-tocopherol, the latter of which is more actively retained in the body than the former. The long hydrophobic tail of vitamin E serves to anchor it in cellular membranes.

- Vitamin E serves as an antioxidant to protect cells from the harmful effects of reactive oxygen species (ROS) generated from free radicals reacting with oxygen. Consequently, vitamin E guards membrane lipids containing polyunsaturated fatty acid chains from peroxidation and protects low-density lipoproteins (LDL) from oxidation. Peroxidation of membrane lipids disrupts membrane integrity, and oxidized LDL are more atherogenic than unaltered LDL.

Therapeutics

Disorders associated with vitamin E

Deficiencies in vitamin E occur due to inadequate dietary intake or conditions that disrupt the absorption of lipids (e.g., cholestasis, cystic fibrosis, abetalipoproteinemia). Without adequate antioxidant protection from vitamin E, erythrocytes are susceptible to rupture (hemolysis), which manifests as hemolytic anemia. Sustained vitamin E deficiency is associated with impaired vision (due to retinal degeneration), muscle weakness (due to myopathy), peripheral neuropathy, ataxia (poor muscle coordination with tremors), areflexia (a loss of reflexes in limbs), poor proprioception (sensation of one's position and movement) and decreased vibratory sensation. Vitamin E toxicity, while rare, is caused by excessive intake of vitamin E supplements. This impairs vitamin K–mediated coagulation and promotes the effects of anticoagulation drugs (e.g., warfarin), which may lead to hemorrhage.

Foundations

Free radicals and antioxidants

Free radicals are atoms, ions, or molecules with an unpaired electron in their outer shell. As such they are extremely reactive and unstable and can damage biological molecules, such as nucleic acids, proteins, and lipids. They are thought to contribute not only to human disease but also to the normal aging process. Superoxide anion (O_2^-) and hydroxyl radical ($\bullet$ OH) are examples of free radicals that contain oxygen, and along with hydrogen peroxide (H_2O_2), constitute the reactive oxygen species (ROS). As part of the immune response, ROS are involved in the killing of pathogens. Antioxidants prevent the formation of ROS, and antioxidant enzymes such as peroxidases, catalase, and superoxide dismutase can eliminate ROS. Vitamins such as C and E act as antioxidants. Minerals such as zinc (Zn) and selenium (Se) act as cofactors of antioxidant enzymes.

Vitamin K

The effects of vitamin K on blood coagulation are attributed to its reduced, active form called vitamin K hydroquinone ($\blacktriangleright$ Fig. 1.8).

- The hydroquinone form of vitamin K serves as a cofactor for γ-carboxylase, an enzyme that carboxylates glutamate residues on precursor clotting factors (e.g., II, VII, IX, X), which turns them into mature active clotting factors. The addition of a carboxyl group to glutamate residues increases the clotting factors' overall negative charge, which allows them to bind to Ca^{2+}. Aided by their chelation of Ca^{2+} ions, clotting factors then bind to phospholipids on the membranes of platelets, endothelial cells, and vascular cells, which leads to blood clotting.

Therapeutics

Disorders associated with vitamin K

Deficiencies in vitamin K occur when (1) the absorption of lipids is disrupted, (2) gut bacterial colonies that synthesize vitamin K are absent (as seen in newborns or due to treatment with broad-spectrum antibiotics), or (3) anticoagulation drugs such as warfarin and dicoumarol are taken. A deficiency in vitamin K makes an individual susceptible to bleeding (bleeding diathesis) and bruising (ecchymosis). Patients with this condition are anemic and weak and present with nose bleeds, bleeding gums, heavy menstrual bleeding, and gastrointestinal bleeding (marked by red/black stool, pink/brown urine, coughing up of blood). A prothrombin time (PT) test measures the time it takes for blood to clot. PT, which normally takes 12 to 14 seconds, is increased in vitamin K–deficient individuals. Excessive intake of synthetic vitamin K (called menadione) causes hemolytic anemia and hepatotoxicity. Individuals taking anticoagulation drugs are advised to consume modest amounts of vitamin K–rich foods because the efficacy of these vitamin K– antagonistic drugs is reduced by high levels of

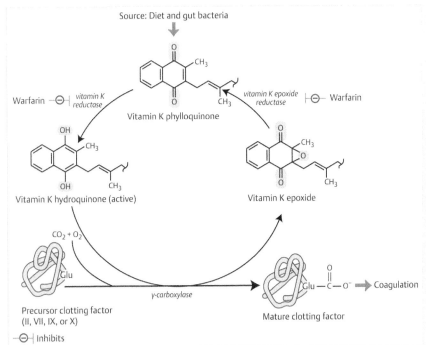

Fig. 1.8 Vitamin K types and role in carboxylation of clotting factors. Vitamin K exists in three forms: vitamin K hydroquinone (the active form), vitamin K phylloquinone, and vitamin K epoxide. Vitamin K hydroquinone serves as a cofactor for g-carboxylase, an enzyme that carboxylates glutamate residues on precursor clotting factors (e.g., II, VII, IX, X), turning them into mature active clotting factors that contribute to blood coagulation. The anticoagulant warfarin exerts its effects by inhibiting enzymes involved in converting vitamin K epoxide and vitamin K phylloquinone into the active vitamin K hydroquinone form. (Note that the partial structure of each vitamin K form is shown.)

I

vitamin K. The international normalized ratio (INR) is calculated to monitor patients taking anticoagulants. The normal INR range with an anticoagulant is 2 to 3. A lower than normal INR indicates that the risk of developing a clot is increased, whereas a higher than normal INR suggests that the risk of bleeding is increased.

1.4.2 Water-soluble Vitamins

Water-soluble vitamins are used in a variety of biochemical reactions either alone or as a cofactor for enzymes. Unlike the lipid-soluble vitamins, the water-soluble vitamins are not stored. Instead, they are excreted in urine; therefore, toxic levels are rarely ever reached. Deficiencies due to inadequate intake of water-soluble vitamins and in some cases as a result of alcoholism do occur and are problematic. The nine water-soluble vitamins, their sources, and their biologically functional forms are listed in ▶ Table 1.4.

Vitamins Involved in Redox Reactions

The biologically relevant forms of vitamins B_2, B_3, and C function in redox (oxidation reduction) reactions, which involve the transfer of electrons, with protons, between two molecules.
- **Vitamin B_2 (riboflavin):** Biologically active vitamin B_2 takes on the form of the electron-carrying molecules flavin mononucleotide (FMN) and flavin adenine dinucleotide (FAD).

Reduction of FMN and FAD generates $FMNH_2$ and $FADH_2$, respectively. Both serve as prosthetic groups of enzymes that catalyze the redox reactions essential for nutrient metabolism and energy production (▶ Table 1.5).
- **Vitamin B_3 (niacin):** Biologically active vitamin B_3 takes on the form of nicotinamide adenine dinucleotide (NAD^+) and nicotinamide adenine dinucleotide phosphate ($NADP^+$). Reduction of NAD^+ and $NADP^+$ generates NADH and NADPH, respectively. Both serve as electron carriers and reducing agents (▶ Table 1.5).
- **Vitamin C (ascorbic acid):** This vitamin functions as an antioxidant, and a reducing agent (▶ Table 1.5).

Therapeutics
Vitamin B_2 (riboflavin)–deficient conditions
A deficiency in vitamin B_2 is caused by consumption of a vitamin B_2– deficient diet, an impaired liver (e.g., from liver disease or chronic alcoholism), or intake of drugs such as oral contraceptives, antibiotics, and antidepressants. Individuals with sickle cell anemia appear to be susceptible to vitamin B_2 deficiency along with deficiencies of vitamins C and E. Riboflavin deficiency results in inflammation of the skin (dermatitis), which becomes irritated (e.g., skin redness, rashes, and swelling). The "mucous lining" of the mouth also becomes inflamed (described as angular stomatitis and cheilosis), which manifests as cracks or splits of areas of the mouth and lips. Another common presentation of vitamin B_2 deficiency is corneal vascularization and lesions of the genitalia.

Therapeutics
Vitamin B_3 (niacin)–deficient conditions
Diets high in untreated corn have low levels of absorbable niacin as well as tryptophan. Pellagra (*pelle* = skin, *agra* = sour) with diarrhea, dermatitis, and dementia are common presentations of vitamin B_3 deficiency or a deficiency of tryptophan, an essential amino acid that can be converted into niacin in the body. Pellagra is treated by supplementation with nicotinic acid.

Therapeutics
Vitamin C–related disorders
Vitamin C (ascorbic acid) is necessary for the formation of collagen (to help oxidize proline to hydroxyproline, and lysine to hydroxylysine) and also carnitine (which functions in fatty acid oxidation). Deficiency of vitamin C causes scurvy with petechiae (purple hemorrhagic spots on the skin), ecchymoses (bruising), spongy and bleeding gums, and poor wound healing. In medieval times, sailors on long voyages were susceptible to developing scurvy. Fresh citrus fruits, which are a rich source of vitamin C, prevent scurvy.

Table 1.4 Water-soluble vitamins: Sources and functional forms

Vitamin	Source	Functional form
Involved in redox reactions		
B_2 (riboflavin)	Milk, eggs	Flavin mononucleotide and flavin adenine dinucleotide (FMN, FAD)
B_3 (niacin)	Meat, yeast products, fruits, vegetables, synthesized from tryptophan	Nicotinamide adenine dinucleotide and nicotinamide adenine dinucleotide phosphate (NAD^+ and $NADP^+$)
C (ascorbic acid)	Fruits, vegetables	Ascorbate
Involved in nonredox reactions		
B_1 (thiamine)	Grain, yeast products, pork	Thiamine pyrophosphate (TPP)
B_5 (pantothenic acid)	Widely distributed	Coenzyme A
B_6 (pyridoxine)	Meat, vegetables, grains	Pyridoxal phosphate
B_{12} (cobalamin)	Meat, liver, milk, eggs	Adenosylcobalamin methylcobalamin
Biotin	Yeast products, legumes, nuts	Biotin
Folate	Fresh green vegetables, liver	Tetrahydrofolate (THF)

Table 1.5 Vitamins involved in redox reactions, their associated enzymes, and functions

Vitamin	Cofactor and its associated enzyme and function
B$_2$ (riboflavin)	FAD is a cofactor for • *Succinate dehydrogenase/complex II:* This enzyme functions in the tricarboxylic acid (TCA) cycle, where it converts succinate to fumarate. It also functions in the electron transport chain to transfer electrons from NADH to coenzyme Q • *Acyl CoA dehydrogenase:* This enzyme catalyzes the first step in the β-oxidation of fatty acids (i.e., inclusion of a double bond) and transfers electrons to FAD • *Retinal dehydrogenase:* This enzyme plays a role in the metabolism of vitamin A by converting retinal into retinoic acid FMN is a cofactor for • *NADH dehydrogenase/complex I:* This enzyme is a component of the electron transport chain that facilitates the transfer of electrons from NADH to coenzyme Q FAD and FMN are cofactors for • *Vitamin-activating enzymes:* These enzymes play a role in the conversion of vitamins A, B$_6$, and folic acid to their active forms, as well as the conversion of tryptophan to vitamin B$_3$
B$_3$ (niacin)	NAD$^+$ serves as a(n) • *Electron carrier:* NADH transfers electrons from the TCA cycle to complex I of the electron transport chain • *Reducing agent:* NADPH is an essential reducing agent used in biosynthesis of lipids. It also protects cells from the damaging effects of reactive oxygen species (ROS) by keeping the antioxidant glutathione in the reduced state
C	Ascorbic acid serves as a(n) • *Antioxidant:* Like vitamin E, vitamin C protects cells from the harmful effects of ROS generated from free radicals reacting with oxygen • *Reducing agent:* Vitamin C keeps iron in its reduced state (Fe^{2+}), which allows it to be effciently absorbed from the intestines

Abbreviations: CoA, coenzyme A; FAD, flavin adenine dinucleotide; FMN, flavin mononucleotide; NAD, nicotinamide adenine dinucleotide; NADH, reduced NAD; NADPH, reduced nicotinamide adenine dinucleotide phosphate.

Vitamins Involved in Nonredox Reactions

The derivatives of the other water-soluble vitamins function in a variety of reactions that primarily involve removal or transfer of chemical groups (▶ Table 1.6).
- **Vitamin B$_1$ (thiamine):** Thiamine pyrophosphate (TPP) is the active form of vitamin B$_1$, which serves as a cofactor of enzymes that remove CO$_2$ in the oxidative decarboxylation of β-ketoacids and that transfer carbon fragments.
- **Vitamin B$_5$ (pantothenic acid):** Vitamin B$_5$ is a key chemical component of coenzyme A which forms thioester bonds with other molecules to activate them.
- **Vitamin B$_6$ (pyridoxine):** The active form of vitamin B$_6$ is pyridoxal phosphate, which functions as a cofactor for a variety of enzymes.
- **B$_{12}$ (cobalamin):** This vitamin exists in two active forms, adenosylcobalamin and methylcobalamin. Enzymes that use these forms of cobalamin as cofactors are described in ▶ Table 1.6.
- **Biotin:** This vitamin serves as a cofactor of enzymes that catalyze carboxylations (i.e., CO$_2$ transfers).
- **Folate:** The active form of folate is tetrahydrofolate (THF) and its derivatives.

Various disorders are attributed to deficiencies in water-soluble vitamins (▶ Table 1.7).

Therapeutics
Antifolates
Analogs of folate (antifolates), such as aminopterin, amethopterin, and methotrexate, are used as anticancer agents. They are structural analogs of folate and act as competitive inhibitors of dihydrofolate reductase, an enzyme that generates dihydrofolate from folate as well as tetrahydrofolate (THF) from dihydrofolate. These compounds are known as antifolates or antimetabolites because their blockage of THF formation interferes with the synthesis of purines and thymidine, which suppresses the growth of rapidly dividing cells such as cancer cells. Normal cells that turn over rapidly, such as oral and intestinal mucosal cells and cells of hair follicles, are also affected.

1.5 Water and Minerals

1.5.1 Water

Water makes up the majority of the human body mass and is used for a variety of purposes.
- It is a critical component of many biological reactions, serving as either a solvent or a reagent.
- It functions as a solvent for components of blood and tissues.
- It serves as a medium for excretion of wastes.
- It regulates body temperature.
- Water comprises 70% of total body weight (e.g., 42 L in a 70 kg adult).

I

Table 1.6 Vitamins involved in nonredox reactions, their associated enzymes, and functions

Vitamin	Cofactor and its associated enzyme and function
B₁ (thiamine)	Thiamine pyrophosphate (TPP) is a cofactor for • *Pyruvate dehydrogenase complex:* This enzyme decarboxylates pyruvate to generate acetyl coenzyme A (CoA) • *α-ketoglutarate dehydrogenase complex:* This tricarboxylic acid (TCA) cycle enzyme decarboxylates α-ketoglutarate to generate succinyl CoA • *Branched chain α-keto acid dehydrogenase:* This enzyme plays a role in the degradation of branched chain amino acids isoleucine, leucine, and valine • *Transketolase:* This enzyme transfers two-carbon fragments between molecules in the pentose phosphate pathway
B₅ (pantothenic acid)	Pantothenic acid is a component of • *Coenzyme A:* This molecule forms high-energy thioester bonds with other molecules to "activate" them and is involved in reactions that transfer fatty acyl groups between molecules • *Fatty acid synthase (FAS) complex:* This enzyme catalyzes the synthesis of fatty acids
B₆ (pyridoxine)	Pyridoxal phosphate is a cofactor for • *Transaminases:* These enzymes, also known as aminotransferases, transfer amino groups between molecules to interconvert amino acids and α-keto acids • *Decarboxylases:* These enzymes catalyze the removal of carboxyl groups. Specific decarboxylases play a critical role in the synthesis of neurotransmitters (e.g., dopamine) • *Glycogen phosphorylase:* This enzyme is involved in the breakdown of glycogen (glycogenolysis) • *Aminolevulinic acid (ALA) synthase:* The rate-limiting step in heme and porphyrin synthesis is catalyzed by this enzyme
B₁₂ (cobalamin)	Adenosylcobalamin and methylcobalamin are cofactors for • *Methylmalonyl CoA mutase:* This enzyme isomerizes methylmalonyl CoA into succinyl CoA in a reaction that is part of the pathway that degrades odd-numbered fatty acids • *Methionine synthase/homocysteine methyltransferase:* This enzyme transfers a methyl group from 5-methyltetrahydrofolate (N⁵-methyl-THF) onto homocysteine to form methionine. Methionine reacts with adenosine triphosphate (ATP) to generate S-adenosyl methionine (SAM), the latter of which regenerates homocysteine when SAM donates a methyl group to target molecules
Biotin	Biotin serves as a cofactor for • *Pyruvate carboxylase:* This enzyme irreversibly carboxylates pyruvate to produce oxaloacetate • *Acetyl CoA carboxylase:* This enzyme irreversibly carboxylates acetyl CoA to form malonyl CoA
Folate	Derivatives of tetrahydrofolate (THF) serve as 'one carbon' donors. Formyl-THF is used in purine biosynthesis, methylene-THF in thymidylate synthesis, and methyl-THF in the conversion of homocysteine to methionine.

Table 1.7 Disorders associated with deficiencies in water-soluble vitamins

Vitamin	Deficiency-associated conditions and symptoms
Involved in redox reactions	
B₂ (riboflavin)	Cheilosis, angular stomatitis, dermatitis
B₃ (niacin)	Pellagra with diarrhea, dermatitis, and dementia
C (ascorbic acid)	Scurvy with petechiae, ecchymoses, bleeding gums
Involved in nonredox reactions	
B₁ (thiamine)	Beriberi, polyneuritis, Wernicke-Korsakof syndrome
B₅ (pantothenic acid)	Deficiency is rare. Fatigue, sleep disturbances, impaired coordination
B₆ (pyridoxine)	Nasolateral seborrhea, glossitis, peripheral neuropathy
B₁₂ (cobalamin)	Pernicious anemia, neurologic disorders, pallor
Biotin	Raw egg whites contain avidin, which binds to biotin, rendering it unabsorbable Fatigue, depression, nausea, dermatitis, muscle pain, fasting hypoglycemia
Folate	Blood-forming tissues are particularly dependent on folate Megaloblastic anemia, mental status changes, glossitis, pallor

Therapeutics

Edema

Edema is the abnormal accumulation of fluid (mainly water) either under the skin (e.g., in arms or legs) or in one or more of the organs or body cavities (e.g., lungs, pericardium). Edema occurs when water either leaks out or is forced out of blood vessels into the interstitial space, usually due to differences in pressure. Conditions such as malnutrition, hypertension, venous insufficiency, liver or kidney diseases, pregnancy, heart failure, and certain drugs (e.g., steroids, thiazolidinediones) are among the causes that result in edema. Treatment usually involves the use of diuretics (e.g., furosemide or Lasix) that cause increased urinary output.

Therapeutics

Dehydration

Dehydration is the result of excessive loss of body water and some electrolytes. It can occur as a result of vigorous physical activity, vomiting, diarrhea, fever, diabetes, or inadequate water intake. The symptoms include thirst, dry mouth, skin turgor (loss of elasticity), decreased urine output, headache and dizziness, and in severe cases, seizures, shock, and coma. It can be treated by fluid and electrolyte replacement and with nonsteroidal anti-inflammatory drugs (NSAIDs).

1.5.2 Minerals

Minerals are a heterogeneous class of inorganic nutrients that function as electrolytes, enzyme cofactors, and signaling molecules. They are divided into two broad categories (▶ Fig. 1.9):

1. **Macroelements:** The most abundant minerals fall into this category because they are required in quantities of over 100 mg/d. They include Na^+, Cl^-, K^+, Ca^{2+}, Mg^{2+}, and PO_4^{3-} (sodium, chloride, potassium, calcium, magnesium, and phosphate, respectively), which have differing concentrations inside and outside a cell. Following are some examples:
   - Na^+, Cl^-, Ca^{2+}: The concentration of these extracellular ions is higher outside relative to inside the cell.
   - K^+, Mg^{2+}, PO_4^{3-}: The concentration of these intracellular ions is higher inside relative to outside the cell.
   - Na^+ and K^+ are the major extra- and intracellular cations, respectively. Cl^- and PO_4^{3-} are the major extra- and intracellular anions, respectively.
2. **Microelements (trace elements):** The minerals that fall under this category are required in quantities less than 100 mg/d. They include Fe, Zn, Cu, Mo, Mn, Co, Cr, S, Se, I, and F (iron, zinc, copper, molybdenum, manganese, cobalt, chromium, sulfur, selenium, iodine, and fluorine, respectively).

K^+, Na^+, and Cl^-

Function

The macroelements K^+, Na^+, and Cl^- (whose sources are described in ▶ Table 1.8) are the three major electrolytes that maintain osmotic pressure and acid–base balance (pH). They create gradients across cell membranes that allow for the maintenance of nerve and muscle excitability. The cations have additional roles in the active and passive transport of molecules across cell membranes, such as the following:

- Na^+ is involved in the absorption of nutrients (e.g., glucose, galactose, and amino acids) in the intestine and reabsorption in the kidneys.
- K^+ is involved in the regulation of insulin secretion.

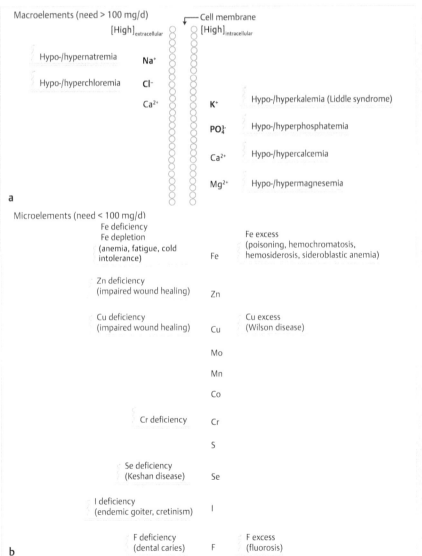

Fig. 1.9 Macroelements and microelements. Disorders and signs associated with deficiencies or excesses in the macroelements (**a**) and microelements (**b**).

Table 1.8 K$^+$, Na$^+$, and Cl$^-$: Sources and normal serum levels

Mineral	Source	Normal serum levels (mEq/L)
K$^+$	Unprocessed foods (meats, vegetables and fruits, nuts and legumes)	3.5–5.0
Na$^+$	Ubiquitous in foods of animal origin and in dietary salt (NaCl in preserved, prepared, and processed foods)	136–145
Cl$^-$	Ubiquitous in dietary salt (ingested as NaCl)	95–105

Regulation

The kidneys play a critical role in maintaining homeostasis by filtering blood so that nutrients, minerals, and water are reabsorbed as metabolic waste products (e.g., urea and ammonia) are excreted in urine. In doing so, the kidneys regulate the concentration of electrolytes and the volume of body fluids (e.g., blood and urine), and they ensure a proper acid–base balance.

• An increase in renal excretion, as well as vomiting and diarrhea, may lead to mineral deficiencies. Excesses have more specific causes, as summarized in ▶ Table 1.9.

Foundations

Other ions: H$^+$ and HCO$_3^-$

Normal blood pH is tightly regulated in a small range (7.35 to 7.45). The sources of protons in blood are both volatile (carbonic acid derived from CO_2) and nonvolatile (SO_4, PO_4, lactic acid, and keto acids). The major buffer system that regulates H$^+$ levels in blood is bicarbonate (HCO_3^-) (and hemoglobin to a lesser extent). A blood pH < 7.35 is termed as acidemia, and that > 7.45 is termed as alkalemia. The physiological causes of the change in blood pH are termed acidosis and alkalosis. Primary acid–base imbalances occur when a single physiological mechanism is not functioning properly or is overwhelmed. These can occur due to either respiratory or metabolic imbalances. Respiratory imbalances

are those in which the primary disturbance is in the concentration of CO_2. Metabolic imbalances are those in which the primary disturbance is in the concentration of bicarbonate.

Foundations

Membrane potentials

Biological membranes (phospholipid bilayers) are impermeable to ions but contain highly regulated ion channels. Ions, like all molecules, move down their concentration gradient (from areas of high concentration to areas of low concentration). However, because ions are charged (+ or -), they have an electrochemical gradient. The concentration of ions (charges) on each side of the membrane therefore becomes an electrical potential. The difference in electrical potentials across a membrane is the membrane potential. Resting cells have a resting membrane potential of -0.05 to -0.09 V (more negative charge inside the membrane than outside).

Foundations

Renin–angiotensin–aldosterone system (RAAS)

In response to a decrease in blood Na$^+$ levels, or blood pressure, the kidneys produce the hormone renin, which is released into the blood. Renin activates angiotensinogen, which is then cleaved to angiotensin I, and finally to active angiotensin II. Angiotensin II induces several activities that cause blood pressure and Na$^+$/water retention to increase. These activities include (1) vasoconstriction, (2) Na$^+$ and water retention, and decreased K$^+$ secretion by the kidneys, (3) increased tonicity and thirst sensation, (4) pituitary gland release of vasopressin (antidiuretic hormone) and corticotrophin, and (5) adrenal cortex release of aldosterone (which increases reabsorption of Na$^+$ and water by the kidneys). A ratio of aldosterone (ng/dL) to renin (ng/(mL·h)) that is greater than 24 is diagnostic of hyperaldosteronism.

Table 1.9 Disorders associated with abnormal levels of K$^+$, Na$^+$, and Cl$^-$

Ion	Disorder	Causes	Symptoms
K$^+$ deficiency	Hypokalemia	Poor intake Use of certain diuretics	Myalgia, myasthenia, cramps, constipation, flaccid paralysis, arrhythmias
K$^+$ excess	Hyperkalemia	Kidney disease, drugs	Palpitations, arrhythmia
Na$^+$ deficiency	Hyponatremia	Increased renal excretion (due to thiazide or loop diuretics or low aldosterone) Excessive water reabsorption from kidneys (due to excessive secretion of antidiuretic hormone, congestive heart failure, or chronic liver disease)	Convulsions and cerebral edema
Na$^+$ excess	Hypernatremia	Decreased renal excretion Decreased water reabsorption from kidneys (insufficient/dysfunctional antidiuretic hormone due to diabetes insipidus)	Convulsions and cerebral edema Dehydration
Cl$^-$ deficiency	Hypochloremia	Vomiting	Chronic respiratory acidosis and also metabolic alkalosis
Cl$^-$ excess	Hyperchloremia	Intravenous saline, diarrhea, drugs	Weakness, labored breathing, intense thirst

Table 1.10 Ca^{2+}, PO_4^{3-}, and Mg^{2+}: Sources and normal serum levels

Mineral	Source	Normal Serum Levels (mg/dL)
Ca^{2+}	Milk and dairy products, soybeans, dark green vegetables (kale, broccoli, spinach)	8.4–10.2
PO_4^{3-}	Dairy products, wheat germ and bran, beans, walnuts	3.0–4.5
Mg^{2+}	Meat, fish, vegetables, nuts and legumes, grains (wheat bran, cereal, and oats)	1.7–2.2

Ca^{2+}, PO_4^{3-}, and Mg^{2+}

Function

Ca^{2+}, PO_4^{3-}, and Mg^{2+} (whose sources are described in ▶ Table 1.10) are all stored as salts deposited on the collagen matrix of bone and teeth. Bone serves as a buffer or reservoir for these ions; its degradation mobilizes the ions to perform other functions in the body. Ca^{2+} constitutes ~1.5 to 2% of the body's mass, whereas PO_4^{3-} constitutes ~1%. Ca^{2+} is found free (as ionized calcium), bound to albumin, or bound to phosphates in the bone mineral hydroxyapatite ($Ca_5(PO_4)_3(OH)$). Ca^{2+} and Mg^{2+} are important intracellular cations with related functions that include the following:

- Ca^{2+} and Mg^{2+} are involved in contraction of skeletal, cardiac, and smooth muscle.
- Ca^{2+} and Mg^{2+} are involved in propagation of nerve impulses.
- Mg^{2+} is an important cofactor for many enzymes, including all enzymes that utilize adenosine triphosphate (ATP). It also plays a role in hormone- receptor binding, neurotransmitter release, and in the gating of transmembrane cation channels (e.g., N-methyl-*d*-aspartate (NMDA) channel in brain).
- Ca^{2+} is an important component of the blood-clotting cascade. It is also an important intracellular transducer of hormone signaling as it acts to stimulate protein kinase C.
- PO_4^{3-} has several important functions:
  - It is a component of nucleic acids (DNA and RNA).
  - It is a component of the high-energy phosphoanhydride bonds of ATP, which are hydrolyzed to power biochemical reactions.
  - It is used to phosphorylate enzymes and small molecules. This is a major mode of activating and inactivating enzymes as well as trapping molecules such as glucose inside the cell.
  - It is used in the phosphorolytic cleavage of molecules such as glycogen and purine nucleosides.

Regulation

Blood levels of Ca^{2+} and PO_4^{3-} are regulated by three key hormones (▶ Fig. 1.10):

1. Calcitriol (1,25-$(OH)_2$D, active form of vitamin D_3): This hormone is produced in the kidneys (▶ Fig. 1.7) and acts on several tissues to cause an increase in blood Ca^{2+} and PO_4^{3-} levels.
2. Parathyroid hormone (PTH): This hormone is produced and secreted by the parathyroid glands in response to low blood Ca^{2+} levels. Its action on various tissues causes blood Ca^{2+} levels to increase. It also increases the excretion of PO_4^{3-} by the kidneys by decreasing its reabsorption (called the phosphaturic effect). Although PTH also increases the absorption of phosphate from the intestines and bones, the net result is a decrease in blood PO_4^{3-} levels.
3. Calcitonin: This hormone is produced by the thyroid gland. Its action on various tissues counters the effects of PTH and causes blood Ca^{2+} and PO_4^{3-} levels to decrease.

Deficiencies or excesses of Ca^{2+}, PO_4^{3-}, and Mg^{2+} result in a host of disorders that are often attributed to abnormal functioning of the thyroid, liver, and kidney and poor nutrient absorption by the intestines (▶ Table 1.11).

Normal

Composition and growth of bone

Osteoblasts secrete the organic matrix of bone (predominantly collagen fibers with some extracellular fluid) to create new bone matter. The structural function of bone is made possible by the deposit of bone salts on the organic matrix, the most important of which is hydroxyapatite, formed from calcium and phosphate.

Certain subsets of calcium salts are exchangeable: they are in equilibrium with calcium in extracellular fluid. Osteoclasts degrade bone to maintain this equilibrium. Normally, resorption (osteoclast activity) and bone deposit (osteoblast activity) are in equilibrium: bone is formed and degraded at the same rate. Bone resorption is promoted by parathyroid hormone (PTH), whereas calcitonin stimulates deposition. Initially, PTH increases phosphate levels in blood due to osteoclast activity. But the overall effect of PTH is a decrease in blood phosphate levels due to its promotion of phosphate excretion by the kidneys.

Fe, Zn, and Cu

The most abundant microelements in the human body are Fe, Zn, and Cu. They are obtained from a variety of animal and plant sources, as summarized in ▶ Table 1.12.

Iron (Fe)

Iron is the most abundant microelement in the human body. The average adult has ~4 g of iron. The majority of the body's iron is found bound to hemoglobin, myoglobin (heme proteins), ferritin (an iron-storing protein), and transferrin (an iron-transporting protein).

Iron function

Iron, an important component of heme, serves to either bind oxygen or participate in redox reactions. Heme-containing proteins include the following:

- Hemoglobin and myoglobin: Iron binds to oxygen in these heme proteins.
- Redox enzymes: These include proteins that function in the electron transport chain (e.g., cytochromes) and those that metabolize hydrogen peroxide (e.g., catalase and peroxidase).

I

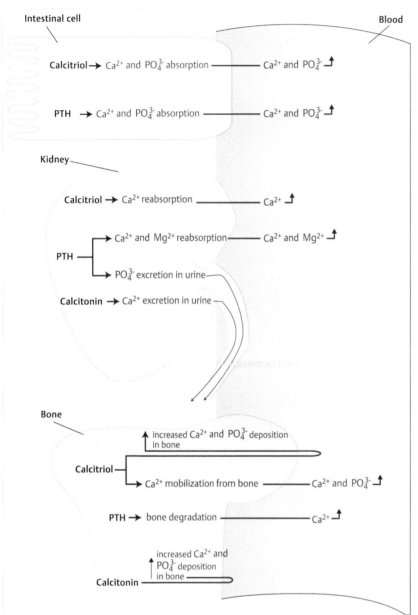

Fig. 1.10 **Calcium metabolism.** The plasma concentration of calcium is regulated by three major hormones: parathyroid hormone (PTH), calcitriol, and calcitonin. Calcitriol stimulates intestinal cells to increase their absorption of Ca^{2+} and PO_4^{3-}. Calcitrol also stimulates the kidneys to reabsorb Ca^{2+}. Calcitonin and calcitriol act to increase the deposition of calcium and phosphate in the bone, whereas PTH causes bone resorption. Calcitonin also increases the excretion of calcium by the kidneys, whereas PTH promotes its retention by reabsorption.

Table 1.11 Disorders associated with abnormal levels of Ca^{2+}, PO_4^{3-}, and Mg^{2+}

Ion	Disorder	Causes	Symptoms
Ca^{2+} deficiency	Hypocalcemia	Hypoalbuminemia or hypomagnesemia Vitamin D deficiency Primary hypoparathyroidism	Rashes, tingling, spasms, arrhythmias, osteoporosis
Ca^{2+} excess	Hypercalcemia	Primary hyperparathyroidism	Constipation, psychosis, bone pain, kidney stones, depression
PO_4^{3-} deficiency	Hypophosphatemia	Refeeding syndrome, respiratory alkalosis, renal loss, malabsorption	Muscle fatigue, mental status changes
PO_4^{3-} excess	Hyperphosphatemia	Hypoparathyroidism, renal failure, drugs	Ectopic calcification, secondary hyperparathy-roidism
Mg^{2+} deficiency	Hypomagnesemia	Alcoholism, diuretics, and drugs (increased renal loss)	Weakness, cramps, irritability, tachycardia
Mg^{2+} excess	Hypermagnesemia	Renal failure	Weakness, hypotension, arrhythmia

Iron is also present in a nonheme form, complexed to sulfur in proteins. Such iron–sulfur proteins function as components of complex I of the mitochondrial electron transport chain.

Disorders associated with deficiencies and excesses in iron are described in ▶ Table 1.13.

Iron absorption, storage, and transport

Iron obtained from animal products in the heme form, which contains iron in the reduced (Fe^{2+}) ferrous state, is efficiently absorbed in the duodenum through the divalent metal ion transporter (DMT). Iron obtained from plant products in the nonheme form exists in the oxidized (Fe^{3+}) ferric state. The absorption of Fe^{3+}, which requires transport proteins, is inefficient. Iron is stored in the cells that line the intestines, as well as in the liver and spleen and in the bone marrow cells. The enzymes and molecules that play important roles in the absorption, storage, and transport of iron are as follows (▶ Fig. 1.11):

- Ferric reductase: This enzyme converts ferric iron (Fe^{3+}) into the more absorbable ferrous iron (Fe^{2+}).
- Vitamin C: Simultaneous intake of vitamin C enhances the efficiency of iron absorption because it keeps iron in the reduced state.
- Certain fibers, antacids, and polyphenols of tea inhibit iron absorption.

Table 1.12 Fe, Zn, and Cu: Sources

Mineral	Source
Fe	Meat, legumes, dark green vegetables (spinach, Swiss chard), whole grains, wheat germ, nuts, legumes
Zn	Grains (oats, cereal, wheat), liver, meat, oysters, nuts, eggs Absorption inhibited by certain minerals and bran
Cu	Cheese, liver, mussels and oysters, poultry, legumes, wheat, cereal, yeast, mushrooms, fruit, nuts, chocolate, cocoa

- Ferritin and hemosiderin: Ferritin is a protein complex that stores iron by binding to multiple ferric (Fe^{3+}) molecules. Hemosiderin, the product of ferritin degradation, also stores iron.
  - Serum ferritin levels (which represent bone marrow iron stores) are measured and used to determine whether iron levels are normal, deficient, or in excess. Normal serum ferritin levels are 15 to 200 ng/mL for males and 12 to 150 ng/mL for females.
- Ferroxidase (ceruloplasmin): This copper-containing enzyme oxidizes ferrous iron (Fe^{2+}) into ferric iron (Fe^{3+}).
- Transferrin: This circulating iron transport protein binds one to two ferric (Fe^{3+}) ions and transports them to various sites either for storage (e.g., liver) or for use in hemoglobin synthesis such as red blood cell development in the bone marrow.
  - The synthesis of transferrin is inversely proportional to the levels of stored iron. When the levels of stored iron are low, the synthesis of transferrin increases, and when stored iron levels are high, the synthesis of transferrin decreases.
  - Total iron-binding capacity (TIBC) is a test that reflects the levels of apotransferrin (i.e., transferrin not bound to iron), which is an indicator of the state of iron stores. A high TIBC is indicative of low iron stores, whereas a low TIBC points to high iron stores.

Normal

Macrophages and iron

Macrophages are phagocytic white blood cells that engulf and digest aged erythrocytes, which allows for the extraction of iron from degraded hemoglobin. The iron is then loaded onto transferrin for transport to the appropriate sites.

Iron regulation

The regulation of the body's iron levels is facilitated by hepcidin, a peptide hormone synthesized by the liver, the levels of which affect the absorption of iron, as follows:

- High levels of dietary iron stimulate an increase in hepcidin synthesis, which suppresses the absorption of iron by

Table 1.13 Disorders associated with abnormal levels of iron

	Disorder description and causes	Symptoms
Iron deficiency	Generally due to insufficient dietary uptake Iron *depletion*, however, can only occur through bleeding (e.g., traumatic blood loss, abnormal menstruation, colon cancer)	Fatigue, anemia
Iron excess/overload	Iron poisoning	Hemorrhagic gastritis and liver necrosis
	Hemochromatosis is an autosomal recessive disease that causes accumulation of iron in the liver, heart, pancreas, and skin. It is caused by unregulated duodenal reabsorption of iron due to low hepcidin levels	Cirrhosis, heart failure, diabetes mellitus, bronzed skin, malabsorption
	Hemosiderosis is a condition in which ferritin is degraded to insoluble hemosiderin, which may accumulate. It is observed in the tissues of alcoholics and patients who have blood transfusions (e.g., hemolytic anemia)	Alveolar hemorrhage
	Sideroblastic anemia is caused by impaired heme synthesis, which results in iron buildup in mitochondria	Pale skin, fatigue, enlarged spleen

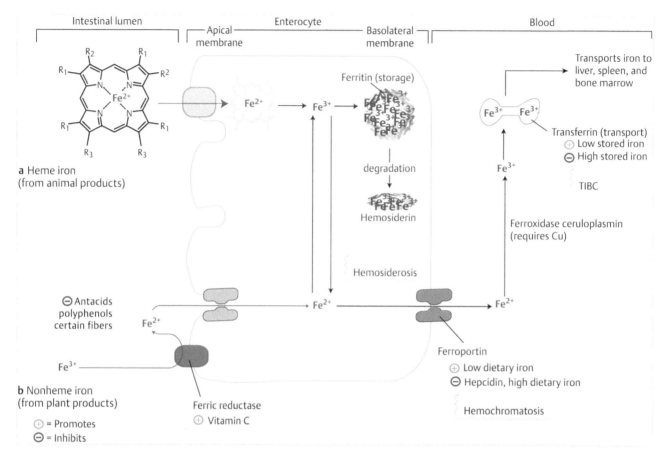

Fig. 1.11 Iron absorption, storage, and transport. (a) Heme iron, which is in the ferrous state (Fe^{2+}), is the most easily absorbable form of iron. Once heme iron enters the enterocyte, it is converted to ferric iron (Fe^{3+}). Ferritin bonds to and stores iron in the ferric form. When ferritin is degraded, it turns into hemosiderin. Hemosiderosis is a disorder marked by hemosiderin accumulation in tissues. **(b)** Nonheme iron, which is in the ferric state, is converted to ferrous iron by ferric reductase via a reaction that requires vitamin C. Ferrous iron (Fe^{2+}) enters the enterocyte and is either converted to ferric iron for storage or exported out of the enterocyte by ferroportin. The amount of available ferroportin is regulated by hepcidin and the levels of dietary iron. Hemochromatosis is a disorder marked by unregulated iron absorption due to low levels of hepcidin. Once in the bloodstream, Fe^{2+} is converted to Fe^{3+} by ferroxidase (a copper-containing enzyme), which gets bound to transferrin for transport to target tissues. Transferrin synthesis is regulated by the levels of stored iron. Total iron-binding capacity (TIBC) is a measure of transferrin levels.

Table 1.14 Enzymes that utilize Zn as a cofactor

Enzyme	Action
Superoxide dismutase	This antioxidant enzyme binds the free radical of molecular oxygen
Collagenases	Belong to the family of matrix metalloproteinases. They are the only enzymes capable of degrading triple helical collagen. They play a major role in tissue repair and remodeling
Alcohol dehydrogenase	Converts alcohol to acetaldehyde
Alkaline phosphatase	Mineralizes bone salts
Transcription factors	Several proteins that contain Zn-finger domains bind to specific sequences on DNA and regulate transcription
Carbonic anhydrase	Interconverts CO_2 and bicarbonate to balance pH

Table 1.15 Enzymes that utilize Cu as a cofactor

Enzyme	Action
Cytochrome-c oxidase	Accepts electrons from cytochrome-c in the electron transport chain
Ferroxidase (ceruloplasmin)	Oxidizes ferrous iron (Fe^{2+}) into ferric iron (Fe^{3+})
Superoxide dismutase	This antioxidant enzyme binds the free radical of molecular oxygen
Lysyl oxidase	Cross-links collagen and elastic tissue during wound healing
Tyrosinase	Synthesizes melanin

increasing the degradation of ferroportin, a membrane-bound iron-transporting protein channel. Conversely, low levels of iron keep hepcidin levels low, which stimulates the absorption of iron due to the elevated levels of ferroportin.

High [Iron] = ↑ Hepcidin = ↓ -Ferroportin = ↓ Iron absorption
Low [Iron] = ↓ Hepcidin = ↑ Ferroportin = ↑ Iron absorption

Foundations

Metalloenzymes

Metalloenzymes are enzymes (proteins or peptides) that require metal ions as cofactors. Metalloenzymes often perform redox reactions (reduction oxidation reactions) in which electrons are transferred from one molecule to another. The metal ion accepts the electron being transferred, and the enzyme therefore becomes temporarily reduced. The electron can then be transferred (oftentimes to another metalloenzyme). This mechanism is important in the electron transport chain. Cytochrome-*c* oxidase receives electrons from cytochrome-*c* in the mitochondria. Cytochrome-*c* oxidase contains two heme

groups and two copper ions. The final electron acceptor in the electron transport chain is molecular oxygen (O_2), which is reduced to form two molecules of water (H_2O).

Zinc (Zn) and Copper (Cu)

The second and third most abundant microelements in the human body are Zn (body content is 2 to 3 g) and Cu (body content is 0.1 to 0.2 g), respectively. They both serve as cofactors for the activity of many enzymes, some of which are listed in ► Table 1.14 and ► Table 1.15). Disorders associated with abnormal levels of Zn and Cu are summarized in ► Table 1.16.

Other Microelements (Trace Elements)

Information about the sources, use, and associated disorders of the remaining eight microelements (Mo, Mn, Co, Cr, S, I, Se, F) are found in ► Table 1.17 (sources), ► Table 1.18 (uses), and ► Table 1.19 (associated disorders).

Table 1.16 Disorders associated with abnormal levels of Zn and Cu

	Disorder description and causes	Symptoms
Zinc deficiency	Alcoholism, rheumatoid arthritis, inflammatory diseases, diarrhea, unleavened bread	Impaired wound healing, loss of taste and smell, growth retardation, hypogonadism, rashes
Copper deficiency	Insufficient copper	Impaired wound healing
Copper excess	Wilson disease, an autosomal recessive disease-causing accumulation of copper in the liver	Liver disease, copper deposits in the eye, dementia, movement disorders

Table 1.17 Sources of other microelements (trace elements)

Trace element		Source
Mo	Molybdenum	Meat, eggs, potatoes, pasta, rice, vegetables, grains, legumes
Mn	Manganese	Fish, meat, cheese, wheat and grains, legumes
Co	Cobalt	Animal foods
Cr	Chromium	Liver, yeast, wheat germ, legumes, vegetables, fruit, cheese, beef, spices
S	Sulfur	Protein (meat, fish), spinach, potatoes, garlic, broccoli, four, wheat, meat, fish, peanuts
I	Iodine	Ubiquitous, especially in fish, also rye, spinach, iodized salt
Se	Selenium	Plants (vegetables, potatoes, fruits), fish, bread, eggs and milk, meat. Selenium is toxic in the mg/d range
F	Fluorine	Occurs in fluorinated drinking water

Table 1.18 Trace elements and their uses

Microelements	Use
Mo	A cofactor for oxidases (xanthine oxidase, aldehyde oxidase, and sulfite oxidase); antagonistic to Cu^{2+}
Mn	A cofactor for pyruvate carboxylase, which converts pyruvate to oxaloacetate
	A cofactor for superoxide dismutase, which binds the free radical of molecules oxygen
	A cofactor for arginase, which catalyzes the formation of urea from arginine
	A cofactor for malic enzyme, which catalyzes the oxidative decarboxylation of malate to pyruvate and CO
Co	Found in cobalamin (vitamin B_{12})
Cr	Involved in the activity of insulin to reduce blood glucose levels
S	Found in coenzyme A, glutathione and S-adenosylmethionine
I	Required for the synthesis of thyroid hormones such as circulating thyroxine (T_4) and the intracellular active hormone tri-iodothyronine (T_3). They play an important role in growth, development, and metabolic processes. Insufficient dietary intake if iodine leads to endemic goiter
Se	A cofactor of glutathione peroxidase, an important antioxidant enzyme that detoxifies hydrogen peroxide; required for the conversion of the thyroid hormone T_4 to T_3
F	Fluorine is not a proper bone salt, but it prevents demineralization of teeth (dental caries)

Table 1.19 Disorders associated with abnormal levels of trace elements

Trace element	Cause	Disorder/Symptoms
Iodine deficiency	Insufficient dietary intake	Endemic goiter, cretinism (congenital hypothyroidism)
Chromium deficiency	Occurs when TPN is used to feed a patient	Impaired glucose tolerance marked by high blood glucose levels (akin to diabetes), confusion, peripheral neuropathy
Selenium deficiency	Occurs when TPN is used to feed a patient	Keshan disease marked by cardiomyopathy, muscle pain, fatigue
Fluorine deficiency	Insufficient intake of fluorinated water	Dental caries
Fluorine excess	Overabundant fluoride in drinking water	Fluorosis

2 Carbohydrate Structure and Chemistry

2.1 Overview

Carbohydrates are organic molecules made up of carbon, hydrogen, and oxygen that have the general formula $C_n(H_2O)_n$, where n is between 3 and 9. Carbohydrates serve as important fuel stores because their metabolism provides a large part of the energy required by an organism. Their carbon skeletons are also used for the biosynthesis of other compounds.

Carbohydrates obtained from the diet come in four forms:
1. **Monosaccharides:** These are the simplest forms of carbohydrates. Examples include glucose, fructose, galactose, and ribose.
2. **Disaccharides:** These carbohydrate chains are composed of two monosaccharides. Examples include maltose, lactose, and sucrose.
3. **Oligosaccharides:** These carbohydrate chains are made up of 3 to 10 monosaccharides. They are often found covalently attached to membrane lipids and proteins, which are referred to as glycolipids and glycoproteins, respectively.
4. **Polysaccharides:** These carbohydrate chains are composed of more than 10 monosaccharides. Examples include glycogen, starch, and cellulose.

2.2 Monosaccharides

2.2.1 Nomenclature

Monosaccharides have the molecular formula $(CH_2O)_x$, where $x \geq 3$. The name assigned to each monosaccharide reflects the number of carbons it contains, its functional group, and its stereoisomeric form, as follows:
1. **Carbon number:** The number of carbons in a monosaccharide is represented in the **pre**fix of its name, which typically ends with -ose. Examples include **tri**ose (three carbons), **tetr**ose (four carbons), **pent**ose (five carbons), **hex**ose (six carbons), and **hept**ose (seven carbons).
2. **Functional group:** Monosaccharides contain a carbonyl group $(C = O)$ as part of either an aldehyde or a ketone (▸ Fig. 2.1a).
   When the carbonyl group is on carbon-1, the monosaccharide is an aldehyde, and when the carbonyl group is on carbon-2, the monosaccharide is a ketone.
3. **Stereoisomeric form:** The asymmetric carbon of a monosaccharide is attached to four different atoms or groups of atoms. Stereoisomers are molecules that have the same molecular formula and bond constituents but differ in the spatial orientation of atoms attached to the asymmetric carbon. For instance, the **D** and **L** designations for monosaccharide stereoisomers are based on the position of the hydroxyl group relative to the asymmetric carbon. The D-form is the most common form observed in cellular metabolism and in biological structures (▸ Fig. 2.1b).
   • The D-form has the hydroxyl group to the right (Latin, *dexter*) of the asymmetric carbon.

• The L-form has the hydroxyl group to the left (Latin, *laevus*) of the asymmetric carbon.

Biologically, these stereoisomers are distinct molecules, and receptors and enzymes can differentiate between them.

2.2.2 Depiction

The two common manners in which the structures of sugars are depicted are the straight-chain and the ring forms (▸ Fig. 2.2).
1. **Straight-chain form (Fischer projection):** This is a linear, open representation of monosaccharides, which shows the carbon chain and functional group(s) and allows for identifcation of the stereoisomeric form (e.g., **D** vs. **L**).
2. **Ring form (Haworth projection):** Monosaccharides do not exclusively exist in the straight-chain form. They may cyclize (form rings) through reactions in which the carbonyl carbon of aldoses and ketose react reversibly with internal alcohol groups (OH) to create hemiacetals and hemiketals, respectively.

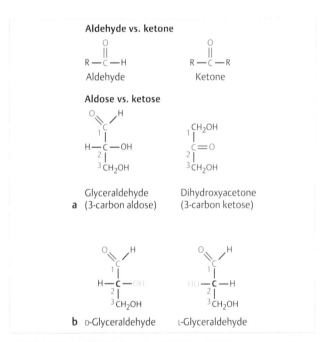

Fig. 2.1 Nomenclature of monosaccharides. (a) The general structure of an aldehyde and a ketone. The carbonyl group (red) of an aldose (e.g., glyceraldehyde) is on carbon-1. The carbonyl group of a ketose (e.g., dihydroxyacetone) is on carbon-2. (b) The D-form of a monosaccharide has the hydroxyl group (blue) to the right of the asymmetric carbon, whereas the L-form has the hydroxyl group to the left. For monosaccharides with multiple asymmetric carbons, the **L** and **D** designations are determined using the asymmetric carbon farthest away from the carbonyl group.

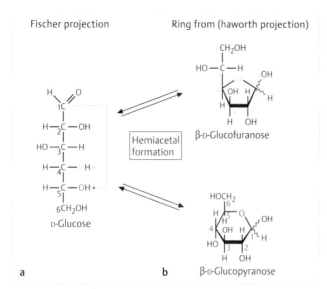

Fischer projection   Ring from (haworth projection)

β-ᴅ-Glucofuranose

Hemiacetal formation

ᴅ-Glucose

β-ᴅ-Glucopyranose

a   b

Fig. 2.2 Depictions of monosaccharide structure. (a) This monosaccharide is D-glucose because the asymmetric carbon (C5), which is farthest from the carbonyl group, has an OH positioned to its right. **(b)** The OH attached to the anomeric carbons (C1 of both β-D-glucofuranose and β -D-glucopyranose) is above the ring. Cyclization of an aldose generates a ring structure in which the anomeric carbon is attached to OH and H groups outside the ring. However, the anomeric carbon of a cyclized ketose is attached to OH and carbon-containing groups (see D-ribulose and D-fructose in ▶ Fig. 2.3). The wavy lines indicate which groups are attached to the anomeric carbon and determine α or β designations.

- Cyclization creates a new asymmetric center (referred to as the anomeric carbon) at the carbonyl carbon of the aldose (C1) or the ketose (C2). This generates a ring that is either five atoms (furanose) or six atoms (pyranose) in size.
- When cyclized sugars are looked at "edge on," the OH group at the anomeric carbon is in one of two positions:
  1. α-Position: OH is below the ring.
  2. β-Position: OH is above the ring.

Foundations

Isomers

Isomers are molecules with the same molecular formula but different structures. Structural isomers have the same atoms arranged in different bonding patterns; stereoisomers have the same bonds but arranged differently in space, making them nonsuperimposable on each other. Stereoisomers are further divided into (1) *enantiomers*, which are mirror images of each other, and (2) *diastereomers*, which are not mirror images. Verapamil is a drug that inhibits the activity of voltage-gated (I-type) calcium channels found in cardiac and smooth muscle. Because it reduces the contractility of muscle by preventing calcium influx, verapamil is prescribed for conditions such as angina, arrhythmias, and hypertension. Research has shown that only one enantiomer, the left mirror image S-verapamil, actively blocks calcium channels, whereas the other, the right mirror image R-verapamil, does not.

2.2.3 Important Monosaccharides

Some monosaccharides play important roles in various metabolic pathways, as described in ▶ Table 2.1 and shown in ▶ Fig. 2.3.

Normal

Blood glucose

Blood glucose levels in normal individuals are strictly regulated through the actions of hormones such as insulin and glucagon. Normal fasting plasma glucose concentration range is 70 to 100 mg/dL and rarely exceeds 140 mg/dL after a meal. When blood glucose drops below 60 mg/dL (hypoglycemia), hunger, sweating, and trembling may be experienced. Levels below 40 mg/dL progressively result in convulsions, coma, brain damage, and death. Fasting levels above 126 mg/dL and postprandial levels above 199 mg/dL (hyperglycemia) are diagnostic of diabetes mellitus.

Table 2.1 Important monosaccharides and their functions

Class	Aldose	Ketose	Function
Triose (3C)	Glyceraldehyde	Dihydroxyacetone	Glyceraldehyde: An important intermediate in glycolysis and the pentose phosphate pathway Dihydroxyacetone: Its phosphate ester is an intermediate in glycolysis
Tetrose (4C)	Erythrose		Erythrose: A pentose phosphate pathway intermediate
Pentose (5C)	D-Ribose	D-Ribulose	D-Ribose: In its furanose form, it contributes to the structure of RNA and nucleotide coenzymes D-Ribulose: Its phosphate ester, which is the most important ketopentose, is an intermediate in the pentose phosphate pathway
Hexose (6C)	D-Glucose D-Galactose D-Mannose	D-Fructose	D-Glucose: The most important aldohexose; it is the building block for glycogen, starch, and cellulose. Free D-glucose is found in blood D-Galactose: A constituent of lactose. It is found in glycolipids and glycoproteins, along with d-mannose D-Fructose: The most widely distributed ketohexose. It is a component of sucrose
Heptose (7C)		Sedoheptulose	Sedoheptulose: An intermediate of the pentose phosphate pathway

Note: l-Arabinose and d-xylose are 5-carbon aldoses and are found in large quantities as constituents of polysaccharides in plant walls.

of ATP in glycolysis when compared to oxidative metabolism, cancer cells have greatly enhanced rates of glucose uptake. This unique property is made use of in clinical detection of cancer by positron emission tomography (PET), where a patient is injected with a glucose analog tracer, fluorodeoxyglucose (FdG). FdG-PET imaging reveals which tissues consume more of this tagged glucose.

Normal
Pentose phosphate pathway

The pentose phosphate pathway (also called the hexose monophosphate shunt) metabolizes glucose to form important by-products, such as the reduced form of nicotinamide adenine dinucleotide phosphate (NADPH), ribose 5-phosphate (R5P), fructose 6-phosphate (F6P), and glyceraldehyde 3-phosphate (G3P). NADPH is necessary for reductive biosynthetic reactions (e.g., fatty acid synthesis), R5P is required for the formation of nucleic acids, and both F6P and G3P are used in glycolysis.

2.2.4 Modifed Monosaccharides

Monosaccharides are chemically modified to create derivatives that are also metabolically important. They include the following (▶ Fig. 2.4):

1. **Deoxyaldoses:** These derivatives are created by replacing an OH group with hydrogen. An example is 2-deoxy-D-ribose, a major component of DNA (▶ Fig. 2.4a).
2. **Acetylated amino sugars:** These are generated when an OH group is replaced by an amino group attached to an acetyl group. Examples include *N*-acetyl-D-glucosamine, *N*-acetyl-D-galactosamine, and *N*-acetylneuraminic acid (sialic acid) (▶ Fig. 2.4b). These modified sugars are components of glycoproteins and glycolipids, which play a major role in cell signaling, cell adhesion, and immune response. Glycosphingolipids are abundant in neural tissue and contribute to my-elin structure.
3. **Acidic sugars:** These are generated via oxidation of the terminal OH of an aldose or ketose, forming a carboxylic acid. Examples include D-glucuronic acid, L-iduronic acid, D-galacturonic acid, ascorbic acid (vitamin C), and the acetylated amino sugar sialic acid (▶ Fig. 2.4c). Acidic sugars are components of glycos-aminoglycans and proteoglycans that are present in plasma membranes of cells and in the extracellular matrix. These macromolecules have a high capacity to bind water and form hydrated matrices that stabilize basement membranes, secretory granules, and zymogens, as well as aid cartilage function.
4. **Sugar esters:** These derivatives are created when a mono-saccharide is attached to a phosphate group (PO_4^{3-}) or a sulfate group (SO_4^{2-}). Examples include glucose 6-phosphate (▶ Fig. 2.4d), ribose 5-phosphate, and galactose 3-sulfate. Glucose 6-phosphate is an important intermediate in glycolysis and glycogen synthesis, ribose 5-phosphate is a precursor of nucleotides, and galactose 6-phosphate is a component of glycosphingolipids that constitute gangliosides in oligodendrocytes of the nervous system. Sulfated galactose and glucuronic acid are also found in glycosaminoglycans.

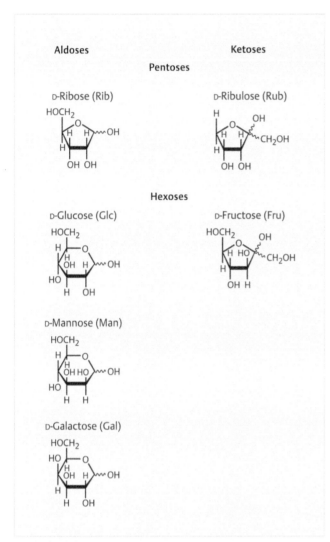

Fig. 2.3 Important monosaccharides. Structures of the important pentoses, D-ribose and D-ribulose, and the important hexoses, D-glucose, D-fructose, D-mannose, and D-galactose, are shown.

Foundations
Glycolysis

Glycolysis, meaning breakdown of glucose, is the process by which most cells generate energy. The six-carbon sugar glucose is metabolized in a series of enzymatic reactions to two molecules of the three-carbon organic acid pyruvate. In this process, there is a net synthesis of two adenosine triphosphate (ATP) molecules. Under aerobic conditions, pyruvate and reducing equivalents from glycolysis can be oxidized in the mitochondria to yield substantially more chemical energy (up to 36 molecules of ATP). Under anaerobic conditions, glycolysis is the only means by which ATP can be generated from glucose. Cells that lack mitochondria (e.g., red blood cells) also rely completely on glycolysis for energy. In other cells, aerobic conditions tend to suppress glycolysis in a phenomenon known as the Pasteur Effect due to allosteric inhibition of glycolytic enzymes by citrate and ATP. However, many cancers exhibit high rates of glycolysis even in the presence of oxygen (Warburg Effect). To compensate for the inefficient production

I

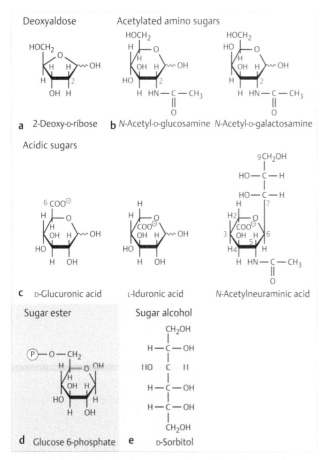

Fig. 2.4 Monosaccharide derivatives. Chemical modifcations of various monosaccharides generate important sugar derivatives, which include (**a**) deoxyaldoses, (**b**) acetylated amino sugars, (**c**) acidic sugars, (**d**) sugar esters, and (**e**) sugar alcohols. N-acetylneuraminic acid (sialic acid) is considered to be both an acetylated amino sugar and an acidic sugar.

5. **Sugar alcohols:** These are created when the carbonyl group is reduced, forming a hydroxyl group. Examples include glyc-erol, xylitol, sorbitol (▶ Fig. 2.4e), and galactitol.
   - Glycerol, a derivative of glyceraldehyde, is also produced from the degradation of triacylglycerols in adipose tissue and is involved in the synthesis of lipids, glycolysis, and gluconeogenesis (production of glucose from noncarbohydrate sources).
   - Xylitol and sorbitol are often used as food additives in processed sugar-free foods.
   - Sorbitol, the sugar alcohol derivative of glucose, is converted to fructose in our body. In uncontrolled diabetics, some glucose is converted to the osmotically active sorbitol, which triggers the movement of water into cells where it accumulates, leading to the destruction of the lens, pericytes, and Schwann cells, which manifest in diabetic patients as cataracts, retinopathy, and peripheral neuropathy, respectively.
   - Galactitol, a derivative of galactose, is also known as dulcitol. Accumulation of galactitol in the lens could lead to cataracts.

Normal

Sweeteners erythritol, xylitol, mannitol, and sorbitol

Erythritol is a four-carbon sugar alcohol used as artificial sweetener. Because little of it is metabolized, it releases little energy when consumed in food. It also does not promote tooth decay. Because it is absorbed in the small intestine and then excreted in urine, it causes less flatulence than other sugar alcohols.

Xylitol is a five-carbon sugar alcohol used as a natural sweetener. It has a low glycemic index (i.e., does not raise blood sugar), does not promote tooth decay, and has somewhat lower energy content than sucrose at about the same sweetness. Unlike many sweeteners, it does not have a bad aftertaste. The only disadvantage is flatulence after excess consumption.

Mannitol is a sugar alcohol used for energy storage by some microorganisms and plants. In medicine it is used to treat head trauma and kidney failure, as a heart–lung machine primer, and to make the blood–brain barrier permeable to drugs. The inhaled solid may be useful for the treatment of cystic fibrosis by osmotically liquefying mucus. Mannitol is also used as a low glycemic index, tooth-friendly sweetener, although it is only about half as sweet as sucrose and in high doses causes flatulence.

The sugar alcohol sorbitol is used as a sweetener in chewing gum, toothpaste, and mouthwash and as a laxative.

Therapeutics

Galactosemias

Through a series of enzymatic reactions, galactose is converted to glucose 6-phosphate (see **Fig. 12.15**), a molecule that is used in both glycolysis and gluconeogenesis. A deficiency in any of the three enzymes that catalyze the metabolism of galactose results in galactosemias—hereditary disorders marked by the damaging accumulation of galactitol in the lens of the eyes. Classic galactosemia occurs when galactose 1-phosphate uridyltransferase (GALT) is deficient and is usually detected by newborn screening. Infants with this condition present with cataracts, hepatomegaly, jaundice, and failure to thrive. A milder form of galactosemia is caused by a deficiency in galactokinase or in uridine diphosphate (UDP)-galactose epimerase. Galactose accumulates in the blood and urine of these patients, particularly when galactose-containing foods are consumed (e.g., milk).

2.3 Disaccharides, Oligosaccharides, and Polysaccharides

2.3.1 Glycosidic Bonds

Carbohydrates can be linked to each other or to other molecules through glycosidic bonds. These bonds are formed between the highly reactive anomeric carbon of the hemiacetal/hemiketal and atoms of a target molecule. Glycosidic bonds are described in terms of two key features:

Table 2.2 Characteristics of major disaccharides

Source	Glycosidase		Disaccharide Monosaccharide components
Maltose	Malt sugars	Maltase	Glucose + glucose (α-linkage)
Lactose	Mammalian milk	Lactase	Galactose + glucose (β-linkage)
Sucrose	Table sugar	Sucrase	Glucose + fructose (α-, β-linkage)

1. **The atom (*O, N,* or *S*) to which the anomeric carbon of a monosaccharide is attached**:
   - *O*-Glycosidic bond: The anomeric carbon is linked via an oxygen atom to another molecule. This is the most common sugar linkage. *O*-Linked glycoproteins have a carbohydrate attached to the oxygen atom of the α-hydroxyl group of serine or threonine in a protein molecule.
   - *N*-Glycosidic bond: The anomeric carbon is linked via a nitrogen atom to another molecule. In nucleosides, for instance, an *N*-glycosidic bond links ribose to a purine or pyrimidine base. *N*-Linked glycoproteins have a carbohydrate attached to the nitrogen atom of the β-amino group of a protein's asparagine residue.
   - *S*-Glycosidic bond: The anomeric carbon is linked via a sulfur atom to another molecule.
2. **The position of the glycosidic bond:** When the glycosidic bond is below the plane of the sugar rings, it is referred to as an α-glycosidic bond. Conversely, if the bond is above the plane of the rings, it is called a β-glycosidic bond.

2.3.2 Disaccharide Composition

Disaccharides are formed from two monosaccharides linked via an *O*-glycosidic bond. The three major disaccharides, maltose, lactose, and sucrose, are found in malt sugars, mammalian milk, and table sugar, respectively. Cleavage of their glycosidic bonds by specific glycosidases releases their monosaccharide constituents (► Table 2.2). The position of the glycosidic bonds in these disaccharides are either α-, β-, or both (► Fig. 2.5).

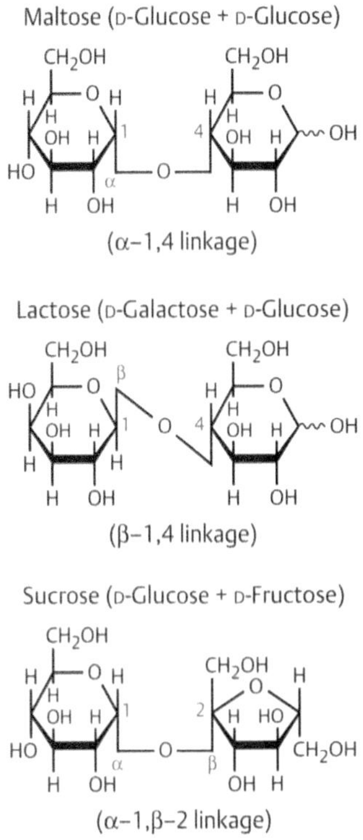

Foundations

Reducing and nonreducing sugars

Sugars are referred to as reducing or nonreducing. In solution, the straight-chain and ring forms are in equilibrium, and if placed in an alkaline solution, the carbonyl group of aldehydes (in the straight-chain form) can reduce Cu^{2+} to Cu_2O, which forms a reddish precipitate. Urinalysis tests performed to detect the levels of reducing sugars in urine exploit this feature to diagnose conditions such as diabetes mellitus and essential fructosuria. Sucrose is a nonreducing sugar because the carbonyl groups of both glucose and fructose are involved in its glycosidic linkage. The reducing sugars include glyceraldehyde, glucose, galactose, maltose, and lactose. Fructose itself (as a ketone) is nonreducing. In the alkaline environment however, it slowly converts to glucose. Hence, in fructosuria, a reducing sugar is found, but tests for glucose using sticks with glucosidase are negative.

Fig. 2.5 Most common disaccharides. Disaccharides are formed by the condensation of two monosaccharides with the elimination of a water molecule. Maltose, lactose, and sucrose are the three most common disaccharides in nature. The chemical bond between the two sugars is called a glycosidic linkage and is designated by the position of the hydroxyl groups involved and their isomeric configurations (α or β). Please note that the fructose structure in sucrose is inverted compared to its orientation in ► Fig. 2.3.

Therapeutics

Lactose intolerance

Lactase (β-galactosidase), an enzyme normally produced by absorptive cells of the small intestine, is responsible for the hydrolysis of the disaccharide lactose into glucose and galactose. A genetic deficiency in lactase gives rise to primary lactose intolerance. Although infants of all races possess sufficient lactase in the intestine, adults of many races lack it. The age-dependent loss of this enzyme after weaning appears to be due to a decrease in the production of the enzyme and may cause secondary lactose intolerance in some adults. Within 2 hours of consuming more than a few ounces of milk, lactose-intolerant individuals will experience diarrhea and intestinal gas caused by microbial fermentation of lactose in the gut. Lactose intolerance may be detected by measuring blood glucose levels after consumption of lactose and by a hydrogen breath test.

2.3.3 Oligosaccharide and Polysaccharide Composition

Oligosaccharides (3 to 10 sugars in length), and polysaccharides (> 10 sugars) exist as linear or branched chains. Polysaccharides are divided into two groups:

1. Homoglycans: composed of one type of monosaccharide
2. Heteroglycans: composed of more than one type of monosaccharide

Polysaccharides function as carbohydrate stores and as structural and mechanical support to cells. When needed, enzymes degrade polysaccharides to their monosaccharide constituents (▶ Table 2.3). There are four important polysaccharides:

1. **Glycogen**, a branched polymer of glucose, is obtained from animal sources or synthesized endogenously from glucose. It is stored in the liver and muscle. It is less osmotically active than glucose and can therefore be stored in large quantities intracellularly.
2. **Starch**, a major dietary polysaccharide, found in plants. Approximately 75% is in the form of amylopectin (a soluble, branched glucose polymer), and 25% is in the form of amylose (an insoluble, linear glucose polymer).
3. **Glycosaminoglycans**, long, linear polysaccharides composed of repeating units of a particular disaccharide. The disaccharide units contain one acetylated amino sugar and one uronic acid—an acidic sugar such as D-glucuronic acid or D-iduronic acid. They are essential components of connective tissue (e.g., cartilage) and synovial fluid (i.e., joint lubricant).
4. **Cellulose**, a plant polysaccharide composed of glucose that cannot be digested by humans because, like many animals (with the exception of ruminants and termites), they lack cellulase, an enzyme that hydrolyzes the β-l,4-glycosidic bonds found in cellulose. Cellulose is a type of dietary fiber that promotes proper functioning of the digestive tract and reduces constipation.

Foundations

Gluconeogenesis

Under fasting conditions, stores of liver glycogen (glucose$_n$), a polymeric storage form of glucose, are sufficient to supply the brain with glucose for only ~12 hours. Gluconeogenesis, the process by which glucose is synthesized from noncarbohydrate precursors such as pyruvate or lactate, amino acids, propionate, and glycerol, must take over. The purpose of gluconeogenesis is to replenish blood glucose levels to provide an energy source for tissues such as brain, erythrocytes, cornea, and testis. Although many of the steps in gluconeogenesis are the reverse of glycolytic reactions, the liver is the only major gluconeogenic organ because most tissues lack two enzymes specific for the pathway.

Therapeutics

Hemorrhoids and cellulose

Hemorrhoids, swollen veins located inside the lower rectum or externally around the anus, are formed due to excessive pressure on the veins of the rectum, which can occur in constipated individuals. A diet that lacks sufficient amounts of fiber (cellulose) and fluid contributes to constipation and is a factor in the development of hemorrhoids.

Table 2.3 Major polysaccharides composed of glucose only

Polysaccharide	Structural description	Degrading enzymes
Glycogen	Linear chains with α-1,4 linkages and branch points with α -1,6 linkages	Glycogen phosphorylase Debranching enzymes
Starch	Amylopectin (75%): linear chains with α-1,4 linkages and the branch points with α-1,6 linkages (water soluble) Amylose (25%): linear chains with α-1,4 linkages (water insoluble)	α -Amylase Amyloglucosidase (debranching enzyme)
Cellulose	Linear chains with β-1,4 linkages	Cellulase (present only in the symbiotic gut bacteria of herbivorous animals)

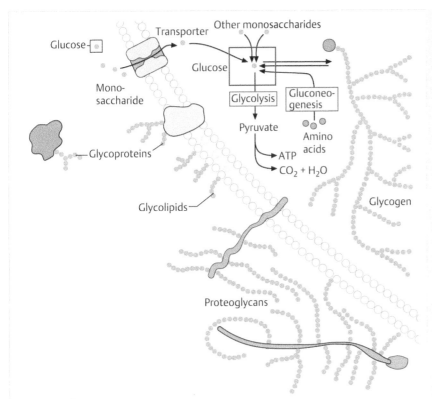

Fig. 2.6 Carbohydrates: Overview.
Carbohydrates are digested to monosaccharides, which can be used as a fuel source (glucose undergoes glycolysis to pyruvate, which can be used to generate ATP). Though carbohydrates are the major fuel source in humans, they are not essential (glucose can be generated through gluconeogenesis from amino acids). Carbohydrates also serve as building blocks and they combine with proteins and lipids to form cell-surface receptors and signaling molecules.

2.3.4 Important Oligosaccharide and Polysaccharide Derivatives

Oligosaccharides and polysaccharides combine with noncarbohydrate molecules to form three extremely important structural molecules (▶ Fig. 2.6):

1. **Glycoproteins** (oligosaccharide + protein): Many proteins on the extracellular surface of plasma membranes (and the majority of secreted proteins) have oligosaccharide residues covalently attached to their polypeptide backbone.

2. **Glycolipids** (oligosaccharide + lipid): They are usually found in membranes with the carbohydrate moieties projecting out into the surrounding environment. Many cell-surface antigens or recognition sites are glycolipids. The oligosaccharide side chains are similar in structure to those found in glycoproteins.

3. **Proteoglycans** (glycosaminoglycan + protein): These protein-carbohydrate compounds are composed of ~ 5% protein and 95% glycosaminoglycan. They are found primarily in connective tissues and joint lubricant.

3 Lipid Structure and Chemistry

3.1 Overview

Lipids are an extremely heterogeneous class of molecules that are all synthesized from acetyl coenzyme A (acetyl CoA), the activated form of acetic acid. They are divided into two broad classes (▶ Fig. 3.1):

1. **Fatty acid derivatives:** These lipids contain fatty acid chains, each made up of a monocarboxylic acid with a long hydrocarbon chain. These chains may be saturated (zero double bonds), monounsaturated (one double bond), or polyunsatu-rated (two or more double bonds). Molecules that fall in this class include glycerides, membrane lipids, and eicosanoids.
2. **Isoprenoids:** These lipids contain multiple units of a fve-carbon molecule, called isoprene, which are linked together to form cyclic structures or linear chains. Molecules such as cholesterol, bile acids, steroid hormones, the lipid-soluble vitamins, and coenzyme Q all fall under this class.

These essential biomolecules are used for the following purposes:

1. **Fuel stores:** Energy is stored in adipose tissue in the form of triacylglycerols (triglyceride). These lipids yield 9 kcal of energy for each gram that undergoes complete combustion. Carbohydrates and proteins, on the other hand, yield only 4 kcal/g.
2. **Structural support:** Lipids are the major structural components of all cellular membranes. As such, they provide mechanical and electrical insulation to cells. Lipids also serve as anchors that tether proteins to membranes.
3. **Signaling events:** Lipids serve as cofactors for enzymes and as direct signaling molecules that regulate cellular processes such as growth and development, the immune response, blood coagulation, vision, and the concentration of key nutrients in the blood.

4. **Miscellaneous:** On the macroscopic level, adipose tissue provides mechanical protection and thermal insulation to organs.

3.2 Fatty Acids

3.2.1 Nomenclature and Classification

The long, unbranched hydrocarbon chains of fatty acids are typically 4 to 24 carbons in length and contain an even number of carbons. Fatty acids have the general formula $CH_3(CH_2)_nCOOH$ and are characterized based on the length of their hydrocarbon chain as follows:

- Short chain: fewer than 6 carbons
- Medium chain: 6 to 12 carbons
- Long chain: 13 to 20 carbons
- Very long chain: more than 22 carbons

The length of a fatty acid's chain influences the method by which it is transported from the gastrointestinal tract to tissues and cellular compartments and the mechanism by which it is metabolized.

- Short- and medium-chain fatty acids from the diet diffuse directly into the hepatic portal vein for transport to the liver.
- Long-chain fatty acids are hardly soluble in aqueous solutions at physiological pH. Therefore, their transport through blood is facilitated by binding to albumin. Additionally, dietary long-chain fatty acids are packaged as triacylglycerols into large lipoproteins, called chylomicrons, for transport to the liver via the lymphatic system and blood. Their transport into and within the cytosol of cells is mediated by fatty acid–binding proteins.
- The catabolism (via β-oxidation) of fatty acids in the mito-chondrial matrix is coupled to energy (ATP) production. Short- and medium-chain fatty acids diffuse directly through

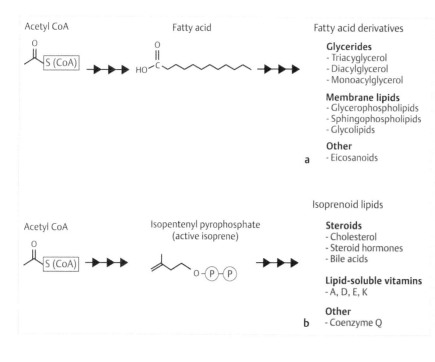

Fig. 3.1 Lipid classes: fatty acid derivatives and isoprenoids. Lipids are formed from acetyl coenzyme A (acetyl CoA), the activated form of acetic acid. (a) Lipids that fall under the category of fatty acid-derived lipids include glycerides such as triacylglycerol, diacylglycerol, and monoacylglycerol; membrane-bound lipids such as the glycerophospho-lipids, sphingophospholipids, and glycolipids; and signaling lipids such as the eicosanoids. (b) Lipids that fall under the category of isoprenoids include steroids such as cholesterol, steroid hormones, and bile acids; lipid-soluble vitamins (A, D, E, K); and others, such as coenzyme Q.

the mitochondrial membranes and into the matrix, whereas long-chain fatty acids can only cross the inner mitochondrial membrane via the carnitine shuttle (see **Fig. 13.7**). Very long chain fatty acids are catabolized in peroxisomes via β-oxidative reactions that are not entirely coupled to ATP production.

Therapeutics

Defects in very long chain fatty acid catabolism

Accumulation of very long chain fatty acids (VLCFAs) in the blood, which is typically attributed to conditions that disrupt the catabolism of VLCFAs, causes demyelinization of nerve axons. For instance, Zellweger syndrome is a condition caused by defects in the biogenesis of peroxisomes, which are the subcellular organelle where VLCFA catabolism occurs. Likewise, X-linked adrenoleukodystrophy, a disorder that results in damage to the myelin sheath that surrounds nerve cells, is caused by defects in the protein that transports VLCFAs into the peroxisome.

Types of Fatty Acids

Fatty acid carbons are normally numbered starting with the α-carbon in the carboxylic acid group (COOH) and ending with the carbon in the terminal methyl group (CH_3). Alternatively, they may be numbered starting with the ω-carbon in the terminal methyl group. The presence or absence of double bonds is the basis for the division of fatty acids into the following three groups (▶ Fig. 3.2):

1. **Saturated fatty acids** contain hydrocarbon chains that lack double bonds. In humans, the most common fatty acids are saturated. Examples include palmitic acid (C16:0), stearic acid (C18:0), and lignoceric acid (C24:0).
2. **Monounsaturated fatty acids** have hydrocarbon chains with one double bond. An example of these monounsaturated fatty acids is oleic acid (C18:1(Δ^9)).
3. **Polyunsaturated fatty acids** contain two or more double bonds in their hydrocarbon chains. Because mammals cannot introduce double bonds beyond carbon-9 in a fatty acid, some polyunsaturated fatty acids must be obtained from the diet and are therefore referred to as essential fatty acids. Examples include linoleic acid (C18:2($\Delta^{9,12}$)), linolenic acid C18:3($\Delta^{9,12,15}$), and arachidonic acid C20:4 ($\Delta^{5,8,11,14}$).

Foundations

ω-3 and ω-6 fatty acids

Omega(ω)-3 fatty acids are essential fatty acids whose final double bonds are located three carbons from the end of their hydrocarbon tails. One common ω-3 fatty acid is α-linolenic acid. Omega-6 fatty acids have a double bond six carbons from the end of their hydrocarbon tails. Linoleic acid and arachidonic acid are examples of ω-6 fatty acids.

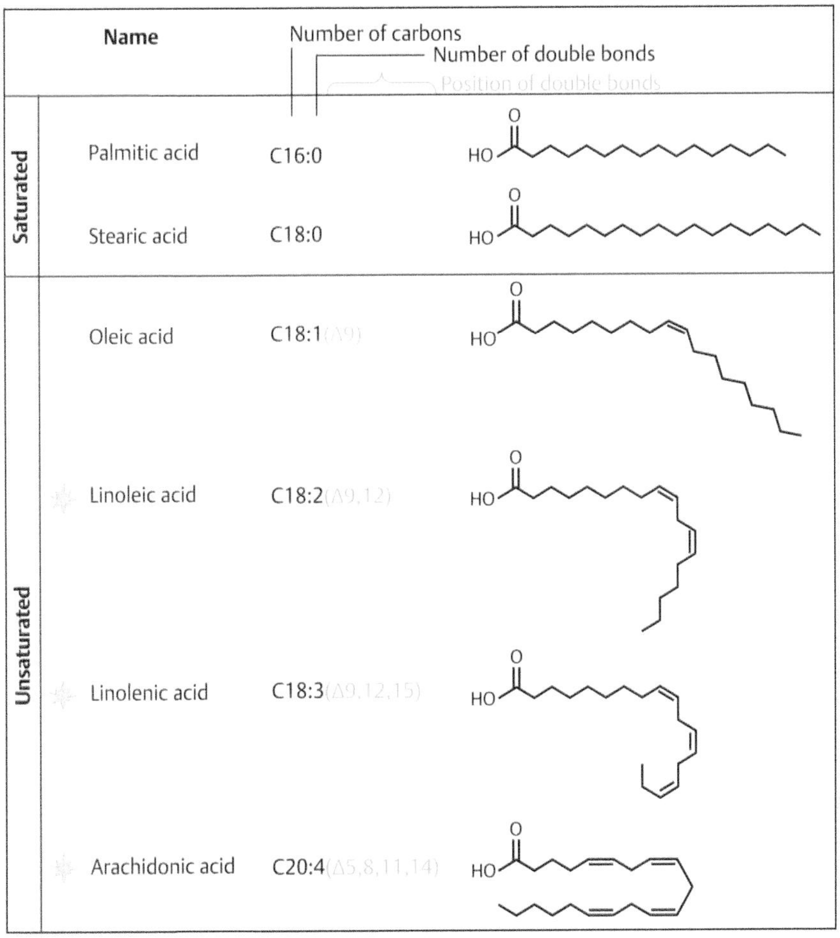

	Name	Number of carbons	
Saturated	Palmitic acid	C16:0	
	Stearic acid	C18:0	
Unsaturated	Oleic acid	C18:1(Δ^9)	
	Linoleic acid	C18:2($\Delta^{9,12}$)	
	Linolenic acid	C18:3($\Delta^{9,12,15}$)	
	Arachidonic acid	C20:4($\Delta^{5,8,11,14}$)	

Fig. 3.2 Fatty acids. Fatty acids are monocarboxylic acids with long hydrocarbon chains. They may be saturated (zero double bonds), monounsaturated (one double bond), or polyunsaturated (two or more double bonds). Fatty acid carbons are normally numbered starting with the carbon in the carboxyl (COOH) group and ending with the terminal methyl group (CH_3). The shorthand format for designating the composition of fatty acids is C#1: #2(Δ#, #,...), where $\#_1$ is the total number of carbons, $\#_2$ is the number of double bonds in the hydrocarbon chain, and the numbers after the delta (Δ) symbol indicate the location of the first carbon involved in each double bond. Stars denote the three essential fatty acids: linoleic, linolenic, and arachidonic acids.

I

β–Oxidation

β-Oxidation is the mitochondrial pathway for the catabolism of saturated fatty acids. In this process, two-carbon units, in the form of acetyl CoA, are successively removed from the carboxyl end of the activated fatty acid (fatty acyl CoA). Complete β-oxidation of the saturated, 16-carbon palmitoyl CoA produces 8 molecules of acetyl CoA, 7 molecules of $FADH_2$, and 7 molecules of NADH, which yield a total of 131 molecules of ATP.

Cis-trans Isomerization

The carbons that flank each double bond of an unsaturated fatty acid can exist in either the *cis-* or *trans-* confguration. Natural unsaturated fatty acids exist only in the *cis-*form. However, when partially hydrogenated, some *cis-*double bonds are converted to *trans-*double bonds. The *cis-* and *trans-*isomers of fatty acids have the following characteristics (▶ Fig. 3.3):

- **Cis-isomer:** These isomers have a kink in their hydrocarbon chains that limits how closely their hydrophobic tails can pack. This causes an increase in the fluidity of membranes in which they reside.
- **Trans-isomer:** These isomers have straight hydrocarbon chains, which strengthens the interactions between molecules in this form and allows them to pack more closely. This characteristic (which is similar to that of saturated fatty acids) reduces their mobility and the fluidity of membranes in which they reside.

3.2.2 Fatty Acid–derived Lipids

Lipids derived from fatty acids are described based on the following three features:

1. **Backbone:** Fatty acids are often attached to a backbone structure, which is typically a molecule of glycerol or sphingosine (▶ Fig. 3.4).
   - Glycerol is a trivalent sugar alcohol (i.e., a three-carbon chain with three hydroxyl groups) derived from the three-carbon carbohydrate glyceraldehyde.

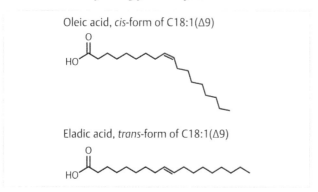

Oleic acid, *cis*-form of C18:1(Δ9)

Eladic acid, *trans*-form of C18:1(Δ9)

Fig. 3.3 Cis- versus trans-isomers of fatty acids. Oleic acid and eladic acid are both composed of 18 carbons and contain one double bond. They differ in that oleic acid is the *cis*-isomer (kink in hydrocarbon tail), and eladic acid is the *trans*-isomer (straight hydrocarbon tail) of the fatty acid.

- Sphingosine is an amino alcohol with an unsaturated alkyl side chain. It is formed from serine and palmitic acid.
2. **Head group:** Certain lipids contain a phosphate residue esterifed to the OH group on carbon-3 of either glycerol or sphingosine. Others have sugars, amino alcohols, or other molecules esterifed to their backbones via either a hydroxyl group or a phosphate residue at carbon-3.
3. **Tail group:** Fatty acid chains attach to the backbone molecules through ester bonds formed with glycerol, or amide bonds formed with sphingosine.

Glycerides

Glycerides are characterized by the presence of a glycerol backbone to which one to three fatty acid (or acyl) residues are esterifed. The three types of glycerides include the following (▶ Fig. 3.5):

1. **Triacylglycerols (fats):** These triglycerides, the major forms of dietary and stored lipids, are made up of a glycerol backbone to which three fatty acid residues (which may differ in chain length and saturation) are esterifed.
2. **Diacylglycerols:** These diglycerides are composed of a glycerol backbone to which two fatty acid residues are esterifed.
3. **Monoacylglycerols:** These monoglycerides are made up of glycerol attached to just one fatty acid residue.

Membrane Lipids

The structural components of cellular membranes are glycerophospholipids, sphingophospholipids, and glycolipids. The former two phosphate-containing lipids are collectively referred to as phospholipids.

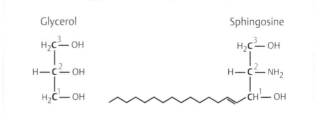

Fig. 3.4 Backbones of fatty acid-derived lipids. The backbone molecules of fatty acid-derived lipids are glycerol and sphingosine.

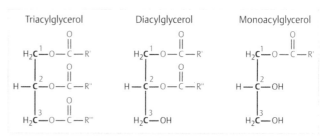

Fig. 3.5 Glycerides. Triacylglycerol, diacylglycerol, and monoacylglycerol are composed of a glycerol backbone to which three, two, and one fatty acid (acyl) residues are esterifed, respectively. R represents the fatty acid residues.

Glycerophospholipids

This group of lipids is derived from phosphatidic acid (PA) (i.e., diacylglycerol with a phosphate residue at carbon-3). Subsequent attachment of certain molecules to PA generates several important membrane lipids, which include the following (▶ Fig. 3.6a):

1. **Phosphatidylcholine** (PA + choline), also known as lecithin, which is the most abundant phospholipid in membranes
2. **Phosphatidylinositol** (PA + inositol), which plays an important role in intracellular signaling
3. **Cardiolipin** (PA + glycerol + PA), which is a component of the inner mitochondrial membrane, and provides stability to the enzyme complexes involved in energy production
4. **Plasmalogens**, which are glycerophospholipids with a fatty acid attached via a vinyl-ether linkage at position 1, a polyunsaturated fatty acid attached via an ester linkage at position 2, and either a phosphoethanolamine or a phosphocholine at position 3, play important roles in membrane structure, signal transduction and in anti-oxidant mechanisms

Sphingophospholipids

These lipids, the main components of membranes of nerve cells in the brain and neural tissue, are composed of ceramide (which is sphingosine attached to an unsaturated fatty acid residue) esterified to a polar head group (▶ Fig. 3.6b).

• **Sphingomyelin** (ceramide + phosphorylcholine) is a major sphingophospholipid in humans. Niemann-Pick disease is an autosomal recessive disorder that causes a defect in acid sphingomyelinase, the enzyme that breaks down sphingomyelin. This leads to lysosomal accumulation of sphingomyelin and cell death.

Glycolipids

These lipids are made up of ceramide attached to sugar molecules. Like the sphingophospholipids, glycolipids are found in myelin sheaths, which insulate the axons of neurons of the central nervous system. Some examples include the following (▶ Fig. 3.6b):

1. **Cerebrosides** (ceramide + 1 sugar): These are found primarily in the brain and contain either glucose or galactose. Gaucher disease and Krabbe disease are autosomal recessive disorders marked by defects in glucocerebrosidase (β-glucosidase), which breaks down glucocerebrosides, and galactocerebro-sidase (β-galactosidase), which breaks down galactocerebro-sides. Gaucher disease causes enlargement and dysfunction of the spleen and liver (hepatosplenomegaly). Krabbe disease affects the central nervous system and affects movement and muscle tone.

2. **Sulfatides** [galactocerebroside + sulfate(s)]: These are also found in the brain. Metachromatic leukodystrophy is an autosomal recessive disorder marked by a defect in arylsulfatase A, the enzyme that removes the sulfate groups on sulfatides. Accumulation of sulfatides causes degeneration of myelin sheaths, leading to Metachromatic leukodystrophy.

3. **Globosides** (ceramide + > 1 sugar): The sugar residues are usually galactose, glucose, or N-acetylgalactosamine. Fabry disease is an X-linked recessive disorder marked by a genetic defect in α-galactosidase, the enzyme that breaks down the globoside, globotriaosylceramide (trihexosylceramide).

4. **Gangliosides** (globoside + acidic sugar): These are globosides that contain one or more acidic sugars (e.g., N-acetylneuraminic acid) and are numbered GM_1, GM_2, and so forth, based on the number and position of the acidic sugar residues. Tay-Sachs disease is an autosomal recessive condition marked by a defect in hexoseaminidase A, the enzyme that breaks down GM_2 gangliosides. Sandhoff disease results from a deficiency of both hexosaminidases A and B leading to an accumulation of GM_2 gangliosides as well as globosides.

Normal
Membrane structure

Membrane lipids are amphipathic; they contain hydrophilic regions in their heads and hydrophobic regions in their tails. This allows them to form membrane bilayers and micelles in which the polar head groups interact with the aqueous environment, and the fatty acid tails interact to form a hydrophobic environment that excludes water. The latter is observed as the center layer of a lipid bilayer or the core of spherical micelles.

Foundations
Glycerides and phospholipids in cell signaling

Diacylglycerol (DAG) is obtained from the hydrolysis of triacylglycerols. It is also generated, along with inositol 1, 4, 5-triphosphate (IP_3), from the hydrolysis of phosphatidylinositol 4, 5-biphosphate (PIP_2), the doubly phosphorylated form of phosphatidylinositol. This hydrolysis is catalyzed by phospholipase C. As a second messenger, DAG activates protein kinase C (PKC), which modulates numerous intracellular processes. IP_3 binds to receptors on the endoplasmic and sarcoplasmic reticula to trigger an increase in the cytoplasmic and sarcoplasmic levels of Ca^{2+}. In addition to activating PKC, calcium binds to the protein calmodulin and activates calmodulin-dependent kinases that are involved in many processes, including neurotransmission, learning and memory.

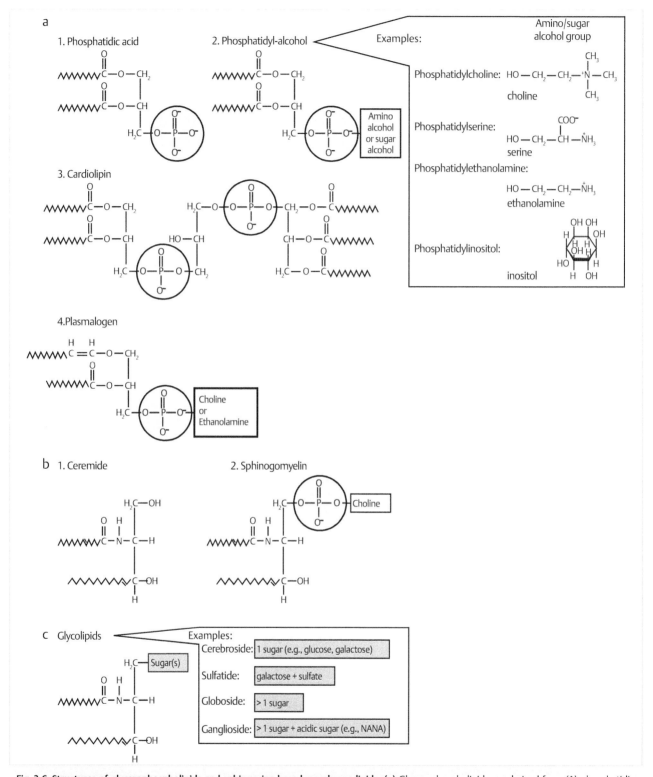

Fig. 3.6 Structures of glycerophospholipids and sphingosine-based membrane lipids. (a) Glycerophospholipids are derived from (1) phosphatidic acid (diacylglycerol + phosphate). (2) Specific phosphatidyl-alcohols are created via the esterification of amino and sugar alcohols (e.g., choline, serine, ethanolamine, inositol) to the phosphate group of phosphatidic acid. (3) Cardiolipin is created from two phosphatidic acids attached to a central glycerol molecule. (4) Plasmalogen is a glycerol with fatty acid in vinyl-ether linkage at position 1, a polyunsaturated fatty acid in ester linkage at position 2 and phosphor-amino alcohol (phosphorylcholine or phosphorylethanolamine) in ester linkage at position 3. **(b)** Sphingosine-based phospholipids are derived from (1) ceramide (sphingosine + 1 fatty acyl residue attached to the amino group at C2). Attachment of a phosphorylcholine group to ceramide generates (2) sphingomyelin. **(c)** Attachment of various sugars to ceramide generates several glycolipids such as cerebrosides, sulfatides, globosides, and gangliosides. NANA, N-acetylneuraminic acid.

Therapeutics
Anticardiolipin antibody test

Antibodies against cardiolipin are seen in individuals with syphilis infections or antiphospholipid syndrome. In the latter case, individuals present with repeat thrombosis (blood clots), and females often have miscarriages.

Therapeutics
Respiratory distress syndrome

Phosphatidylcholine (lecithin), sphingomyelin, and phosphatidylglycerol are components of lung surfactant, which serves as a lubricant that lowers the surface tension of alveoli, making it easier for the lung to expand. The immature lungs of a preterm infant often fail to produce sufficient surfactant, which leads to respiratory distress syndrome (RDS), impairing gas exchange and increasing the risk for partial lung collapse. A test that measures the lecithin to sphingomyelin ratio (L:S) in amniotic fluid allows for the maturity of a fetus's lungs to be determined. An L:S ratio of less than 2:1 indicates a deficiency in lecithin, which increases the risk of an infant developing RDS. An L/S ratio greater than 2:1 coupled with the presence of phosphatidylglycerol is indicative of mature lungs.

Foundations
Myelination in the central nervous system

Gross visual inspection of the central nervous system (brain and spinal cord) reveals two types of tissue: gray matter and white matter. Gray matter contains the cell bodies of neurons, whereas white matter contains the axons of neurons that are coated with lipid-based myelin sheaths. Myelination insulates axons electrically, allowing nerve conduction to proceed at higher velocities. Conditions that disrupt myelination manifest as neurologic disorders. Glial cells are responsible for insulating neuronal axons by producing myelin. In the central nervous system, these glial cells are called oligodendrocytes, whereas those of the peripheral nervous system are called Schwann cells.

Eicosanoids

Eicosanoids are signaling molecules derived from the 20-carbon, polyunsaturated fatty acids, such as arachidonic acid. The latter is obtained directly from the diet or via synthesis from two essential fatty acids, linoleic acid and linolenic acid. Upon its excision and release from membrane lipids by phospholipase A_2, arachidonic acid is converted to various eicosanoids with the aid of two key enzymes, cyclooxygenase (COX, also known as prostaglandin synthase), and lipoxygenase (▶ Fig. 3.7).

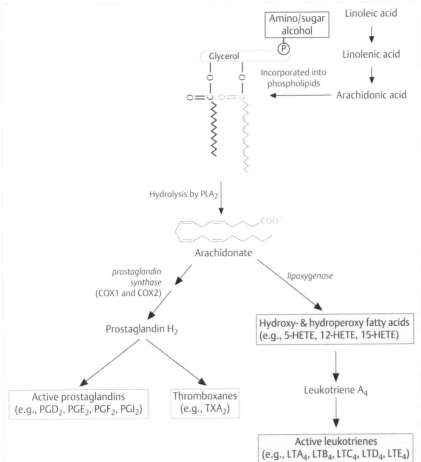

Fig. 3.7 Eicosanoids. The essential fatty acid arachidonic acid is synthesized from linoleic and linolenic acids. It is also obtained from phospholipase A2 (PLA_2) catalyzed hydrolysis of arachidonic acid-containing phospholipids. The human body incorporates arachidonic acid into phospholipids or uses it to synthesize eicosanoids. In the latter, arachidonic acid is converted to prostaglandin H_2 (via the action of prostaglandin synthase), which serves as the precursor for the generation of active prostaglandins and thromboxanes. Alternatively, via the action of lipoxygenase, arachidonic acid is converted to leukotriene A_4, which serves as the precursor for the generation of active leukotrienes. COX, cyclooxygenase; HETE, hydoxyeicosatraenoic acid; LTB_4, leukotriene B_4; LTC_4, leukotriene C_4; LTD_4, leukotriene D_4; LTE_4, leukotriene E_4; PGD_2, prostaglandin D_2; PGE_2, prostaglandin E_2; PGF_2, prostaglandin F_2; PGI_2, prostaglandin I_2 (prostacyclin); TXA_2, thromboxane A_2.

I

Eicosanoids are short-lived signaling molecules that are locally produced and communicate with small neighboring groups of cells. They play a major role in the body's response to damage and infection and are divided into four groups:

1. **Prostaglandins** promote inflammatory responses in tissue. Individual prostaglandins may promote or inhibit contraction of smooth muscles by interacting with different receptors. For instance, prostaglandin I_2 (PGI_2) causes vasodilation and bronchodilation, whereas prostaglandin E_2 (PGE_2) causes contraction of intestinal and uterine muscle and is used to induce labor or abortion.
2. **Thromboxanes** are important mediators of thrombocyte (platelet) aggregation in the hemostatic pathway. For instance, platelets produce thromboxane A_2 (TXA_2), which promotes platelet aggregation as well as vasoconstriction in arterioles.
3. **Hydroxyeicosatetraenoic** acids affect neutrophils and eosinophils.
4. **Leukotrienes** are important in inflammatory responses and immediate hypersensitivity reactions, in particular asthma.

Normal
Inflammatory response
The body's response to damage or infection (in an attempt to heal) is called the inflammatory response. It is driven by vasodilation, increased blood vessel permeability, movement of fluids and white blood cells (e.g., neutrophils) to the damaged site, and platelet aggregation. Signs and symptoms of this response include pain, redness, swelling, and heat at the site of damage/infection. Persistent inflammation causes disorders such as rheumatoid arthritis and atherosclerosis.

Therapeutics
Nonsteroidal antiinflammatory drugs (NSAIDs)
Nonsteroidal antiinflammatory drugs (NSAIDs), such as aspirin and ibuprofen, are used in conjunction with anticoagulants to prevent strokes. The antiinflammatory effects of NSAIDs are achieved through inhibition of prostaglandin synthase, the enzyme that catalyzes the first step in the conversion of arachidonic acid to prostaglandins. Thromboxane synthase, an enzyme that converts prostaglandins to thromboxane A_2, is a target of the antiplatelet drug picotamide, which also inhibits thromboxane A_2 receptor activity. In clinical trials, picotamide appears to inhibit platelet aggregation and reduce the complications of peripheral arterial disease in diabetes.

3.3 Isoprenoids

Isoprenoids are a class of lipids that are synthesized from acetyl CoA via a five-carbon, "active isoprene" intermediate called isopentenyl pyrophosphate (IPP). Condensation of multiple units of IPP produces lipids that include the steroids, lipid-soluble vitamins, and coenzyme Q.

3.3.1 Steroids
Cholesterol
The most important steroid, cholesterol, is found in all cells and tissues of higher organisms. It is especially abundant in nervous tissue and egg yolk. Its 27-carbon structure, which includes a characteristic four-ringed gonane and a side chain, is derived from six IPP units (▸ Fig. 3.8). Cholesterol has three major functions:

1. It is a component of membranes.
2. It is a precursor of many important biological molecules including bile acids, steroid hormones, and vitamin D.
3. It is a component of bile, a heterogeneous solution stored in the gallbladder that aids in the digestion of lipids.

Steroid Hormones
Steroid hormones are signaling molecules that alter gene transcription. They do so by first binding to intracellular receptors called transcription factors located in the cytoplasm or nucleus of cells. Then the hormone-receptor complex binds to selected regions of DNA to induce, or repress, the expression of particular genes.

An enzyme called 20, 22 desmolase (cytochrome P-450$_{scc}$), which is found in all steroid-producing tissues, cleaves the side chain of cholesterol to form the 21-carbon pregnenolone—the most important intermediate in the synthesis of other steroid hormones, such as the following (▸ Fig. 3.8a):

1. **Progesterone** (21-carbon), a gestation-supportive hormone
2. **Aldosterone** (21-carbon), a mineralocorticoid that increases Na^+ and water retention and raises blood pressure
3. **Cortisol** (21-carbon), a glucocorticoid "stress" hormone that increases gluconeogenesis and blood pressure and has anti-inflammatory effects
4. **Testosterone** (19-carbon), an androgen, the principal male sex hormone
5. **Estradiol** (18-carbon), an estrogen, the principal female sex hormone, which is involved in female sexual development and the maintenance of bone structure

Bile Acids
Bile acids are derivatives of cholesterol that are produced in the liver, stored in the bile mixture of the gallbladder, and delivered to the intestines for use. Bile acids function as detergents that emulsify lipids to promote their digestion and absorption in the intestine. They are divided into the following categories (▸ Fig. 3.8b):

1. **Primary bile acids:** The two primary bile acids (cholic acid and chenodeoxycholic acid) have three fewer carbon atoms than cholesterol (24 instead of 27) and contain a carboxylic acid group in the side chain and additional hydroxyl groups that are absent in cholesterol.
2. **Conjugated bile acids:** These are bile acids that contain an amino acid (e.g., glycine or taurine) attached to their carboxyl carbon via an amide bond. Examples include glycocholic and taurocholic acids, and glycochenodeoxycholic and taurochenodeoxycholic acids.

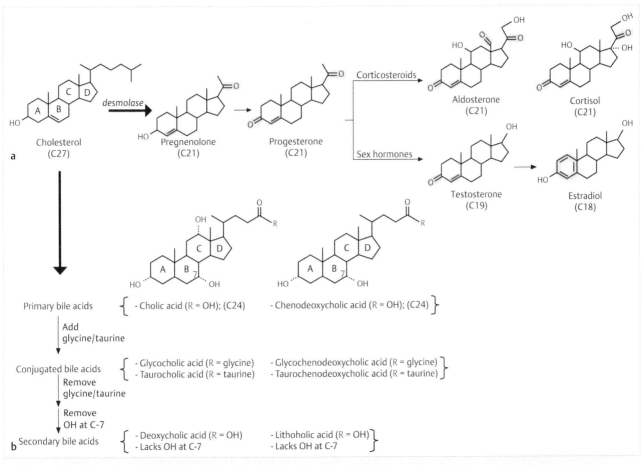

Fig. 3.8 Steroids: cholesterol, steroid hormones, and bile acids. Cholesterol, the most important steroid, is converted to various steroid hormones (**a**) and bile acids/salts (**b**). Hydroxyl groups are highlighted in blue. Alkenes and carbonyl groups are highlighted in brown.

3. **Secondary bile acids:** These are created when intestinal bacteria remove the amino acid group from conjugated bile acids and the hydroxyl group at carbon-7. Examples include deoxycholic and lithocholic acids.
4. **Bile salts:** These are the ionized forms of both free and conjugated bile acids.

Therapeutics
Gallstones
The gallbladder is a pear-shaped organ that stores bile, a lipid-emulsifying liquid, which is pumped from the gallbladder into the intestines to aid in the digestion and absorption of lipids. The cholesterol normally found in bile needs bile salts to stay in solution. When bile contains too much cholesterol and too little bile salts, the cholesterol hardens into pebble-like solids called gallstones. Continued disturbance of bile salt metabolism can lead to malabsorption syndromes such as steatorrhea and, in extreme cases, a deficiency in fat-soluble vitamins. Oral chenodeoxycholic acid has been useful as replacement therapy to supplement the bile acid pool and can in some cases help dissolve gallstones.

3.3.2 Lipid-soluble Vitamins

Vitamins A, D, E, and K are hydrophobic molecules whose structures are characterized by the presence of one or more rings and long, methyl-branched tails created from varying amounts of IPP (▶ Table 3.1). Additional details about the source, function, and metabolism of lipid-soluble vitamins are included in Chapters 1 and 14.

Table 3.1 Structures of lipid-soluble vitamins and the number of isopentenyl pyrophosphate (IPP) units used to create yhem

Vitamin	Structure	No. of IPP Units
A	C20	4
D	C27	6*
E	C29	4
K	C31	4

*Vitamin D is derived from cholesterol, which is created with 6 IPP units.

3.3.3 Other

Coenzyme Q (ubiquinone) is a lipid-soluble molecule that is primarily found in the mitochondrial membrane of eukaryotic cells. It is a member of the electron transport chain and transports electrons from complexes I and II to complex III. Coenzyme Q also serves as an important antioxidant that protects the mitochondrial DNA and membrane lipids from the damaging effects of reactive oxygen species. The side chain of coenzyme Q is created with 6 to 10 IPP units (▶ Fig. 3.9).

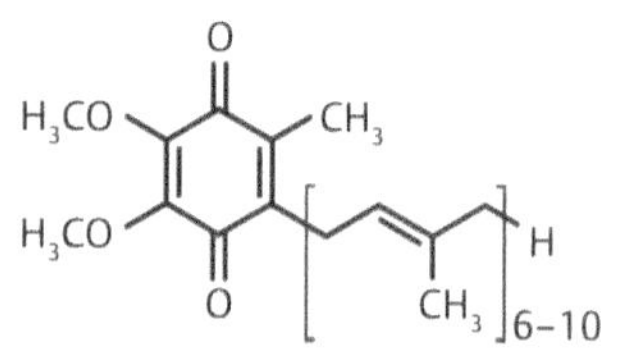

Fig. 3.9 Coenzyme Q. Coenzyme Q is an isoprenoid that is in part created from 6 to 10 isopentenyl pyrophosphate units.

4 Amino Acids and Proteins

4.1 Amino Acids

Amino acids are nitrogen-containing carboxylic acids. Twenty of them, known as proteinogenic amino acids, serve as the basic building blocks of peptides and proteins and are incorporated in them in the particular order specifed by the genetic code for that peptide or protein. Ten of these are considered essential because they cannot be synthesized or are not synthesized in adequate amounts by the human body and must therefore be obtained from the diet. In addition, amino acids function as precursors for the production of biologically important molecules, which include the following:

- **Peptides and proteins:** Amino acids are linked to each other via peptide bonds formed between the carboxyl group of one amino acid and the amino group of another. When the molecule formed contains fewer than 50 amino acids, it is usually considered a peptide; when it contains more than 50 amino acids, it is a protein. Examples of peptides include the hormones insulin and glucagon, both of which bind to target receptors.
- **Nitrogen-containing molecules:** Amino acids are precursors for many nitrogen-containing molecules, such as those that bind O_2 in blood (e.g., heme), biogenic amines (e.g., dopamine, epinephrine, norepinephrine, and serotonin), the skin pigment melanin, and genetic material (e.g., purines and pyrimidines).
- **Metabolically relevant molecules:** Acetyl CoA, which enters the tricarboxylic acid (TCA) cycle to generate adenosine triphosphate (ATP), is produced from pyruvate, which can be generated from amino acids. Several TCA cycle intermediates (e.g., α-ketoglutarate, succinyl CoA, oxaloacetate, and fumarate) can also be generated from amino acids.

4.1.1 Structure and Classification

Amino acids are made up of a central α-carbon that is attached to a carboxyl group, an amino group, a hydrogen, and an R-group or side chain (▶ Fig. 4.1). Each amino acid's identity is defined by its unique R-group, which contains C, H, S, O, and N atoms in various combinations and structural arrangements.

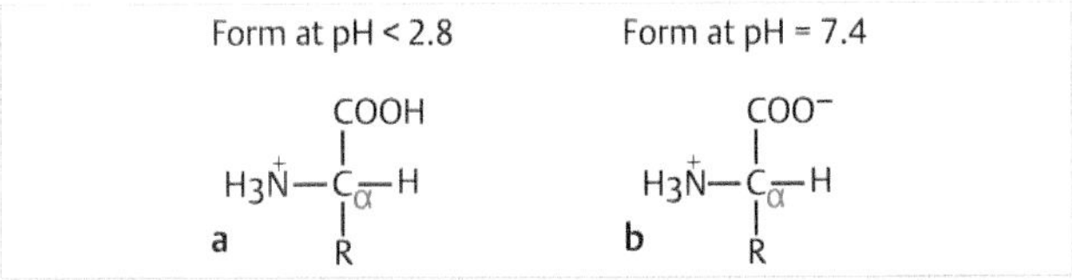

Fig. 4.1 Structure of amino acids. Amino acids contain a central carbon atom bound to four groups: an α-carboxyl group, an α-amino group, a hydrogen atom, and an R-group or side chain. Amino acids difer only in the composition of the R-group. (**a**) At a low pH (< 2.8), the fully protonated form of amino acids predominates. (**b**) At physiological pH (7.4), the α-carboxyl group's proton dissociates to form a negatively charged carboxylate ion. Note that the α-amino group remains protonated at both of these pH values.

The following are important features of amino acid structure and behavior:

- With the exception of glycine, the smallest amino acid where R = H, all protein-forming amino acids have an asymmetrical α-carbon and can therefore exist in the L- or D-forms. In humans, most amino acids are in the L-form. One notable exception is D-serine, which functions as a neurotransmitter. D-Amino acids are also found in the cell walls of bacteria and in peptide antibiotics.
- The pK_a of the ionizable α-carboxyl and α-amino groups are in the range of 1.8 to 2.8 and 9.1 to 9.7, respectively. This means that these groups lose a proton in environments where the pH is higher than the pK_a of their ionizable groups. Additional ionizable groups are contained within the side chains of some amino acids.

Nonpolar Amino Acids

Nonpolar amino acids are characteristically hydrophobic because they contain side chains that are insoluble in water (▶ Fig. 4.2a). Therefore, these amino acids are found in the hydrophobic interior of globular/spherical proteins placed in aqueous environments or on the surface of proteins that interact with the hydrophobic layer of cellular membranes.

- These amino acids have only two pK_a values, which are attributed to their ionizable α-carboxyl and α-amino groups. Therefore, at neutral pH, the net charge of these amino acids will be zero because the α-carboxyl group will be deprotonated (-1 charge), and the α-amino group will be fully protonated (+ 1 charge).

Polar Amino Acids

Polar amino acids are characteristically hydrophilic because they contain water-soluble side chains (▶ Fig. 4.2b). Therefore, they are found in regions of proteins that make contact with aqueous solutions, such as the cytosol or extracellular environment. These polar amino acids are further classifed based on the nature of their charge.

- **Uncharged (neutral):** Like their nonpolar counterparts, these six uncharged amino acids have a net charge of zero at neutral pH. Cysteine and tyrosine each have an ionizable R-group with pK_a values of 8.3 and 10.1, respectively. The side chains of these polar amino acids are known to form noncovalent and covalent bonds, such as the following:
  - Hydrogen bonds: The carbonyl and amide groups of asparagine and glutamine, as well as the hydroxyl groups of serine, threonine, and tyrosine, form hydrogen bonds (H-O, H-N) with other polar molecules.
  - Disulfide bonds: The sulfhydryl (SH) group of cysteine forms disulfide bonds (S-S) with other cysteine residues.
  - Phosphoester bonds: The phosphorylation of proteins creates a phosphoester bond between hydroxyl-containing amino acids and phosphate.
  - Glycosidic bonds: Glycosylation of proteins occurs when an oligosaccharide is attached to the hydroxyl groups of serine and threonine or the amide group of asparagine.

Nonpolar amino acids

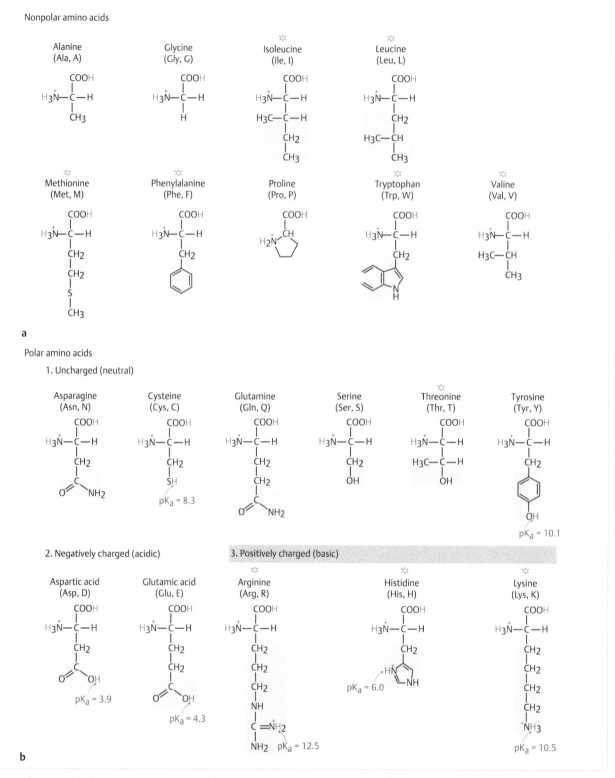

a

Polar amino acids

1. Uncharged (neutral)

2. Negatively charged (acidic)   3. Positively charged (basic)

b

Fig. 4.2 Proteinogenic amino acids. There are 20 proteinogenic amino acids; 8 are nonpolar, and 11 are polar. (**a**) Nonpolar amino acids possess hydrophobic side chains. (**b**) Polar amino acids contain hydrophilic side chains and are further divided into three groups based on their charge at neutral pH: (1) uncharged amino acids are neutral, (2) negatively charged amino acids are acidic, and (3) positively charged amino acids are basic. Stars indicate the essential amino acids.

- **Negatively charged (acidic):** Aspartic acid and glutamic acid each have an ionizable side chain with pK_a values of 3.9 and 4.3, respectively. As a result, they will have a negative charge (-1) at neutral pH, which explains why they are referred to as aspartate and glutamate, respectively.
- **Positively charged (basic):** Arginine, lysine, and histidine each have an ionizable side chain with pK_a values of 12.5, 10.5, and 6.0, respectively. At neutral pH, both arginine and lysine will have a positive charge. Histidine, on the other hand, is a weak base and will have a charge of zero at neutral pH. However, certain ionic environments of a protein may cause histidine to donate the dissociable proton on its imidazole ring, leaving it with a positive charge.

Normal
Histamine

Histamine is a biogenic amine that functions as a neurotransmitter and plays a role in the local immune response. It is created by the decarboxylation of histidine via a reaction catalyzed by histidine decarboxylase. This enzyme requires the cofactor pyridoxal phosphate—a derivative of vitamin B_6—for its activity.

4.1.2 Acid–Base Characteristics of Amino Acids

Amino acids contain a weakly acidic α-carboxyl group whose proton dissociates as the pH of its environment is raised above 2.8. Because amino acids behave according to the same principles that apply to any weak acid, the dissociation constant (K_a) of the proton (H^+) at the α-carboxyl group, and the resulting conjugate base (A^-), is described as follows:

Standard reaction: $HA \leftrightarrow H^+ + A^-$

Proton dissociation equation: $K_a = ([H^+] \cdot [A^-])/[HA]$

This relationship can be expressed in a manner that directly relates the concentrations of the acid, proton, and conjugate base to the pH of the environment by using the Henderson-Hasselbalch equation:

$$pH = PK_a + \log \frac{[A^-]}{[HA]}$$

This equation shows that the pH is equal to the pK_a when the concentration of the conjugate base and acid are equal (remember, if their ratio is 1, then the log of the ratio is 0). Thus, the pH of a solution containing an acid is best buffered—that is, it changes very little upon addition of a strong base or acid—when the solution's pH is near the pK_a.

Titration Curve

When an amino acid in solution is titrated by the addition of a strong base (e.g., NaOH), its acid–base behavior is represented as a titration curve in a graph where the pH (x-axis) is plotted against the equivalents of NaOH added (y-axis). Examination of the titration curve allows for the identifcation of the amino acid based on the number of pK_a points and their values. The titra-tion curves of glycine, aspartic acid, and arginine are depicted in ▶ Fig. 4.3.

Isoelectric Point

Amino acids are zwitterions because they possess both positive and negative charges at neutral pH. The sum of the charges varies with pH such that an amino acid that has one α-carboxyl group and one α-amino group will be positively charged at low pH values (<2.8). As the pH of the environment is elevated, the net charge of the amino acid becomes zero. At even higher pH, the charge becomes negative. The pH at which the charge is zero is called the isoelectric point (pI). The pI of an amino acid is obtained by calculating the average of its two pK_a values that are closest in value to each other. Importantly, the pI defines the pH at which molecules in solution will not migrate in an electric field. This behavior is observed in amino acids with uncharged side-groups.

Foundations
Protein charge

A protein's overall charge at a particular pH is directly related to its amino acid composition. Proteins are composed of neutral, hydrophilic, and charged (both positive and negative) amino acids. The net electrical charge of a protein is determined by a combination of charges on its component amino acids at a given pH. The isoelectric point (pI) of a protein is defined as the pH at which the protein has no net charge. A protein carries a net positive charge at pH values below its pI and a net negative charge at values above its pI. The property of protein charge can be used to separate the proteins in a complex mixture using an electrical field. For example, native gel electrophoresis is employed to resolve the major serum proteins such as the albumin and the α_1-, α_2-, β-, and γ-globulins.

4.1.3 Derivatives of Amino Acids

Amino acids are converted into nonproteinogenic amino acids, as well as biogenic amines (biologically active amine-containing compounds), via modifications to their chemical structures (▶ Table 4.1).

4.2 Proteins

Proteins are biomolecules that are built from amino acids and are critical to cells as they contribute to the following:

1. **Fuel supply:** Proteins are important in the generation of ATP through the TCA cycle because they are degraded to their constituent amino acids, the latter of which are converted to several TCA cycle intermediates.
2. **Structural support:** Certain proteins, such as elastin, keratin, and collagen, are key components of connective tissue found in physical structures such as tendons, cartilage, hair, bone, and skin, which provide structural support.
3. **Activity:** Some proteins act as enzymes to catalyze chemical reactions in the body. Others play a crucial role in cell signaling by binding to and transporting molecules both in the bloodstream and across the cell membrane. Additional proteins such as actin, tubulin, and myosin mediate the motion of cells.

a Nonpolar amino acid glycine: two ionizable groups

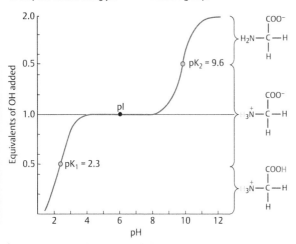

b Acidic amino acid aspartic acid: three ionizable groups

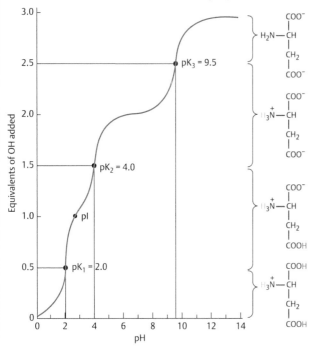

c Basic amino acid arginine: three ionizable groups

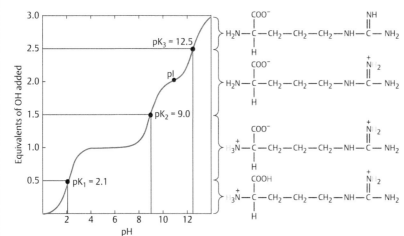

Fig. 4.3 Titration curves of amino acids. At the indicated pK_a points, the concentration of an amino acid prior to and after the loss of a proton at an ionizable group is equal. At the indicated pI points, the sum of the charges of an amino acid is zero. As such, when the pH of the environment is less than the pI, the net charge of the amino acid is positive. Conversely, when the environment's pH is greater than the pI, then the amino acid's net charge is negative. The titration curves presented are for (**a**) glycine, a polar amino acid that has two ionizable groups; (**b**) aspartic acid, an acidic amino acid that has three ionizable groups; and (**c**) arginine, a basic amino acid that has three ionizable groups. *Note:* Some titration curves have the pH on the *y*-axis and the NaOH equivalents on the *x*-axis.

Table 4.1 Derivatives of amino acids

Molecule	Structural details	Function/Relevance
Nonproteinogenic amino acids		
Cystine	A dimer of two cysteines attached via a disulfide bond	It forms stones in the kidneys, ureter, and bladder when its reabsorption is disrupted
Homocysteine	It is derived from methionine and similar in structure to cysteine except that it has an extra methylene group ($-CH_2$) in its R-group	It can be converted to cysteine or methionine via mechanisms that utilize vitamins B_6 (pyridoxine), B_9 (folate), and B_{12} (cobalamin) and hyperhomocysteinemia is a risk factor for coronary artery disease
Homocystine	A dimer of two homocysteines attached via a disulfide bond	It can be reduced to homocysteine and then converted to cystathionine by mechanisms using vitamin B_6 (pyridoxine)
S-adenosylmethionine (SAM/ AdoMet)	It is a derivative of methionine and is made up of methionine attached to the ribose group of adenosine via a carbon–sulfur bond	It serves as a donor of methyl groups
Taurine	A derivative of cysteine	It is added (conjugated) to bile acids to improve the latter's solubility in the intestines, which makes them better lipid emulsifers
Selenocysteine	It is structurally similar to cysteine, but the sulfur atom is replaced with selenium (Se)	It is a component of the antioxidant enzyme glutathione peroxidase and several others
Ornithine and citrulline	Ornithine is derived from arginine, and it serves as a precursor for citrulline	Both are intermediates in the urea cycle
L-dopa	It is derived from tyrosine	It is a precursor for melanin and the "fight or fght" hormones dopamine, norepinephrine, and epinephrine
Biogenic amines		
Cysteamine	It is derived from cysteine	It is a component of coenzyme A (CoA)
Histamine	It is derived from histidine	It plays a role in activating the infammatory response
Dopamine, norepinephrine, epinephrine	These catecholamines are synthesized from l-dopa	They play a role in activating the "flight or fight" response
Carnitine	It is derived from lysine and methionine	It plays a role in the transport of fatty acids into the mitochondria for degradation
Creatine	It is derived from arginine, glycine, and methionine	In its phosphorylated form (phosphocreatine), it serves as an energy store

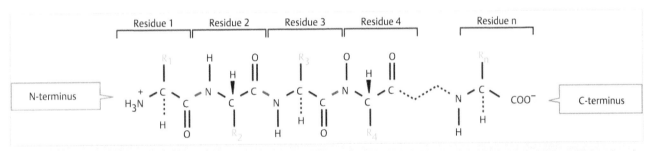

Fig. 4.4 Primary structure of proteins. Protein sequences are written from the left to right starting with the N-terminus (identified by the NH_3 group) and ending with the C-terminus (identified by its COO^- group). R-groups alternate between positions that are above or below the linear arrangement of amino acid residues. Color legend: peptide bonds are red; R-groups are green; N-terminus is shaded blue; C-terminus is shaded pink.

4.2.1 Structure

The structures of proteins are divided into four levels: primary, secondary, tertiary, and quaternary.

Primary Structure

The primary structure is the linear arrangement of amino acid residues. The amino acids are linked to each other by peptide bonds formed between the α-carboxyl group of one amino acid and the α-amino group of another. The conventional way of writing a protein's primary sequence is to list the amino acid residues in order from left to right, starting with the N-terminus (which has an amino group, NH_3^+), and ending with the C-terminus (which has a carboxylate ion, COO^-) (▶ Fig. 4.4).

Foundations

Rotation around the polypeptide backbone

Although no rotation is possible around the peptide bond (due to its partial double bond character), rotation is allowed along the polypeptide backbone at the bonds attached to the α-carbons of the amino acid residues. This rotation, however, is extremely limited due to steric hindrance between the different R-groups and the carbonyl oxygens.

I

Secondary Structure

The secondary structure is created by coiling and/or pleating of peptide/protein chains into the following conformations (▶ Fig. 4.5):

1. **Helices:** These take on a screwlike conformation and exist as α-helices or collagen helices. The shape of α-helices, which are tightly coiled in a right-handed manner, is stabilized by hydrogen bonds between nonadjacent amino acid residues. The shape of collagen helices, which are loosely coiled in a left-handed manner, is too stretched out to allow the formation of hydrogen bonds between amino acid residues.

2. **β-Pleated sheets:** These structures are composed of two or more straight (noncoiled) strands of amino acids that associate with each other via hydrogen bonds to create a pleated plane. β-Pleated sheets have alternate carbonyl oxygens pointing in opposite directions within the plane and alternate R-groups pointing above and below this plane. β-Pleated sheets are stabilized by hydrogen bonds between amino acids of neighboring strands and exist in two forms:
   - Parallel: Neighboring peptide strands run in the same direction (i.e., their N- and C-termini run in the same direction).
   - Antiparallel: Neighboring peptide strands run in opposite directions (i.e., their N- and C-termini run in opposite directions).

3. **β-Turns:** These segments, which are typically four amino acids in length, are found in turns that help to change the direction of a peptide chain. At least one of the amino acids found in β-turns is proline. β-Turns are stabilized by hydrogen bonds and are found at turns of antiparallel β-pleated sheets or at the junction between sheets and a-helices.

Foundations

Hydrogen bonds

Hydrogen bonds in proteins are noncovalent interactions between hydrogen and electronegative atoms such as nitrogen, oxygen, and fluorine. In proteins, the hydrogen in an NH group forms hydrogen bonds with the oxygen atom in the carbonyl group of a nearby amino acid. Although a single hydrogen bond is quite weak (1 to 6 kcal/mol), multiple hydrogen bonds have an additive strength, which makes them an important determinant of secondary structure. Hydrogen bonds also play a major role in the DNA double helical structure.

Tertiary Structure

The tertiary structure is the specific three-dimensional conformation of a particular peptide chain. For instance, most proteins assume a globular or spherical conformation that is stabilized by four types of interactions (▶ Fig. 4.6):

1. **Hydrophobic interactions:** Nonpolar amino acid residues fold into the center, away from the aqueous solvent, forming a hydrophobic core. This is the most important stabilizing component of a compact protein.

2. **Disulfide bonds:** The oxidation of cysteine residues forms covalent disulfide bonds between sulfhydryl (SH) groups.

3. **Metal ions:** The tertiary conformation of proteins supports the formation of complexes with metal ions such as Mg^{2+} and Cu^{2+}.

4. **Hydrogen bonding:** Hydrogen bonding occurs between the R-groups of nearby amino acid residues.

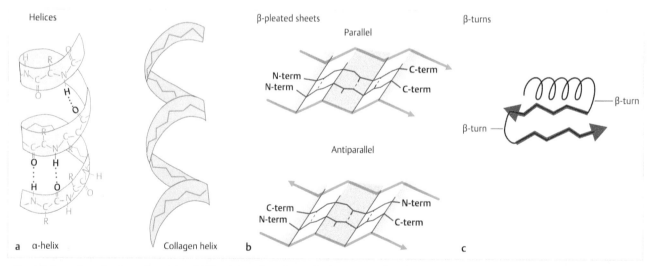

Fig. 4.5 Secondary structure of proteins. (a) The tight coiling of peptide chains in a right-handed direction forms an α-helix, which is stabilized by hydrogen bonds between nonadjacent amino acids. Loose coiling in the left-handed direction creates a collagen helix in which hydrogen bonding cannot take place. **(b)** The pleating of peptide chains forms β-pleated sheets. They are stabilized by hydrogen bonds between amino acid residues on neighboring strands, which are either parallel or antiparallel to each other. **(c)** β-Turns are observed at the junction between α-helices and β-pleated sheets or at the turns of antiparallel β-pleated sheets.

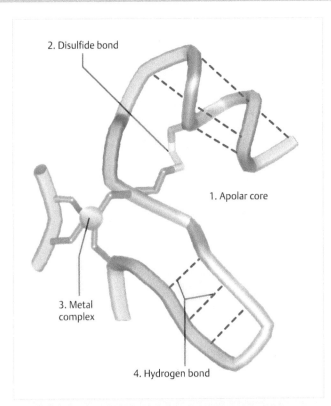

Fig. 4.6 Tertiary structure of proteins. The three-dimensional, tertiary structure of a protein is stabilized by (**1**) hydrophobic interactions between nonpolar amino acid residues that form a hydrophobic (apolar) core, (**2**) disulfide bonds between cysteine residues, (**3**) complexes with metal ions, and (**4**) hydrogen bonds between amino acid residues.

Quaternary Structure

Quaternary structure is the arrangement of more than one protein chain (subunit) into complexes (see ▶ Fig. 4.9, Hemoglobin). The subunits are held together by noncovalent associations that include the following:

1. **Hydrogen bonds:** Hydrogen bonding occurs between polar R-groups of amino acids from individual subunits.
2. **Salt bridges:** Also known as ionic bonds, salt bridges are formed due to the electrostatic attractions that take place between ions of opposite charge. It typically forms between the NH_3^+ and COO^- groups in the R-groups of basic and acidic amino acids, respectively.
3. **Hydrophobic interactions:** These interactions take place between the nonpolar R-groups of the amino acid residues.
4. **Van der Waals forces:** These are weak forces of attraction that occur between atoms, molecules, and surfaces. They include induction, dispersion, and electrostatic interactions.

Foundations
Disulfide bonds
Oxidation of the sulfhydryl (–SH) group of cysteine residues in the lumen of the rough endoplasmic reticulum creates covalent disulfide bonds, usually in secreted proteins. The oxidizing environment necessary for the formation of disulfide bonds, however, does not exist within the cytoplasm due to high concentrations of the antioxidant glutathione. Keratin, which is a major protein in hair, has a high cysteine content and tends to form disulfide bonds. Manipulating such bonds is key to curling or straightening in hairstyling.

Normal
Protein turnover
A typical 70 kg (154 lb) person consumes ~100 g of protein daily. This protein is hydrolyzed to its component amino acids by proteolytic enzymes in the stomach and duodenum prior to absorption. Further metabolism of amino acids occurs to provide energy or to create other important biomolecules. Approximately 400 g of protein is degraded per day in the tissues, and ~ 400 g of new proteins are synthesized daily. The nitrogen atoms contained in proteins are channeled into the urea cycle of the liver. Nitrogen may then be excreted as urea in urine or sweat.

Normal
Kidney and nitrogen levels (BUN), nitrogen balance
Normally, healthy adults have a nitrogen balance (NB) equaling zero (intake = output), in which the amount of ingested nitrogen is equal to that excreted in urine, feces, and sweat. Nitrogen imbalances may be either physiologic or pathophysiological:
Positive (+) NB: Nitrogen intake exceeds nitrogen excretion. A positive NB coincides with situations in which protein is being synthesized:
• Growing children and pregnant/nursing women
• Patients recovering from surgery or traumatic injury

Negative (–) NB: Nitrogen loss exceeds nitrogen intake. A negative NB coincides with situations in which tissue is being degraded:
• Patients suffering from malnutrition or starvation (tissue degraded for fuel)
• Patients suffering from third-degree burns
• Patients suffering from cachexia (muscle wasting) due to terminal cancer

4.2.2 Post-translational Protein Modifications

Many polar amino acid residues are altered once they have been incorporated into the peptide or protein. These post-translational modifications are crucial to a protein's function, regulation, subcellular localization, interaction with other molecules, and degradation (▶ Table 4.2, ▶ Fig. 4.7).

Table 4.2 Posttranslational protein modification

Modification	Description	Examples and their biological relevance
Acetylation	Attachment of an acetyl group ($COCH_3$ e.g., to SH group on a Cys or NH_2 group on a Lys)	Acetylation of histone relaxes its association with DNA, making the latter available for transcription
Acylation	Attachment of an acyl group (e.g., fatty acids)	Acylation of small G-proteins with palmitic acid or myristic acid affects their attachment to subcellular membranes
ADP ribosylation	Attachment of an ADP-ribose group donated by NAD^+	Several bacterial toxins exert their effect by ADP ribosylating target proteins, such as G-proteins
Carboxylation	Attachment of a carboxyl group (COOH)	Vitamin K–dependent clotting factors (e.g., VII, IX, X) are activated by carboxylation
Disulfde bonds	Attachment of two cysteine residues to each other via oxidation of their sulfhydryl (SH) bonds into a disulfide bond (S-S)	This modification stabilizes protein structures
Glycation and glycosylation	Nonenzymatic attachment of glucose (glycation), or enzymatic attachment of a number and variety of sugars (glycosylation)	High levels of glycated hemoglobin are observed in patients with poorly controlled diabetes; glycosylation of erythrocyte membrane proteins defines an individual's blood type
GPI (glycosylphosphatidylinositol)	Attachment of a glycolipid	GPI-linked proteins are attached to the plasma membrane's outer surface.
Hydroxylation	Attachment of an OH group	Vitamin C–dependent hydroxylation of proline and lysine are essential for the structural stability of collagen
Methylation	Attachment of a methyl group (CH_3) donated by SAM (S-adenosylmethionine)	Methylation of histones tightens their association with DNA, which inhibits DNA transcription
Phosphorylation	Attachment of a phosphate group (PO_4^{3}) via an ester bond	Phosphorylation of several proteins activates or inhibits their functions
Prenylation	Attachment of isoprenoids (e.g., farnesyl, geranyl)	Prenylation of proteins anchors them to the inner leaflet of the cell membrane
Sulfation	Attachment of a sulfate group (SO_4^{2-}) from PAPS (phosphoadenosine phosphosulfate)	Sulfation is performed on fibrinogen (a protein involved in coagulation) and gastrin (a hormone that promotes gastric acid secretion in the stomach)
Ubiquitination	Attachment of a small protein called ubiquitin	Ubiquitination tags proteins for degradation by the proteasome

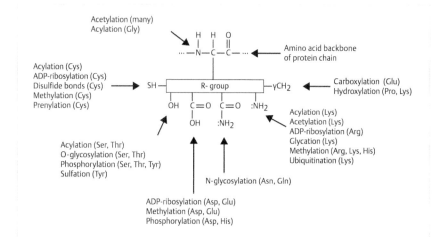

Fig. 4.7 Posttranslational protein modifications. The posttranslational modification of proteins takes place on specific sites of certain amino acid residues. The relevant sites, and the modifications that occur on them, are summarized in this figure.

Therapeutics

Drug-induced lupus erythematosus

The body metabolizes certain drugs by acetylating them. This action detoxifies or reduces the potency of drugs such as hydralazine (antihypertensive), procainamide (antiarrythmic), and isoniazid (antituberculosis medication). Drug-induced lupus erythematosus is seen in individuals who have genetic mutations in enzymes that carry out acetylation reactions. As such, these individuals show a slow rate of drug acetylation, which confers a longer half-life to these drugs. Consequently, these drugs are converted to by-products that are toxic to the body, and they trigger the production of antinuclear (e.g., antihistone) antibodies. Affected individuals present with lupus-like signs and symptoms, such as muscle and bone pain, rashes, inflammation of the lungs and heart, fever, and fatigue.

4.2.3 Physical Dynamics of Proteins

Protein Folding

The folding of proteins into a unique "native" secondary, tertiary, or quaternary structure is essential for their function. Protein folding is a kinetically and thermodynamically controlled process that ensures that a protein's native structure has one of the lowest free energies possible. Although some proteins fold spontaneously in solution, others do so with the help of other proteins called chaperones and chaperonins, which have the following characteristics:

1. The interaction of chaperones with proteins prevents the latter from misfolding into incorrect structures and thus prevents them from aggregating with each other before folding is completed.
2. Chaperones are also known as heat shock proteins (HSPs), whose cellular levels are elevated at high temperatures.

Amyloidosis

Amyloidosis is a family of disorders characterized by the aggregation of improperly folded proteins (amyloids), which causes them to accumulate in organs and tissues (▶ Table 4.3).

Foundations

Diagnosing amyloidosis

Amyloid proteins are those proteins whose structure has been modified in a manner that causes them to aggregate into deposits in a variety of organs and tissues, with a shape characteristic of β strands. Determination of the presence of amyloid proteins in plaques or deposits is performed using Congo red, a dye that intercalates between β strands. When Congo red is applied to tissues, they stain red-orange. However, when viewed under polarized light, the amyloid deposits appear green due to apple-green birefringence. Alternatively, the dye thioflavin T can also bind to amyloid fibrils to produce yellow-green fluorescence.

Protein Denaturation

A protein's native conformation can be disrupted or denatured, causing it to lose its secondary, tertiary, and quaternary

Table 4.3 Types of amyloidoses and their characteristics

Amyloidosis	Characteristics
Primary amyloidosis	Deposits of amyloid light chain (AL) in organs, such as the kidneys • AL contains the light chains of antibodies (Ig) synthesized by plasma cells • It is sometimes observed in patients with multiple myeloma (cancer of plasma cells)
Secondary amyloidosis	Accumulation of serum amyloid A protein (SAA), which is secreted during the initial phases of the inflammatory response triggered in conditions such as rheumatoid arthritis, Crohn disease, and tuberculosis
Alzheimer disease	Deposits of β-amyloid in the brain • β-Amyloid is derived from the degradation of amyloid precursor protein (APP)
Diabetes mellitus (type 2)	Deposits of amylin in the pancreas • Amylin is a peptide hormone synthesized by the insulin-releasing β cells of the pancreas
Dialysis-associated amyloidosis	Accumulation of β_2-microglobulins in the blood, often seen in long-term dialysis patients

structure, as well as its function. Although the peptide bonds remain intact in a denatured protein, the noncovalent bonds are broken. Protein denaturation can be achieved by altering a protein's environment in the following manners:

1. Increasing or decreasing the pH
2. Altering the ionic strength of a protein's environment with high salt concentrations. This causes dehydration of proteins (salting out).
3. Increasing the temperature (heating), which weakens the noncovalent bonds that contribute to the tertiary and secondary structure
4. Adding salts of heavy metals, such as mercury (Hg), lead (Pb), and silver (Ag). They disrupt salt bridges in proteins and cause precipitation of insoluble metal protein salt.
5. Adding chaotropic (denaturing) agents, such as urea and guanidine salts. They disrupt hydrogen bonds and hydrophobic interactions.
6. Adding surface active detergents, such as sodium dodecyl sulfate (SDS). SDS disrupts hydrophobic interactions and causes unfolding of the protein.
7. Adding organic solvents that tend to weaken the hydrophobic interactions and alter the dielectric constant of the system.

4.3 Noteworthy Proteins

4.3.1 Collagen

Collagen is the most abundant protein in the human body. It is an important structural constituent of tendons, ligaments, cartilage, bone, skin, and the interstitial matrix. There are numerous types of collagens, some of which assemble into structures such as fine fibers (fibrils), or mesh networks, to support their intended function. The four types of collagens (out of 28 types identified so far) are listed here from strongest to weakest:

• **Type I:** This is the most common type of collagen. It assembles into fibrils and is found in the skin, bone, tendons, blood vessels, and cornea.

- **Type II:** It forms fibrils and is found in cartilage and the vitreous body of the eye.
- **Type III:** It also forms fibrils and is found in blood vessels and fetal skin.
- **Type IV:** It assembles into a mesh/sheet network and is found in the lens of the eye, capillaries, and basement membrane to provide support for epithelial cells.

Structure

Collagen is composed of three individual left-handed helical polypeptides that are wound tightly around each other to form a long, rope-like triple helix molecule called procollagen (▶ Fig. 4.8). The latter is stabilized by intra-chain hydrogen bonds and by disulfide bonds at both N- and C-termini. Procollagen is cleaved into tropocollagen in the extracellular matrix. Multiple tropocollagen molecules assemble into fibrils that are stabilized by covalent linkages between tropocollagen molecules. Key features of collagen are as follows:

1. **Amino acid composition:** Each individual left-handed collagen peptide contains roughly 33% glycine (G), 13% proline (P), and 9% hydroxyproline (Hyp). Glycine is found in repeating sequences of Gly-X-Y, where the X position is occupied by proline, and the Y position is filled by either proline or lysine.
   - Prolines are often found at the turns of the left-handed helix. Because glycine is the smallest amino acid, it is placed in positions where the three left-handed helices meet in the triple helical procollagen molecule.
2. **Posttranslational modifications:** The proline and lysine residues (at the Y position) are hydroxylated into hydroxyproline and hydroxylysine, respectively. These modifed amino acids serve to stabilize the collagen triple helix by increasing the number of intrachain hydrogen bonds.
   - The hydroxylations are catalyzed by hydroxylases that require ascorbic acid/vitamin C as a cofactor.
3. **Cross-linking:** Some of the lysine residues on tropocollagen molecules are oxidized to allysine by lysyl oxidase, which requires copper as a cofactor. Lysines and allysines on adjacent tropcollagens covalently cross-link with each other to increase the overall stability of collagen fibrils.

Therapeutics
Disorders attributed to defects in collagen

Ascorbic acid (vitamin C) deficiency leads to scurvy, a condition characterized by abnormal integrity of connective tissues and skin, which manifests as easy bruising. Ehlers-Danlos syndrome is a family of inherited disorders caused by genetic defects in the genes of fibril-forming collagen (Type I and III), or of enzymes involved in its processing (e.g., lysyl oxidase), or in the availability of copper. Individuals with this condition present with thin, stretchy skin and abnormally loose/bendable joints. Osteogenesis imperfecta is a family of inherited conditions marked by deficiencies in Type I collagen. Their severity varies and often manifests as brittle bones, loose joints, and blue sclerae.

4.3.2 Hemoglobin

Hemoglobin is a protein found in red blood cells. It serves to transport oxygen and aids in the buffering of blood by performing the following actions:

1. Hemoglobin binds up to four molecules of O_2 and transports them from the lungs to tissues.
2. Hemoglobin transports protons (H^+) and CO_2 from tissues to the lungs.

Structure

Hemoglobin is a tetramer composed of four helical peptide chains: two α-globin chains and two β-globin chains (▶ Fig. 4.9). Each chain (or subunit) possesses a heme group with a reduced iron (Fe^{2+}) at its center that reversibly binds O_2. The following are other relevant structural features of hemoglobin:

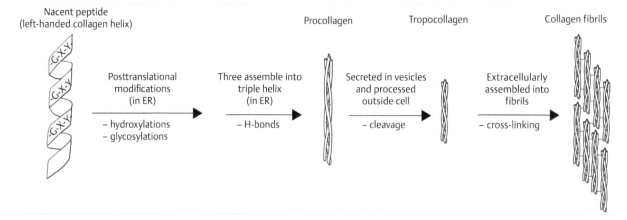

Fig. 4.8 Structure and synthesis of collagens. Collagen is first synthesized as a pre-propeptide and undergoes posttranslational modifications such as proline and lysine hydroxylations that are dependent on vitamin C and glycosylation of specific hydroxylysine residues. Procollagen containing the triple helix is formed inside the lumen of the endoplasmic reticulum (ER) and then exported to the Golgi apparatus for packaging and secretion by exocytosis. Outside the cell, cleavage of staggered ends by procollagen peptidase leads to the formation of tropocollagen. Action of lysyl oxidase generates oxidized lysines (allysines) which are cross-linked to lysines on adjacent chains to yield mature collagen fibrils. Several fibrils can be packed together to form collagen fibers.

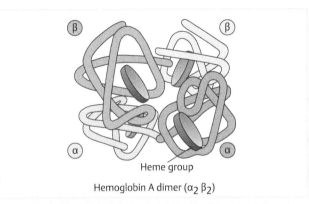

Heme group

Hemoglobin A dimer ($\alpha_2 \beta_2$)

Fig. 4.9 Hemoglobin structure. Hemoglobin is a protein whose major function is to transport oxygen from lungs to the tissues in the body and transport CO_2 back to the lungs. A molecule of hemoglobin is a tetramer of two identical α polypeptide chains and two identical β polypeptide chains. Each of the four subunits contains iron in the form of a heme prosthetic group. Hemoglobin is contained in red blood cells.

- **$\alpha\beta$ Dimers:** Hemoglobin's subunits are arranged into identical $\alpha\beta$ dimers [$(\alpha \beta)_1$ and $(\alpha \beta)_2$]. These dimers associate with each other via polar bonds.
- **T and R forms:** When O_2 is absent from hemoglobin (deoxyhemoglobin), its structure is said to be in the tense or taut (T) form, which restricts the movement of the $\alpha\beta$ dimers relative to each other. However, when O_2 is bound to hemoglobin (oxyhemoglobin), its structure is said to take on a relaxed (R) form, which gives the $\alpha\beta$ dimers more freedom to move relative to each other.

Foundations
Methemoglobinemia
Methemoglobin is a type of hemoglobin that contains the oxidized form of iron (Fe^{3+}) in its heme group. As such, it cannot bind O_2. Unlike its red counterpart hemoglobin, methemoglobin is bluish/brownish in color. As such, it confers a bluish/chocolate brown color to blood when it is in high amounts. Elevated levels of methemoglobin (methemoglobinemia) may be due to genetic mutations or caused by oxidizing compounds, such as nitrates, nitrites, sulfonamides, and aniline dyes used to produce blue-colored jeans.

Therapeutics
Hemoglobinopathies versus thalassemias
Hemoglobinopathies are disorders caused by genetic mutations in one of the globin chains of hemoglobin that results in an *abnormally structured* protein (e.g., sickle cell anemia). Thalassemias, on the other hand, are conditions caused by the *inadequate synthesis* of normal globin chains.

Therapeutics
Sickle cell anemia
Sickle cell anemia is a disorder caused by a point mutation (single base substitution) that causes a glutamic acid to be replaced with valine in the β-globin chain of hemoglobin (HbS). This change from a polar, acidic amino acid to one that is nonpolar and neutral causes deoxyhemoglobin to aggregate in red blood cells. This gives erythrocytes a distorted (sickled) shape and rigid structure, which contributes to their aggregation as they pass through capillaries. Sickled erythrocytes also turn over more rapidly than normal red blood cells.

O_2–Hemoglobin Dissociation Curve

The degree to which O_2 binds to the four heme groups of hemoglobin (Hb) is referred to as hemoglobin saturation with O_2—ranges from 0% (meaning no O_2 is bound to Hb) to 100% (meaning four O_2 are bound to Hb). When hemoglobin's saturation with O_2 is plotted against the partial pressure of O_2 (Po_2), the resulting curve is referred to as the O_2–hemoglobin dissociation curve (▶ Fig. 4.10a). Specific characteristics about hemoglobin's behavior are garnered from this curve, as follows:

1. **Hb cooperatively binds to O_2:** The binding of O_2 to one heme group increases the affinity of the remaining heme groups to O_2. This feature is known as the cooperative binding of hemoglobin to O_2 and is reflected in the sigmoidal shape of the dissociation curve. Likewise, the dissociation of O_2 from Hb is also cooperative.
   - Myoglobin is an O_2-binding heme protein that serves to store O_2 in heart and skeletal muscle. It is composed of a single peptide chain (similar to an individual hemoglobin subunit), and its O_2 dissociation curve takes on a hyperbolic shape. The latter indicates that myoglobin is saturated at the partial pressure of O_2 (Po_2) in heart and skeletal muscle and will therefore only release O_2 under hypoxic or oxygen-depleted conditions.
   - Hemoglobin's (and myoglobin's) affinity for carbon monoxide (CO) is more than 200 times greater than that for O_2. The tight yet reversible binding of CO to any of the heme groups increases the affinity of O_2 for the remaining heme groups. The bound O_2, however, cannot be released to tissues. The effect of CO on hemoglobin's saturation with O_2 is reflected in the formation of a more hyperbolic-shaped curve instead of a sigmoidal-shaped curve (left shift).
2. **O_2 affinity and Po_2:** Hemoglobin is 100% saturated at a Po_2 of ~100 mm Hg. This means that all four heme groups are bound to O_2 at the Po_2 observed in the lungs. This condition supports efficient O_2 loading onto hemoglobin. Alternatively, hemoglobin is 50% saturated at a Po_2 of ~26 mm Hg. This means that half of hemoglobin's heme groups are bound to O_2 at the Po_2 (referred to as P_{50}) observed in tissues. This condition supports efficient O_2 unloading from hemoglobin.

I

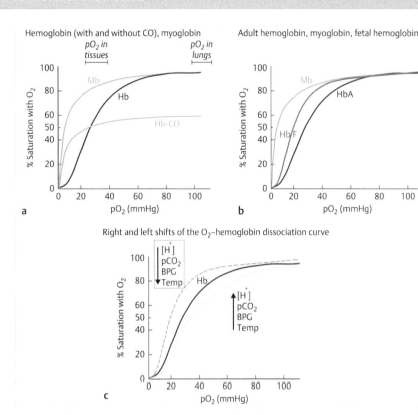

Fig. 4.10 O$_2$-hemoglobin dissociation curves.
(**a**) Binding of O$_2$ to the monomeric myoglobin (Mb) yields a hyperbolic saturation curve. The partial pressure of oxygen (Po$_2$) at which myoglobin is 50% saturated with O$_2$ (P$_{50}$) is quite low. This characteristic allows myoglobin to hold on to O$_2$ tightly until the Po$_2$ in the muscle drops to very low levels. Because the subunits of hemoglobin (Hb) exhibit cooperativity in the binding of O$_2$, the saturation curve is sigmoidal, with the steepest slope of the curve at Po$_2$ levels present in tissues. The competitive inhibitor, carbon monoxide (CO), not only lowers the total binding capacity but also abolishes the cooperativity among the subunits of hemoglobin (note the decreased P$_{50}$). (**b**) Fetal hemoglobin (HbF) has a higher affinity for oxygen than the adult hemoglobin (HbA), as indicated by the lower P$_{50}$ value. This feature allows for efficient transfer of oxygen from maternal blood to fetal blood. (**c**) Effectors such as [H$^+$], CO$_2$, Cl$^-$, 2,3-bisphosphoglycerate (BPG) and higher temperature shift the O$_2$ dissociation curve to the right (causing an increase in P$_{50}$ that signifies decreased affinity for O$_2$). As a result, such effectors facilitate the release of O$_2$ from hemoglobin. Pco$_2$, partial pressure of carbon dioxide.

A molecule's P$_{50}$ is an indicator of its affinity for O$_2$. For instance:

- The P$_{50}$ for myoglobin, fetal hemoglobin, and adult hemoglobin are 1, 19, and 26 mm Hg, respectively (▶ Fig. 4.10b). The higher a molecule's P$_{50}$, the lower its affinity for O$_2$ and the better its ability to unload O$_2$ to target tissues. Therefore, the order of molecules, listed in decreasing order of affinity to O$_2$, is myoglobin, fetal hemoglobin, adult hemoglobin.

3. **Right and left shifts in the standard O$_2$–hemoglobin dissociation curve:** When hemoglobin encounters conditions that decrease its affinity for O$_2$, the O$_2$–hemoglobin dissociation curve shifts to the right, and the P$_{50}$ increases. Conditions that cause such an effect include the following (▶ Fig. 4.10c):
   - An increase in [H$^+$] (i.e., decrease in pH) and an increase in the partial pressure of CO$_2$ (Pco$_2$). Both are collectively referred to as the Bohr effect.
   - An increase in 2,3-bisphosphoglycerate (BPG). BPG is normally generated from the glycolytic intermediate, 1,3-bisphosphoglycerate, by the action of bisphosphoglycerate mutase in red blood cells. Levels of BPG increase under conditions such as chronic hypoxia (e.g., emphysema) and high altitude. BPG binds with a higher affinity to deoxyhemoglobin (T state) than to fully oxygenated

hemoglobin (R state). Thus, BPG helps the transition of hemoglobin from R to T state.
   - An increase in [Cl$^-$]
   - An increase in body temperature

Conversely, a decrease in the aforementioned molecules and conditions causes the curve to shift to the left. This results in a decrease in the P$_{50}$ and an increase in hemoglobin's affinity for O$_2$. It is important to know the following:

- The shifting of the O$_2$–hemoglobin dissociation curve reflects the body's attempt to maintain homeostasis under stressful conditions. Thus, a right shift allows hemoglobin to unload O$_2$ more efficiently to target tissues, and a left shift allows hemoglobin to load O$_2$ more effectively.
- Metabolically active tissues contain higher concentrations of CO$_2$ and H$^+$ than the alveolar capillaries of the lungs (where CO$_2$ is exhaled).
- Hypoxic conditions caused by high altitudes, narrow pulmonary airways, chronic hypoxia, or anemia cause an increase in the concentration of BPG.

A summary of the mechanism by which hemoglobin plays a role in the exchange of O$_2$ and CO$_2$ between the lungs and tissues is detailed in ▶ Fig. 4.11.

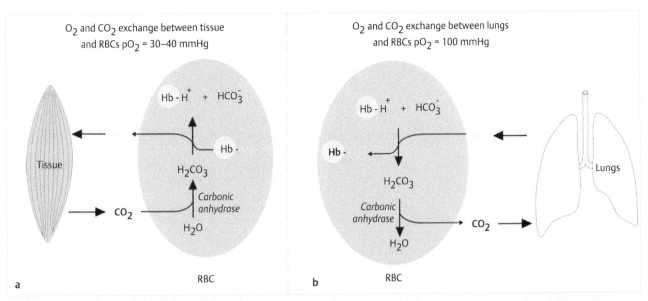

Fig. 4.11 Hemoglobin-mediated O_2 and CO_2 transport/exchange. (a) In the tissues, the partial pressure of oxygen (Po_2) is low, and CO_2 is produced. The CO_2 is converted by carbonic anhydrase to carbonic acid H_2CO_3, which ionizes to form bicarbonate (HCO_3^-) and H^+. The protons bind to hemoglobin and cause the release of O_2 by decreasing its affinity. **(b)** On the other hand, the Po_2 is high in the lungs, which facilitates its binding to hemoglobin, forcing out the protons. The protons combine with bicarbonate to form carbonic acid, which is converted to CO_2 by the reverse reaction of carbonic anhydrase. RBC, red blood cells.

Foundations

Fetal hemoglobin

Adult hemoglobin (HbA, $\alpha_2\beta_2$) and fetal hemoglobin (HbF, $\alpha_2\gamma_2$) differ in that the latter cannot efficiently bind to 2,3-bisphosphoglycerate because HbF lacks positively-charged amino acids (e.g., histidine) at the interface of β subunits that bind to 2,3-bisphosphoglycerate in HbA. This feature gives HbF a stronger affinity for O_2 and allows it to draw O_2 from the maternal blood. While 2,3-bisphosphoglycerate decreases HbA's affinity for O_2, it has little effect on HbF's affinity for O_2.

5 Biochemical Reactions and Enzymes

5.1 Principles of Biochemical Reactions

Metabolism is the all-encompassing term for the intracellular biochemical reactions that harness energy from nutrients to sustain life. It begins with the ingestion of food, which is then broken down into molecular components that can be transported into cells, where they are used to do the following:
- Produce energy via reactions that occur in the catabolic pathways
- Synthesize molecules via reactions that occur in the anabolic pathways

Those biochemical reactions that release energy are called exergonic, whereas those that consume energy are called endergonic.

5.1.1 Free Energy Change (ΔG)

The dynamics of a biochemical reaction is described using free energy change (ΔG), which is an indication of the spontaneity of a reaction and the amount of "useful" energy the reaction can produce to do work. For the reaction

$$A + B \rightleftarrows C + D$$

the following equation describes the relationship between ΔG and the energy status of the reaction:

$$\Delta G = \Delta G^{\circ\prime} + RTln\frac{[C][D]}{[A][B]} \tag{5.1}$$

where $\Delta G^{\circ\prime}$ is the free energy change at standard conditions (pH 7, 1 M concentrations of reactants and products at 298° K), $\frac{[C][D]}{[A][B]}$ is the ratio of products to reactants, R is the gas constant, and T is the absolute temperature of a reaction. As such, the following are true:
- When $\Delta G = 0$, the reaction is at equilibrium, and no useful energy is produced or consumed.
- When $\Delta G < 0$, the reaction occurs spontaneously, and energy is released that can be harnessed to do "useful" work (exergonic reaction).
- When $\Delta G > 0$, the reaction cannot occur spontaneously (endergonic reaction).

5.1.2 Equilibrium Constant (K_{eq}) and Standard Free Energy Change ($\Delta G^{\circ\prime}$)

Because $\Delta G = 0$ at equilibrium, and K_{eq} is the ratio of the concentrations of products to reactants at equilibrium, substituting these into Eq. 5.1 yields the following.

$$\Delta G^{\circ\prime} = -RTlnK_{eq} \tag{5.2}$$

According to this equation, the standard free energy change ($\Delta G^{\circ\prime}$) of a reaction is directly related to K_{eq}, and like $\Delta G^{\circ\prime}$, K_{eq} is an indicator of the spontaneity of a reaction such that the following are true:

- When $K_{eq} = 1$, then $\Delta G^{\circ\prime} = 0$, which means that the reaction is at equilibrium.
- When $K_{eq} > 1$, then $\Delta G^{\circ\prime} < 0$, which means that the reaction is spontaneous and will proceed to the right.
- When $K_{eq} < 1$, then $\Delta G^{\circ\prime} > 0$, which means that the reaction is not spontaneous and will proceed to the left.

Please note that the standard free energy change ($\Delta G^{\circ\prime}$) is a theoretical constant, whereas ΔG is the free energy change under actual reaction conditions. This means that ΔG can vary with changing values for A, B, C, and D in Equation 5.1.

Foundations

Reaction velocity

The numerical values of the standard free energy change ($\Delta G^{\circ\prime}$) of a reaction indicate whether the reaction will proceed without the input of energy but are not indicative of the velocity at which the reaction takes place. Reaction velocity can be increased by the presence of a biological catalyst called an enzyme.

5.1.3 Reaction Drivers

A biochemical reaction can be driven against an "unfavorable" equilibrium through the principle of mass action or by the input of energy, as described next:

Mass action (Le Chatelier's principle) states that because K_{eq} is a ratio of the concentrations of products to reactants, it can be manipulated by altering the concentrations of products and reactants. Therefore, a reaction ($A + B \rightleftarrows C + D$) that is strongly favored to the left (i.e., $K_{eq} < 1$), can be driven to the right by either or both of the following:
- Increasing the concentration of the reactants via addition of A and B
- Decreasing the concentration of products via removal of C and D

Input of energy (coupled reactions) allows an endergonic reaction to be coupled to an exergonic reaction in order for the former to occur. The coupling of reactions is possible if they share a common intermediate. When reactions are coupled, the $\Delta G^{\circ\prime}$ of each reaction is added to obtain an overall $\Delta G^{\circ\prime}$, which determines whether the process as a whole will occur spontaneously. For instance, in biological systems, most energy is stored in adenosine triphosphate (ATP). Because the hydrolysis of ATP to adenosine diphosphate (ADP) is extremely exergonic ($\Delta G^{\circ\prime} = -7.4$ kcal/mol), it can be used to power endergonic biochemical reactions.

This is illustrated using the reaction that condenses ammonia (NH_3) and glutamate to produce glutamine:

Reaction 1: Glutamate + NH₃ → Glutamine + H₂O
($\Delta G^{\circ\prime} = + 3.35$ kcal/mol)
Reaction 2: ATP + H₂O → ADP + Phosphate
($\Delta G^{\circ\prime} = - 7.4$ kcal/mol)

Reaction 3: (coupled): Glutamate + NH₃ + ATP →
Glutamine + ADP + Phosphate
(ΔG°' = - 4.05 kcal/mol)

Water (H_2O) is the common intermediate for reactions 1 and 2. When these reactions are coupled, the sum of their standard free energy change is negative.

5.2 Biochemical Reaction Classes

All biochemical reactions are transfer reactions, which involve the movement of either electrons, atoms, or groups of atoms from within molecules or from one molecule to another via one of five major mechanisms listed here.

5.2.1 Additions/Eliminations

Additions involve the transfer of an atom or group of atoms to a multiple bond (e.g., a double bond). Eliminations involve the removal of an atom or group of atoms that results in the formation of a multiple bond.

5.2.2 Substitution Reactions

Substitution reactions involve the replacement of one functional group with another. For example, hydroxyl groups of sugars can be replaced by amino groups.

5.2.3 Rearrangements (Isomerizations)

Rearrangements (isomerizations) involve the shifting of functional groups within the same molecule to produce isomers (i.e., molecules with the same molecular formula but different arrangements of atoms). There are two main types of isomers:
1. Structural isomers, which have the same atoms but different bonds
2. Spatial isomers (stereoisomers), which have the same atoms and bonds but different spatial arrangements and are nonsuperimposable

5.2.4 Oxidation-Reduction Reactions

The most general description of oxidation-reduction (redox) reactions is that they involve the transfer of electrons from one molecule (the reducing agent) to another (the oxidizing agent). Oxidation may also involve the addition of oxygen or the removal of hydrogen. The affinity of a molecule for electrons is reflected in its standard redox potential (E_o') such that
• The molecule with the more negative E_o' is the stronger electron donor (reducing agent), and it will therefore reduce (or be oxidized by) the electron acceptor (oxidizing agent).

Foundations
Relationship between K_{eq} and $\Delta E_o'$
A large K_{eq} is associated with a large positive $\Delta E_o'$. Thus, $\Delta E_o'$ is mathematically related to $\Delta G_o'$, but the two are opposite in sign.

5.2.5 Acid-Base Reactions

These types of reactions involve acids (compounds that donate protons) and bases (compounds that accept protons). In the human body, combinations of acids and corresponding bases function as buffering agents that maintain the pH of blood at physiological levels (pH 7.37 to 7.43) and behave as follows:
• When a weak acid dissociates in water, it produces a proton and its conjugate base. For example, acetic acid dissociates into a proton (H^+) and acetate.

$$CH_3COOH \rightleftharpoons H^+ + CH_3COO^-$$

Acetic acid   Acetate

(acid)   (conjugatebase)

• When a weak base combines with protons in the presence of water, its conjugate acid is formed. For example, bicarbonate combines with H^+ to form carbonic acid.

$$HCO_3^- + H^+ \rightleftharpoons H_2CO_3$$

Bicarbonate   Carbonicacid

(base)   (conjugateacid)

Dissociation constants and acidity

The dissociation constant (K) is an equilibrium constant that indicates the tendency of a larger compound to dissociate (or separate) into smaller components. Subsequent calculations using K provide valuable information about the acidity of a solution (pH) and the strength of an acid (pK_a).
• pH defines the acidity of a solution, and ranges in value from 0 to 14. Neutral solutions have a pH of 7, acidic solutions have a pH that is less than 7, and basic solutions have a pH that is greater than 7.
• The dissociation of water is often used to show how pH is derived mathematically because it dissociates into H^+ and hydroxide ion (OH^-), as depicted in the reaction $H_2O \rightleftharpoons H^+ + OH^-$.

At equilibrium, the dissociation constant of pure water (K_w) is commonly expressed as Eq. 5.3, whose value is 10^{-14}. At equilibrium, the [H^+] is known to be equivalent to that of the [OH^-] (Eq. 5.4), both of which are equal to 10^{-7} M. The pH is then calculated by determining the negative $\log_{10}$ of [H^+] (Eq. 5.5). Thus, the pH of pure water is determined to be 7, indicating that it is a neutral solution.

$$K_W = [H^+][OH^-] = 10^{-14} \tag{5.3}$$

$$[H^+] = [OH^-] = 10^{-7} M \tag{5.4}$$

$$pH = -\log_{10}[H^+] = -\log_{10}(10^{-7}M) = 7 \tag{5.5}$$

• pK_a is an indicator of the strength of an acid such that the stronger the acid, the lower its pK_a. Likewise, the weaker the acid, the larger its pK_a. The derivation of pK_a begins with a commonly written expression for the dissociation of a weak acid (HA $\rightleftharpoons$ H$^+$ + A$^-$), where HA is the acid, and A$^-$ is its conjugate base.

The resulting acidic dissociation constant (K_a) is expressed as Eq. 5.6, and the pK_a is determined by calculating the negative $\log_{10}$ of $[K_a]$ (Eq. 5.7).

$$K_a = \frac{[H^+][A^-]}{[HA]} \qquad (5.6)$$

$$pK_a = -\log[K_a] \qquad (5.7)$$

Buffers

A solution that contains a mixture of a weak acid and its conjugate base functions as a buffer because it resists changes to its pH when strong acids or bases are added. To that end, the Henderson-Hasselbalch equation (Eq. 5.8) is used to predict the optimal pH of buffered solutions. The buffering capacity of an acid–conjugate base solution is optimal when its pH is equal to its pK_a (with a range of ±1 pH unit). This occurs when the concentration of the acid is equal to that of its conjugate base.

$$pH = pK_a + \log\frac{[A^-]}{[HA]} \qquad (5.8)$$

The normal pH range for blood is 7.37 to 7.43, and it is maintained primarily by the carbonic acid/bicarbonate (H_2CO_3/HCO_3^-) buffer system. When the blood's pH is lower or higher than normal, it leads to acidosis and alkalosis, respectively. These conditions can be caused by hypoventilation, hyperventilation, and metabolic disturbances, as summarized in ▶ Fig. 5.1.

Foundations

Biological oxidation

Redox reactions are the most important class of biochemical reactions given that biological oxidation provides most of the

energy for aerobic metabolism. Energy is released when electrons are transferred from fuel molecules through the electron transport chain (down the redox potential) to oxygen. Energy released from these electron transfers is used to pump hydrogen ions across the mitochondrial membrane. The resulting proton gradient powers the phosphorylation of ADP to ATP.

Normal

Acid–base balance and the kidneys

One of the major roles of the kidneys is to regulate the pH of blood. The kidneys can do so because of their ability to remove protons (H$^+$) from the blood in the form of ammonium ion (NH$_4^+$) and to reabsorb bicarbonate (HCO$_3^-$). Therefore, low blood pH triggers an increase in both the removal of protons and the reabsorption of bicarbonate. When the pH of blood is too high, fewer protons are removed and less bicarbonate is reabsorbed.

Therapeutics

Diabetic ketoacidosis

Diabetic ketoacidosis (DKA) is a condition marked by hyperglycemia and low blood pH that often afflicts individuals with uncontrolled type 1 diabetes. The lack of insulin prevents glucose from being taken up by cells to produce energy. Consequently, the body switches to degrading fatty acids for energy. The degradation (via β-oxidation) of fatty acids promotes the formation of acidic compounds called ketone bodies. They include acetone, acetoacetic acid, and β-hydroxybutyric acid. The dissociation of the latter two ketone bodies releases H$^+$, which causes the pH of blood to decrease. The symptoms of DKA include dehydration, vomiting, confusion, and coma and may lead to death. Treatment involves administration of insulin (to treat hyperglycemia) and fluids (to treat dehydration).

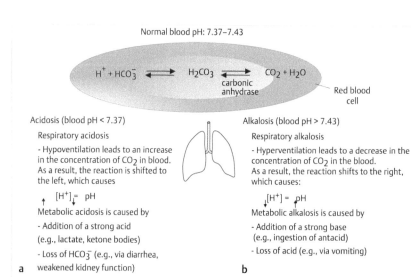

Fig. 5.1 Disorders associated with acid-base imbalances. (a) Respiratory acidosis may be caused by hypoventilation, which leads to elevated levels of blood CO_2. The latter effect contributes to respiratory acidosis because the elevated levels of CO_2 cause an increase in [H$^+$] in the blood and therefore decrease its pH. Metabolic acidosis is caused by conditions in which a strong acid is added to the blood or bicarbonate (HCO$_3^-$) is lost. (b) Respiratory alkalosis is caused by hyperventilation, which lowers blood CO_2 levels. The latter effect decreases [H$^+$] in the blood and therefore increases its pH. Metabolic alkalosis is caused by conditions in which a strong base is ingested, or acids are lost.

5.3 Enzymes

5.3.1 Overview

Enzymes are proteins that act as biological catalysts to speed up the rate of biochemical reactions. They do so by binding to substrates and converting them to products. Enzymes are not consumed in reactions though they may be temporarily altered. The acceleration of biochemical reactions is attributed to the effects that enzymes have on specific reaction parameters as follows (▶ Fig. 5.2):

- Enzymes lower the reaction's activation energy (E_a)—that is, the minimum amount of energy required to transform the substrate into an activated intermediate.
- Enzymes do not alter the concentration of substrates and products at equilibrium (K_{eq}) or a reaction's net free energy change (ΔG). In ▶ Fig. 5.2, ΔG is the difference between the free energies of the product(s) and the substrate(s).

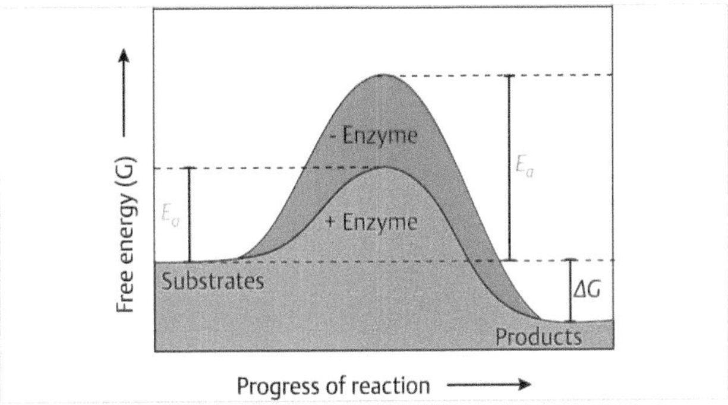

Fig. 5.2 Energetics of enzyme catalysis. An enzyme speeds up a reaction by lowering the activation energy (E_a). The E_a of a reaction without enzyme (purple) is higher than that of the same reaction with enzyme (orange). The presence of an enzyme does not change the concentration of the substrates or products, or the reaction's net free energy change (ΔG) at equilibrium.

Enzyme Classes

There are six major classes of enzymes that are named for the type of reactions they catalyze (▶ Fig. 5.3).

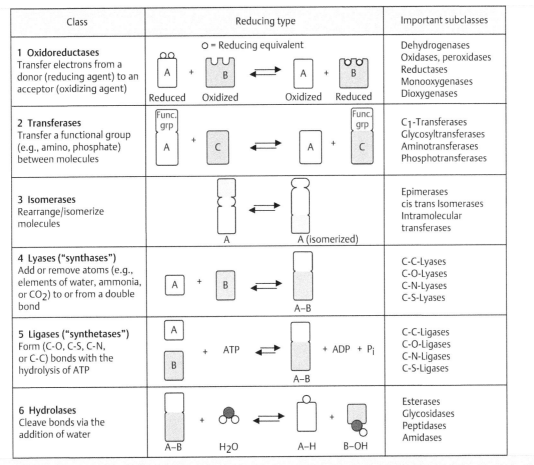

Class	Reducing type	Important subclasses
1 Oxidoreductases Transfer electrons from a donor (reducing agent) to an acceptor (oxidizing agent)	○ = Reducing equivalent	Dehydrogenases Oxidases, peroxidases Reductases Monooxygenases Dioxygenases
2 Transferases Transfer a functional group (e.g., amino, phosphate) between molecules		C_1-Transferases Glycosyltransferases Aminotransferases Phosphotransferases
3 Isomerases Rearrange/isomerize molecules		Epimerases cis trans Isomerases Intramolecular transferases
4 Lyases ("synthases") Add or remove atoms (e.g., elements of water, ammonia, or CO_2) to or from a double bond		C-C-Lyases C-O-Lyases C-N-Lyases C-S-Lyases
5 Ligases ("synthetases") Form (C-O, C-S, C-N, or C-C) bonds with the hydrolysis of ATP		C-C-Ligases C-O-Ligases C-N-Ligases C-S-Ligases
6 Hydrolases Cleave bonds via the addition of water		Esterases Glycosidases Peptidases Amidases

Fig. 5.3 Enzyme classes. The enzyme classes, the type of reactions they catalyze, and the various subclasses to which they belong are summarized here.

5.3.2 Enzyme Structure and Function

Some enzymes are composed of a single polypeptide chain, whereas others are made up of two or more polypeptide chains that can be either identical or different. The folding of these polypeptide chains into tertiary or quaternary structures creates a pocket, called the active site, in which biochemical reactions are catalyzed. Some enzymes also contain regions for nonprotein partners, known as cofactors and coenzymes, to bind.

Active Site

The three-dimensional cleft or pocket in enzymes that serves as the active (catalytic) site to which the substrate binds is relatively small compared with the overall size of the protein. The amino acid residues that inhabit the active site may be far apart in the protein's primary sequence but are brought into close proximity of each other through the folding of the enzyme. These active site residues are critical for the proper functioning of the enzyme because they play a role in the following:

• **Substrate binding:** The substrate binds to the enzyme's active site through multiple weak interactions with certain amino acids. Substrate binding may then trigger a conformational change in the active site that facilitates interactions between the enzyme and the substrate.

• **Catalytic reaction:** Specific amino acid residues within the enzyme's active site directly participate in the making or breaking of chemical bonds.

Cofactors and Coenzymes

Some enzymes must associate with nonprotein organic or inorganic molecules to catalyze their reactions. These nonprotein molecules bind loosely or tightly to their target enzymes and may be reversibly altered during the enzymatic reaction. An inactive enzyme that lacks its nonprotein partner is referred to as an apoenzyme; an active enzyme that is bound to its nonprotein partner is referred to as a holoenzyme. These nonprotein molecules are divided into two categories:

1. **Cofactors:** These are metal ions that associate with enzymes via noncovalent interactions. Examples include copper (Cu), iron (Fe), magnesium (Mg), and zinc (Zn). See ▶ Table 5.1 for a summary of enzymes that require metal ion cofactors for their activity.

2. **Coenzymes:** These are small organic molecules mostly derived from vitamins. These coenzymes, the enzymes with which they associate, and the vitamins from which some of them are derived are found in ▶ Table 5.2.

Coenzymes are further divided into two groups based on the strength of their association with the enzyme:

• **Cosubstrate:** These are coenzymes that associate with enzymes temporarily. They bind in one state and detach in an altered state. For instance, nicotinamide adenine dinucleotide (NAD^+) binds to complex I of the electron transport chain in the reduced state as NADH and leaves in the oxidized state as NAD^+. ▶ Fig. 5.4 illustrates the position of NAD^+ within the active center of lactate dehydrogenase.

• **Prosthetic group:** These are coenzymes that associate permanently with enzymes. Examples include flavin adenine dinucleotide (FAD), flavin mononucleotide (FMN), and heme.

Optimal pH and Temperature

Each enzyme has an optimal pH and temperature at which its activity is maximal. Such restrictive parameters ensure that enzymes will function only in specific locations. Enzymes are denatured and rendered nonfunctional in environments where the pH or temperature is beyond that which is optimal.

1. **Optimal pH:** The activity of the majority of human enzymes is maximal at pH values between 4 and 8. Gastric enzymes, however, are most active at pH values around 2. These enzymes (e.g., pepsin) will therefore cease to function once they enter more neutral pH environments, such as that of the duodenum (▶ Fig. 5.5a).

2. **Optimal temperature:** Most enzymes in the human body function best at 37 °C (body temperature). A rise in

Table 5.1 Metal ions and examples of proteins that require them for activity

Cu

Cytochrome c oxidase: Accepts electrons from cytochrome-c in the electron transport chain
Ferroxidase: Oxidizes ferrous iron (Fe^{2+}) into the less absorbable ferric iron (Fe^{3+})
Superoxide dismutase (antioxidant): Binds the free radical of molecular oxygen
Lysyl oxidase: Cross-links collagen and elastic tissue during wound healing *Tyrosinase:* Synthesizes melanin

Fe

Heme proteins (hemoglobin and myoglobin): Require Fe^{2+} to bind O_2
Cytochromes: Function in the electron transport chain
Catalases and peroxidases: Metabolize hydrogen peroxide

Mg

ATPases: Hydrolyze ATP to ADP and use the released energy to do mechanical work (e.g., ion transport)
Adenylate cyclase: Converts ATP to cyclic adenosine monophosphate (AMP)
Kinases: Transfers phosphate groups to target molecules

Se

Glutathione peroxidase (antioxidant): Detoxifies hydrogen peroxide

Zn

Superoxide dismutase (antioxidant): Binds the free radical of molecular oxygen
Collagenase: Replaces Type III collagen with the stronger Type I collagen during wound healing
Alcohol dehydrogenase: Converts alcohol to acetaldehyde
Alkaline phosphatase: Mineralizes bone salts
Transcription factors (proteins that contain Zn-finger domains): Bind to Specific sequences on DNA to regulate gene transcription
Carbonic anhydrase: Interconverts CO_2 and bicarbonate (HCO^-_3) to balance blood pH

Table 5.2 Coenzymes: Sources and some enzymes that require them for activity

Coenzyme	Vitamin source	Enzyme/Protein/Function
Adenosylcobalamin, methylcobalamin	B_{12} (cobalamin)	• Methylmalonyl coenzyme A (CoA) mutase • Methionine synthase
Ascorbate	C (ascorbic acid)	• Hydroxylases (e.g., lysyl hydroxylase)
Biotin	Biotin	Carboxylases, such as • Pyruvate carboxylase • Acetyl CoA carboxylase
Flavin nucleotides: flavin mononucleotide (FMN), flavin adenine dinucleotide (FAD)	B_2 (riboflavin)	Redox enzymes, such as • NADH dehydrogenase/complex 1 • Succinate dehydrogenase/complex II • Acyl CoA dehydrogenase • Retinal dehydrogenase • Vitamin-activating enzymes • α-Ketoglutaratedehydrogenase complex • Branched-chain α-keto acid dehydrogenase • Pyruvate dehydrogenase complex
Heme	–	• Hemoglobin, myoglobin • Cytochromes • Catalases and peroxidases
Lipoic acid	–	• α-Ketoglutaratedehydrogenase complex • Branched-chain α-keto acid dehydrogenase • Pyruvate dehydrogenase complex
Nicotinamide adenine dinucleotides (NAD$^+$, NADP$^+$)	B_3 (niacin)	• α-Ketoglutaratedehydrogenase complex • Branched-chain α-keto acid dehydrogenase • Pyruvate dehydrogenase complex • Redox enzymes, such as those found in the tricarboxylic acid (TCA) cycle, and enzymes involved in the biosynthesis of lipids
Pantothenic acid, coenzyme A (CoA)	B_5 (pantothenic acid)	• α-Ketoglutarate dehydrogenase complex • Branched-chain α-keto acid dehydrogenase • Pyruvate dehydrogenase complex • Fatty acid synthase complex
Pyridoxal phosphate	B_6 (pyridoxine)	• Transaminases • Decarboxylases • Glycogen phosphorylase • Aminolevulinic acid (ALA) synthase
Tetrahydrofolate (THF)	Folate	• A source of one-carbon groups for enzymes that transfer them between molecules (e.g., thymidylate synthetase)
Thiamine pyrophosphate (TPP)	B_1 (thiamine)	• α-Ketoglutarate dehydrogenase complex • Branched-chain α-keto acid dehydrogenase • Pyruvate dehydrogenase complex • Transketolase

Note: The following five coenzymes—coenzyme A, NAD$^+$, FAD, lipoic acid, and thiamine pyrophosphate—are all found in the following three enzyme complexes—α-ketoglutarate dehydrogenase, branched-chain α-keto acid dehydrogenase, and pyruvate dehydrogenase.

temperature causes the collisions between the molecules to increase and thus increases the chances that the substrate will collide with the active site of its target enzyme. The rate of most enzymatic reactions approximately doubles for each 10 °C rise in temperature as it approaches the optimal temperature for function. At temperatures above that, proteins become less active due to heat-induced denaturation. ▶ Fig. 5.5b depicts the activity profile of an enzyme whose optimal temperature is 37 °C.

Normal
Gastric proton pump inhibitors
The gastric proton pump (also known as the H$^+$/K$^+$ ATPase), located in the parietal cells that line the gastric lumen, pumps protons (H$^+$) into the gastric lumen, where they combine with

Cl$^-$ to create HCl, a key component of gastric acid. When a patient's condition warrants a reduction in the secretion of gastric acid (e.g., due to duodenal ulcers, indigestion, and heartburn), drugs are prescribed that inhibit the gastric proton pump. Such inhibitors include omeprazole (e.g., Prilosec, AstraZeneca, Wilmington, DE), lansoprazole (e.g., Prevacid, Takeda Pharmaceutical, Chuo-ku, Osaka, Japan), and esomeprazole (e.g., Nexium, AstraZeneca). A reduction in HCl production, however, causes hypochlorhydria, which leads to a decrease in the absorption of nutrients (e.g., vitamin B_{12} and Ca^{2+}), an increase in sensitivity to food poisoning, and a reduction in the efficacy of gastric enzymes (e.g., pepsin, gastric amylase, and gastric lipase) that digest proteins, carbohydrates, and lipids, respectively.

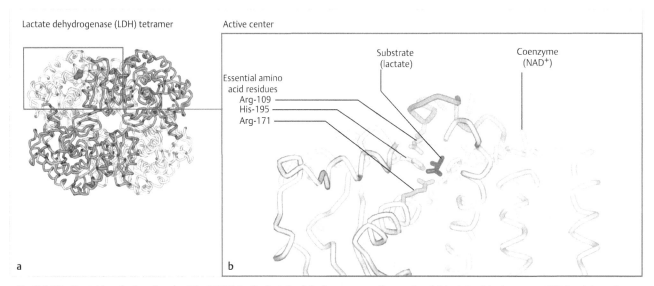

Lactate dehydrogenase (LDH) tetramer

Active center

Essential amino
acid residues
Arg-109
His-195
Arg-171

Substrate
(lactate)

Coenzyme
(NAD$^+$)

a

b

Fig. 5.4 Nicotinamide adenine dinucleotide (NAD$^+$) in the lactate dehydrogenase active center. (a) Lactate dehydrogenase (LDH) catalyzes the NADH-dependent reduction of pyruvate to lactate, or NAD$^+$-dependent oxidation of lactate to pyruvate. The active form of LDH exists as a tetramer composed of four subunits. **(b)** This illustration shows the active center of LDH, which is found in each of its subunits. The essential amino acid residues, substrate, and coenzyme are identified.

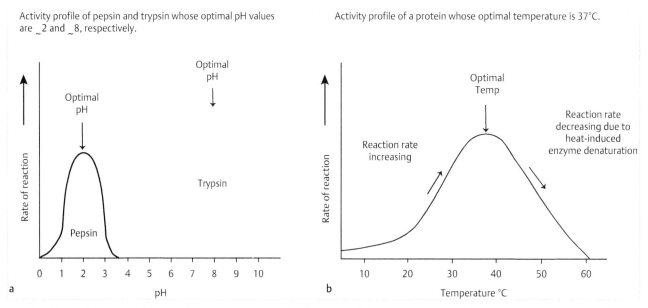

Activity profile of pepsin and trypsin whose optimal pH values are ~2 and ~8, respectively.

Activity profile of a protein whose optimal temperature is 37°C.

Optimal
pH

Optimal
pH

Trypsin

Pepsin

Rate of reaction

0 1 2 3 4 5 6 7 8 9 10
pH

a

Optimal
Temp

Reaction rate
increasing

Reaction rate
decreasing due to
heat-induced
enzyme denaturation

Rate of reaction

10   20   30   40   50   60
Temperature °C

b

Fig. 5.5 Enzyme activity as a function of pH and temperature. (a) The activity of the gastric enzyme pepsin is optimal at around pH 2, and the activity of the duodenal enzyme trypsin is optimal at around pH 8. **(b)** The activity of the enzyme depicted here increases on approach to 37 °C, its optimal temperature. Above 37 °C, this enzyme's activity decreases due to heat-induced denaturation.

Covalent Modifications and Enzyme Activity

The activity of some enzymes is affected by covalent modifications such as protein phosphorylation, such as the following:
- Phosphorylation of glycogen synthase inactivates this ratelimiting enzyme and prevents it from synthesizing glycogen chains from glucose (see **Fig. 12.12**).
- Phosphorylation of glycogen phosphorylase activates this rate-limiting enzyme, which degrades glycogen polymers to ultimately regenerate glucose (see **Fig. 12.12**).

5.4 Enzyme Kinetics

5.4.1 Overview

K$_m$, velocity (v), and V$_{max}$

To understand the kinetics of enzyme-catalyzed reactions, it is important to know how relationships between various components of an enzyme-catalyzed reaction are used to deduce information about the velocity of the reaction and the affinity of the enzyme for its substrate. A typical enzyme-catalyzed reaction is written as

$$E + S \underset{k_2}{\overset{k_1}{\rightleftharpoons}} ES \overset{k_3}{\longrightarrow} E + P$$

where E is the enzyme, S is the substrate, ES is the enzyme-substrate complex, P is the product, and k_1, k_2, k_3 are the rate constants. Using the aforementioned components, the velocity (v) of the reaction and the affinity (K_m) of the enzyme for its substrate are expressed via Eqs. 5.9 to 5.13:

$$v = k_3[ES] \tag{5.9}$$

$$K_m = \frac{k_2 + k_3}{k_1} \tag{5.10}$$

$$v = \frac{V_{max}[S]}{K_m + [S]} \text{ (Michaelis – Menten equation)} \tag{5.11}$$

$$\text{When } v = \frac{1}{2}V_{max}, K_m = [S] \tag{5.12}$$

$$\frac{1}{v} = \frac{1}{V_{max}} + \left[\frac{1}{[S]} \times \frac{k_m}{V_{max}}\right] \text{ (Lineweaver – Burk equation)} \tag{5.13}$$

From these equations, the Michaelis-Menten and Lineweaver-Burk graphs are drawn, and important information about the kinetics of enzyme-catalyzed reactions is derived:

1. **Reaction velocity:** The velocity, v, of a reaction is directly proportional to the concentration of the enzyme-substrate [ES] complex. In the presence of a fixed concentration of enzyme, [ES] increases with increasing substrate concentration [S] until the enzyme is saturated.
2. **Enzyme-substrate affinity:** K_m, the Michaelis constant, reflects the enzyme's affinity for its substrate; a high K_m indicates weak binding between enzyme and substrate, and a low K_m indicates strong binding.
3. **Maximal velocity:** When the concentration of enzyme is kept constant and that of substrate is increased, it allows for the identification of the enzyme's maximal velocity, V_{max}. V_{max} is reached when the enzyme is saturated with substrate (i.e., when all enzymes are bound to a substrate). The larger the V_{max}, the more efficient the enzyme. V_{max} is directly

proportional to enzyme concentration as long as there is enough substrate.

4. **Michaelis-Menten graph:** This graph is created by plotting the velocity, **v**, against the substrate concentration, [S] (▶ Fig. 5.6a). The resulting hyperbolic curve allows for the V_{max} and K_m to be estimated. For instance, the velocity that the curve approaches—as indicated by the asymptote parallel to the x-axis—is identified as the V_{max}. K_m is equivalent to the substrate concentration at which the reaction rate is one half of V_{max}.

5. **Lineweaver-Burk graph:** Rearrangement (i.e., the double reciprocal) of the Michaelis-Menten equation generates the Lineweaver-Burk equation. When the reciprocal of velocity (1/v) is plotted against the reciprocal of the substrate concentration (1/[S]), it generates a straight-line graph (▶ Fig. 5.6b). Using this line allows for values of V_{max} and K_m to be determined: the line's x-intercept is $-1/K_m$, the y-intercept is $1/V_{max}$, and the slope is K_m/V_{max}.

5.4.2 Enzyme Inhibition and Inactivation

Inhibitors are molecules that block the activity of enzymes. Many poisons, insecticides, metal ions, and drugs used in medicine function as inhibitors, which either prevent the enzyme from binding to its substrate or stop the enzyme from catalyzing its biochemical reaction (even though it may bind to its substrate). The inhibition of an enzyme may be reversible or irreversible, but the irreversible loss of enzyme function is called inactivation (suicide inhibition).

Enzyme Inhibition (Reversible)

The reversible inhibition of an enzyme occurs when the inhibitor attaches to the enzyme via noncovalent bonds. There are two major types of reversible inhibitors.

1. **Competitive inhibitors:** These inhibitors may resemble the substrate and compete with it for binding to the active site of the free enzyme. Other competitive inhibitors may bind to non-active sites but cause a conformational change in the enzyme that prevents substrate binding. Competitive inhibitors form enzyme-inhibitor (EI) complexes and have the following effects on the kinetics of their target enzymes (▶ Fig. 5.7a):

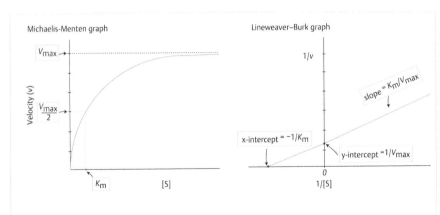

Fig. 5.6 Michaelis-Menten and Lineweaver-Burk graphs. (a) The Michaelis-Menten graph is obtained by plotting an enzyme's reaction velocity (v) against the concentration of its substrate [S]. The V_{max} is the velocity the curve approaches (but never really reaches), and K_m is the substrate concentration at which the reaction velocity is at V_{max}. **(b)** The Lineweaver-Burk graph is obtained by plotting the inverse of velocity (1/v) against the inverse of substrate concentration (1/[S]) to generate a straight-line graph. The point at which the line intercepts the x-axis is identified as $-1/K_m$, and that at which it intercepts the y-axis is $1/V_{max}$, and the slope of the line is K_m/V_{max}.

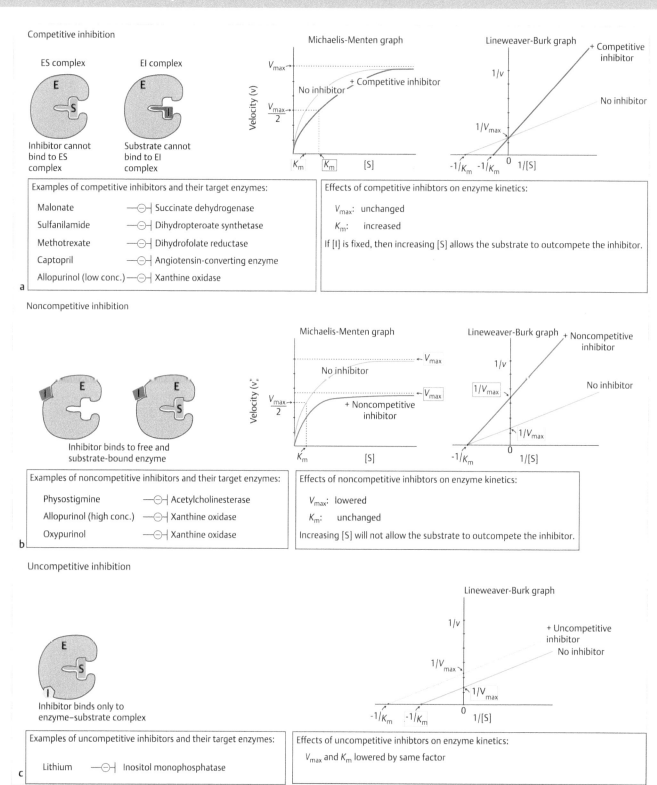

Fig. 5.7 Enzyme inhibition (reversible). Agents that reversibly inhibit enzymes do so by forming noncovalent bonds with the enzyme. **(a)** Some competitive inhibitors compete with the substrate for binding to an enzyme's active site. Others (not shown) bind to regions outside of the active site and cause a conformational change in the enzyme that prevents substrate binding. The competitive inhibitor and substrate cannot bind the enzyme at the same time. **(b)** Noncompetitive inhibitors do not resemble the substrate and bind to either the free or the substrate-bound enzyme at a region other than the active site. **(c)** Uncompetitive inhibitors only bind to the enzyme-substrate complex. EI, enzyme-inhibitor; ES, enzyme-substrate.

Table 5.3 Competitive inhibitors

Inhibitor	Enzyme target and catalytic reaction	Inhibitor effect/Use
Malonate	Succinate dehydrogenase *Reaction:* Succinate → fumarate	Inhibits the TCA cycle and the e⁻ transport chain
Sulfanilamide	Dihydropteroate synthetase *Reaction:* PABA → diphosphate + dihydropteroate	Inhibits prokaryotic nucleic acid synthesis; has limited use as an antibiotic due to bacterial resistance
Methotrexate	Dihydrofolate reductase *Reaction:* Dihydrofolic acid → tetrahydrofolic acid	Inhibits eukaryotic nucleic acid synthesis

Abbreviations: PABA, para-aminobenzoic acid; TCA, tricarboxylic acid.

- The V_{max} is not affected because the inhibitor disrupts the binding of the enzyme to its substrate and not the catalytic activity of the enzyme itself.
- The apparent K_m, which is the Michaelis constant measured in the presence of a competitive inhibitor, is increased. This means that in the presence of the inhibitor, a higher substrate concentration is needed to reach ½ V_{max}.
- If the inhibitor is at a fixed concentration, however, its effects can be overcome by increasing the substrate's concentration, which has the effect of diluting or outcompeting the inhibitor.
- Examples of competitive inhibitors (and their target enzymes) include malonate (which inhibits succinate dehydrogenase), sulfanilamide (which inhibits dihydropteroate synthetase), and methotrexate (which inhibits dihydrofolate reductase) (▶ Table 5.3). Because both substrate and inhibitor cannot bind at the same time, the species at the active site is determined by Le Chatelier's principle (mass action).

Therapeutics

Allopurinol: suicide inhibitor/inactivator

Allopurinol is a pharmaceutical agent used for the treatment of chronic gout—a condition caused by the accumulation of uric acid (a product of purine degradation) in the synovial fluids surrounding joints and marked by throbbing pain due to the inflammation of joints. Individuals suffering from chronic gout have persistent joint pain and reduced ability to move the affected joints, typically of the hands, wrists, shoulders, knees, and feet (especially the big toe). Xanthine oxidase, an enzyme that first converts hypoxanthine to xanthine and then to uric acid in purine degradation, is the target of allopurinol.

Allopurinol is often described as a suicide inhibitor/inactivator because its mechanism of action involves binding to the active site of xanthine oxidase, which then converts allopurinol into its active metabolite, oxypurinol (alloxanthine). The latter binds tightly to the active site and is only slowly released from it.

At low concentrations, allopurinol is described as a competitive inhibitor, but at high concentrations, it is described as a noncompetitive inhibitor. Oxypurinol is described as a noncompetitive inhibitor also.

1. **Noncompetitive inhibitors:** These types of inhibitors do not resemble the substrate. They bind to the free and substrate-bound enzyme at a region other than the substrate binding site. Because the inhibitor binds to a constant fraction of the enzyme regardless of the substrate concentration, the resulting effect on the enzyme's kinetics are as follows (▶ Fig. 5.7b):
   - The apparent V_{max} is lowered because the inhibitor disrupts the enzyme's ability to catalyze its reaction.
   - K_m appears unchanged because the affinity of the enzyme for its substrate is not affected. The inhibitor's effects, therefore, cannot be overcome by increasing the substrate concentration.
   - Physostigmine is a noncompetitive inhibitor used for the treatment of myasthenia gravis. It inhibits acetylcholinesterase (an enzyme that breaks down acetylcholine into choline and acetate), so that acetylcholine levels are elevated.
2. **Uncompetitive inhibitors:** These types of inhibitors bind only to the enzyme-substrate complex at a site other than the active site. The binding of the inhibitor appears to decrease both K_m and V_{max} by the same factor.
   - Lithium, which is used to treat bipolar disorder, is thought to exert its effects through uncompetitive inhibition of inositol monophosphatase, thereby preventing the recycling of inositol and polyphosphoinositide formation (▶ Fig. 5.7c).

Therapeutics

Physostigmine treatment for myasthenia gravis

Myasthenia gravis is an autoimmune disease caused by an inhibition of acetylcholine signaling by antibodies that bind to and thus block acetylcholine nicotinic receptors from binding to their cognate ligand, acetylcholine. It is marked by muscle weakness, inability to hold one's gaze, and fatigue. Treatment involves administration of acetylcholinesterase inhibitors such as physostigmine, neostigmine, and pyridostigmine. Physostigmine binds to the active site of acetylcholinesterase and slowly carbamoylates the enzyme. The covalent bond formed inactivates acetylcholinesterase, thus preventing the breakdown of acetylcholine in the synaptic cleft. Because this bond can be hydrolyzed (it takes 30 minutes to 6 hours), physostigmine is described as a reversible inhibitor.

Normal

Captopril treatment for hypertension

Blood pressure is regulated by the renin–angiotensin–aldosterone system (RAAS). When blood pressure or the body's extracellular fluid volume is too low, the kidneys respond by secreting renin, an enzyme that converts the liver-secreted peptide angiotensinogen to angiotensin I. Angiotensin I is then converted to angiotensin II by angiotensin-converting enzyme (ACE), a dipeptidase. Angiotensin II increases blood pressure by stimulating both vasoconstriction and the release of aldosterone by the adrenal glands. Aldosterone increases blood volume and thus blood pressure because it stimulates the kidneys to increase the reabsorption of sodium and water. Conversely, blood pressure is decreased by bradykinin, a peptide that stimulates vasodilation but whose degradation is catalyzed by ACE. Captopril is used to treat hypertension because it competitively inhibits ACE and thus reduces the levels of angiotensin II and elevates the levels of bradykinin.

Foundations

Inhibition of metalloenzymes

Metalloenzymes (enzymes that require metal cofactors such as Mg^{2+} and Zn^{2+} for activity) are inhibited by chelating agents that bind to and remove these metals from their metalloenzymes. One such chelator, ethylenediaminetetraacetic acid (EDTA), inhibits metalloenzymes.

Therapeutics

Chelating agents for lead poisoning

Lead (Pb) inhibits δ-aminolevulinic acid (ALA) dehydratase and ferrochelatase, enzymes involved in the biosynthesis of heme, a coenzyme of hemoglobin. A patient suspected of lead poisoning may present with abdominal pain, sideroblastic anemia, irritability, headaches, and signs of impaired nervous system development and encephalopathy. Treatment includes administration of Ca-EDTA with dimercaprol. Because lead has a higher affinity for EDTA than does calcium, it displaces calcium from Ca-EDTA to create Pb-EDTA, which is excreted in urine. Alternatively, lead poisoning in children can be treated with the chelating agent succimer (dimercaptosuccinic acid).

Enzyme Inactivation (Irreversible)

The irreversible inactivation of an enzyme involves destruction or covalent modification of one or more of the functional groups of the key amino acids in the active site (▶ Fig. 5.8). Because irreversible inactivators reduce the enzyme's ability to catalyze a chemical reaction, the kinetics of their effects mirror that of noncompetitive inhibitors as follows:

- V_{max} is lowered.
- K_m appears unchanged because the affinity of the enzyme for its substrate is not affected.
- The inhibitor's effects cannot be overcome by increasing the substrate's concentration.
- Examples of irreversible enzyme inactivators include the heavy metal ions lead and mercury, organophosphates, cyanide, sulfide, and aspirin (▶ Table 5.4).

Enzyme inactivation by suicide inhibitors can only be overcome by the synthesis of new enzyme protein molecules. Thus, because the irreversible inactivation of cyclooxygenases in platelets by aspirin can impair clotting mechanisms, patients are withdrawn from the aspirin regimen for at least a week prior to surgery to enable restoration of platelet function through synthesis of new platelets.

Therapeutics

Treating organophosphorus poisoning

Poisoning from organophosphorus inhibitors of acetylcholinesterase, such as nerve gas (e.g., sarin) and insecticides, presents as excessive/uncontrolled salivation (acetylcholine promotes the flow of saliva), diarrhea, urination, teary eyes, and vomiting. Early treatment consists of the administration of pralidoxime (in conjunction with atropine and diazepam). Pralidoxime removes the organophosphorus inhibitor from acetylcholinesterase, permitting the enzyme to function again.

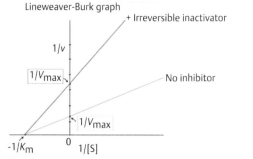

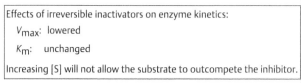

Examples of irreversible inactivators and their target enzymes:	
Organophosphates	—⊖⊣ Acetylcholinesterase
Cyanide, sulfides	—⊖⊣ Cytochrome- c oxidase (complex IV)
Aspirin	—⊖⊣ Prostaglandin synthase (COX1/2)

—⊖⊣ Inhibits

Effects of irreversible inactivators on enzyme kinetics:

V_{max}: lowered

K_m: unchanged

Increasing [S] will not allow the substrate to outcompete the inhibitor.

Fig. 5.8 Enzyme inactivation (irreversible). Agents that irreversibly inactivate enzymes do so by destroying or covalently modifying key amino acid residues.

Table 5.4 Irreversible inhibitors

Inhibitor	Enzyme target and catalytic reaction	Inhibitor effect/Use
Lead (Pb)	Aminolevulinic acid (ALA) dehydratase, ferrochelatase *Reaction:* δ-Aminolevulinic acid → heme	Lead poisoning blocks the production of heme
Organophosphates (e.g., nerve gas, insecticides)	Acetylcholinesterase *Reaction:* Acetylcholine → choline + acetate	Poisonous due to excessive levels of acetylcholine
Cyanide, sulfide	Cytochrome oxidase (complex IV) *Reaction:* Transfers e$^-$ from cytochrome-c to O_2	Inhibits the e$^-$ transport chain and thus oxidative phosphorylation
Aspirin	Cyclooxygenase (COX) (prostaglandin synthase) *Reaction:* Arachidonic acid → prostaglandin H_2	Inhibits the synthesis of eicosanoids such as prostaglandins, prostacyclins, and thromboxanes to relieve pain and inflammation

Abbreviation: e$^-$, electron.

Table 5.5 Positive (+) and negative (−) allosteric effectors

Effector	Enzyme target and catalytic reaction	Effector outcome/Use
(+) Acetyl CoA	Pyruvate carboxylase *Reaction:* Pyruvate → oxaloacetate	A positive effector that stimulates gluconeogenesis
(+) Fructose 2,6-BP (−) Citrate	Phosphofructokinase-1 *Reaction:* Fructose 6-P → fructose 1,6-BP	Positive and negative effectors that respectively stimulate and inhibit glycolysis
(−) Glucose 6-P	Hexokinase *Reaction:* Glucose → glucose 6-P	A negative effector that inhibits glycolysis
(+) ATP (−) CTP	Aspartate carbamoylase *Reaction:* Carbamoyl-P + aspartate → carbamoyl aspartate	Positive and negative effectors that stimulate and inhibit pyrimidine synthesis, respectively

Abbreviations: ATP, adenosine triphosphate; BP, bisphosphate; CoA, coenzyme A; CTP, cytidine triphosphate; P, phosphate.

5.5 Allosteric Enzymes, Isozymes, and Proenzymes

5.5.1 Allosteric Enzymes

An allosteric enzyme is one whose activity is modulated through the noncovalent binding of a specific metabolite (called an allosteric effector molecule) at a site other than the catalytic site. The following are characteristics of allosteric enzymes and their behavior:

- Allosteric enzymes are usually composed of two or more polypeptide subunits. However, monomeric enzymes (e.g., glucokinase) may also exhibit allosteric properties.
- Binding of an effector molecule to the allosteric site affects either the binding of the substrate to the catalytic site or the efficiency of the catalytic site by changing the conformation of the allosteric enzyme. This effect can be either positive (e.g., to increase the binding of substrate) or negative (e.g., to decrease the binding of substrate).
- Allosteric enzymes usually catalyze either the first or the committed reaction step of a metabolic pathway. The pathway's final product then serves as a negative effector

that inhibits the allosteric enzyme. This mechanism is referred to as end-product, or feedback inhibition.

Allosteric Enzyme Kinetics

Allosteric enzymes do not follow Michaelis-Menten kinetics. When the reaction velocity (v) is plotted against substrate concentration ([S]), a sigmoidal curve rather than a hyperbolic curve is obtained. This sigmoidal curve is analogous to that of the O_2–hemoglobin dissociation curve whose S shape reflects positive cooperativity—that is, binding of the first substrate molecule enhances the binding of subsequent molecules at other sites. (Note: oxygen binding to myoglobin, however, follows Michaelis-Menten kinetics because it only has a single binding site for oxygen.) The effects of allosteric activators and inhibitors on an allosteric enzyme's kinetics are as follows (▶ Fig. 5.9):

- An allosteric activator has the effect of shifting the sigmoidal curve to the left; an allosteric inhibitor shifts it to the right. Examples of enzymes whose activities are regulated by positive and negative allosteric effector molecules are summarized in ▶ Table 5.5.

I

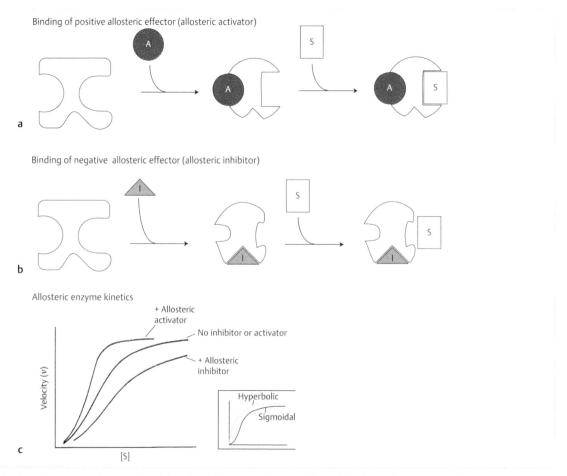

Fig. 5.9 Monomeric allosteric enzyme characteristics. (**a**) Binding of a positive allosteric effector (A) induces the enzyme to adopt a conformation that has a greater affinity for the substrate (S). (**b**) Binding of the negative allosteric effector (I) induces a conformational change that decreases the enzyme's affinity for the substrate. (**c**) When the velocity (*v*) and the substrate concentration [S] of a reaction catalyzed by an allosteric enzyme are plotted against each other, a sigmoidal curve is generated. The presence of an allosteric activator shifts the curve to the left, while that of an allosteric inhibitor shifts the curve to the right. (Inset: comparison between a hyperbolic curve and a sigmoidal curve.)

- The sigmoidal response of allosteric enzymes facilitates a more vigorous control of enzyme activity compared with enzymes displaying Michaelis-Menten kinetics.

5.5.2 Isozymes

Isozymes are enzymes that catalyze the same chemical reaction but differ in amino acid sequence. As a result, they have different kinetic properties (V_{max}, K_m, allosteric binding sites), subunit composition, and optimal temperature and pH, and the substrate specificity of isozymes may also differ. Isozymes can be made up of multiple polypeptide subunits of two or more differing types. Isozymes of lactate dehydrogenase, creatine kinase, and aspartate aminotransferase serve as markers for myocardial infarction when their blood levels are elevated beyond those that are normal (▶ Table 5.6, ▶ Fig. 5.10).

1. **Lactate dehydrogenase (LDH):** LDH is an enzyme that catalyzes the conversion of pyruvate to lactate, and lactate back to pyruvate. It is a tetramer composed of various combinations of two types of subunits—M (muscle) and H (heart)—that generates five isozymes (LDH-1 to LDH-5).

Normal blood LDH levels range from 45 to 90 U/L, and various mixtures of the LDH isozymes are found in different tissues, as follows:
- LDH-1 (HHHH) is found predominantly in cardiac muscle and red blood cells.
- LDH-2 (HHHM) is the form predominantly found in serum.
- LDH-5 (MMMM) is found predominantly in skeletal muscle and the liver.

2. **Creatine kinase (CK):** Creatine kinase is an enzyme that transfers energy-rich phosphate groups between ATP and phosphocreatine. Phosphocreatine serves to store high-energy phosphates, which it donates to ADP when ATP is needed. Creatine kinase is a dimeric enzyme composed of two types of subunits—M (muscle) and B (brain)—which assemble to form the three isozymes CK-BB (CK1), CK-MB (CK2) and CK-MM (CK3). Normal levels of CK in blood range from 25 to 90 U/L, and different isozymes are found in different tissues.
- CK-BB (CK1) is prevalent in the brain, smooth muscle, and lungs.
- CK-MB (CK2) is predominantly found in cardiac muscle.
- CK-MM (CK3) is predominantly found in skeletal muscle.

Table 5.6 Enzymes and proteins used in diagnosing myocardial infarction (MI)

Enzyme/Protein	Time of increase	Peak of increase	Special notes
LDH-1	10–12 hours after MI	2–3 days after MI	Levels return to normal after 7–10 days
CK-MB	4–8 hours after MI	12–24 hours after MI	Levels return to normal after 3–4 days
Troponin (cTn-I)	4–6 hours after MI	12–24 hours after MI	Levels stay elevated for 3–10 days
AST/SGOT1	12–16 hours after MI	1–2 days after MI	Levels return to normal after 4–5 days

Abbreviations: AST, aspartate aminotransferase; CK-MB, creatine kinase muscle–brain; LDH, lactate dehydrogenase; SGOT, serum glutamate oxaloacetate transaminase.

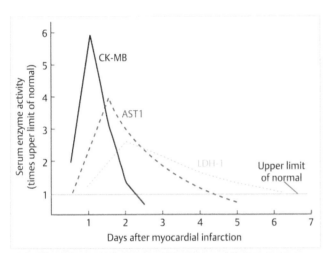

Fig. 5.10 Key enzyme activities after myocardial infarction. Serum activity of creatine kinase muscle-brain (CK-MB), aspartate aminotransferase 1 (AST1), and lactate dehydrogenase 1 (LDH1) after a myocardial infarction.

3. **Aspartate aminotransferase (AST):** This enzyme, also known as glutamate oxaloacetate transaminase (GOT), plays a role in amino acid metabolism; it catalyzes the reversible transfer of the α-amino group between aspartate and glutamate. It exists as two isozymes, which are found in different tissues and subcellular locations, as follows:
- AST1 (GOT1) is found in the cytosol of cardiac muscle and red blood cells.
- AST1 (GOT2) is found in the mitochondria of liver cells.

Therapeutics
Troponin in myocardial infarction
Troponin is a protein complex that plays a role in muscle contraction and relaxation triggered by elevated or depressed levels of intracellular Ca^{2+}, respectively. This trimeric protein complex is composed of three types of subunits—the tropomysin-binding subunit (Tn-T), the calcium-binding subunit (Tn-C), and the inhibitory subunit (Tn-I). Upon calcium binding, the protein changes its conformation. This change is transmitted to tropomysin, which then allows myosin to bind

to actin filaments, and hence muscle contraction occurs. The Tn-I subunit comes in three isoforms that are found in different tissues. For instance:
- cTn-I is found in cardiac muscle. Its serum levels increase after a myocardial infarction.
- sTn-I (of which there are two forms) is found in skeletal muscle.

Therapeutics
Enzymes useful for medical diagnoses
Enzymes normally found in various tissues and organs can be used as markers of damage when they are found in blood. These enzymes, although always present in blood at low levels, are elevated far above normal in pathological conditions. The following are examples of diseases and the enzymes whose serum levels are measured to determine a diagnosis:

Bone disease	Alkaline phosphatase
Obstructive liver disease	Sorbitol dehydrogenase Lactate dehydrogenase (LDH-5)
Prostatic cancer	Acid phosphatase
Acute pancreatitis	Amylase
Muscular dystrophy	Aldolase and aspartate aminotransferase (AST)
Liver disorder	Alanine aminotransferase (ALT) CK-MM isoform of creatine kinase

5.5.3 Proenzymes

A proenzyme (or zymogen) is the inactive precursor form of an enzyme. Cleavage of a specific peptide bond within the proenzyme generates the active mature enzyme. Examples of inactive proenzyme/active enzyme pairs are pepsinogen/pepsin, trypsinogen/trypsin, and chymotrypsinogen/chymotrypsin. The aforementioned active enzymes are proteolytic (i.e., they digest proteins). However, they originate from, and function in, different organs and environments, as follows:
- Pepsinogen is released by chief cells of the stomach, where the high acidic environment aids in its self-cleavage

(autocatalysis) into pepsin. Pepsin is only active in low pH (1.5 to 2.0) environments, such as that of the stomach.

• Trypsinogen is synthesized by the pancreas and released into the duodenum, where it is cleaved into active trypsin by enteropeptidase (enterokinase). Enteropeptidase is an

enzyme that is secreted by the mucosal cells that line the duodenum.

• Chymotrypsinogen is synthesized by the pancreas and released into the duodenum, where its conversion to active chymotrypsin is aided through cleavage by trypsin.

Review Questions: Nutrition and Biomolecules

1. The diagram below shows the free energy as a function of reaction progress. If a catalyst were introduced into this system, which parameter would change?

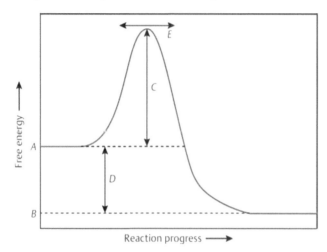

A) A
B) B
C) C
D) D
E) E

2. Vitamin D, either obtained through diet or produced endogenously must undergo a series of biological transformations before it becomes potent. Several organs are required to achieve this. The most potent vitamin D metabolite is 1,25-dihydroxycholecalciferol (calcitriol) and is synthesized in the
A) Intestinal mucosal cell
B) Skin
C) Liver
D) Kidney
E) Blood

3. Inorganic minerals, including sodium, chloride, potassium, magnesium, and zinc, serve as important electrolytes and enzymatic cofactors that maintain proper bodily function. Which of the following minerals is the major intracellular cation?
A) Magnesium
B) Zinc
C) Sodium
D) Potassium
E) Chloride

4. Serum calcium levels are usually normal despite suboptimal calcium absorption and vitamin D deficiency because serum calcium is being maintained by
A) Low parathyroid hormone (PTH) levels inhibiting calcium excretion
B) An increase in calcitonin
C) Increased bone resorption stimulated by PTH
D) Lack of 1,25-dihydroxy vitamin D, which prevents bone from taking calcium from blood
E) Calcitriol (1, 25-dihydroxylcholecalciferol), decreases intestinal calcium absorption

5. Iron is an essential trace metal required for proper oxygen transport, energy metabolism, cell proliferation, and host defense. It is a crucial component of many important biological proteins, including hemoglobin, myoglobin, the cytochromes, the P-450 enzymes, and the lysosomal enzyme myeloperoxidase. While it is absolutely essential for life, iron is also toxic. Which of the following best describes iron absorption?
A) The presence of reducing agents such as ascorbic acid decreases the bioavailability of iron.
B) Iron obtained from plant products is in the most efficiently absorbed form.
C) The low pH of the stomach favors production of Fe^{2+} and thus enhances absorption.
D) Simultaneous intake of fiber with iron enhances the efficiency of its absorption.
E) Ceruloplasmin is the major protein responsible for transporting iron from the intestine to the bloodstream.

6. In a Dutch family, three out of five siblings whose parents were fourth cousins were found to have osteoarthritis-like degenerative joint disease, prominent interphalangeal joints, midface prominence, a short, upturned nose, prominent supraorbital ridges, and protruding eyes. All three were deaf from birth. If you sequenced their *COL11A2* gene, which contains the sequence for one of the α chains of type XI collagen, what type of mutation are you likely to find?
A) A glycine → arginine missense mutation in the triple-helical region
B) A tryptophan → arginine missense mutation in the triple-helical region
C) A selenocysteine → arginine missense mutation in the triple-helical region
D) A nonsense mutation in an intron
E) Loss of a TATA box

7. A 56-year-old alcoholic man, who lives alone, is admitted to the hospital for evaluation of a leg wound that is not healing well. On physical examination, numerous ecchymoses are noted on the posterior aspect of his legs and thighs. Careful examination of the man's skin reveals minute hemorrhages around hair follicles and splinter hemorrhages in the nail beds. Laboratory examination is remarkable for a low hemoglobin level; no other hematologic abnormalities are noted. The biochemical defect underlying the above clinical condition is likely to be decreased activity of
A) lactase
B) methemoglobin reductase
C) γ-carboxylase
D) 1-α-hydroxylase
E) prolyl hydroxylase

8. A deficiency of which of the following elements is associated with teeth that have defects in the enamel, white mineral deposits, yellow-brown discoloration and pitting?
A) Chromium
B) Fluorine
C) Iodine
D) Selenium
E) Zinc

9. Chymotrypsin is a serine protease, with Ser-195, His-57, and Asp-102 forming the catalytic triad. In serine proteases, the ring nitrogen of histidine's side chain in the catalytic triad acts as a proton acceptor during the enzymatic reaction sequence. If the pH were lowered below the pK_a of the His-57 side chain, what would happen to the enzymatic activity?
A) The enzyme would be activated because His-57 needs to be protonated to be active.
B) The enzyme would be activated because His-57 needs to be deprotonated to be active.
C) The enzyme would be inactivated because His-57 needs to be protonated to be active.
D) The enzyme would be inactivated because His-57 needs to be deprotonated to be active.
E) There would be no effect because His-57 can fulfill its role in both the protonated and deprotonated state.

10. You went to the grocery store intending to pick up a snack for yourself and your roommate, but greed got the better of you, and you ate the whole thing. Feeling guilty, you read the package label (as shown below) to see how much trouble you will be in with your dietitian. Unfortunately, in your haste to open the package, you have torn through the part of the label that lists calories. Using other information from the label, how many calories did you consume?
A) 36
B) 66
C) 102
D) 82
E) 615

Serving size	2 ounces
Servings per package	3
Calories per serving	
Carbohydrates	20 g
Protein	5 g
Fat	11 g
Calcium	400 mg
Ascorbic acid	20 mg

11. Fluoride bulb, which contains a mixture of anticoagulant and sodium fluoride, is used for blood glucose estimation. Addition of this fluoride to the blood inhibits glucose utilization by which of the following mechanisms?
A) It inhibits phosphofructokinase and hence glycolysis.
B) It inhibits enolase and hence glycolysis.
C) It binds calcium and hence inhibits blood clotting.
D) It acts as a buffer to keep the blood pH in the normal range.
E) It inhibits tricarboxylic acid cycle in the erythrocytes during storage.

12. The following diagram shows an enzyme-catalyzed reaction. Which among the following statements best describes this reaction?

A) It is catalyzed by an oxidoreductase.
B) It involves only a transfer of functional group.
C) It requires water for the removal of functional groups.
D) It requires water to form a double bond.
E) It involves the transfer of a functional group within the molecules.

13. Trypsinogen is synthesized and released into the duodenum where it is cleaved to form active trypsin by enteropeptidase (enterokinase). Trypsin has pH-optimum near 8 corresponding to the environment found in the intestine. A mutation in the trypsinogen gene that increases its rate of self-cleavage will most likely result in a defect in
A) Stomach
B) Pancreas
C) Peripheral joints
D) Prostrate
E) Cardiac muscle

14. You prescribe omeprazole to a patient with ulcus ventriculi. Because omeprazole inhibits the gastric proton pump, H^+/K^+-ATPase, it will indirectly decrease the activity of which of the following digestive proteases?
A) Pepsin
B) Trypsin
C) Chymotrypsin
D) Carboxypeptidase A
E) Alanine-aminopeptidase

15. A 55-year-old man works on a farm. He is accidentally exposed to organophosphate pesticides and presents to the clinic with headache, nausea and dizziness, vomiting, excessive sweating and tightness of chest. Further enzyme kinetic studies reveal that organophosphates are a noncompetitive inhibitor of enzyme acetylcholine esterase in the body. What is the effect of this inhibitor on K_m and V_{max} of the enzyme?
    A) Low V_{max} and a near normal K_m.
    B) Altered V_{max} and K_m.
    C) Near normal V_{max} and high K_m.
    D) Low V_{max} and low K_m.
    E) Near normal V_{max} and K_m.

16. The enzyme succinate dehydrogenase converts the metabolic intermediate succinate (–OOC – CH2 – CH2 – COO-) to fumarate (–OOC – CH = CH – COO-). Based on their molecular structure, a compound (–OOC – CH2 – COO-) is most likely to act as an inhibitor of succinate dehydrogenase and the effects of the inhibitor can be offset by higher substrate concentrations. The type of inhibition is
    A) Allosteric
    B) Competitive
    C) Noncompetitive
    D) Irreversible
    E) Uncompetitive

17. There are 20 proteinogenic amino acids, 10 of which are considered essential. Which one of the following groups consists entirely of amino acids that need to be supplemented in the diet of an individual with negative nitrogen balance?
    A) Valine, isoleucine, tyrosine, arginine
    B) Leucine, methionine, isoleucine, alanine
    C) Glutamic acid, arginine, cysteine, tryptophan
    D) Valine, isoleucine, tyrosine, lysine
    E) Lysine, tryptophan, phenylalanine, threonine

18. Roughly 70% of the body's total energy expenditure is due to regulation of basal physiological processes, including those found in the liver, brain, heart, and kidneys, among others. Most of this energy is consumed by maintaining fluid homeostasis, with only ~10% consumed for mechanical work (e.g., breathing, cardiac activity, digestion). Which of the following statements about the basal metabolic rate (BMR) is correct?
    A) It is higher in people with hyperthyroidism.
    B) It is often expressed as a function of the amount of food consumed.
    C) It is lower in children than in adults.
    D) It cannot be calculated from the rate of oxygen consumption.
    E) It cannot be altered by administration of exogenous hormones.

19. In hyperventilation syndrome, patients have the feeling that they do not get enough air. As a result, they breathe faster. This leads to chest pain, paresthesia (prickling or burning sensation in skin), and panic attacks. Regarding blood pH, such patients will have
    A) metabolic acidosis with respiratory compensation
    B) metabolic alkalosis with respiratory compensation

C) respiratory acidosis with metabolic compensation
D) respiratory acidosis without metabolic compensation
E) respiratory alkalosis without metabolic compensation

20. Which of the following effects is produced in sickle hemoglobin (HbS) upon unloading of oxygen?
    A) Movement of heme iron into the plane of the heme ring system
    B) A cooperative effect that is different from that of "normal" hemoglobin
    C) An increase in the probability of aggregation
    D) A decrease in polymerization
    E) Release of protons

21. Increase in the concentration of which of the following in the blood will favor oxygen delivery in the peripheral tissues?
    A) pO_2
    B) pH
    C) HbF
    D) H^+
    E) CO

22. The structure of soluble proteins is held together by hydrophobic interactions between amino acids in the core, whereas hydrophilic amino acids on the surface allow interactions with the environment. Which of the following amino acids would you expect to find in the core of a protein?
    A) Lysine
    B) Arginine
    C) Glutamate
    D) Leucine
    E) Aspartate

23. Which among the following would you expect to be in negative nitrogen balance?
    A) A 25-year-old male following a balanced diet
    B) A 29-year-old pregnant female with no known illness
    C) A 25-year-old athlete
    D) A refugee in a camp after a famine
    E) A 35-year-old coach in a school

24. Which of the following enzymes would need Cu^{2+} as a cofactor?
    A) Carbonic anhydrase
    B) ATPases
    C) Metalloproteases
    D) Lysyl oxidase
    E) Cytochrome P450

25. Gangliosides are primarily found highly concentrated in ganglion cells of the central nervous system. Which of the following will be absent from gangliosides extracted from ganglion cells?
    A) Neuraminic acid
    B) Galactose
    C) Fatty acid
    D) Sphingosine
    E) Phosphate

26. The primary function of digestion is the hydrolysis of starch, protein, and fats from the diet into readily absorbable units.

This is accomplished by a well-orchestrated gastrointestinal system, including the mouth, stomach, and small and large intestines, as well as accessory organs such as the liver, pancreas, and gallbladder. Which of the following represents the major site of absorption and the type of carbohydrate?

A) the mouth; Disaccharides
B) the stomach; Polysaccharides
C) the small intestine; Monosaccharides
D) the large intestine; Disaccharides
E) the pancreas; Monosaccharides

27. Coenzymes are small organic molecules that are often required to assist catalysis by enzymes. Each coenzyme helps catalyze a specific type of reaction for a given class of substrates. The coenzyme involved in the biochemical transfer of methyl, formyl, or hydroxymethyl groups from one molecule to another is a derivative of

A) biotin
B) pyridoxine
C) lipoic acid
D) folic acid
E) ascorbic acid

28. The phosphate ion (PO_4^{3-}) is an anion that constitutes ~ 1% of the body's mass. It can be found in the body as a free phosphate ion or as part of many different phosphate esters. Which of the following is a function or role of phosphate?

A) A constituent of bone
B) A part of some heme proteins
C) A component of blood clotting cascade
D) A cofactor for antioxidant enzyme
E) A part of the structure of adenosine

29. A 55-year-old man with congestive heart failure is treated with furosemide (a diuretic). The patient complains about muscle weakness. You would add which of the following drugs to his regimen?

A) Amiloride (a potassium-sparing diuretic)
B) Caffeine (a diuretic)
C) Hydrochlorothiazide (a diuretic)
D) Mannitol (a diuretic)
E) Methazolamide (a carbonic anhydrase inhibitor)

30. Gallstones are formed within the gallbladder from the buildup of bile components such as cholesterol, calcium salts, bilirubin, and other bile pigments. A person with a gallstone blocking the bile duct is at some risk of developing

A) scurvy
B) night blindness
C) pellagra
D) Wernicke disease
E) ariboflavinosis

31. Fructose is a ketose sugar. Which one of the following is an endogenous source of fructose in the body?

A) Table sugar
B) Honey
C) Milk
D) Sorbitol
E) Fiber

32. The apparent K_m of an enzyme for its substrate is increased by which of the following?

A) Competitive inhibitor
B) Uncompetitive inhibitor
C) Noncompetitive inhibitor
D) Suicide inhibitor

33. Deficiency of which of the following nutrients produces dermatitis, diarrhea, dementia, and if untreated, death?

A) Ascorbic acid
B) Niacin
C) Thiamine
D) Cobalamin
E) Folic acid

34. Which of the following statements concerning dietary fiber is correct?

A) Fiber binds to certain substances, such as bile acids, and increases their absorption.
B) Fiber decreases stool bulk.
C) Fiber promotes absorption of certain nutrients, such as iron.
D) Fiber decreases the transit time of intestinal contents.
E) Fiber increases the rate of carbohydrate absorption.

35. Excessive intake of which mineral may trigger hypertension in sensitive people?

A) Magnesium
B) Molybdenum
C) Fluoride
D) Zinc
E) Sodium

36. A 45-year-old woman comes to the emergency room with severe right-upper-quadrant abdominal pain. History: Her stool has been light colored and claylike for a few days, and her urine has been unusually dark. There was some pain during that time, but it became much stronger 2 hours ago. $G_3 P_{2+1+0+3}$ (i.e., 3 pregnancies, 1 term infant, 0 abortions, 3 living children), intrauterine device for 3 years, one pack of cigarettes per day for 25 years, little alcohol, no street drugs. Physical examination: overweight, body temperature 37.3 °C (normal), blood pressure 130/80 mm Hg (prehypertensive), pulse 96/min, respiration 20/min (normal), sclerae icteric (yellow sclera) and a positive Murphy sign highlighting pain in the upper right abdomen, indicative of obstructive jaundice due to gallstones. The uptake of which of the following vitamins will be reduced in this patient?

A) Retinal
B) Thiamine
C) Ascorbate
D) Biotin
E) Folate

37. A 6-year-old boy is found to be at the 10th percentile of height during a routine school entry medical exam. His skin is rough, and his nails are spoon shaped. His parents are of Middle Eastern origin, and unleavened bread is a staple food in their family. The child says that he has lost appetite because food no longer tastes and smells appetizing. His parents add that they have noticed that their child

occasionally eats soil, and he has suffered frequently from upper respiratory tract infections. Further examination reveals night blindness, patchy hair loss, and an ataxic gait. This child should be supplemented with which of the following minerals?
A) Iron
B) Zinc
C) Copper
D) Selenium
E) Iodine

38. A 60-year-old man comes to a family physician because of wheezing and cough. History: two packs of cigarettes per day since the age of 16, two glasses of beer per day, nutrition high in saturated fat, low in fresh fruits and vegetables. Patient works as a driver and his physical activity is limited by shortness of breath. Physical exam: BP 142/93 mm Hg (normal is 120/80 mm Hg), absent pedal pulses and gallop rhythm indicate cardiovascular disease. Fine crackles in lower lung fields and reduced lung function not improved by inhaled bronchodilator. How will the patient's condition affect erythrocyte 2,3-bisphosphoglycerate (2,3-BPG) concentration and the structure of hemoglobin (Hb) molecules?[1]
A) Hypoxemia will lead to an increase in 2,3-BPG, shifting the Hb to the T-state.
B) Hypoxemia will lead to an increase in 2,3-BPG, shifting the Hb to the R-state.
C) Hypoxemia will lead to a decrease in 2,3-BPG, shifting the Hb to the T-state.
D) Hypoxemia will lead to a decrease in 2,3-BPG, shifting the Hb to the R-state.

39. Two siblings, a male now 23 years old and a female now 14 years old, were noted in early infancy with failure to thrive, vomiting, and progressive neurologic dysfunction. They were born to first-cousin Algerian parents after normal pregnancy and vaginal delivery at term. They have two normal brothers, but a third brother died from unknown causes as a neonate. By age 2 they had developed cataracts, and at age 12 they could no longer walk. Both have an IQ around 50 (average is 90 to 109), hyperelastic skin, lax joints, and hypotonia. Laboratory: Hyperammonemia, low serum levels of ornithine, citrulline, arginine, and proline. Both were found homozygous for an R84Q mutation in Δ[1]-pyrroline-5-carboxylate synthase (P5CS, an enzyme involved in the synthesis of proline). The skin and joint problems in these patients are most likely caused by their inability to produce a protein with
A) a triple helix
B) α-helix
C) antiparallel β-strands
D) mostly random coil regions
E) the lack of any stable conformation

40. P.S., a 24-year-old man, is a patient of yours. Five years ago, he had jaundice, which cleared after a couple of weeks. Since then he has had increasing difficulties walking, getting up, or raising his arms, combined with worsening pain in the legs. Analgesics are ineffective; he is now

bedridden. There is no muscle weakness. X-ray shows general demineralization of bones, which somewhat improved with vitamin D and Ca^{2+}. Laboratory: hemoglobin, white blood cell, cholesterol, blood urea nitrogen, bilirubin, and alkaline phosphatase were all normal; alanine aminotransferase (ALT) and aspartate aminotransferase (AST) elevated; ceruloplasmin low. Twenty-four-hour urine excretion of Ca^{2+} and HPO$^{2-}_4$ is elevated. Patient refused a transcutaneous liver biopsy. Slit lamp exam shows Kayser-Fleischer rings in both eyes, and the patient is diagnosed with Wilson disease. This patient should be treated with
A) Cu supplementation
B) Zn supplementation
C) Penicillamine (Cu chelation therapy)
D) Deferoxamine (Tx for iron poisoning)
E) Multivitamin

41. An 18-year-old male patient comes to you for nutritional advice. His intake of vitamin A is on average 950 µg/d. The DRI of vitamin A for his age group is EAR 625 µg/d, RDA 900 µg/d, and UL 2,800 µg /d. He will suffer from vitamin A
A) poisoning with a probability of ~ 50%
B) poisoning with a probability of ~ 98%
C) deficiency with a probability of ~ 98%
D) deficiency with a probability of ~ 50%
E) deficiency with a probability of ~ 2%

42. A.B., a 56-year-old man, had an acute myocardial infarct (AMI) 30 hours ago, for which he had been treated in your hospital. He was recovering in the intensive care unit when he suddenly started to complain about chest pain again. Which of the following enzymes would be most suitable to determine whether he had a second infarct?
A) Cardiac troponin inhibitory subunit (cTn-I)
B) Cardiac troponin tropomyosin binding subunit (cTn-T)
C) Total creatine kinase (CK)
D) Myoglobin
E) Lactate dehydrogenase

43. James Gillray, the grandfather of all political cartoonists, created an illustration of an inflamed and swollen joint of the big toe into which a fire-breathing demon digs its fangs and talons. This piece of art, called The Gout, depicted the severe pain associated with a condition of the same name. Gout can be diagnosed by the presence of which of the following in the aspirated synovial fluid examined by the polarized microscopy?
A) Cystine
B) Calcium oxalate
C) Cholesterol
D) Starch
E) Mono Sodium Urate

44. A 17-year-old male patient presented to the emergency room in July after an episode of syncope (loss of consciousness) lasting several seconds. He had a previous history of 2 months of fatigue, muscle cramping, and spasms after manual labor outdoors in hot weather. This had also occurred the previous summer. There was no fever, vomiting, diarrhea, constipation, asthma, or cough. Physical exam: Patient alert but fatigued, BP 94/60 mm Hg (normal

is 120/80 mm Hg), pulse 80/min, respiration 15/min (normal), temperature 37 °C, height 183 cm (6 ft), weight 96 kg (211.6 lb). Laboratory: blood pH 7.56 (normal is 7.35 to 7.45), serum K^+ 2.2 mEq/L (normal is 3.5 to 5.0 mEq/L), Cl^- 75 mEq/L (normal is 95 to 105 mEq/L), P CO_2 6.16 kPa (normal is 4.4 to 5.9 kPa), HCO_3- 39.6 mEq/L (normal is 22 to 28 mEq/L), BUN 56 mg/dL (normal is 7 to 18 mg/dL), creatinine 2.3 mg/dL (normal is 0.6 to 1.2 mg/dL), uric acid 12.2 mg/dL (normal is 3.0 to 8.2 mg/dL). Fractional excretion of Na^+, Cl^-, and K^+ were 0.2, 0.2, and 29.2%, respectively. The patient was hospitalized for 3 days and received oral fluids and potassium, which improved his azotemia (high blood levels of nitrogen-containing compounds), but total CO_2 in serum remained high and serum K^+ low. Genetic analysis revealed that he was compound heterozygous for the ΔF508 and R117 H mutations of cystic fibrosis transmembrane conductance regulator protein (CFTR). This patient is in

A) metabolic acidosis with respiratory compensation
B) metabolic alkalosis with respiratory compensation
C) respiratory acidosis with metabolic compensation
D) respiratory acidosis without metabolic compensation
E) respiratory alkalosis without metabolic compensation

45. A 40-year-old male is brought to the emergency room (ER) in a confused state after falling from a bar stool. His movements are uncoordinated, and he has no memory of the evening. The patient's friends state that his nutrition is mostly of the alcoholic kind. Upon investigation, the patient has edema and tachycardia and is emaciated and cyanotic. He vomits several times during his stay in the ER. Laboratory: Low oxygen saturation of blood, high serum pyruvate. The patient requires immediate supplementation with

A) retinal
B) thiamine
C) cobalamin
D) ascorbate
E) menaquinone

46. A 20-year-old woman meets with her gynecologist after not having a period for 5 months. A pregnancy test comes back positive. Her history revealed that she works out regularly, eats a healthy diet, and only takes medication to control her acne. Ultrasound reveals a ~ 22-week-old fetus with heart defects and a cleft palate. Upon questioning, she denies any family history of cleft palates and informs the doctor that she has been controlling her acne by taking the contraceptive Seasonique (Duramed Pharmaceuticals, Cincinnati, OH), which had reduced her periods to four times per year, topical antibiotics, and oral isotretinoin. She added that she was obtaining these medications from a friend with insurance, for whom the medications were prescribed. The patient was not covered and had not seen a physician for over a year. What is the most likely cause of the anatomical defects observed on the fetus?

A) Use of oral contraceptives
B) Inadequate intake of ascorbic acid
C) Use of topical antibiotics
D) Spontaneous genetic abnormality
E) Use of oral isotretinoin

47. A 10-month-old-male infant was brought to your clinic for genetic and metabolic workup. He was born as the first child to nonconsanguineous parents after a 9-month gestation by vaginal delivery. Initially he appeared healthy. However, from 4 months of age his development slowed, even regressed, and his health deteriorated. None of the treatments his local pediatrician tried seemed to have much beneficial effect. Physical exam: dermatitis, alopecia, low blood pressure, loss of hearing. Parents report occasional seizures. Laboratory: metabolites of leucine and isoleucine, such as 3-OH isovaleric acid, β-methylcrotonylglycine, and 3-OH propionic acid, were elevated in urine. However, in fibroblast cultures, propionyl CoA carboxylase, β-methylcrotonyl CoA carboxylase, and pyruvate carboxylase activities were normal. The child is suffering from biotinidase deficiency and should be treated with high dose of biotin. The metabolite of isoleucine which is elevated in the urine is propionic acid.
Which other amino acid pair also metabolizes to propionic acid in the body?

A) Valine and methionine
B) Valine and leucine
C) Valine and phenylalanine
D) Phenylalanine and tyrosine
E) Glycine and phenylalanine

48. A 24-year-old patient was diving and blacked out when he rose to the water's surface. His instructor believes he did not hyperventilate before diving. Hyperventilating before diving brings down blood CO_2 concentration and thereby reduces the urge to breathe. How will the reduced CO_2 concentration affect oxygen delivery to the tissues?

A) Oxygen delivery is decreased because of a reduced Bohr effect.
B) Oxygen delivery is decreased because of an increased Bohr effect.
C) Oxygen delivery is increased because of a reduced Bohr effect.
D) Oxygen delivery is increased because of an increased Bohr effect.

49. A 45-year-old Mexican American man was sent to a family physician by his wife because he had to visit the restroom several times per night, which interfered with her sleep. Family history: Father died of acute myocardial infarction (AMI) at age 55, and a paternal aunt died from stroke. Physical examination reveals height 1.73 m (5 ft, 8 in), weight 89 kg (195.8 lb), waist and hip circumference 107 (42.1 in) and 102 cm (40.2 in), respectively; pulse 90/min, BP 140/90 mm Hg (hypertensive), urine glucose 1 +. An appointment is made for phlebotomy; the results (mg/dL) are fasting glucose 140 (normal is 70 to 110 mg/dL), total cholesterol 220 (normal is < 200 mg/dL), HDL (high-density lipoproteins) 35 (low, therefore risk for heart disease is high), LDL (low-density lipoproteins) 140 (elevated, therefore risk of developing heart disease is high), triglycerides 180 (elevated, therefore the risk of developing heart disease is also elevated). Over the next 15 years, the patient returns repeatedly, complaining about numbness of feet, poor wound healing, impotency,

and renal failure. However, he does not take medicines regularly, and his weight increases steadily to 120 kg (264 lb). Finally, he dies suddenly in his home and is found 2 days later by his wife and son upon return from a family visit. During the autopsy, tissue samples are taken from several organs and processed for histology. The pancreas, stained with Congo red and observed under polarized light, shows birefringence caused by Congo red staining of

A) amylin

B) apolipoprotein AI

C) immunoglobulin light chain

D) lysozyme

E) crystallin α

50. A 17-year-old male patient came to the emergency room of a local hospital with complaints of bilateral flank pain, hematuria, and bleeding from the nasal and oral mucosa. He admitted being in an altercation. Since it was difficult to stop his bleeding, laboratory investigations were instigated that showed prolonged prothrombin and activated partial thromboplastin times and elevated levels of PIVKA-II antigen (uncarboxylated factor II). His parents, searching his bedroom, found marijuana, hallucinogenic mushrooms, a large tube of glue, empty bottles of several prescription drugs, hypodermic needles, alcoholic beverages, and a three-fourths empty bottle of d-CON (a rodenticide containing brodifacoum, a second-generation super-warfarin). Upon questioning, the patient admitted habitually lacing his marijuana with d-CON before smoking it, a practice he had picked up from friends at a party. The patient needs treatment with

A) retinoids

B) cholecalciferol

C) phylloquinone

D) tocopherol

E) ascorbic acid

51. A patient consuming corn as a staple diet, presents to the clinic with diarrhea. On examination, he appears to be pale and has light sensitive dermatitis. Further examination reveals sores in the oral cavity and glossitis. His tongue appears red and swollen. Because of the painful sores in his mouth, he prefers liquid food. His behavior appears aggressive and unpredictable. This patient will respond to treatment with:

A) thiamine

B) ascorbate

C) niacin

D) folate

E) cobalamin

52. An irritable 10-month-old infant is brought to the hospital by her parents because they suspect that a caregiver may have handled the child too roughly. Upon examination, the physician determines that the "bruises" observed by the parents are signs of petechiae and ecchymoses. Further examination reveals bleeding gums and bilateral lower limb tenderness. As suspected, laboratory tests come back indicating severely low serum levels of a water-soluble

vitamin. Why does a deficiency in this vitamin cause the aforementioned symptoms?

A) The deficient vitamin is needed for the function of γ-carboxylase.

B) The deficient vitamin is needed for the function of prolyl hydroxylase.

C) The deficient vitamin is needed for the function of serine hydroxymethyltransferase.

D) The deficient vitamin is needed for the function of lysyl oxidase.

E) The deficient vitamin is needed for the function of glycogen phosphorylase.

53. In 1860 the explorers Burke, Gray, King, and Wills started on an expedition to cross Australia for the first time in a south–north direction (Melbourne to the Gulf of Carpentaria). On their return journey they ran short of food and had to supplement their diet with local freshwater mussels (*Velesunio ambiguous* Philippi,) and sporocarps of an aquatic fern known as nardoo (*Marsilea drummondii* A. Braun). After a few weeks on this diet they fell ill, suffering from a weakness that made it difficult and painful to get up or walk, tachycardia, confusion, convulsions, vomiting, and emaciation. Gray, Burke, and Wills died; the only survivor, King, never recovered from peripheral neuropathy. Like many mussels and sea food, *Velesunio ambiguus* contains thiaminase, which destroys the vitamin B_1 (thiamine) in the diet. The explorers were suffering from which hypovitaminosis?

A) Beriberi

B) Pellagra

C) Scurvy

D) Rickets

E) Pernicious anemia

54. A 55-year-old man was admitted to the hospital for severe flaccid weakness of proximal muscles on all limbs. History: Treatment of hypertension started 2 weeks earlier with prescription of amlodipine (Ca channel blocker), benzylhydrochlorothiazide (diuretic), and valsartan (angiotensin receptor blocker), and a 4-year history of recurrent limb muscle weakness attributed to transient ischemic attacks. Current condition started after heavy alcohol consumption. Physical examination: blood pressure 138/68 mm Hg (prehypertensive), pulse 68 bpm. Laboratory: K^+ 1.4 mEq/L (normal range is 3.5 to 5.0 mEq/L), creatine kinase 15,000 U/L (normal range is 25 to 90 U/L), indicating rhabdomyolysis, blood pH 7.54 (normal range is 7.35 to 7.45), HCO_3^- 38 mM (normal range is 22 to 28 mM). The diuretic was discontinued, and potassium substitution initiated. His symptoms resolved within 2 weeks, and creatine kinase returned to normal, but hypokalemia persisted with high potassium excretion in urine. Hyperaldasteronism was indicated by an aldosterone:renin activity ratio (ARR) that was almost 10 times higher than the maximum normal value of 30. Your diagnosis would be[2]

A) Conn syndrome

B) Cushing syndrome

C) Addison disease

D) Liddle syndrome

E) Congenital adrenal hyperplasia

55. Lipids are the primary constituents of cellular membranes. They can be oxidatively damaged when free radicals are allowed to persist within the membrane, especially lipids containing polyunsaturated fatty acids. Such damage can lead to the loss of membrane integrity and the formation of mutagenic or carcinogenic moieties. Many vitamins can act as antioxidants; however, not all are protective against membrane damage. Which of the following functions primarily as an antioxidant to prevent polyunsaturated fatty acids from undergoing peroxidation?
   A) Vitamin A
   B) Vitamin D
   C) Vitamin E
   D) Vitamin K

56. A medical student was on a weight loss regimen and successfully lost 2 lb in 1 week through changes in diet and exercise. Which statement below could explain her success?
   A) Her caloric intake exceeded that of her total energy expenditure over that 1-week period.
   B) Her total energy expenditure exceeded that of her total caloric intake by 3,500 kcal.
   C) There was an increase in her physical activity level (PAL) and a decrease in her basal metabolic rate (BMR) due to these lifestyle changes.
   D) Her total energy expenditure exceeded that of her total caloric intake by 7,000 kcal.
   E) There was a decrease in her PAL and an increase in her BMR due to these lifestyle changes.

57. Iron is the most abundant microelement found in the body; its transport and storage are highly regulated. It is stored in the liver, spleen, and bone marrow and in the cells that line the intestine. There are two ionic iron species found in the body, ferrous iron (Fe^{2+}) and ferric iron (Fe^{3+}). Which of the following proteins is involved in the transport of ferric ions?
   A) Ferritin
   B) Lactoferrin
   C) Ceruloplasmin
   D) Transferrin
   E) Hemosiderin

58. Pantothenic acid is used as a component of
   A) pyruvate carboxylase.
   B) acyl coenzyme A (acyl CoA) dehydrogenase.
   C) malate dehydrogenase.
   D) fatty acid synthase.
   E) complex III.

59. Although several hundred amino acids have been characterized in nature, only 20 of them are coded for by DNA and therefore end up in peptides and proteins. Additionally, amino acids serve as precursors for the production of important biomolecules. There are 10 essential amino acids, so described because
   A) they do not serve as substrates for aminotransferases (transaminases).
   B) their carbon chains cannot be synthesized by the body.
   C) they are found only in animal protein.

   D) they are important intermediates in metabolic pathways.
   E) their carbon chains cannot be completely degraded by the body.

60. Hemoglobin is an iron-containing tetrameric protein found in erythrocytes, with each of its four subunits containing a nonprotein heme group. Each heme group is able to bind a single molecule of oxygen. The binding of O_2 is part of normal physiology; however, the binding of CO or CN^- can lead to death. The major reason that carbon monoxide poisoning is fatal is because
   A) the oxygen-binding capacity of hemoglobin is reduced.
   B) less 2,3-bisphosphoglycerate (BPG) can be bound.
   C) iron in hemoglobin is oxidized to the ferric state.
   D) oxygen affinity is decreased.
   E) oxygen affinity is increased.

61. The kinetics of most Michaelis-Menten enzyme reactions can be described in terms of K_m or V_{max}. Which of the following best describes K_m?
   A) The concentration of an inhibitor required to produce 50% inhibition
   B) The velocity of the reaction at saturating levels of substrate
   C) The half maximal velocity
   D) The concentration of a substrate at half maximal velocity
   E) The concentration of the enzyme at which half of all substrate molecules are enzyme bound.

62. Eicosanoids are short-lived signaling molecules that may be derived from arachidonic acid. The latter can be obtained upon excision and release from membrane lipids by
   A) Desmolase
   B) Phospholipase C
   C) Lipoxygenase
   D) Cyclooxygenase
   E) Phospholipase A_2

63. You are working on a research project to elucidate the reaction mechanism of an enzyme. You think that a particular serine (Ser) residue in the protein is required for catalytic activity. To test this hypothesis, you want to genetically replace this Ser by another amino acid, and then test whether the enzyme is still active. Which amino acid would you choose to replace the Ser?
   A) Threonine (Thr)
   B) Alanine (Ala)
   C) Tryptophan (Trp)
   D) Glutamic acid (Glu)
   E) Histidine (His)

64. The rod-shaped bacterium, *Helicobacter pylori*, frequently infects the stomach and is the common etiological agent of antral gastritis (antral inflammation), gastric ulcers, duodenal ulcers and stomach cancer. Patients with *H. pylori*-associated antral gastritis have increased basal and meal-stimulated serum gastrin concentrations (hypergastrinemia) as well as hypersecretion of acid. A treatment regimen of bismuth subsalicylate, metronidazole, and tetracycline four times a day for 14 days has been

shown to resolve gastritis and eliminate *H. pylori* in some patients. What system does the body have in place to counter the effects of *H. pylori* on the G cells of the antral mucosa?
A) The release of acid by parietal cells of the gastric mucosa.
B) The release of pepsinogen by chief cells of the stomach.
C) The release of somatostatin by D cells of the antral mucosa.
D) The release of cholecystokinin by the I-cells of the duodenum.
E) The release of trypsinogen by the cells of the pancreas.

65. Vitamins play many roles in normal metabolism and are often found as coenzymes in metabolic enzymes. Which of the following vitamins regulates key processes such as inhibition of cell proliferation, differentiation, apoptosis, shaping of the embryo, and organogenesis and has the mechanism of intracellular signaling?
A) Thiamine
B) Riboflavin
C) Ascorbic acid
D) Retinoic acid
E) Niacin

66. Sialic acid is
A) found only in mammalian tissues.
B) the major carbohydrate found in heparin.
C) a normal constituent of gangliosides and glycoproteins.
D) an ε-carboxyl amino acid.
E) a cofactor for sialidase.

67. Which one of the following sugars is found exclusively in glycosaminoglycans?
A) *N*-Acetylglucosamine
B) *N*-Acetylgalactosamine
C) Sialic acid
D) L-Iduronic acid
E) L-Arabinose

68. Proteins emerge as a random coil following translation of a sequence of mRNA by the ribosome and must then fold properly. Which of the following determines all levels of protein structure?
A) Primary structure
B) Secondary structure
C) Tertiary structure
D) Quaternary structure
E) Domain

69. Methotrexate is a folate analogue that binds to the active site of dihydrofolate reductase and inhibits it. How will increasing concentrations of methotrexate affect the V_{max} and apparent K_m of the enzyme?
A) V_{max} will be decreased and K_m increased.
B) V_{max} will be decreased and K_m decreased.
C) V_{max} will be decreased, and K_m will stay constant.
D) V_{max} will stay constant, and K_m will increase.
E) V_{max} will stay constant, and K_m will decrease.

70. The enzyme phosphoglucose isomerase catalyzes the reaction glucose 6-phosphate → fructose 6-phosphate, $\Delta G^{0\prime}$= -0.43 kcal/mol. For this reaction to proceed in the physiological direction (toward fructose 6-phosphate), one has to
A) remove Glu-6 P in a second reaction.
B) remove Fru-6 P in a second reaction.
C) do nothing, as reactions proceed toward positive ΔG.
D) increase the Fru-6 P concentration.
E) increase the enzyme concentration.

71. Enteropeptidase deficiency is a rare autosomal recessive disorder (observed in six families described worldwide) that is life-threatening in infants, but patients improve spontaneously once they get older. Which of the following enzymes can still be converted into active form in infant patients with enteropeptidase deficiency?
A) Pepsinogen
B) Trypsinogen
C) Chymotrypsinogen
D) Procarboxypeptidase
E) Proelastase

72. The turnover number (k_{cat}) is the general rate constant of an enzyme-catalyzed reaction at saturation. It reflects the number of substrate molecules that are converted into product on a single catalytic site (saturated with substrate), in a given amount of time. If you are peacefully digesting a hefty meal, most of the glucose arriving at your liver will be phosphorylated within the cells to be directly proportional to glucose concentrations in the blood by
A) hexokinase, because this enzyme has a very high affinity for glucose.
B) hexokinase, because this enzyme has a low k_{cat}.
C) glucokinase, because this enzyme has a very high affinity for glucose.
D) glucokinase, because this enzyme has a high k_{cat}.
E) glucokinase, because this enzyme has a high i_m.

73. The graph below shows the velocity of an enzymatic reaction as a function of the substrate concentration. The K_m is marked in green. The V_{max} of this reaction is

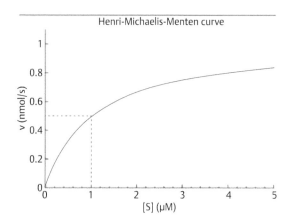

A) 0.5 nmol/s.
B) 0.75 nmol/s.
C) 1.0 nmol/s.
D) 1.25 nmol/s.
E) 1.5 nmol/s.

74. If an enzyme is turning over at 75% of its maximal velocity at a substrate concentration of 1.0 mM, the K_m is
A) 0.25 mM.
B) 0.33 mM.
C) 0.50 mM.
D) 0.75 mM.
E) 1.00 mM.

75. The free energy of the reaction $H_2SO_4 + NaCl \rightarrow 2\ HCl$ (g) $+ NaHSO_4$ is $\Delta G°' = -1.04$ kcal/mol. Under standard conditions, this reaction is
A) exergonic
B) endergonic
C) nonspontaneous
D) proceeds toward the left
E) at equilibrium

76. Protein structure can be described on four levels: primary, secondary, tertiary, and quaternary. Correct functioning of a protein relies on the proper conformation in all four levels. Which of the following causes an alpha helix to beta pleated sheet conformation change, leading to aggregates?
A) Denaturation
B) Ubiquitination
C) Posttranslational modification
D) Side-chain phosphorylation
E) Reorganization of hydrogen bonds

77. The image below is the Lineweaver-Burk plot of the interaction of a new pharmaceutical inhibitor, an enzyme, and its substrate. Inhibitor concentrations are indicated in the legend.
The inhibitor binds

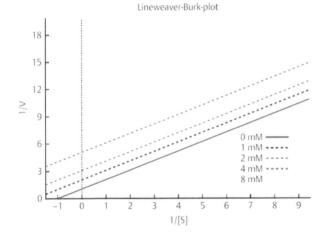

A) the free enzyme only.
B) the enzyme–substrate complex only.
C) both the free enzyme and the enzyme–substrate complex.
D) neither the enzyme nor the enzyme–substrate complex.

78. Hemoglobin is a heme protein whose polypeptide chains are folded into stretches of alpha helix. Which among the following statements is true about this protein?
A) The alpha-helix found in hemoglobin is an example of protein tertiary structure.

B) The primary structures of hemoglobin are stabilized by H-bonding.
C) The secondary structure of hemoglobin is stabilized by disulfide bonds.
D) Hemoglobin has no quaternary structure because it is a monomeric protein.
E) Cooperative binding allows hemoglobin to deliver more oxygen to the tissues.

79. An excerpt from the first clinical trial in history published in 1753 titled "A Treatise" by a ship's doctor, James A. Lind:
On the 20th of May 1747, I took 12 patients on-board the *Salisbury* at sea. Their cases were familiar as I could have them. They all in general had putrid gums, the spots of lassitude, with weakness of their knees ... and had one diet common to all, viz., water-gruel sweetened with sugar in the morning; fresh mutton-broth often times for dinner; at other times puddings, boiled biscuit with sugar, etc; and for supper, barley and raisins, rice and currants, sago and wine, or the like.
Two of these ... had each two oranges and one lemon given them every day. ... They continued but 6 days under this course, having consumed the quantity that could be spared. The consequence was, that the most sudden and visible good effects were perceived ...; one of those who had taken them, being at the end of 6 days fit for duty. ... The other was the best recovered of any in his condition; and being now deemed pretty well, was appointed nurse to the rest of the sick.
The patients were lacking which of the following?
A) Retinol
B) Niacin
C) Ascorbate
D) Cholecalciferol
E) Iodine

80. γ-Carboxyglutamate is most commonly found in proteins of the coagulation cascade and provides a binding site for calcium ions. This posttranslational modification of glutamic acid requires the use of which of the following vitamin as a cofactor?
A) Vitamin A
B) Vitamin D
C) Vitamin E
D) Vitamin K
E) Vitamin C

81. The folding of a protein is generally coincident with its biosynthesis and is a reflection of the specific amino acid sequence it contains (primary structure). Higher order protein structure is primarily determined by noncovalent interactions between side chains. In an alpha helix secondary structure, the stability arises from the formation of the maximum possible number of which of the following noncovalent interactions?
A) Peptide bonds
B) Hydrogen bonds
C) Disulfide bonds
D) Hydrophobic interactions
E) Van der Waals forces

82. Which among the following best describes cholesterol?
    A) It is made up of more than 30 carbons.
    B) It is one of the major components of plasma membrane.
    C) It is a precursor for prostaglandin synthesis.
    D) It is catabolized for energy in the body.
    E) It is especially abundant in citrus fruits.

83. Enzymes may alter the
    A) free energy (ΔG) of a reaction.
    B) equilibrium constant (K_{eq}) of a reaction.
    C) enthalpy (ΔH) of a reaction.
    D) entropy (ΔS) of a reaction.
    E) activation energy (ΔE_a) of a reaction.

84. Glycine to serine conversion in the body requires transfer of a methyl group and a vitamin cofactor. Which of the following vitamins is required for this reaction?
    A) Folic acid
    B) Niacin
    C) Pantothenic acid
    D) Riboflavin
    E) Ascorbic acid

85. Shown below is the structure of a lipid obtained from the diet. Which of the following statements about this lipid is true? $CH_3-CH_2-CH=CH-CH_2-CH=CH-CH_2-CH=CH-CH_2-CH_2-CH_2-CH_2-CH_2-CH_2-COOH$
    A) It is a nonessential fatty acid.
    B) It is an ω-3 fatty acid.
    C) It will tend to increase serum triglyceride levels.
    D) It is a precursor to the formation of arachidonic acid.
    E) It is oleic acid.

86. Monosaccharides may be linked together via glycosidic bonds to create disaccharides, oligosaccharides, and polysaccharides. In each of these, the individual monosaccharides that comprise the entire unit may or may not be the same. Among the sundry monosaccharides found in nature, glucose is perhaps one of the most ubiquitous. Which one of the following carbohydrates contains a monosaccharide unit other than glucose?
    A) Glycogen
    B) Cellulose
    C) Maltose
    D) Lactose
    E) Starch

87. Which fatty acid is essential and a precursor of arachidonic acid?
    A) Palmitic acid (C16:0)
    B) Lignoceric acid (C24:0)
    C) Linoleic acid (C18:2(Δ9, 12))
    D) Oleic acid (C18:1(Δ9))
    E) Myristic acid (C14:0)

88. A 10-year-old boy is brought to the office of a pediatrician with a stuffy nose and red, watery, itchy eyes. He had the same signs every spring for several years. The pathomechanism of this case involves a small molecule produced from an amino acid by the patient's mast cells. The enzyme that makes this molecule requires which of the following vitamins as cofactor?
    A) Riboflavin

B) Niacin
C) Biotin
D) Pyridoxine
E) Ascorbate

89. To buffer the rapid pH changes during anaerobic exercise, muscle cells contain large amounts of carnosine, a dipeptide composed of β-alanine (β-Ala) and histidine (His) as shown in the image below. Which of the following groups are mainly responsible for the buffering ability of carnosine?

β-Alanine   Histidine

A) α-amino group of His
B) α-carboxyl group of His
C) imidazole nitrogen of His
D) β-amino group of β-Ala
E) α-carboxyl group of β-Ala

90. In our body, alcohol dehydrogenase converts ingested methanol into formaldehyde, which destroys the optic nerve. Methanol poisoning therefore leads to blindness. To protect their vision, patients with methanol poisoning may be infused with ethanol, which is also oxidized by alcohol dehydrogenase to acetaldehyde. The methanol will then be slowly excreted by the kidneys. If you were to plot the effect of ethanol on the rate of oxidation of methanol by alcohol dehydrogenase in a Lineweaver-Burk plot, you would see a
    A) decrease of the slope and unchanged y-intercept.
    B) increase of the slope and unchanged y-intercept.
    C) increase of the slope and decrease of the y-intercept.
    D) decrease of the slope and increase of the y-intercept.
    E) decrease of both the slope and the y-intercept.

91. A 32-month-old girl was transferred to a large children's hospital because of rickets that was refractory to vitamin D treatment. She was the second child of parents who were first cousins. X-ray of hands, wrists, and knees revealed florid changes of rickets. Ophthalmology slit lamp examination showed corneal crystals. Blood and urine lab tests (e.g., glucose in urine and aminoaciduria) indicated that her condition is caused by an accumulation of an amino acid–derived compound that forms stones in the kidneys, ureter, and bladder when its reabsorption is disrupted. What compound is it?
    A) Cysteine
    B) Cystine
    C) Homocysteine
    D) Urate
    E) Methionine

Answers and Explanations: Nutrition and Biomolecules

1. C A catalyst changes the activation energy (ΔE_a), which is shown in parameter C. Activation energy is the energy required for the substrate to reach the transition state and is the difference between the free energy of the substrate (parameter A) and the free energy of the transition state (peak of the curve).

A Parameter A is the free energy of the substrate (G_s). It is not changed by a catalyst.

B Parameter B is the free energy of the product (G_p). It is not changed by a catalyst.

D Parameter D is the change in free energy (ΔG), which is the difference between G_s and G_p (G_p - G_s). The free energy change is not altered by a catalyst.

E Parameter E (the width of the peak in the energy diagram) is not a relevant thermodynamic parameter.

2. D 1,25-Dihydroxycholecalciferol (calcitriol) is the final, fully potent form of vitamin D. It is formed in the proximal tubule of the nephron by the action of 1-α-hydroxylase.

A Ergocalciferol, also called vitamin D_2, is obtained through the diet primarily from plant sources but can also be found in some vitamin D supplements. It is converted to cholecalciferol by intestinal cells.

B Cholecalciferol, the inactive form of vitamin D, is obtained through the diet or endogenously produced by UV irradiation of 7-dehydrocholesterol in the skin.

C 25-Hydroxylase is a liver enzyme that hydroxylates cholecalciferol (vitamin D_3) to form 25-hydroxycholecalciferol (25-OH-D_3).

E 25-Hydroxycholecalciferol is the primary storage form of vitamin D and is the predominant form found in serum. As such, the concentration of 25-hydroxycholecalciferol in the blood is used clinically as an indicator for overall vitamin D regulation.

3. D Potassium (K^+) is the major intracellular cation. Aside from its use in maintaining osmotic pressure, K^+ is used to help generate electrical potentials in nervous tissues, is required as a cofactor for some enzymes, and is involved in the regulation of insulin secretion.

A Magnesium (Mg^{2+}) is also a key intracellular cation; however, its concentration in comparison with K^+ is much lower. Mg^{2+} itself is an important cofactor for ATPases and for adenylate cyclase.

B Zinc (Zn^{2+}) is an essential trace element that is not the major intracellular cation but is required in over 100 known enzymes. It is typically not found in the free state but rather is bound to the serum transport proteins albumin, transferrin, and metallothionein, when not incorporated into an enzyme.

C Sodium (Na^+) is a major extracellular cation. In addition to its role in maintaining osmotic pressure and pH balance, Na^+ plays a key role in the absorption of glucose, galactose, and amino acids in the intestine.

E Chloride (Cl^-) is the major extracellular anion. Along with Na^+ and K^+, Cl^- helps maintain osmotic pressure and pH balance.

4. C Parathyroid hormone (PTH) is released in response to low serum calcium levels and stimulates bone marrow osteoclastic activity to release calcium ion into the blood.

A Parathyroid hormone is released in response to low serum calcium levels. The high PTH promotes calcium reabsorption throughout the tubules.

B An increase in calcitonin decreases blood calcium levels opposing the effects of PTH hormone.

D Lack of 1,25-dihydroxy vitamin D will prevent bone osteoclastic activity and not prevents bone from taking calcium from blood.

E Calcitriol (1, 25-dihydroxycholecalciferol), through interaction of the calcitriol-receptor complex, affects the production of mRNAs that code for proteins involved with intestinal calcium absorption (e.g., calbindin).

5. C Nonheme iron is most easily absorbed in the Fe^{2+} state. At physiological pH, ferrous (Fe^{2+}) iron is rapidly oxidized to the insoluble ferric iron (Fe^{3+}). Gastric acid allows iron to remain in its soluble Fe^{2+} form and thus enhances its absorption in proximal duodenum.

A Simultaneous intake of reducing agents, specifically ascorbic acid, increases the bioavailability of iron. It does so by helping to keep iron in the Fe^{2+} state, it's most easily absorbable form.

B The iron in plants is generally in the nonheme Fe^{3+} state. Absorption of Fe^{3+} requires the use of specific transport proteins and is inefficient. Iron obtained from animal products is predominantly in the heme form (Fe^{2+}) and is absorbed via iron channels in the duodenum.

D The phytates commonly found in fiber-containing foods (e.g., wheat bran) chelate iron. But unlike other chelation agents such as ascorbic and citric acid, phytates impede iron uptake by the absorption machinery.

E Ceruloplasmin (ferroxidase), plays a small role in iron transport because it oxidizes Fe^{2+} to Fe^{3+} so that the latter can be bound and transported by transferrin, the major protein responsible for transporting iron from the intestine to the bloodstream. Ceruloplasmin is primarily responsible for transporting copper.

6. A The triple helix is formed by Gly-Xxx-Pro repeats; only the small glycine (Gly) in the first position allows the tight packing of the protein chains around each other, which is responsible for the high tensile strength of collagen (stronger than steel rope!). Any other amino acid in this place would weaken the triple helix. The proline (Pro) (which may be hydroxylated posttranslationally) causes a sharp angle so that the chains wrap around each other.

B The triple helix is formed by Gly-Xxx-Pro repeats, where Xxx can be any amino acid except tryptophan (Trp), which is too large to fit into collagen.

C Selenocysteine (Sec) is a very rare amino acid found in the catalytic center of some enzymes, where the more acidic selenol-group (pK_a = 5.2) fulfills functions that the thiol-group in Cys (pK_a = 10.3), the alcoholic OH-group in Ser and Thr (pK_a = 13.6), or the phenolic OH-group in Tyr (pK_a = 10.1) could not perform. There is no Sec in collagen.

D Nonsense mutations are caused by deletion or insertion of one or two base pairs into the DNA, which introduces a premature stop signal. However, such mutations are relevant only in exons because introns are cut from the final mRNA.

E TATA boxes are the place where the transcription of genes into mRNA starts. Loss of the TATA box therefore would result in the complete loss of an α chain of type XI collagen.

7. E Vitamin C is an essential co factor for the hydroxylases required for collagen synthesis and processing. Collagen undergoes post translational modification such as proline and lysine hydroxylation which is dependent on Vitamin C. Low activity of these hydroxylases results in weak collagen. Vitamin C deficiency presents with superficial hemorrhages with no other hematological abnormalities.

A Lactase, an enzyme normally produced by absorptive cells of the small intestine, is responsible for hydrolysis of disaccharide lactose into glucose and galactose. A genetic deficiency in lactase leads to primary lactose intolerance. Lactose intolerant individuals experience diarrhea and flatulence on lactose consumption.

B Methemoglobin is a type of hemoglobin that contains oxidized form of iron (Fe^{3+}) in its heme group and is unable to bind O_2. Elevated levels of methemoglobin (methemoglobinemia) may be due to a genetic mutation in Methemoglobin reductase and may present as bluish brown cyanosis.

C Vitamin K serves as a cofactor for Gamma carboxylase, an enzyme that carboxylates glutamate residues on precursor clotting factors (II,VII,IX,X) converting them into mature clotting factors. Low vitamin K availability may lead to gastrointestinal bleeding and prolonged prothrombin time (PT).

D Cholecalciferol, an inactive form of Vitamin D, is first hydroxylated in the liver and then hydroxylated second time in the kidney by 1-α-hydroxylase to convert into active form of Vitamin D (Calcitriol). Calcitriol is responsible for proper bone mineralization. Low 1-alpha-hydroxylase activity (e.g., renal failure) can present as poor bone mineralization.

8. B The primary function of fluorine (as fluoride) in the body is to strengthen bone and prevent tooth decay by preventing demineralization. Fluoride is part of calcium fluorapatite [Ca_5(PO_4)$_3$ F], an important part of tooth enamel.

A Some studies have shown that chromium aids in the regulation of blood sugar levels by helping to potentiate insulin action.

C Iodine is needed by the thyroid to synthesize the thyroid hormones thyroxine (T_4) and triiodothyronine (T_3).

D Selenium is a cofactor in several enzymes, one being glutathione peroxidase, an important antioxidant enzyme that detoxifies hydrogen peroxide and heavy metals. It is also important for the normal functioning of the immune system and thyroid gland.

E Zinc is an essential part of more than 100 enzymes involved in key biological processes, including digestion, metabolism, reproduction, and wound healing.

9. D Because the ring nitrogen of histidine (His) in the catalytic triad of serine proteases acts as a proton acceptor during the enzymatic reaction sequence, it needs to be unprotonated to begin with. If the pH is lowered below its pK_a, the His side chain would be constantly protonated and hence unable to function.

A Lowering the pH below the pK_a would indeed protonate the His side chain. However, His in the catalytic triad of serine

proteases acts as a proton acceptor and needs to be deprotonated to fulfill this role.

B Because His acts as a proton acceptor in the catalytic triad of serine proteases, it needs to be unprotonated to function. Lowering the pH below its pKa, however, would protonate it.

C Lowering the pH below the pK_a would indeed protonate the His side chain. However, because His in the catalytic triad of serine proteases acts as a proton acceptor, it would not be able to fulfill its role if it were protonated.

E Because His acts as a proton acceptor in the catalytic triad of serine proteases, it needs to be unprotonated to function. Lowering the pH below its pKa, however, would protonate it.

10. E The total number of Calories can be calculated by knowing that carbohydrates provide 4.1 Cal/g → 82 Cal; proteins provide 4.1 Cal/g → 20.5 Cal; and lipids provide 9.3 Cal/g → 102.3 Cal. Adding these together gives roughly 205 Cal/serving. 3 servings × 205 Cal/serving = 615 Calories.

A More than 36 Calories were consumed.

B More than 66 Calories were consumed.

C 102 is the number of Calories coming from one serving of fat.

D 82 is the number of Calories coming from one serving of carbohydrates.

11. B Fluoride (used as sodium fluoride) is a strong competitive inhibitor of Enolase, blocking glycolysis. Addition of an enzyme inhibitor to the blood inhibits glucose utilization in vitro and prevents false low values for blood glucose

A While citrate inhibits phosphofructokinase, it can do so only when present in the cytosol. As a charged molecule, it cannot easily cross the plasma membrane when added to blood.

C Citrate is used when tests require whole blood rather than serum. Its three carboxylic acid groups chelate metal ions, including Ca^{2+}, which is required for blood clotting as "factor IV."

D Blood is highly buffered already; adding additional buffer is not necessary.

E Fluoride inhibits Glycolysis. The tricarboxylic acid cycle occurs in mitochondria; erythrocytes do not have these.

12. A Transfer of hydrogen is a redox reaction, catalyzed by oxidoreductases. One of the important subclasses of oxidoreductases is dehydrogenase. This particular reaction is the oxidation of ethanol to ethanal (acetaldehyde), catalyzed by alcohol dehydrogenase.

B It is a redox reaction catalyzed by oxidoreductase. Transferases catalyze the transfer of functional groups between molecules.

C It is a redox reaction catalyzed by oxidoreductase. Hydrolases catalyze the removal of functional groups by hydrolysis.

D It is a redox reaction catalyzed by oxidoreductase. Lyases form double bonds by removing functional groups from a molecule.

E It is a redox reaction catalyzed by oxidoreductase. Isomerases catalyze the transfer of functional groups within a molecule.

13. B Trypsinogen is synthesized by the pancreas and released into the duodenum where it is cleaved into trypsin, a gastrointestinal protease. Mutation in the trypsinogen gene that increases its rate of self-cleavage will most likely result in pancreatitis.

A Pepsinogen is released by chief cells of the stomach and is cleaved into pepsin. Pepsin is also one of the gastrointestinal proteases.

C Trypsinogen is synthesized by pancreas.

D Trypsin is a gastrointestinal protease.

E Trypsinogen is synthesized by the pancreas and released into the duodenum.

14. A Because omeprazole is an inhibitor of the stomach H^+/K^+-ATPase, it will increase the pH of gastric juice. Pepsin has a low pH-optimum and will no longer be fully active.

B Trypsin is an enzyme produced by the pancreas and is active in the small intestine. Omeprazole is a gastric proton pump inhibitor and will increase the pH in the stomach, not in the small intestine.

C Chymotrypsin is an enzyme produced by the pancreas and active in the small intestine. Omeprazole is a gastric proton pump inhibitor and will increase the pH in the stomach, not in the small intestine.

D Carboxypeptidase A is an enzyme produced by the pancreas and active in the small intestine. Omeprazole is a gastric proton pump inhibitor and will increase the pH in the stomach, not in the small intestine.

E Alanine-aminopeptidase is an enzyme of the mucosal membrane in the small intestine. Omeprazole is a gastric proton pump inhibitor and will increase the pH in the stomach, not in the small intestine.

15. A(E)-Noncompetitive inhibitors do not resemble the substrate. They bind to free or substrate bound enzyme at a region other than substrate binding site. K_m remains unchanged because the affinity of the enzyme for its substrate is not affected. The apparent V_{max} is lowered because the inhibitor disrupts the enzyme's ability to catalyze its reaction.

C Competitive inhibitors may resemble the substrate and compete with it for binding to the active site of the free enzyme. The effects of the inhibitor can be offset by higher substrate concentrations; hence V_{max} will stay the same. However, the apparent affinity of the enzyme for the substrate decreases, so the K_m will increase.

D, B Uncompetitive inhibitors bind only to enzyme-substrate complex at a site other than active site. The binding on the inhibitor will decrease both V_{max} and K_m by the same factor.

16. B If an inhibitor has a structural similarity to the substrate and binds to the active site of an enzyme, it will result in competitive inhibition because substrate and inhibitor cannot bind to the same site at the same time. (Note that the converse of that statement is not necessarily true: not all competitive inhibitors bind to the active site.) In competitive inhibition, the effects of the inhibitor can be offset by higher substrate concentrations.

A Allosteric negative effectors bind to the enzyme at a site different from the catalytic site. Binding of effector causes conformational changes that are transmitted through the bulk of the protein to the catalytically active site(s).

C Noncompetitive inhibition cannot be offset by increasing substrate concentrations.

D Inhibitor binds to the enzyme inactivating it by covalent modification of enzyme structure.

E. Uncompetitive inhibition would cause changes in both V_{max} and K_m.

17. E There are 20 proteinogenic amino acids, 10 of which are considered essential and must be obtained from the diet. The mnemonic PVT TIM HALL can be used to help remember the essential amino acids: **P**henylalanine- **V**aline- **T**ryptophan, **T**hreonine- **I**soleucine- **M**ethionine, **H**istidine-**A**rginine- **L**ysine-**L**eucine. Only selection **E** contains amino acids within this mnemonic.

A Tyrosine is not an essential amino acid. It is synthesized from phenylalanine (an essential amino acid) by the enzyme phenylalanine hydroxylase in a reaction requiring molecular oxygen and the coenzyme tetrahydrobiopterin.

B Alanine is not an essential amino acid and is primarily synthesized from pyruvate via transamination reactions catalyzed by the enzyme alanine aminotransferase (ALT). Like all aminotransferases, ALT requires the coenzyme pyridoxal phosphate.

C Glutamic acid is not an essential amino acid and is primarily synthesized from α-ketoglutarate via transamination reactions catalyzed by aminotransferases. Cysteine is not an essential amino acid and is synthesized from serine by two consecutive reactions.

D Tyrosine is not an essential amino acid. It is synthesized from phenylalanine by the enzyme phenylalanine hydroxylase in a reaction requiring molecular oxygen and the coenzyme tetrahydrobiopterin.

18. A BMR is higher in people with hyperthyroidism, including people with Graves disease. The overproduction of thyroid hormones increases O_2 consumption and ATP hydrolysis.

B BMR is generally measured in the morning after a 12-hour fast, with the patient in the prone position. The measurement is taken at a temperature that minimizes both sweating and shivering.

C Infants and children require higher basal energy expenditure due to their rapid growth and development. In adults, there is roughly a 2% drop in BMR every decade as muscle tissue is replaced with fat and water due to normal aging processes.

D The processes that make up the BMR require an intake of oxygen to run the TCA cycle and electron transport chain. Therefore, one method to measure BMR is to measure the rate at which oxygen is taken up and then calculating the energy equivalent.

E BMR can be elevated by exogenous thyroxine, human growth hormone, epinephrine, cortisol, and several sex hormones or derivatives thereof.

19. E Fast and deep breathing leads to loss of CO_2, and hence increased blood pH. The loss of buffering capacity will be so large that the kidneys cannot compensate in time. This is a clinical emergency because it prevents the Bohr effect and thus oxygen release from hemoglobin in the tissues. The patient's feeling of hypoxia (despite normal oxygen saturation) will increase, and breathing will accelerate further, leading to a vicious circle with a potentially fatal outcome. Treatment is by encouraging the patient to slow the breathing (7 seconds in, 11 seconds out). Initially a bag held in front of the patient's mouth can be helpful in restoring blood CO_2 levels.

A There is no metabolic problem, but the rapid loss of CO_2 will disturb the carbonate/bicarbonate buffer system and lead to alkalosis.

B The alkalosis is caused not by a metabolic problem, but by the loss of CO_2 with rapid breathing, which disturbs the carbonate/bicarbonate buffer system.

C There is no acidosis here, but alkalosis. Loss of CO_2 will increase the pH.

D There is no acidosis here, but alkalosis. Loss of CO_2 will increase the pH.

20. C The probability of sickling is increased under anoxia. Replacement of the Glutamic acid (E) residue at position 6 in the beta chain by valine (V) creates a "sticky" hydrophobic contact point, on the outer surface of the molecule and decreases the solubility of the mutant Hb (HbS). HbS aggregates under low O_2 tension; polymerizes in rod shaped form and distorts shape of the red blood cell to sickle shape.

A The quaternary structure of hemoglobin changes upon the binding of O_2 due to movement of heme iron into the plane of the heme ring system. The iron is also bound to a proximal histidine, which moves as well, causing a conformational shift in the globin chains.

B A cooperative effect is seen on oxygen loading. Sickle cell hemoglobin has the same O_2-binding properties as "normal" hemoglobin, including its property of cooperative binding.

D HbS aggregates under low O_2 tension, polymerizes in rod shaped form, distorts the shape of the red blood cell to sickle shape.

E Deoxyhemoglobin has a higher affinity for protons than oxyhemoglobin. Protonation of deoxyhemoglobin allows for its stabilization due to salt bridge formation. The binding of O_2 disrupts these salt bridges and causes protons to be released. Dissociation of O_2, concomitant with the binding of CO_2 and protons, is referred to as the Bohr effect.

21. D Protons (H^+) protonate the terminal His residue (His 146) of the β subunit of hemoglobin due to which formation of salt bridges are favored. Reformation of the salt bridges facilitates the release of oxygen from oxygenated (R form) hemoglobin and the reformation of the Taut structure of hemoglobin and hence Deoxy form of hemoglobin is stabilized. Overall, an increase in proton concentration stabilizes the deoxy form and promotes oxygen release.

A Increasing pO2 will favor R form which promotes oxygen binding rather than release.

B Increasing pH will decrease protons and favors the R form.

C HbF has γ chains wherein residue 143 is serine instead of histidine and hence cannot form a salt bridge with BPG. It binds BPG only weakly resulting in higher oxygen affinity.

E When CO binds to one or more sites in hemoglobin, the latter shifts to the relaxed configuration. This change in conformation causes the remaining sites to bind oxygen with higher affinity, shifting the O_2-hemoglobin dissociation curve to the left, thus preventing oxygen from being properly delivered to the tissues.

22. D The side chain in leucine is a branched hydrocarbon without polar groups.

A The ε-amino group of lysine is positively charged at neutral pH and hence is hydrophilic.

B The guanidine-group of arginine is positively charged at neutral pH and hence is hydrophilic.

C The carboxylic acid group of glutamate has a negative charge at neutral pH and hence is hydrophilic.

E The carboxylic acid group of aspartate has a negative charge at neutral pH and hence is hydrophilic.

23. D Nitrogen balance is achieved when nitrogen intake is equal to the combined nitrogen losses in urine, feces, milk (lactating females only), and "other losses." Nitrogen balance (whether negative or not) is a reflection of the amount of nitrogen taken in compared with the amount lost. Nitrogen balance is not associated with the intake of essential versus nonessential amino acids. In the starved patients of the camp, muscle protein would be broken down for gluconeogenesis; thus, nitrogen loss would exceed dietary intake, resulting in a negative nitrogen balance. The nitrogen loss exceeds dietary nitrogen intake in negative nitrogen balance.

A,B,C,E Nitrogen balance is achieved when nitrogen intake is equal to the combined nitrogen losses in urine, feces, milk (lactating females only), and "other losses." Dietary nitrogen intake exceeds nitrogen loss in positive nitrogen balance.

24. D Lysyl oxidase has Cu^{2+} in its active center. Fibrillar array of collagen molecules serves as substrate for lysyl oxidase.

A Carbonic anhydrase contains a catalytic Zn^{2+}, which can be blocked with acetazolamide, a diuretic drug.

B In the cytosol, nucleotides, as well as inorganic phosphate and pyrophosphate, are complexed with Mg^{2+}. Enzymes handling these compounds — such as ATPases — have binding sites for Mg^{2+} and do not function without it.

C Most metalloproteases contain Zn^{2+}, and some contain Co^{2+}. Examples include the digestive carboxypeptidases, or endoproteases involved in cellular protein maturation (e.g., matrix metalloprotease).

E Cytochromes contain heme-iron in their active center.

25. E Gangliosides are a type of glycolipid that contain ceramide (sphingosine and fatty acid) and at least one or more acidic sugars (typically N-acetylneuraminic acid, NANA). Gangliosides are similar to sphingomyelin in having ceramide; however, they do not contain a phosphate group, and the polar head is provided by saccharides attached directly to the ceramide via an O-glycosidic bond.

A The inclusion of neuraminic acid is one of the key distinguishing characteristics of gangliosides. Their location and quantity on the ganglioside determines its specific name (e.g., G_{M2}, G_{D3}).

B Galactose is found in the polar carbohydrate head group. In all gangliosides the ceramide is linked to glucose, which is then linked to galactose.

C Fatty acids comprise part of the hydrophobic tail of gangliosides and are linked via an amide bond to sphingosine to complete the ceramide core structure.

D Gangliosides are composed of sphingosine linked to a fatty acyl residue via an amide bond and to a carbohydrate via an O-glycosidic bond.

26. C Pancreatic α-amylase is secreted into the duodenum of the small intestine, where it acts to hydrolyze the α-1 → 4 glycosidic bonds of carbohydrates. Other enzymes found in the small intestine include lactase, sucrase, and maltase. The combination of these enzymes allows for a majority of carbohydrates to be digested and absorbed as monosaccharides.

A Although the mouth contains salivary α-amylase, allowing for the initial breakdown of polysaccharides into oligosaccharides and disaccharides, it is not the major site of carbohydrate digestion. The main function of salivary α-amylase is to keep our teeth clean.

B The stomach is the primary site for the digestion of proteins. The acidic pH of the stomach denatures proteins, making them more susceptible to degradation by pepsin and later by pancreatic peptidases. The amino acids that are released travel to the small intestine, where they are absorbed.

D The function of the large intestine is to absorb water from any remaining indigestible material. Food is no longer broken down once it reaches the large intestine; however, vitamins and other nutrients produced by intestinal flora can be absorbed.

E The pancreas is the source of the digestive enzymes that are responsible for the breakdown of carbohydrates, lipids, and proteins. Once formed, these enzymes are secreted into the duodenum, where digestion occurs.

27. D Folic acid plays a major role in one-carbon metabolism. The derivative, N^5-methyltetrahydrofolate, is used for the synthesis of methionine from homocysteine, in a reaction requiring vitamin B_{12}. Another derivative, N^{10}-formyltetrahydrofolate, is used in the biosynthesis of purines, contributing carbons 2 and 8 to the purine ring system. N^5, N^{10}-methylenetetrahydrofolate is used by serine hydroxymethyl transferase to transfer hydroxymethyl groups between serine and glycine and for the synthesis of deoxythymidine monophosphate.

A Biotin is a coenzyme found in carboxylation reactions where it functions as a carrier of activated carbon dioxide. It is covalently bound to the ε-nitrogen of lysine residues found in biotin-dependent enzymes.

B Pyridoxine is a precursor to pyridoxal phosphate, a coenzyme involved in all aminotransferase reactions. Other roles for pyridoxal phosphate include deamination, decarboxylation, and condensation reactions.

C Lipoic acid is one of several coenzymes found in the pyruvate dehydrogenase, branched chain keto acid dehydrogenase, and α-ketoglutarate dehydrogenase complexes. It acts as a carrier of activated acyl groups and is involved in acyl transfer reactions.

E The main function of ascorbic acid is as a reducing agent. Its most well-known role is to regenerate Fe^{2+} from Fe^{3+} in the catalytic center of hydroxylases, especially those that hydroxylate the proline and lysine residues found in collagen.

28. A Phosphate, along with calcium, constitutes the bone salt hydroxyapatite. This salt is deposited on the collagenous matrix of bone, giving it its strength.

B Iron is a component of heme containing proteins include cytochromes of electron transport chain.

C Ca^{++} is an important component of blood clotting cascade.

D Selenium is a cofactor for glutathione peroxidase, an important antioxidant enzyme that detoxifies hydrogen peroxide.

E Adenosine is a nucleoside consisting of the purine, adenine, linked to ribose. Phosphorylation of adenosine is required for the formation of the high-energy molecule ATP and for the biosynthesis of nucleic acids.

29. A Muscle weakness and arrhythmia are symptoms of hypokalemia. Amiloride is a potassium-sparing diuretic, which inhibits the epithelial sodium channels (ENaC) of the kidneys. It can be used to prevent the potassium loss caused by other diuretics.

B The patient is suffering from hypokalemia as a result of furosemide treatment. Treatment must be complemented with a potassium-sparing diuretic, either an ENaC-blocker like amiloride or an aldosterone antagonist like spironolactone or eplerenone. Caffeine acts as a diuretic only in people not used to it; it is therefore unsuitable for long-term treatment.

C The patient is suffering from hypokalemia as a result of furosemide treatment. Treatment must be complemented with a potassium-sparing diuretic, either an ENaC-blocker like amiloride or an aldosterone antagonist like spironolactone or eplerenone. Thiazides increase potassium loss.

D The patient is suffering from hypokalemia as a result of furosemide treatment. Treatment must be complemented with a potassium-sparing diuretic, either an ENaC-blocker like amiloride or an aldosterone antagonist like spironolactone or eplerenone. Mannitol must be given by intravenous injection because it would act as a laxative in the intestine. That limits its use as a diuretic to acute oliguric renal failure.

E The patient is suffering from hypokalemia as a result of furosemide treatment. Treatment must be complemented with a potassium-sparing diuretic, either an ENaC-blocker like amiloride or an aldosterone antagonist like spironolactone or eplerenone. Methazolamide is a carbonic anhydrase inhibitor and therefore increases potassium loss by inhibiting proton excretion.

30. B Blockage of biliary flow (cholestasis) may cause malabsorption syndrome, leading to a deficiency of lipid-soluble vitamins because bile is required for their proper absorption. Among the lipid-soluble vitamins, vitamin A deficiency can lead to xerophthalmia, a condition that includes milder stages of night blindness. (Note that most people have considerable amounts of vitamin A stored in their liver, which suffice for weeks. A blocked bile duct is so painful that patients would hardly wait long enough for a deficiency in vitamin A to occur.)

A Scurvy is a collagen disease caused by inadequate levels of vitamin C. In the synthesis of collagen, vitamin C is a required cofactor for the proper hydroxylation of both proline and lysine by prolyl hydroxylase and lysyl hydroxylase, respectively. Hydroxylation allows collagen to maintain its triple helix structure.

C Pellagra is a disease involving the skin, gastrointestinal tract, and central nervous system caused by a chronic lack of niacin (B_3). It is characterized by dermatitis, diarrhea, dementia, and possibly death if untreated. Niacin can be obtained directly from the diet, or indirectly via biosynthesis from the amino acid tryptophan. Although tryptophan is an essential amino acid, neither it nor niacin's absorption is dependent on bile.

D Wernicke disease is a brain disorder caused by a deficiency in the water-soluble vitamin thiamine (B_1). Sometimes seen in alcoholics, it is characterized by apathy, memory loss, and nystagmus. Thiamine is a water-soluble vitamin and therefore is not dependent on the effects of bile for proper absorption.

E Ariboflavinosis, caused by a deficiency in the water-soluble vitamin riboflavin (B_2), is marked by cheilosis, angular stomatitis, and dermatitis.

31. D Monosaccharides are the simplest forms of carbohydrates and can exist in either linear or cyclic form. Cyclization occurs when the carbonyl carbon of aldoses and ketoses reversibly react with an internal hydroxyl group, forming a hemiacetal or hemiketal, respectively. D-Fructose is a ketose sugar. Sorbitol, the sugar alcohol derivative of glucose formed intracellular with the help of the enzyme aldose reductase. Sorbitol is converted to fructose in the body by sorbitol dehydrogenase. In uncontrolled diabetes, sorbitol accumulation is also linked with diabetic complications like cataracts, retinopathy, and peripheral neuropathy.

A, B Fructose is the most widely distributed ketohexose. It can be found alone (honey) or as a component of sucrose (including glucose) in the diet. Sucrose is found in table sugar.

C d-Glucose is the most important aldohexose. It is the primary energy source of the body and the only source that can be directly utilized by the brain. It can be as a component of lactose (including galactose) in the diet. d-Galactose is an aldohexose that is used in the body for the synthesis of glycolipids and glycoproteins. Lactose is found in milk and milk products.

E Dietary fiber consists of non-starch polysaccharides and other plant components, one such as cellulose.

32. A Competitive inhibitors increase the apparent K_m (lower the apparent affinity) of an enzyme for its substrate. This is because a substrate cannot bind to an enzyme when a competing inhibitor is bound, and vice versa.

B Uncompetitive inhibitors lower the K_m (increase the affinity) of an enzyme for its substrate.

C A noncompetitive inhibitor decreases the V_{max} without altering the K_m.

D A suicide inhibitor decreases the V_{max} without altering the K_m.

33. B Niacin deficiency can lead to pellagra, which is classically described by "the four D's": dermatitis, diarrhea, dementia, and death. Untreated pellagra can kill within 4 to 5 years; treatment is with nicotinamide.

A A deficiency in ascorbic acid can lead to a destabilization of the collagen triple helix due to improper hydroxylation of proline and lysine. Extended deficiency can lead to scurvy, with clinical symptoms including bleeding gums, anemia, osteoporosis, and slow wound healing.

C A deficiency in thiamine can lead to beriberi (with loss of appetite, constipation, irritability, depression, and fatigue), polyneuritis, and Wernicke-Korsakoff syndrome (with confusion, nystagmus, anisocoria, ataxia, amnesia, confabulations, and hallucinations).

D A deficiency in cobalamin (vitamin B_{12}) is associated with a buildup of abnormal fatty acids due to the inability to properly degrade odd-number fatty acids. Low cobalamin can also cause a secondary deficiency in folic acid, leading to megaloblastic anemia.

E Thought to be the most common vitamin deficiency in the United States, low levels of folic acid are associated with loss of appetite, weight loss, weakness, and irritability, with extreme deficiency leading to megaloblastic anemia. The fetus of pregnant women with folic acid deficiency is at risk for spina bifida, due to incomplete closure of the neural tube.

34. D Dietary fiber consists of those compounds that cannot be broken down by the human digestive system, such as cellulose, lignin, and pectin. Although humans are unable to break these materials down, a small portion can be digested due to the action of intestinal flora. Several forms of fiber, particularly cellulose and hemicellulose, decrease intestinal transit time. This has been associated with the effects of fiber on regularity.

A Fiber, especially lignins, are able to adsorb organic substances such as cholesterol and bile salts, helping to lower plasma cholesterol levels. This ability is also believed to help remove potential carcinogens taken in from dietary sources.

B Fiber increases stool bulk. Furthermore, the increase in stool bulk has a diluting effect on potential carcinogens, and coupled with decreased transit time, helps reduce the risk of colon cancer.

C Fiber decreases the efficiency of absorption of some nutrients, particularly minerals that may bind to it. The binding of iron (and other minerals) to fiber reduces its availability for transport, therefore decreasing absorption efficiency.

E Fiber aids in the regulation of blood sugar. The consumption of fiber, especially soluble fiber, slows the rate of carbohydrate absorption from the gut, effectively modulating the corresponding rise in blood sugar. This can be especially helpful to patients with diabetes, who often have high blood sugar due to either underproduction of insulin or the inability to fully utilize the insulin that is produced.

35. E About 20% of the US population is at risk for sodium-dependent hypertension. In Hispanics and African Americans, this condition is particularly frequent. Note that sodium is not only contained in table salt but also as bicarbonate, glutamate, citrate, phosphate, saccharinate, benzoate, sorbate, propionate, and nitrite in processed food. These account for ~ 10% of daily Na^+ intake in the average diet in the United States and other industrialized countries. Processed food may also contain high amounts of sodium chloride.

A Magnesium toxicity is seen almost exclusively in patients with renal problems, where elimination no longer works. Hypermagnesemia leads to a (potentially serious) fall in blood pressure.

B Molybdenum is an ultra-trace element. Toxicity has not been described in humans and is known only from animal studies, either deliberately induced in the laboratory or in animals grazing on polluted soil. It generates histological changes in the liver and kidney.

C Chronic high doses of fluoride (usually from contaminated wells) cause mottled teeth. In even higher doses, it causes skeletal problems (e.g., joint pain, osteoporosis).

D Excess zinc can come from acidic food stored in galvanized containers, but nowadays it is usually associated with excess supplementation. Zinc is relatively nontoxic, and excessive intakes of it causes diarrhea and vomiting.

36. **A** The patient is suffering from a gallstone, which has blocked the bile duct. This diagnosis is supported by the positive Murphy sign, which suggests she has an inflamed gallbladder (cholecystitis), or a blocked bile duct (choledocholithiasis). Her jaundice (sclera icteric), light- or clay-colored stool, and dark urine, all point to an obstruction of the bile duct. Because bile can no longer reach the intestine, the uptake of dietary fat and fat-soluble vitamins will be inhibited. Of the vitamins listed, only retinal is fat soluble. Note, however, that because of the intense pain, this problem will usually be surgically corrected long before body stores of fat-soluble vitamins are depleted.

B The patient is suffering from gallstone blockage of the bile duct, which prevents bile from reaching the small intestine. As a result, the uptake of fat and fat-soluble vitamins is inhibited. Thiamine (vitamin B_1), however, is a water-soluble vitamin.

C The patient is suffering from gallstone blockage of the bile duct, which prevents bile from reaching the small intestine. As a result, the uptake of fat and fat-soluble vitamins is inhibited. Ascorbate (vitamin C), however, is a water-soluble vitamin.

D The patient is suffering from gallstone blockage of the bile duct, which prevents bile from reaching the small intestine. As a result, the uptake of fat and fat-soluble vitamins is inhibited. Biotin, however, is a water-soluble vitamin.

E The patient is suffering from gallstone blockage of the bile duct, which prevents bile from reaching the small intestine. As a result, the uptake of fat and fat-soluble vitamins is inhibited. Folate, however, is a water-soluble vitamin.

37. **B** This patient is suffering from zinc (Zn) deficiency as a result of the unleavened bread in his diet. Unleavened bread contains phytate (inositol hexakisphosphate, IP6), which binds Zn (and other metal ions), inhibiting their absorption. During the process of leavening bread, the phosphate groups are removed from the phytate by microorganisms such as yeast and bacteria, rendering it inactive. Zn deficiency causes growth retardation (leading to dwarfism), lack of bone maturation (as marked by epiphyses that do not close), lack of sexual maturation in males (as marked by hypogonadism), rashes, lack of appetite, reduced ability to taste (hypogeusia) and smell (hyposmia) things, an appetite for nonnutritive substances (pica), and depressed immune function, which increases susceptibility to infection, night blindness, hair loss, and unsteady walk (ataxic gait).

A Although a relative iron (Fe) deficiency (as suggested by his spoon-shaped nails) may be a confounding factor in this child's problems, his are not the classical signs of Fe deficiency, which are hypochromic, microcytic anemia leading to pale mucus membranes, cyanosis, and exertional fatigue.

C Although a relative copper (Cu) deficiency may be a confounding factor in this child's problems, his are not the classical signs of Cu deficiency, which are pancytopenia (reduction in all types of blood cells), depigmentation, hypercholesterolemia, glucose intolerance, and bone fractures.

D Selenium (Se) deficiency leads to Keshan disease (named after a region in China with Se-poor soil), which is marked by cardiomyopathy. It may also be involved in Kashin-Beck disease, marked by osteoarthritis.

E Iodine (I) deficiency would lead to goiter or even cretinism (congenital hypothyroidism).

38. **A** The patient is suffering from chronic obstructive pulmonary disease (COPD) and cardiovascular disease as a result of poor nutrition, little exercise, and years of smoking. The lack of oxygen will increase the 2,3-BPG concentration in his erythrocytes, which binds into a small pocket between the β-subunits of hemoglobin. This pocket is lined with positive charges that can interact with the phosphate groups of 2,3-BPG. In the R-state, this pocket is too small to accept 2,3-BPG, and 2,3-BPG-binding will therefore stabilize the T-state of hemoglobin, which has a lower affinity for oxygen than the R-state. Even at this late stage, smoking cessation can significantly improve the prognosis for this patient.

B 2,3-BPG shifts Hb to the T-state.

C 2,3-BPG will increase due to low O2.

D 2,3-BPG will increase due to low O2 and shift Hb to the T-state.

39. **A** P5CS deficiency prevents the synthesis of proline, arginine, and ornithine. Proline is required for collagen synthesis. Proline's presence causes the tight wrapping of the three protein strands around each other that is responsible for the high tensile strength of collagen. Many of these prolines are hydroxylated posttranslationally, which stabilizes the triple helix against thermal dissociation. Inability to hydroxylate proline in collagen leads to a melting temperature below 37 °C and weak connective tissue, for example, in scurvy.

B The hyperelasticity of the skin and the lax bone joints point to a problem with collagen formation here because of the inability to make proline, which is required for collagen synthesis. Proline is rare in α-helices. Where it does occur in helices, it will introduce a kink.

C The hyperelasticity of the skin and the lax bone joints point to a problem with collagen formation here because of the inability to make proline, which is required for collagen synthesis. Proline does not occur in β-strands.

D, E The hyperelasticity of the skin and the lax bone joints point to a problem with collagen formation, here because of the inability to make proline, which is required for collagen synthesis.

40. **C** The patient is suffering from Wilson disease (hepatolenticular degeneration), an inherited failure of Cu excretion. The Kayser-Fleischer rings (copper deposition in the Descemet membrane) are characteristic. Excess Cu needs to be removed by chelation therapy with penicillamine. The derangement in Ca and P_i metabolism results from kidney damage, via failure to produce calcitriol. Ceruloplasmin is low despite elevated [Cu] because it is produced in the liver.

A Because the patient is suffering from Wilson disease (inherited Cu poisoning), Cu supplementation would make matters worse.

B The patient is not suffering from Zn deficiency, which would cause acrodermatitis.

D Deferoxamine is used to treat Fe, rather than Cu poisoning.

E The patient's condition is not caused by a vitamin deficiency.

41. **E** Because the patient's intake is above the recommended daily allowance and way below the upper limit (UL) of intake, the risk of deficiency would be minimal and the risk for poisoning is essentially zero.

A Because the dose is way below the upper limit of intake, the risk for poisoning is essentially zero.

B Because the dose is way below the upper limit of intake, the risk for poisoning is essentially zero.

C The dose is just above the RDA; thus, the risk for deficiency is much lower than 98%.

D The dose is just above the RDA; thus, the risk for deficiency is much lower than 50%.

42. **D** Myoglobin rises within 2 to 3 hours and returns to baseline within 24 hours after an infarct. Thus, an increased level in your patient would indicate a second infarct if other causes for myoglobin release (i.e., skeletal muscle disease) can be excluded. All other enzymes take longer to rise, and, more importantly, decline over several days. Thus, in the patient, these other enzymes would be elevated, independent of whether he had or had not suffered a second infarct.

A Cardiac troponins reach peak concentrations ~ 24 hours after an AMI and stay elevated for ~ 10 days. In your patient, therefore, cTn-I would be elevated irrespective of whether he had or had not suffered a second infarct.

B Cardiac troponins reach peak concentrations ~ 24 hours after an AMI and stay elevated for ~ 10 days. In your patient, therefore, cTn-T would be elevated irrespective of whether he had or had not suffered a second infarct.

C Total CK reaches peak levels ~ 24 hours after an AMI and stay elevated for ~ 3 days. In your patient, therefore, CK would be elevated irrespective of whether he had or had not suffered a second infarct.

E Lactate dehydrogenase 1 (LDH-1) rises and falls very slowly, reaching a peak after ~ 48 hours and returning to baseline after a week or so. In your patient, therefore, LDH-1 would be elevated irrespective of whether he had or had not suffered a second infarct.

43. **E** Gout is associated with hyperuricemia that leads to precipitation of long needle shaped sodium urate crystals in the synovial fluid of joints and connective tissue. Monosodium urate crystals elicit an inflammatory response leading to red, swollen and tender joints mainly involving the great toe. Gout can be diagnosed by the presence of monosodium urate negatively birefringent crystals in the aspirated synovial fluid examined by the polarized microscopy.

A Cystinuria is one of the most common inherited disease due to a genetic error of amino acid transport. It is the defect in transporter responsible for the uptake of amino acids cysteine, ornithine, arginine, lysine and is associated with presence of cystine.

B, C, D Gout is associated with hyperuricemia that leads to precipitation of long needle shaped sodium urate crystals in the synovial fluid of joints and connective tissue.

44. **B** The patient is suffering from a mild cystic fibrosis. The ΔF508 mutation results in a functional but slow-folding CFTR protein, the majority of which are degraded before reaching the plasma membrane. The R117 H mutation results in a partially functional protein. Under usual environmental conditions these patients can function normally, but in a hot climate the salt loss due to inability to reclaim Cl⁻ from the isotonic primary

sweat leads to massive salt depletion, extracellular volume contraction, secondary hyperaldosteronism, and potassium wasting in both sweat and urine. The kidneys will excrete protons and reabsorb more bicarbonate. Ammonia production by the kidney will be increased. The result is metabolic alkalosis. This will be partially compensated by reduced respiration, resulting in an increased plasma CO_2 concentration.

A The blood pH indicates that there is alkalosis, not acidosis (normal pH is 7.35 to 7.45).

C The blood pH indicates that there is alkalosis, not acidosis (normal pH is 7.35 to 7.45).

D The blood pH indicates that there is alkalosis, not acidosis (normal pH is 7.35 to 7.45).

E The elevated PCO_2 indicates some respiratory (not metabolic) compensation.

45. **B** Patient is suffering from wet beriberi and Wernicke encephalopathy due to his nutrient-poor diet, which lacks sufficient amounts of vitamin B_1, thiamine. Without the latter, Wernicke encephalopathy may progress to Korsakoff disease, which is irreversible. In the ER, it is essential that thiamine is given to any patient with even a remote possibility of beriberi (including alcoholics) before intravenous glucose is started. Beriberi is still a major health problem in developing countries. In the Philippines it is the fourth leading cause of infant death (75 deaths per 100,000 live births). This is caused by the use of polished (white rather than brown) rice.

A Retinal (vitamin A) deficiency would result in eye problems (e.g., xerophthalmia, photophobia, or reduced night vision).

C A lack of cobalamin (vitamin B_{12}) would result in megaloblastic anemia.

D Ascorbate (vitamin C) deficiency results in scurvy, with petechiae and weak gums.

E Menaquinone (vitamin K) deficiency would result in a bleeding disorder.

46. **E** Isotretinoin closely resembles retinoic acid, a natural vitamin A derivative that plays a major role in normal embryonic development. It is a well-known teratogen, listed by the FDA as pregnancy category X (for drugs whose risk to the fetus outweighs any possible benefit). There is a strong association of a group of birth defects and isotretinoin use during the first several weeks of pregnancy. Among these are external ear malformation, cleft palate, ventricular septal defects, conotruncal heart defects, aortic arch malformation, and several brain malformations.

A Fetal abnormalities have rarely been reported in women who have remained on oral contraceptives throughout early pregnancy, but a clear association has not been firmly established. More commonly, the fetus will show signs of modified sexual organ development.

B Lack of ascorbic acid causes scurvy and is not known to be associated with birth defects.

C The topical antibiotics most commonly used for the treatment of acne are clindamycin and erythromycin. Animal studies have failed to indicate teratogenicity, and the FDA has assigned these drugs to pregnancy category B (no evidence of risk to the human fetus). There have been no controlled studies in humans, although no reports of fetal abnormalities have been disclosed.

D Certain genetic abnormalities have been shown to cause cleft palate, although this accounts for less than 25% of cases. The most common cause is an environmental factor that affects one or more genes, such as smoking, alcohol use, malnutrition, and use of teratogenic drugs.

47. A (B,C,D,E) The child is suffering from biotinidase deficiency (late-onset multiple carboxylase deficiency, MCD), which prevents biotin recycling and causes late-onset multiple carboxylase failure. In cell culture, when supplied with biotin, the carboxylases have normal activity. Onset of the disease is after weaning, when biotin in the mother's milk is replaced by biocytin (biotin linked to the ε-amino-group of lysine) in normal food. Neonatal MCD is caused by a reduced biotin affinity of holocarboxylase synthetase (an enzyme that attaches biotin to biotin-dependent enzymes), which prevents the utilization of biotin. The metabolite of isoleucine which is elevated in the urine is propionic acid. Methionine, threonine, valine and odd chain fatty acid metabolism also contributes to propionic acid in the body.

48. A CO_2 reacts with water, forming bicarbonate and hydrogen ions. In addition, CO_2 reacts with the amino-termini of all four subunits of hemoglobin, forming carbamino-hemoglobin and hydrogen ions. Both mechanisms therefore increase H^+ concentration, resulting in (among others) protonation of His-146 in the β-subunits, which then forms salt bridges with Asp-94, thereby stabilizing the T-conformation of hemoglobin (Bohr effect). Thus, CO_2 lowers the affinity of hemoglobin for O_2 and increases the amount of oxygen that is released in the tissues. Lowering the plasma CO_2 concentration will prevent this effect.

B, C, D Reduction of plasma CO_2 leads to alkalosis and a decrease in the Bohr effect. That increases the affinity of hemoglobin for O_2 and hence reduces the amount of O_2 released in the tissues.

49. A Amylin (islet amyloid protein) is co-secreted with insulin. In diabetes mellitus type 2, insulin and amylin secretion are increased, and some of the amylin forms amyloid between the β-cells and the capillaries. This leads to the death of β-cells and insulin dependence in long-term diabetes type 2. Congo red stains amyloid reddish, with a green birefringence in polarized light. This patient is an archetypical case of metabolic syndrome. He inexorably develops from overweight to morbidly obese (judged either by body mass index (BMI) or, according to newer guidelines, by waist circumference), despite increasing medical problems and a positive family history of cardiovascular accidents. He does not follow medical advice, be it about diet, lifestyle, or pharmaceuticals. Management of these patients requires great psychological skill.

B Amyloid formation from mutated apolipoprotein AI is often clinically silent but may lead to nephropathy and cardiomyopathy. This is one of the Ostertag familial visceral amyloidoses. The patient's problem, however, is metabolic syndrome.

C Excess immunoglobulin light chain (Bence-Jones protein) is produced in monoclonal plasma cell disorder. This may be excreted but also forms amyloid throughout the body. This patient had metabolic syndrome, not cancer.

D Mutated lysozyme can form amyloid in lens and kidneys, leading to keratoconjunctivitis sicca, xerostomia, and progres-

sive nephropathy. The patient's problem, however, is metabolic syndrome.

E Crystallin αA (and αB) are small heat shock proteins that keep proteins soluble in the eye lens, preventing cataracts. High blood sugar leads to glycation of these proteins, and they then precipitate as amyloid. This causes about half of the $45 \times - 10^6$ cases of blindness per year worldwide. The patient's death, however, was not related to this.

50. C The warfarin analog inhibits vitamin K epoxide reductase and prevents recycling of vitamin K. That prevents the introduction of γ-carboxyglutamate (Gla) into several blood-clotting factors and some other Ca-dependent proteins. Note that because of the long biological half-life of super-warfarins, treatment must continue for several months.

A Deficiency of retinoids (vitamin A, retinol and retinal) leads to night blindness, photophobia, and xerophthalmia.

B Deficiency of cholecalciferol (vitamin D) leads in severe cases to rickets and osteomalacia and in milder ones to immune problems.

D Tocopherol (vitamin E) deficiency leads to hemolysis, skin problems, and nutritional muscular dystrophy.

E Ascorbic acid (Vitamin C) deficiency leads to swollen, bleeding gums, loose teeth, pinpoint hemorrhages around hair follicles (petechiae), gums, nails, soreness and stiffness of joints & lower extremities, slow wound healing, anemia and fatigue.

51. C-The patient is suffering from pellagra ("the four D's": diarrhea, dermatitis, dementia, death). Corn contains plenty of niacin, but in a bound form unavailable to humans unless the corn is nixtamalized (treated with alkali). This leads to pellagra.

A Thiamine deficiency would lead to beriberi.

B Ascorbate deficiency would lead to scurvy.

D Folate deficiency would lead to megaloblastic anemia.

E Cobalamin deficiency would lead to pernicious anemia.

52. B The infant has scurvy (also called Barlow disease), caused by a deficiency in vitamin C. Vitamin C is a cofactor for hydroxylases, such as prolyl hydroxylase and lysyl hydroxylase, which hydroxylate collagen at proline and lysine residues, respectively. These hydroxylation reactions are essential for collagen's structural integrity and proper function in connective tissue and blood vessels.

A γ-Carboxylase is a key enzyme found in the coagulation cascade and requires adequate levels of vitamin K to function correctly. Although a deficiency in this vitamin can cause several of the observed symptoms, including petechiae and ecchymoses, it can be ruled out here because it is not water soluble.

C Serine hydroxymethyltransferase is an important enzyme found in one-carbon metabolic pathways. It simultaneously converts serine to glycine and tetrahydrofolate to 5,10-methylene tetrahydrofolate. A deficiency in this water-soluble vitamin can lead to folate deficiency anemia, a symptom of which can be irritability. Even with adequate dietary intake of folic acid, it is possible to have a deficiency if there is a defect in the enzyme homocysteine methyltransferase or a deficiency in vitamin B_{12} When either of these situations arises, folate gets shunted to methyl tetrahydrofolate and is effectively trapped there in an unusable state.

D Lysyl oxidase is an important enzyme used in the stabilization of collagen. It converts lysine or hydroxylysine to reactive intermediates that allow fibril cross-linking to occur and requires copper as a cofactor. A deficiency in this enzyme can lead to lathyrism, with symptoms including poor bone formation and strength.

E Glycogen phosphorylase requires pyridoxal phosphate, a derivative of the water-soluble vitamin pyridoxine (vitamin B_6) and is involved in the rate-limiting step of glycogen degradation. Mutations in this enzyme have been associated with the glycogen storage disorders: McArdle disease (muscle isoform) and Hers disease (liver isoform). Whereas McArdle disease can often cause muscle weakness and myalgia as a consequence of low glucose levels in the muscles, it has not been associated with, nor should it be expected to be, a cause of the other symptoms in this patient.

53. A Destruction of vitamin B_1 by thiaminase led to the typical signs of (in this case, dry) beriberi. Remember that there is also a wet form with edema and congestive heart failure. Incidentally, nardoo also contains a thiaminase, which unlike that contained in seafood is heat resistant and hence cannot be destroyed by cooking. Aborigines soak the sporocarps in water to remove the thiaminase; the water is then consumed well after the meal, when the thiamine in the diet has been absorbed. That way, water-soluble vitamins and minerals of the sporocarps are not wasted.

B Pellagra is caused by a deficiency of niacin and characterized by the "4Ds": diarrhea, dermatitis, dementia, and death. The dermatitis is limited to sun-exposed parts of the body (Casal necklace, named after the Spanish physician who first described the disease in the Western medical literature). Pellagra is derived from the Italian pelle agra, "rough skin."

C Scurvy is a vitamin C (ascorbate) deficiency characterized by weak connective tissue leading to petechia, bleeding gums, and lost teeth, combined with apathy. It occurred mainly on long sea voyages, where sailors had no access to fresh produce.

D Rickets is caused by a deficiency in vitamin D (calcitriol) and leads to disturbances in calcium and phosphate equilibrium. In children, this results in weak long bones that bend under the weight of the patient and in a small rib cage that crowds inner organs (pigeon breast). In adults, the results are osteoporosis and osteomalacia. Because of the paracrine functions of calcitriol in the immune system, there is also an increased sensitivity to infections and cancer.

E Pernicious anemia is caused by an autoimmune gastritis, which prevents the uptake of vitamin B_{12} (cobalamin). The result is a progressive megaloblastic anemia that leads to death unless treated.

54. A The patient was suffering from Conn syndrome, and his aldosterone-secreting adrenal adenoma was responsible for the high blood pressure, hypokalemia, and high K+ excretion in urine. Treating him for primary hypertension 2 weeks prior to his current condition was a dangerous error. His hypokalemia worsened and caused a bout of rhabdomyolysis. Alcohol-induced dehydration may have been a contributing factor.

B Cushing syndrome is caused by high levels of cortisol, adrenocorticotropic hormone (ACTH), or corticotropin-releasing hormone (CRH). This patient, on the other hand, had elevated aldosterone and aldosterone:renin activity ratio.

C Addison disease (chronic primary adrenocortical insufficiency) is characterized by reduced concentrations of adrenal

hormones. This patient had elevated aldosterone and aldosterone:renin activity ratio.

D Liddle syndrome is a rare, autosomal dominant mutation in the epithelial sodium channel (ENaC) in the kidney, which prevents the ubiquitination and destruction of this protein. This leads to increased sodium reabsorption and hypokalemia, resulting in high blood pressure. In industrialized countries, this should be detected in routine childhood exams, not in a 55-year-old.

E Congenital adrenal hyperplasia is caused by one of several autosomal recessive mutations in enzymes involved in steroid synthesis from cholesterol, most commonly 21-hydroxylase. Genetically female patients are born with ambiguous genitalia and show masculinization. There can also be salt-wasting and dehydration. The disease is usually diagnosed in newborn screening, not in a 55-year-old man.

55. C The compounds that comprise the vitamin E family, γ- and α-tocopherol, contain long hydrophobic tails that promote insertion into cellular membranes. Here they function as antioxidants, scavenging free radicals, including the reactive oxygen species (ROS) often formed as by-products of the electron transport chain, and protecting cellular components (e.g., polyunsaturated fatty acids) from unregulated, noncatalyzed oxidation.

A Vitamin A (retinol) is essential for vision; its aldehyde form (retinal) is a component of the pigments that comprise the rod and cone cells. Although vitamin A is not an antioxidant that protects polyunsaturated fatty acids from oxidative damage, its provitamin form, β-carotene, serves as a general antioxidant.

B Vitamin D (cholecalciferol, D_3) is the inactive form of the vitamin. It must undergo two hydroxylation reactions to become fully active (calcitriol). Neither the active nor the inactive form of vitamin D is an antioxidant. Calcitriol is a nuclear hormone that controls the absorption and metabolism of Ca^{2+} and PO_4^{3-}.

D Vitamin K (phylloquinone) is stored in both liver and fat tissues and is an essential cofactor for the synthesis of prothrombin and several clotting factors (e.g., II, VI, IX, and X). It is not considered an antioxidant.

56. D A deficit of 3,500 kcal results in the loss of 1 lb of body weight. The loss of 2 lb requires a cumulative deficit of 7,000 kcal during the week.

A If caloric intake exceeds total energy expenditure, one would expect an increase in weight rather than a decrease.

B A difference between energy expenditure and total caloric intake of 3,500 kcal would account for a weight loss of only 1 lb.

C An increase in the amount of exercise for the week (i.e., increasing PAL) would cause an increase in the BMR.

E Although an increase in her BMR is expected due to an increase in the amount of exercise, the exercise would also effectively raise her PAL.

57. D Transferrin is a glycoprotein responsible for the delivery of ferric iron from absorption centers in the body, namely, the duodenum and macrophages, to all other tissues. It is predominantly used to transport ferric ions to the bone marrow for either storage or use in the synthesis of hemoglobin.

A Ferritin is a protein complex that is used to store iron in the ferric (Fe^{3+}) state. Serum ferritin levels are indicative of the amount of iron stored in the body.

B Lactoferrin is a member of the transferrin family of iron transport proteins. It is present in milk, plasma, neutrophils, and nearly every exocrine secretion (e.g., tears, saliva, gall, and pancreas).

C Ceruloplasmin (ferroxidase) oxidizes Fe^{2+} to Fe^{3+} but does not carry iron.

E Hemosiderin is a poorly characterized iron storage protein formed from the proteolysis of ferritin. It is most commonly found in macrophages, with high levels often seen following a hemorrhagic event.

58. D Pantothenic acid is used to make CoA and the acyl-carrier protein (ACP) of fatty acid synthase.

A Pyruvate carboxylase requires biotin as cofactor, not pantothenic acid.

B Acyl CoA dehydrogenases (for which there are versions for short, medium, long, and very long chain fatty acids) contain flavin adenine dinucleotide (FAD) as a prosthetic group, which is derived from riboflavin, not pantothenic acid.

C Malate dehydrogenase requires NAD^+ as cofactor. NAD^+ is derived from nicotinamide (niacin), not pantothenic acid.

E Complex III requires cytochrome b. All cytochromes have iron in their active center, either as heme or as an Fe-S center. They are involved in redox reactions, transferring electrons to and from that iron.

59. B Amino acids that cannot be synthesized in the body, or not synthesized in adequate quantity, are considered essential and must be obtained through the diet. The carbon skeletons are critical; amino groups can usually be added by transamination.

A Aminotransferases (transaminases) are enzymes that catalyze the transfer of the α-amino group from an amino acid to an α-keto acid. These enzymes are important in the biosynthesis of several amino acids, as well as in their catabolism. The two most important aminotransferases are alanine aminotransferase (which transfers its amino group from alanine to α-ketoglutarate, thus forming pyruvate and glutamate) and aspartate aminotransferase (which transfers an amino group from glutamate to oxaloacetate, thus forming α-ketoglutarate and aspartate). The only two amino acids that do not serve as substrates for aminotransferases are lysine and threonine.

C The 10 essential amino acids are also found in plant proteins.

D Many amino acids, both essential and nonessential, have important roles in metabolism. Examples of these include acetyl CoA (produced from alanine, by way of pyruvate) and several intermediates in the tricarboxylic acid (TCA) cycle (e.g., α-ketoglutarate is produced from glutamate; oxaloacetate is produced from aspartate) or the urea cycle (fumarate is produced from aspartate).

E Although not every carbon of each amino acid will end up as carbon dioxide (CO_2), all amino acids can be catabolized and eliminated.

60. E Although CO is a competitive inhibitor of oxygen binding, this is not the primary reason for its toxicity. When CO binds to one or more sites in hemoglobin, the latter shifts to the relaxed configuration. This change in conformation causes the remaining sites to bind oxygen with higher affinity, shifting the O_2-hemoglobin dissociation curve to the left, thus preventing oxygen from being properly delivered to the tissues. Consequently, even small amounts of CO in the blood can cause toxic effects. Other toxic effects of CO include binding to myoglobin and the inhibition of cytochrome-c oxidase activity of the mitochondrial electron transport chain.

A Although CO competes with oxygen for the heme-binding site and binds roughly 25,000 times more strongly (in an isolated system), the oxygen-binding capacity of hemoglobin is not significantly reduced. Under physiological conditions, the heme-CO bond is not able to assume its preferred perpendicular orientation, causing the affinity to drop to just ~200 times that of heme O_2.

B BPG binds to deoxyhemoglobin and stabilizes the taut confirmation, effectively shifting the O_2-haemoglobin dissociation curve to the right and decreasing oxygen affinity. The binding of CO does not directly affect the binding of BPG; however, chronic exposure to low levels of CO (e.g., cigarette smoking) will increase levels of BPG. This presumably counteracts the left shift of the O_2-hemoglobin dissociation curve caused by the binding of CO.

C Although the ferrous iron found in hemoglobin can be oxidized to the ferric state under times of oxidative stress (e.g., methemoglobinemia), the binding of CO or other competitive inhibitors, such as cyanide, sulfur monoxide, and nitric oxide, does not induce a change in iron's oxidation state. Protective enzymes such as cytochrome-b_5 reductase (methemoglobin reductase) are able to reverse spontaneous oxidation when it does occur.

D CO causes an increase of O_2 affinity. Factors that decrease affinity are those that shift the O_2-hemoglobin dissociation curve to the right, such as increasing body temperature, CO_2 levels, and BPG concentration, or decreasing pH (acidosis).

61. D K_m is the substrate concentration that gives a rate equal to one-half of V_{max}.

A K_m and V_{max} are measured in the absence of inhibitors. The concentration of an inhibitor that leads to 50% inhibition is the IC_{50}.

B The reaction velocity at saturating (i.e., infinite) substrate concentration is V_{max}.

C K_m is the substrate concentration at which the reaction velocity is half maximal, not the velocity at this concentration.

E K_m is the substrate concentration at which the reaction velocity is half maximal. At this substrate concentration, one half of the enzyme molecules contain bound substrate.

62. E Arachidonic acid upon excision and release from membrane phospholipids by phospholipase A_2 is converted into various eicosanoids (prostaglandins, thromboxanes, and leukotrienes) by the action of cyclooxygenases and lipoxygenases.

A Desmolase is cytochrome p450 side chain cleavage enzyme essential for steroid hormone biosynthesis.

B Ligand stimulated G_q signaling causes phospholipase C to cleave inositol 4, 5-bisphosphate (PIP_2) into IP_3 and diacylglycerol (DAG).

C, D Arachidonic acid is converted into eicosanoids with the aid of the two key enzymes prostaglandin synthase (cyclooxygenase 1 and 2) and lipoxygenase.

63. B Ala looks very much like Ser, except that the OH-group that makes Ser reactive is replaced by hydrogen. Thus, it forms a perfect control in this situation.

A Thr has almost the same structure as Ser; its side chain is just one carbon longer. Both Ser and Thr have an OH group. Because of this, replacing Ser with Thr may well result in a working enzyme. This would lead you to the possibly erroneous conclusion that the Ser is unimportant.

C Of all amino acids, Trp is the bulkiest. Thus, there is a high likelihood that it disrupts the secondary and tertiary structure of the enzyme because it simply does not fit in. It would then be impossible to tell whether the inactivity of the mutant enzyme is due to the lack of the catalytic Ser or the disruption of the enzyme's structure.

D This would replace a polar amino acid (Ser) with a negatively charged one (Glu), with unpredictable effects for enzyme structure. It would then be impossible to tell whether the inactivity of the mutant enzyme is due to the lack of the catalytic Ser or the disruption of the enzyme's structure.

E This would replace a polar amino acid (Ser) with a positively charged one (His), with unpredictable effects for enzyme structure. It would then be impossible to tell whether the inactivity of the mutant enzyme is due to the lack of the catalytic Ser or the disruption of the enzyme's structure.

64. C *H. pylori*-associated gastritis, due to an infection of the antral mucosa, results in an increase in the release of gastrin (by G cells of the antral mucosa), which stimulates the secretion of acid by the parietal cells of the stomach. The D cells of the antral mucosa normally release somatostatin which acts to inhibit gastrin and acid release.

A Release of acid would further potentiate the effects of *H. pylori*.

B Pepsinogen does not counter the effects of gastrin release and acid secretion. Instead, pepsinogen benefits from the acidic environment of the stomach that allows it to cleave itself into active pepsin.

D Cholecystokinin causes the release of pancreatic enzymes but does not inhibit, nor help neutralize, gastric acid secretion.

E Trypsinogen does not counter the effects of gastrin release. Trypsinogen is synthesized by the pancreas and released into the duodenum where it is cleaved into Trypsin, a gastrointestinal protease.

65. D Retinoic acid, a biologically active form of Vitamin A regulates key processes such as inhibition of cell proliferation, differentiation, apoptosis, shaping of the embryo, and organogenesis and has the mechanism of intracellular signaling.

A Thiamine is a component of thiamine pyrophosphate (TPP), a coenzyme that functions as a carrier of an activated aldehyde group formed from the decarboxylation of α-keto acids. The most notable enzymes that require TPP are the pyruvate dehydrogenase and α-ketoglutarate dehydrogenase complexes.

B Riboflavin is a part of flavin mononucleotide (FMN) and flavin adenine dinucleotide (FAD). These compounds play important roles in the redox chemistry of the electron transport chain and are cofactors in vitamin-activating enzymes.

FAD has additional roles in the redox chemistry of the enzymes acetyl CoA dehydrogenase and retinal dehydrogenase.

C Ascorbic acid is utilized by prolyl hydroxylase and lysyl hydroxylase, enzymes that catalyze the hydroxylation of collagen.

E Niacin is part of nicotinamide adenine dinucleotide (NAD), which serves as an electron carrier or as a reducing agent, when phosphorylated.

66. C Sialic acid (neuraminic acid) is a common moiety often found at the termini of the oligosaccharide side chains of complex glycoproteins and gangliosides.

A Sialic acids are found in all animal tissues and many species of plants, fungi, yeast, and bacteria.

B Heparin is a highly sulfated glycosaminoglycan. The major carbohydrates found in heparin are sulfated derivatives of glucuronic acid and glucosamine.

D Although a few sialic acid derivatives are technically amino acids, conventional nomenclature does not include an ε-carbon. This nomenclature is typically used for α-amino acids.

E Sialic acid is a product of the action of sialidase on gangliosides.

67. D l-Iduronic acid is found in humans only in the glycosaminoglycans heparin, heparan sulfate, and dermatan sulfate.

A *N*-Acetylglucosamine is a component of the carbohydrate domain of many glycoproteins and is typically the carbohydrate that connects to asparagine in *N*-linked glycoproteins.

B *N*-Acetylgalactosamine is typically the carbohydrate that connects to serine or threonine in *O*-glycosylated proteins. It is also found as the terminal carbohydrate in the blood group A antigen.

C Sialic acids are found in numerous glycoproteins, glycolipids, proteoglycans, and gangliosides.

E L-Arabinose is a five-carbon sugar produced in plants, primarily in the polymers hemicellulose and pectin.

68. A Proteins contain all the information to correctly fold up given proper conditions, so the primary structure is sufficient to produce all other levels of structure.

B A protein's secondary structure arises from the coiling and/or pleating of its primary structure into helices, β-sheets, and/or β-turns. Often, a random coil will be present to connect each of these conformations in a given protein.

C Tertiary structure is the specific three-dimensional conformation a protein takes. The interaction of elements in the secondary help determine the tertiary structure. These interactions can be hydrophobic in nature, result from the formation of disulfide and/or hydrogen bonds, or occur upon complexation of metal ions.

D A protein's quaternary structure is the arrangement of more than one tertiary structure held together by noncovalent interactions, including hydrogen bonds, salt bridges, hydrophobic interactions, or van der Waals forces.

E A domain is part of the protein that can function independently of the rest of the protein chain. Protein domains have their own three-dimensional structure and can often form an individual functional unit.

69. D If an inhibitor binds to the active site of an enzyme, it will result in competitive inhibition because substrate and inhibitor cannot bind to the same site at the same time. (Note that the reversal of that statement is not necessarily true: not all competitive inhibitors bind to the active site.) In competitive inhibition, the effects of the inhibitor can be offset by higher substrate concentrations; hence V_{max} will stay the same. However, the apparent affinity of the enzyme for the substrate decreases, so the K_m will increase.

A The V_{max} will not increase, but the K_m will.

B The V_{max} will not decrease, and the K_m will not decrease.

C The V_{max} will not decrease, and the K_m will not stay constant.

E The V_{max} will stay constant, but the K_m will not decrease.

70. B Removing the product of a reaction lowers its concentration and forces more substrate to be turned into product in order to maintain the equilibrium constant. This is an application of the Le Chatelier principle.

A Removing the substrate of a reaction would actually reduce the amount of product formed.

C Reactions proceed toward negative ΔG.

D Increasing the product's concentration would drive the reaction toward the substrate.

E Increasing the enzyme's concentration has no effect on the equilibrium; it only reduces the time required to attain it.

71. A Pepsinogen is an enzyme in the stomach and is not activated by the duodenal enteropeptidase. It autoactivates in the low pH of gastric juice.

B C D E Trypsinogen is activated by enteropeptidase and then activates the other pancreatic zymogens (Chymotrypsinogen, pro carboxypeptidase and pro elastase). In adult patients, but not in infants, autoactivation of trypsin is sufficient to cover nutritional needs; hence the spontaneous improvement with age.

72. D Hexokinase has a high affinity (low K_m) for glucose and therefore can handle glucose uptake for the liver's metabolic needs even when blood glucose concentration is moderately low. However, its turnover number k_{cat} is low, so it is not able to handle glucose quickly enough to lower blood glucose levels after a meal. That is the job of glucokinase, which has a low affinity (high K_m) but a very high k_{cat}. It therefore works only when blood glucose is high, but then it works very fast. This allows glucose to be removed from the blood quickly and stored as liver glycogen.

A Hexokinase's high affinity for glucose allows it to work well at low blood glucose concentration. However, because the turnover number k_{cat} is low, flux through this enzyme is too small to effectively control blood glucose after a meal. That is the job of glucokinase.

B The k_{cat} of hexokinase is much smaller than that of glucokinase; therefore, after a meal most of the glucose is handled by the latter.

C Glucokinase has a low affinity for glucose, much lower than that of hexokinase. However, glucokinase has a much higher k_{cat} than hexokinase and therefore will handle most of the glucose after a meal when blood glucose concentrations are high.

E Glucokinase has a low affinity and hence a high K_m for glucose (compared to hexokinase).

73. C (A, B, D, E) K_m is the substrate concentration [S] at which $v=1/2\ V_{max}$; here [S] = 1 mM, and v= 0.5 nmol/s. V_{max} must be 2×0.5/nmol/s = 1 nmol/s.

74. B (A, C, D, E) We have to rearrange the Michaelis-Menten equation $v= V_{max}$ [S]/(K_m + [S]) to $K_m = V_{max}$ [S]/ v - [S]. Substituting 1.0 mM for [S] and 3/4 V_{max} for v generates a K_m of 0.33 mM.

75. A $\Delta G^{\circ\prime}$ is negative, so the reaction is exergonic and will spontaneously progress to the right under standard conditions.

B, C, D, E Because the reaction is exergonic (because $\Delta G^{\circ\prime}$ is negative), it will progress toward the right under standard conditions.

76. E Alpha helices are tightly coiled in a right-handed manner and stabilized by hydrogen bonds between nonadjacent amino acid residues. Beta pleated sheets are composed of two or more straight (noncoiled) that associate with each other via hydrogen bonds to create a beta pleated plane. Beta pleated sheets are stabilized by hydrogen bonds between amino acid residues of neighboring strands and exists in two forms, parallel and antiparallel. Conformation change of alpha helix into beta pleated sheets thus requires reorganization of hydrogen bond. Higher order of this conformational change may lead to beta pleated sheet aggregates.

A Unfolding or other radical conformational changes that convert the enzyme to inactive forms is referred to as denaturation and is often irreversible.

B Ubiquitination is a posttranslational modification that tags proteins for degradation by the proteasome.

C Posttranslational modification is often a critical requirement for the proper functioning, regulation, trafficking, degradation, and interaction with other molecules.

D Phosphorylation can lead to inactivation of proteins. This is not due to a loss in tertiary structure, but rather is often due to the induction of a conformational change in the tertiary structure.

77. B Parallel lines in a Lineweaver-Burk plot indicate uncompetitive inhibition, which results from the inhibitor (I) binding only to the enzyme–substrate complex (ES) but not to the free enzyme (E).

A Interaction of the inhibitor with only E but not ES would result in competitive inhibition, characterized by lines intersecting on a common point on the 1/ v-axis.

C Interaction of the inhibitor with both E and ES would result in noncompetitive inhibition, characterized by all lines intersecting in a common point to the left of the 1/ v-axis.

D If there was no interaction of the inhibitor with either E or ES, there would be no inhibition, and all data would fall onto the same line, irrespective of the inhibitor concentration.

78. E Cooperative binding allows hemoglobin to deliver more oxygen to the tissues in response to relatively small changes in the partial pressure of oxygen.

A The alpha-helix found in hemoglobin is an example of protein secondary structure.

B The primary structures of hemoglobin are stabilized by disulfide bonding.

C The secondary structure of hemoglobin is stabilized by Hydrogen (H-bonding) bonding.

D Hemoglobin has a quaternary structure because it is a tetrameric protein.

79. C The sailors were suffering from scurvy because the diet on board was devoid of fresh fruits and vegetables, which are the source of vitamin C (ascorbate). The sailors "putrid gums" might have appeared spongy and bleeding, and their lack of energy manifested as 'spots of lassitude, with weakness of their knees." They would have also had petechiae (purple hemorrhagic spots on the skin) and ecchymoses (bruising). Lind discovered that lime juice could prevent the disease and would not spoil during long journeys. To this day, British servicemen are nicknamed "limeys."

A Lack of retinol (vitamin A) leads to night blindness, keratomalacia and Bitot spots, possibly leading to loss of the eye.

B Lack of niacin leads to pellagra, characterized by the four Ds: diarrhea, dermatitis, dementia, and death.

D Cholecalciferol (vitamin D) is required for calcium and phosphate metabolism and also as a paracrine hormone. Gross deficiency leads to rickets and osteomalacia. In less severe cases you see immune problems (increased incidence of cancer and autoimmune disease, preterm deliveries in pregnant women, reduced ability to fight bacterial infections such as tuberculosis), and triggering of winter metabolism, contributing to metabolic syndrome.

E Iodine deficiency would lead to goiter or even cretinism.

80. D Vitamin K (phylloquinone) is required for the successful posttranslational carboxylation of glutamic acid by the enzyme. The key step involves the conversion of vitamin K hydroquinone to the vitamin K epoxide by vitamin K epoxidase. In the process, one mole of O_2 is consumed, and a glutamate residue of the substrate protein (e.g., a clotting factor) is "activated" as a carbanion. This carbanion then proceeds to react nonenzymatically with CO_2 to form the γ-carboxylglutamate.

A Vitamin A (retinol) is essential for vision and not associated with γ-carboxylation of glutamic acid. Its aldehyde form (retinal) is a component of the visual pigments present in the rod and cone cells of the eyes. Its provitamin form (β-carotene) serves as a general antioxidant.

B The main function of the active form of vitamin D (calcitriol) is the regulation of calcium absorption and metabolism. It is not associated with the formation of γ-carboxylglutamate. Calcitriol acts primarily through nuclear receptors, regulating gene expression.

C Vitamin E functions primarily as a lipid-soluble antioxidant and is not involved in the carboxylation of glutamic acid. Vitamin E is predominantly found in cell membranes and plasma lipoproteins, where it can react with lipid peroxide radicals formed by the peroxidation of polyunsaturated fatty acids by reactive oxygen species (ROS).

E Vitamin C (ascorbate) plays a role as an antioxidant and Fe^{3+}/Cu^{3+} reducing agent whose action contributes to the function of enzymes that, for instance, catalyze the hydroxylation of proline and lysine residues in collagen.

81. B (D, E) – In an alpha helix secondary structure, the stability arises from the formation of the maximum possible number of hydrogen bonds. Hydrogen bond are formed between each carbonyl oxygen atom of a peptide bond and the hydrogen attached to the amide nitrogen of the peptide bond 3.6 amino acid residues further along the polypeptide chain.

A, C Peptide and disulfide bonds are covalent bonds.

82. B Plasma membrane is a lipid bilayer and is rich in cholesterol.

A. Cholesterol is a 27-carbon structure. It is an amphipathic compound with hydroxy functional (-OH) group.

C Cholesterol is a precursor for bile acid, steroid hormones and vitamin D and not prostaglandins.

D Cholesterol is not catabolized for energy in the body.

E It is abundant in egg yolk and not citrus fruits.

83. E Enzymes, like all catalysts, act by lowering the activation energy of a reaction, thereby reducing the time required to reach the equilibrium of a reaction. They do not change the position of the equilibrium and therefore do not change the free energy, enthalpy, and entropy of the reaction.

A Enzymes do not change the equilibrium, so the free energy of a reaction does not change.

B Enzymes do not change the equilibrium of a reaction.

C Enzymes do not change the enthalpy of a reaction.

D Entropy, or disorder of a system, is related to the number of particles (e.g., in the reaction $A \rightarrow B + C$, the number of particles increases, and so does the system's disorder) and their aggregate state (e.g., conversion of a solid substrate to gaseous products during gunpowder burning results in an increase in entropy). None of these parameters are changed by the presence of enzymes.

84. A The enzyme serine hydroxymethyltransferase catalyzes the conversion of glycine into serine and requires the folic acid derivative N^5N^{10}-methylenetetrahydrofolate as a cofactor.

B Niacin is part of nicotinamide adenine dinucleotide (NAD), which serves as an electron carrier or as a reducing agent when phosphorylated.

C Pantothenic acid is a component of coenzyme A (CoA), an important molecule that activates carbonyl groups by forming high-energy thioester bonds, and fatty acid synthase, a multifunctional enzyme that catalyzes the synthesis of fatty acids.

D Riboflavin is part of flavin mononucleotide (FMN) and flavin adenine dinucleotide (FAD). These compounds play important roles in the redox chemistry of the electron transport chain and are cofactors in vitamin-activating enzymes. FAD has additional roles in the redox chemistry of the enzymes acetyl-CoA dehydrogenase and retinal dehydrogenase.

E Ascorbic acid is utilized by prolyl hydroxylase and lysyl hydroxylase, enzymes that catalyze the hydroxylation of collagen.

85. B The shown compound is α-linolenic acid. The structure of α-linolenic acid includes an 18-carbon chain, with three conjugated *cis* double bonds starting 3 carbons away from the terminus of the carbon chain.

A Alpha-linolenic acid is one of two essential fatty acids, the other being linoleic acid (an ω-6 fatty acid). These fatty acids are required to maintain the fluidity of membranes and for synthesis of the eicosanoids. Their deficiency leads to scaly dermatitis, hair loss, and poor wound healing.

C Numerous human clinical trials have shown increased intake of α-linolenic acid significantly lowers serum triglyceride levels.

D Alpha-linolenic acid is a precursor to the formation of eicosapentanoic acid (EPA) and docosahexanoic acid (DHA), the ω-3 fatty acids that play a role in ocular health.

E The shown compound is α-linolenic acid, an essential ω-3 fatty acid shown to lower serum triglyceride levels and decrease the incidence of thrombosis. Oleic acid is a monounsaturated ω-9 fatty acid and is the most abundant fatty acid in human adipose tissue.

86. D Most notably found in milk, lactose is a disaccharide formed via condensation of galactose and glucose through a β-1,4 glycosidic linkage. The enzyme β-D-galactosidase (lactase) is required to cleave lactose into its individual subunits so that absorption can occur. Lack of this enzyme in the digestive system (alactasia) is the primary cause of lactose intolerance.

A Glycogen is the long-term energy storage polysaccharide in animals. Through the action of the enzymes glycogenin (initiation), glycogen synthase (elongation), and glucosyl (4:6) transferase (branching), it is primarily made in the liver and muscle by the polymerization of glucose. The primary chain of glycogen consists of α-1,4 linkages, whereas the branch points consist of α-1,6 linkages.

B Cellulose is found in the primary cell wall of green plants, where it serves as the main structural component of the cell. It is an unbranched glucose polymer made up of β-1,4 linkages.

C Maltose is a disaccharide of two glucose units joined by an α-1,4 glycosidic bond. It is produced by the hydrolysis of starch by the enzyme amylase and can be further hydrolyzed to glucose by maltase.

E Starch is the long-term energy storage polysaccharide in green plants. A polymer of glucose, it can exist in either linear (amylose) or branched (amylopectin) form. Like glycogen, the primary chain consists of α-1,4 linkages, whereas the branch points consist of α-1,6 linkages.

87. C Essential fatty acids are linoleic and α-linolenic acid (C18:3(Δ9,12,15)) because the introduction of double bonds beyond position Δ9 is possible for plant but not mammalian desaturases. Of these two, linoleic acid is elongated and desaturated to arachidonic acid (C20:4(Δ5,8,11,14)).

A Palmitic acid is saturated and a product of fatty acid synthase; thus, it is not essential. It cannot be converted to linoleic acid in humans and is not a precursor of prostaglandins.

B Lignoceric acid is saturated and not essential.

D Oleic acid is not essential; humans can make it by desaturating stearate. In addition, oleic acid cannot be desaturated to linoleic acid, which is the precursor for arachidonic acid and prostaglandins.

E Myristic acid is saturated and not essential.

88. D The boy has hay fever, which is mediated by histamine. Decarboxylation of histidine to histamine requires pyridoxal phosphate, which is the active form of pyridoxine (vitamin B_6).

A Riboflavin occurs in enzymes as FAD and contributes to electron transfer reactions. The mediator in question is not produced by a redox reaction.

B Niacin in the form of NAD or $NADP^+$ contributes to electron transfer reactions. The mediator in question is not produced by a redox reaction.

C Biotin, bound to a lysine in the active center of an enzyme as biocytin, is a cofactor of carboxylases. The mediator (histamine) is not produced by carboxylation.

E Ascorbate is used in our body as an antioxidant. No antioxidant is required to make the mediator (histamine).

89. C In carnosine, the imidazole nitrogen of His has a pK_a of 6.83. His is the only one of the proteinogenic amino acids that has a pK_a near neutral. Remember that buffer substances work best no more than ± 1 pH unit away from their pK_a.

A The α-amino group of His is in a peptide linkage and is not ionizable. Therefore, it does not contribute to the buffering capacity of carnosine.

B The α-carboxyl group of His has a pK_a value in the range of 1.8 to 2.8. It cannot buffer around neutral pH.

D The β-amino group has a pK_a value of approximately 10.31. It cannot buffer around neutral pH.

E The α-carboxyl group of β-Ala is in a peptide linkage and is not ionizable.

90. B (A, C, D, E) Because ethanol and methanol are both substrates of alcohol dehydrogenase, both bind to the same site. Thus, one inhibits the turnover of the other competitively. In a Lineweaver-Burk plot, this results in lines that have the same y-intercept ($1/V_{max}$) but slopes that increase with increasing inhibitor concentration.

91. B The patient is suffering from cystinosis marked by an accumulation of cystine due to a defect in cystinosin, the protein that transports cystine out of lysosomes. Cystine is formed by joining two cysteines via a disulphide bond. The patient should be treated with cysteamine, which converts cystine into a mixed disulphide that can leave the lysosome passively. The rickets is secondary to kidney damage indicated by the glucose in urine and aminoaciduria.

A The patient has cystinosis, and the accumulating substance is not the amino acid cysteine but cystine. The latter is formed by joining two cysteines via a disulphide bond.

C Homocystinuria (defective cystathionine β synthase), marked by an accumulation of homocysteine, results in mental retardation, lens dislocation, bone elongation, osteoporosis, and thrombosis.

D Gout is associated with accumulation of monosodium urate in the body fluids.

E Hypermethioninemia is a result of methionine adenosyltransferase deficiency, marked by an accumulation of methionine in the blood. This is a rare defect in amino acid metabolism that does not lead to clinical problems apart from a cabbage-like smell to the breath. Patients are usually detected serendipitously in newborn screening for homocystinuria.

References

[1] Harris M. A smoking related triad: PAD, COPD and CCF. Aust Fam Physician. 2004; 33(4):207–210

[2] Goto A, Takahashi Y, Kishimoto M, et al. Intern Med. 2009; 48(4):219–223

Part II

Membranes, Transport, and Signaling

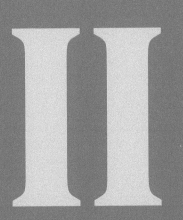

6 Membranes and Transport

6.1 Membrane Structure and Composition

6.1.1 Membrane Structure

Biological membranes are physical structures that create a protective physical barrier (called a plasma membrane) between cells and their external environments and compartmentalize organelles within cells. These membranes are composed of lipids, proteins, and carbohydrates. The primary components of membranes are phospholipids, which are amphipathic molecules that contain a hydrophilic head group and a hydrophobic tail. In membranes, phospholipids are arranged in two layers or sheets to form a lipid bilayer in the following manner (▶ Fig. 6.1):
- The hydrophilic heads face the aqueous environments outside and inside the cell and thus make up the outer and inner surfaces of cellular membranes.

- The hydrophobic tails are directed toward the interior of the membrane and thus make up the hydrophobic core of the lipid bilayer.

6.1.2 Membrane Composition

A membrane's lipid bilayer serves as the foundation in which a variety of lipids and proteins are embedded or to which they are anchored. Additionally, carbohydrate molecules are found covalently attached to some membrane lipids and proteins (▶ Fig. 6.2).

Membrane Lipids

Membranes contain three types of lipids that contribute to the structural integrity and function of the cells and organelles they enclose. These lipids fall into three categories: phospholipids, glycolipids, and cholesterol.

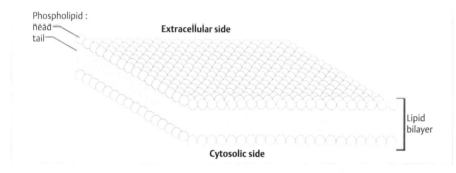

Fig. 6.1 Model of a lipid bilayer. Biological membranes are bilayers composed of amphipathic phospholipids. The polar heads (blue) of the phospholipids form the outer surface (extra-cellular side) and inner surface (cytosolic side) of the membrane, whereas the nonpolar hydrophobic tails (yellow) form the interior.

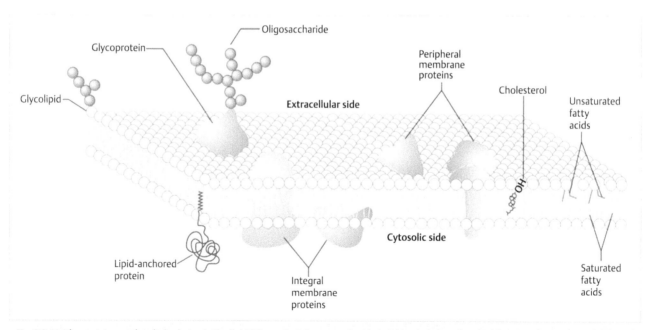

Fig. 6.2 Lipids, proteins, and carbohydrates in the lipid bilayer. Proteins are embedded within or anchored to the bilayer. Both membrane lipids and membrane proteins are frequently glycosylated (attached to carbohydrate molecules) on the extracellular side of the lipid bilayer.

Table 6.1 Location of membrane lipids

Outer sheet (faces the extracellular environment)	Inner sheet (faces the intracellular environment)
Phosphatidylcholine	Phosphatidylinositol
Sphingomyelin	Phosphatidylserine
Glycolipids	Phosphatidylethanolamine

1. **Phospholipids:** These are the most abundant types of lipids found in biological membranes. Their hydrophilic heads contain a phosphate group, and their hydrophobic tails are composed of fatty acid chains. Phospholipids are further categorized as glycerophospholipids and sphingophospholipids based on the identity of their backbone as follows:

   • Glycerophospholipids are made up of a glycerol backbone to which a polar phosphate residue (which forms the hydrophilic head group) and the two nonpolar fatty acid chains (which form the hydrophobic tails) are esterified. Esterification of the phosphate residue with amino or sugar alcohols (e.g., choline or myo-inositol) generates unique glycerophospholipids, such as phosphatidylcholine and phosphatidylinositol, which are located in different sheets of the lipid bilayer (▶ Table 6.1). The chemical structures of these lipids are depicted in **Fig 3.6**.

   • Sphingophospholipids are made up of a sphingosine backbone. Whereas glycerol is a sugar alcohol, sphingosine is an amino alcohol that contains a long unsaturated hydrocarbon chain. Attachment of a long-chain fatty acid and phosphorylcholine to sphingosine generates sphingomyelin, the most abundant lipid found in the membranes of nerve tissue. Like phosphatidylcholine, sphingomyelin is located in the outer sheet ("leaflet") of the lipid bilayer. The chemical structure of sphingomyelin is depicted in **Fig 3.6**.

2. **Glycolipids:** Like sphingophospholipids, glycolipids are generally made up of a sphingosine backbone. Unlike sphingophospholipids, however, glycolipids contain carbohydrate (oligosaccharide) residues rather than a phosphate residue. Glycolipids are found in the outer sheet of the lipid bilayer.

3. **Cholesterol:** The steroid alcohol cholesterol is embedded within the lipid bilayer, where its hydroxyl group interacts with the polar heads of neighboring membrane lipids, and its sterol ring and methyl branched chain associate with the hydrophobic tails of membrane lipids. The chemical structure of cholesterol is depicted in **Fig 3.8**.

Normal

Phosphatidylserine as a marker for apoptosis

In healthy cells, phosphatidylserine (PS) is found in the intracellular sheet of the lipid bilayer. When cells undergo apoptosis (programmed cell death), PS is displayed on the extracellular surface of the plasma membrane. This labels the dying cell for recognition and removal by phagocytes (white blood cells).

Therapeutics

Niemann-Pick disease

Niemann-Pick disease is a rare hereditary disease caused by a deficiency in sphingomyelinase, the enzyme that breaks down sphingomyelin. As a result, sphingomyelin accumulates in the lysosomes of the liver, spleen, central nervous system, and bone marrow. This autosomal recessive disorder leads to enlargement of the liver and spleen (hepatosplenomegaly), and neurologic damage that manifests as mental retardation, seizures, ataxia, and spasticity. An additional hallmark of this disease is a "cherry red spot" in the macula of the eye of these patients. Children with the type A form of this disorder rarely live past 18 months.

Membrane Proteins

Proteins found in membranes are identified by the manner in which they associate with the phospholipid bilayer.

1. **Integral proteins** are firmly embedded in the membrane and stabilized through hydrophobic interactions with membrane lipids. Integral proteins that span the entire lipid bilayer and interact with both the internal and the external environments are referred to as transmembrane proteins. Those that do not span the lipid bilayer are referred to as integral monotopic proteins.

   • Transmembrane proteins include transport proteins, ion channels, and receptors whose functions regulate the flow of certain molecules into and out of cells and receive and transmit extracellular signals to the intracellular environment.

   • Integral monotopic proteins are firmly attached to one sheet of the lipid bilayer. Some, such as carnitine palmitoyltransferase I (CPT I, see Chapter 13, section "Phase I: Transport of Long-Chain Fatty Acids into Mitochondrial Matrix via the Carnitine Shuttle" and **Fig. 13.7**), possess enzymatic activity and catalyze a variety of important biochemical reactions.

2. **Peripheral proteins** are loosely bound to the membrane surface through electrostatic interactions with lipids or other proteins (e.g., phospholipases—enzymes that cleave lipids).

3. **Lipid-anchored proteins** are so called because they are tethered to membranes via a covalent attachment to a lipid molecule. Such proteins include the small G proteins, which are anchored to the inner sheet of the bilayer, and proteins attached to the outer sheet of the bilayer through glycosylphosphatidylinositol (GPI)-anchors.

Carbohydrate Residues

Carbohydrate (oligosaccharide) molecules are found covalently attached to some membrane lipids and proteins that face the extracellular space. As such, the outer sheet of many biomembranes is covered with a carbohydrate shell called a glycocalyx due to the presence of glycolipids and glycosylated proteins (glycoproteins).

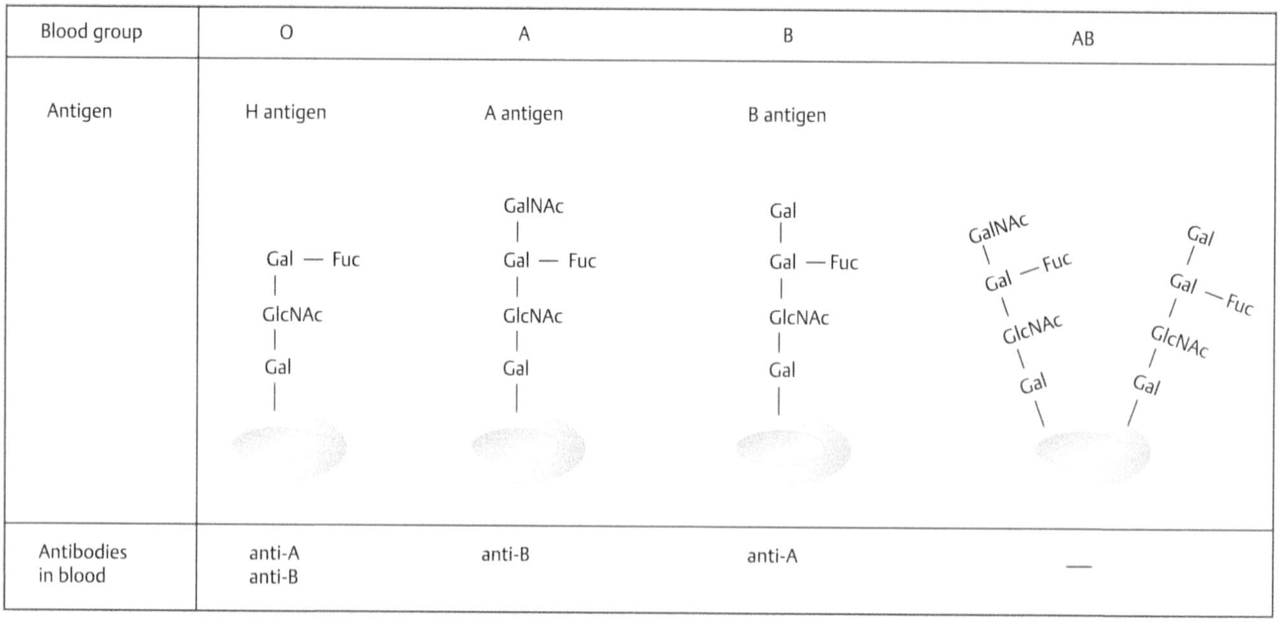

Blood group	O	A	B	AB
Antigen	H antigen	A antigen	B antigen	
	Gal — Fuc GlcNAc Gal	GalNAc Gal — Fuc GlcNAc Gal	Gal Gal — Fuc GlcNAc Gal	GalNAc Gal — Fuc GlcNAc Gal / Gal Gal — Fuc GlcNAc Gal
Antibodies in blood	anti-A anti-B	anti-B	anti-A	—

Fig. 6.3 **The ABO blood system.** The carbohydrate components of glycolipids or glycoproteins act as antigens. There are four blood groups in the ABO blood system: O, A, B, and AB. The O blood group is identified by its H antigen, which lacks both of the terminal sugar residues found in the A and B antigens. The A and B blood groups contain A and B antigens, respectively, which differ in the identity of their terminal sugar residue (galactose vs. N acetylgalactosamine). The AB blood group contains both A and B antigens. Fuc, fucose; Gal, galactose; GalNAc, N-acetyl-D-galactosamine; GlcNAc, N-acetyl-D-glucosamine.

The glycocalyx has three key functions:
1. **Protection:** The carbohydrate shell protects membrane components from mechanical injury or premature enzymatic degradation.
2. **Cell adhesion:** The glycocalyx enables cells to make stable contacts with other cells, an important function for tissue formation and fertilization.
3. **Cell identification:** The glycocalyx allows the body to differentiate its own healthy cells from foreign or diseased cells. For instance, the glycocalyces of red blood cells of individuals with A, B, AB, or O blood types differ in the carbohydrate composition of their oligosaccharide residues (▶ Fig. 6.3).

Normal

ABO blood group system

Blood transfusion routinely involves the transfer of packed red blood cells from a donor to a recipient. Because the plasma of the recipient may contain antibodies to one or more ABO (and Rh) antigens, it is important to cross-match the donor and recipient blood to ensure that the donor blood cells do not react with the recipient plasma. An incompatible transfusion could result in acute hemolysis, renal failure, and shock. The best-case scenario is when the donor and recipient blood groups are the same. Persons with type O are considered universal donors because their erythrocytes do not express any blood group antigens. Similarly, persons with type AB are universal recipients because their plasma does not contain antibodies to either A or B antigen. Patients with type O blood can receive only type O blood because the recipient plasma contains both anti-A and anti-B antibodies and is therefore incompatible with other blood types.

Therapeutics

Rh factor and hemolytic disease of the newborn

In addition to the carbohydrate antigens of the ABO blood group, red blood cells express protein antigens called Rh factors, which also must be cross-matched for compatibility during transfusions. The Rh system is named after rhesus monkeys, which were used in the initial research on blood group typing. Although there are many Rh antigens, the term *Rh factor* applies only to the D antigen, which is inherited in an autosomal dominant fashion. Individuals that are Rh + express the D antigen on their erythrocytes, whereas those that are Rh – do not. Rh factor also plays a role in the hemolytic disease of the newborn (erythroblastosis fetalis), which occurs due to incompatibility of Rh blood types between the mother and the fetus. When the mother is Rh – and the fetus is Rh + , the mother can produce Rh antibodies during pregnancy that can cross the placental barrier and attack the fetus. The risk of the disease is much greater in subsequent pregnancies. The newborns have severe jaundice, edema, and failure of liver and spleen. The disease can be prevented by injecting the pregnant Rh– mothers at ~28 weeks of gestation with anti-RhD immunoglobulin, which destroys any fetal erythrocytes that may have crossed over into maternal circulation, before the mother's immune system is activated.

6.2 Membrane Fluidity

The ability of proteins and lipids to rotate and move laterally within the membrane is critical for their function. The relatively mobile characteristic of membrane lipids and proteins imparts a fluid-like quality to the bilayer and is often described as a fluid mosaic. Optimal membrane fluidity allows proteins and lipids to move to specific areas within the membrane to carry out their functions. However, this movement is restricted in rigid, semicrystalline membranes, and it is disordered in membranes that are too fluid. Factors such as temperature, lipid composition, and cholesterol affect membrane fluidity.

1. **Temperature:** The temperature at which membranes switch from a fluid to a rigid semicrystalline state is called the transition (or melting) temperature (T_m). At temperatures below the T_m, membrane lipid molecules tend to exhibit ordered packing, which keeps the membranes in a rigid semicrystalline state. Above the T_m, membranes become fluid. At temperatures significantly higher than the T_m, membranes become too fluid.

    Temp $> > > T_m$=too fluid
    Temp $> T_m$ = optimal fluidity
    Temp $< T_m$ = rigid, semicrystalline

2. **Lipid composition:** Lipids that contain long, saturated (zero double bonds) fatty acid chains decrease membrane fluidity. This occurs due to the tighter packing of these straight-chain lipids, which strengthens the interactions between them and thus reduces their mobility. Conversely, lipids that contain short, unsaturated (one or more double bonds) fatty acid chains increase membrane fluidity because the kinks in their fatty acid chains do not allow for tight packing between lipids.

    Saturated lipids = decreased fluidity
    Unsaturated lipids = increased fluidity

3. **Cholesterol:** Cholesterol decreases membrane fluidity by intercalating in between and thereby reducing the mobility of fatty acyl tails of membrane phospholipids. In a membrane that is too rigid due to a high content of saturated fatty acids or due to temperatures below the T_m, cholesterol increases membrane fluidity by preventing close packing of fatty acid chains. In a fluid membrane, one with a high proportion of lipids with unsaturated fatty acyl chains, cholesterol stabilizes membrane fluidity by fitting into the gaps created by the kinks in these lipid tails. It dampens large changes in fluidity that can occur at temperatures above and below the T_m.

    Cholesterol in a fluid membrane = decreased fluidity
    Cholesterol in a rigid membrane = increased fluidity

Foundations
Lipid flip-flop
Although membrane lipids and proteins can float around easily and rapidly within one sheet of a lipid bilayer, a flip-fop of membrane proteins between the two sheets of a membrane does not occur. However, the flip-fop of certain lipids does occur, but quite slowly, and appears to require special translocators called flippases.

Normal
Alterations in membrane lipid content in response to changes in temperature
In response to certain conditions (e.g., cold temperatures), cells alter the relative amounts of certain lipids in their cell membranes to maintain an optimal fluid state. For instance, when cells are exposed to temperatures below the T_m, they respond by increasing the amounts of lipids containing unsaturated fatty acids in the cell membrane. This lowers the T_m and allows the membrane to remain fluid at a lower temperature, instead of transitioning to a rigid semicrystalline state.

Normal
Spur cell anemia
Spur cell anemia—a type of hemolytic anemia—is characterized by elevated levels of cholesterol in the erythrocyte membrane, which decrease the fluidity and flexibility of the membranes. Consequently, these erythrocyte membranes break/lyse as they pass through the capillaries of the spleen (where red blood cells are stored). Spur cell anemia is associated with abetalipoproteinemia and with advanced stages of alcoholic cirrhosis.

6.3 Passive and Active Membrane Transport

Membranes regulate the flow of biomolecules into and out of cells. Some biomolecules diffuse directly through membranes, whereas others require the assistance of proteins embedded within the membrane. The transport of molecules from one side of a membrane to the other side is divided into two categories based on their dependence on energy.

1. **Passive transport** is an energy-independent mechanism that moves molecules down their concentration gradient ("downhill") from areas of high concentration to those of low concentration.
2. **Active transport** is an energy-dependent mechanism that moves molecules against their concentration gradient ("uphill") from areas of low concentration to regions of high concentration.

6.3.1 Passive Transport

The energy-independent movement of molecules down their concentration gradient can occur unaided (simple diffusion) or with the assistance (facilitated diffusion) of transmembrane proteins (▶ Fig. 6.4).

1. Simple diffusion: Molecules that are small, nonpolar and uncharged polar, freely diffuse across membranes via simple diffusion. Molecules diffuse faster down a steep concentration gradient.
2. Facilitated diffusion: Molecules that are large and charged and ions cross membranes with the help of transmembrane proteins that function as channels and transporters. As a result, the rate at which a molecule is transported across a membrane is greatly increased.

Simple diffusion
(movement from high to low concentration; energy-independent)

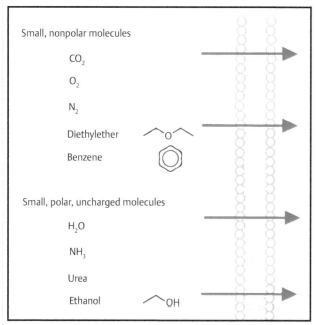

Facilitated diffusion
(movement from high to low concentration; energy-independent)

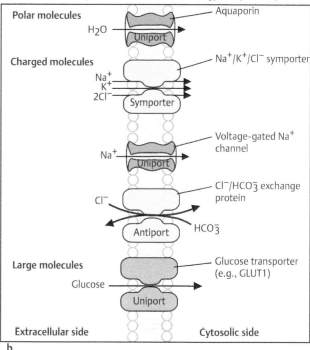

Fig. 6.4 Passive transport: Simple and facilitated diffusion. Passive transport, the energy-independent movement of molecules from an area of high concentration to one of lower concentration, occurs with and without the involvement of proteins. (**a**) Only small, nonpolar, and small uncharged polar molecules pass through the lipid bilayer without help (simple diffusion). (**b**) Channel proteins and transporters are required for polar and charged molecules to move across the lipid bilayer (facilitated diffusion). Transporters bind the transported molecule and undergo a conformational change to issue it across the membrane. Uniport is the unilateral downhill movement of a molecule across a channel or transporter. Symport involves the concurrent transport of two or more different types of molecules in the same direction. Antiport involves the concurrent transport of two different types of molecules in opposite directions. HCO_3^-, bicarbonate.

- Channels contain a core of polar residues that allow charged and polar molecules (e.g., ions and water) to move across membranes rapidly. Transporters, on the other hand, bind to a molecule on one side of the membrane and undergo a conformational change to issue the molecule to the other side of the membrane. The conformational changes are induced either by binding of the transported molecule or by hydrolysis of ATP.
- Channels and transporters are further characterized by the direction and number of the molecules they transport. A uniporter transports one substance in one direction (downhill). A cotransporter transports two different substances in the same direction (symporter) or opposite directions (antiporter).
- Channels and transporters are reversible, and because they are limited in number, they are saturable.

Foundations

Defective amino acid transporter leads to cystinuria

Cystinuria is an autosomal recessive disease caused by a defect in the transport system responsible for the uptake of the dimeric amino acid cystinex, and dibasic amino acids Arg, Lys, and ornithine. (Cystine is formed when two cysteines are oxidized and linked by a disulfide bond.) This results in the formation of cystine crystals or stones in the kidneys (renal calculi), which can

be identified via a positive nitroprusside test. Patients with this condition present with renal colic (abdominal pain that comes in waves and is linked to kidney stones).

Therapeutics

Defective amino acid transporter leads to Hartnup disease

Hartnup disease is an autosomal recessive disorder caused by a defect in a transporter for nonpolar or neutral amino acids (e.g., tryptophan), which is primarily found in the kidneys and intestine. It manifests in infancy as failure to thrive, nystagmus (abnormally rapid and repetitive eye movement), intermittent ataxia (lack of muscle coordination), tremor, and photosensitivity.

Foundations

Ligand-gated ion channels

Ligand-gated ion channels admit specific ions in a manner regulated by the opening/closing of the channel. Binding of a ligand (e.g., neurotransmitters or hormones) to the ion channel opens it, allowing the rapid transport of ions across the membrane down their concentration gradient. Dissociation of the neurotransmitter or hormone from the channel closes it.

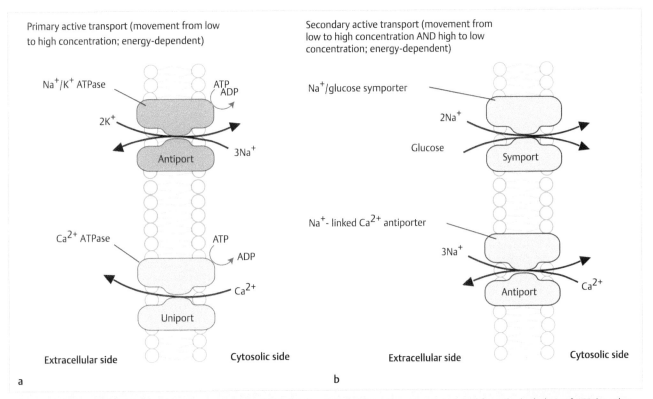

Primary active transport (movement from low to high concentration; energy-dependent)

Na$^+$/K$^+$ ATPase

ATP ADP

2K$^+$

Antiport

3Na$^+$

Ca^{2+} ATPase

ATP

ADP

Ca^{2+}

Uniport

Extracellular side   Cytosolic side

a

Secondary active transport (movement from low to high concentration AND high to low concentration; energy-dependent)

Na$^+$/glucose symporter

2Na$^+$

Glucose

Symport

Na$^+$- linked Ca^{2+} antiporter

3Na$^+$

Antiport

Ca^{2+}

Extracellular side   Cytosolic side

b

II

Fig. 6.5 Primary active and secondary active transport. Primary active transport uses the energy generated from the hydrolysis of ATP (or other energy-rich metabolites) to move molecules against their concentration gradient. (a) The Na$^+$/K + ATPase moves Na$^+$ and K + ions against their concentration gradient via a conformational change induced by ATP hydrolysis. The net movement of three Na$^+$ out of the cell in exchange for two K + ions causes an accumulation of positive charge on the outer surface of the membrane. (b) The transport of Na$^+$ (via the sodium-glucose transporter 1) down its concentration gradient into cells provides the energy needed to simultaneously transport a different molecule (e.g., glucose) in the same direction but against its concentration gradient.

Foundations

Voltage-gated ion channels

Voltage-gated ion channels open/close in response to changes in the membrane potential—the electrical voltage across the lipid bilayer that is created by the large excess of negative charge inside the cell. Depolarization (an increase in membrane potential due to an influx of positively charged ions) triggers the opening of voltage-gated ion channels, permitting specific ions to cross the lipid bilayer down their concentration gradient. These types of channels are found in excitable cells such as neurons.

6.3.2 Active Transport

Primary active transport. Primary active transport is the protein-assisted, energy-dependent movement of molecules against their concentration gradient (▶ Fig. 6.5a). This process is mediated by transmembrane protein transporters, which bind to a specific molecule on one side of the bilayer. Chemical energy (e.g., ATP) is used to induce a conformational change in the transporter, allowing the molecule to be released on the other side of the membrane. Two examples of transporters involved in primary active transport are the Na$^+$/K$^+$ ATPase and the Ca^{2+} ATPase.

- **Na$^+$/K$^+$ ATPase:** Found in the plasma membrane of all cells, this antiporter is responsible for maintaining high intracellular concentrations of K$^+$ and low intracellular concentrations of Na$^+$ relative to the extracellular

environment. The Na$^+$/K$^+$ ATPase couples the hydrolysis of one ATP with the movement of two K$^+$ ions into and three Na$^+$ ions out of the cell. This helps in the maintenance of normal membrane potential.

- **Ca^{2+} ATPase:** This transporter is responsible for maintaining low cytoplasmic Ca^{2+} levels. It is found in the plasma membrane of most cells and the sarcoplasmic reticulum (SR) of muscle cells. The Ca^{2+} ATPase rapidly removes Ca^{2+} from the cytoplasm, allowing muscles to relax. This ATPase either expels Ca^{2+} into the extracellular environment or transports it into the SR for storage.

Secondary active transport: Secondary active transport also moves molecules (e.g., glucose or amino acids) against their concentration gradient in an energy-dependent, protein-assisted manner. However, the required energy is not supplied by the hydrolysis of ATP but rather by the facilitated diffusion of a different molecule (e.g., Na$^+$ or H$^+$) down its concentration gradient (▶ Fig. 6.5b). This gradient is typically established and maintained by primary active transport mechanisms. Two examples of transporters involved in secondary active transport are the sodium-glucose transporter 1 (SGLT1) and the Na$^+$- linked Ca^{2+} antiporter.

- **Sodium-glucose transporter 1:** The unidirectional movement of both Na$^+$ and glucose into the epithelial cells that line the small intestine is mediated by SGLT1. The transport of two Na$^+$ ions downhill provides the energy needed to transport one glucose molecule uphill. The

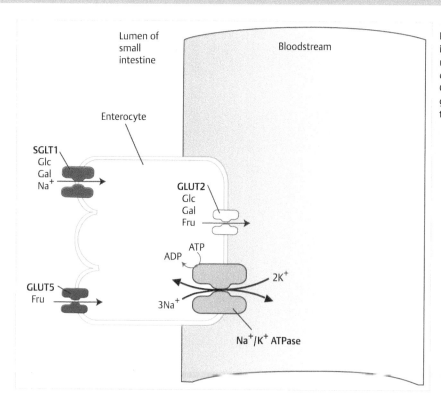

Fig. 6.6 Glucose transport from lumen of intestines to blood. The uptake of dietary monosaccharides is mediated by facilitated diffusion via glucose transporter 2 (GLUT2) and GLUT5, secondary active transport via sodium-glucose transporter 1 (SGLT1), and primary active transport via Na$^+$/K$^+$ ATPase.

movement of Na$^+$ down its concentration gradient is possible because of the low intracellular Na$^+$ levels that are maintained by the Na$^+$/K$^+$ ATPase pump.
- **Na$^+$- linked Ca^{2+} antiporter (Na$^+$- Ca^{2+} exchanger):** The Na$^+$-Ca^{2+} exchanger is an antiporter that, similar to the Ca^{2+} ATPase pump, maintains low levels of cytosolic Ca^{2+}. It imports three Na$^+$ ions down their concentration gradient, generating the energy needed to simultaneously export one Ca^{2+} ion.

6.3.3 Transport Mechanisms in the Uptake of Dietary Monosaccharides

Monosaccharides derived from the digestion of polysaccharides such as starch and disaccharides such as sucrose and lactose in the diet need to be transported from the intestinal lumen, across the enterocyte, into the bloodstream. This process is accomplished by utilizing both facilitated diffusion and active transport mechanisms, as follows (▶ Fig. 6.6):
- **D**-Glucose and D-galactose enter the intestinal epithelial cells from the lumen along with Na$^+$ by secondary active transport mediated by SGLT1 in the apical surface.
- D-Glucose and D-galactose are transported across the cell's basal surface into the bloodstream by facilitated diffusion using glucose transporter 2 (GLUT2).
- Fructose, on the other hand, is transported only by facilitated diffusion down its concentration gradient, using GLUT5 transporters on the apical side and GLUT2 transporters on the basal side of the enterocyte.
- The Na$^+$ transported in by SGLT1 is delivered to the bloodstream using a primary active transport process mediated by Na$^+$/K$^+$ ATPase in the basolateral membrane.

Therapeutics
Cardiotonic drugs

Cardiac glycosides, like ouabain and the more lipophilic digoxin, act as cardiotonic (contraction-inducing) drugs by virtue of their inhibition of the Na$^+$/K$^+$ ATPase pump on cardiac myocyte plasma membranes. Such inhibition leads to an increase in intracellular Na$^+$ and a secondary increase in intracellular Ca^{2+} (due to a slowing down of the Na$^+$/Ca^{2+} exchanger). Increased sarcoplasmic Ca^{2+} results in a stronger contraction of heart muscle with each action potential.

Therapeutics
Defective Cl$^-$ transport leads to cystic fibrosis

Cystic fibrosis (CF) is an autosomal recessive disorder affecting mainly the lungs, salivary glands, pancreas, intestine, and reproductive tract. Thick mucus secretions in the lungs interfere with breathing and lead to secondary microbial infections. CF causes scarring (fibrosis) and cysts in the pancreas. The disease is the result of mutations in the CF transmembrane conductance regulator (*CFTR*) gene, the most common being a deletion of three nucleotides in the coding region resulting in a loss of a phenylalanine residue at position 508 (ΔF^{508}) in the protein. The CFTR protein is an ion channel that mediates active transport of Cl$^-$ ions from inside cells to outside in the airways using the energy of hydrolysis of ATP. In the sweat ducts, CFTR normally mediates the reuptake of Cl$^-$ into the cells. Na$^+$ then flows into airway cells due to the increased negative electric potential and is followed by water. In CF, a defective CFTR prevents the uptake of Cl$^-$ and as a result leads to very high levels of salt in the sweat. Pancreatic secretion of HCO$_3^-$ is also mediated by CFTR and is defective leading to pancreatic insufficiency in CF patients.

7 Cell Signaling

7.1 Overview

All living cells respond to their environment through a set of mechanisms known as cell signaling. This ability is the basis for normal cellular homeostasis, cell growth, division, and differentiation. Errors in cell signaling contribute to the development of diseases such as cancer, autoimmunity, and diabetes. Hence a clear understanding of cell signaling is vital to effectively treating such diseases. Cell signaling operates through an intricate network of biochemical pathways. However, the following four steps are common to all signaling pathways (▶ Fig. 7.1):

• In response to a stimulus, a signaling cell synthesizes and secretes a signaling molecule. These are typically small lipid-soluble and water-soluble molecules (e.g., hormones and growth factors).
• The signaling molecule is transported to the target cell, where it binds to a specific receptor protein either at cell surface or inside the cell.
• The signaling molecule–receptor complex activates or inhibits cellular pathways in the target cell that control cellular functions such as metabolism and gene expression.
• The signal is terminated by removal of the signaling molecule or receptor, or inactivation of the signaling events triggered by the signaling molecule–receptor complex.

7.2 Types of Signaling

There are four types of cell signaling mechanisms (▶ Fig. 7.2):

1. **In endocrine signaling**, the molecule secreted by the signaling cell is transported to the target cell via the bloodstream. For instance, epinephrine, a hormone released by the adrenal medulla, acts on heart muscle to increase the heart rate.
2. **In paracrine signaling**, the molecule released by the signaling cells diffuses to neighboring target cells of a different cell type. For instance, testosterone, produced in Leydig cells of the testis, induces spermatogenesis by acting on Sertoli cells and germ cells in neighboring seminiferous tubules.
3. **In autocrine signaling**, the secreting cells themselves express cell surface receptors for the signaling molecule. Autocrine loops tend to occur with chemokines (small signaling proteins such as interleukins). For instance, interleukin-1, produced by T-lymphocytes, acts to promote their own replication and is important for the immune response.

4. **In juxtacrine signaling**, the molecule stays attached to the signaling cell and binds to a receptor on an adjacent target cell, establishing physical contact between the two cells. For instance, membrane-bound heparin-binding epidermal growth factor–like growth factor (HB-EGF), which binds to the EGF receptors of neighboring cells, is involved in wound healing.

7.3 Types of Signaling Molecules and Their Receptors

Signaling molecules are classified as either lipophilic or hydrophilic based on their solubility properties. The localization of their receptors is also a reflection of the solubility properties of the signaling molecules (▶ Table 7.1).

7.3.1 Lipophilic Signaling Molecules and Their Receptors

Lipophilic signaling molecules are lipid-soluble (hydrophobic) molecules that freely diffuse through the lipid bilayer of plasma membranes to interact with specific receptors inside the target cell (▶ Fig. 7.3a). Lipophilic signaling molecules such as steroid hormones, thyroid hormones, and retinoids (derivatives of vitamin A) share certain common characteristics:

• Because they are not water soluble, these signaling molecules must be bound to carrier proteins such as albumin or specific globulins to be transported in the bloodstream.
• They tend to have long half-lives (hours to days).
• Their intracellular receptors are located in the cytosol or nucleus.

Receptors for lipophilic signaling molecules are members of a large family of DNA-binding transcription factors that share sequence and structural similarities. Binding of the signaling molecule to its receptor leads to alterations in gene transcription, but the mechanism of action depends on whether the receptor is located in the cytosol or in the nucleus.

• **Cytoplasmic receptors** exist in the cytoplasm in an inactive complex with heat shock proteins (HSPs), such as HSP 90. Upon binding to a signaling molecule, the receptor dissociates from the HSP. The signaling molecule–receptor complex then translocates to the nucleus, where it binds as a dimer to a specific DNA sequence—called the hormone response

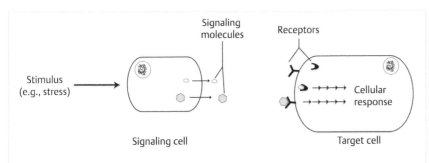

Fig. 7.1 General signaling steps. In response to a stimulus, a signaling cell synthesizes and secretes a signaling molecule. The signaling molecule is transported to the target cell, where it binds to a specific receptor protein. The signaling molecule-receptor complex activates or inhibits cellular pathways that elicit a particular cellular response. The signal is terminated by removal of the signaling molecule and/or receptor or inactivation of the signaling events triggered by the signaling molecule-receptor complex.

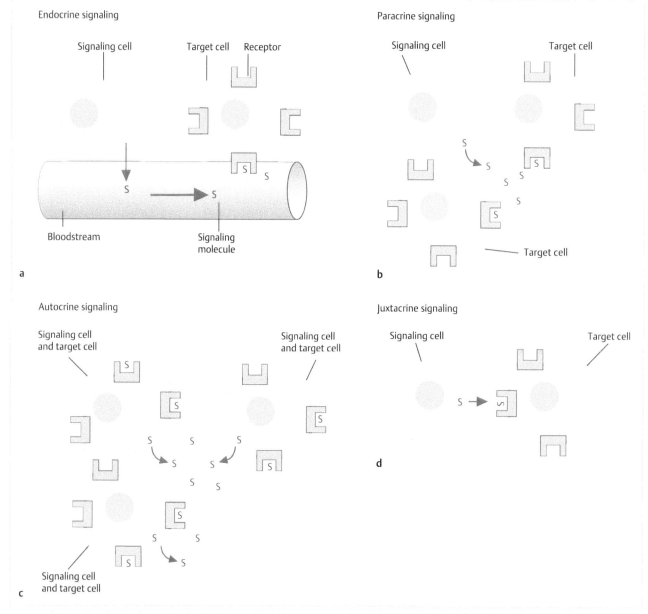

Fig. 7.2 Endocrine, paracrine, autocrine, and juxtacrine hormone signaling. (a) In endocrine signaling, the signaling molecule (S) is released by a cell distant from the target cell and transported via the bloodstream to the target cell. **(b)** In paracrine signaling, the signaling molecule is released by one cell type and diffuses to a neighboring target cell of a different cell type. **(c)** In autocrine signaling, the signaling molecule acts on the same cell type as the secreting cells themselves. **(d)** In juxtacrine signaling, the signaling molecule stays attached to the secreting cell and binds to a receptor on an adjacent target cell. Some signaling molecules participate in more than one type of signaling.

Table 7.1 Signaling molecules and features of their receptors

Signaling molecules	Receptor location and type
Lypophilic ("lipid-loving")	• Found in the cytoplasm and nucleus
• *Steroid hormones:* progesterone, estradiol, testosterone, cortisol,	• Family of DNA-binding transcription factors
• aldosterone, vitamin D	
• *Thyroid hormone:* thyroxine	
• *Retinoids:* retinol, retinoic acid	
Hydrophilic ("water-loving")	• Found on the surface of plasma membranes
• *Amino acid derived:* histamine, serotonin, melatonin, dopamine, norepinephrine, epinephrine	• Includes transmembrane proteins such as G protein–coupled receptors and receptor tyrosine kinases
• *From lipid metabolism:* acetylcholine	
• *Polypeptides:* insulin, glucagon, cytokines, thyroid-stimulating hormone	

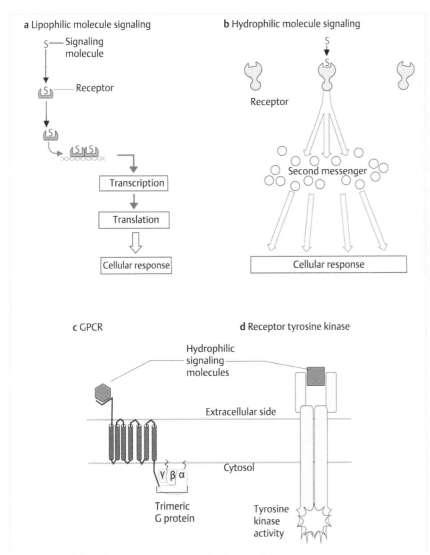

a Lipophilic molecule signaling

b Hydrophilic molecule signaling

Fig. 7.3 Lipophilic and hydrophilic signaling molecule action. (a) Lipophilic signaling molecules pass through the membrane of the target cell and bind to specific receptor proteins inside the cell. The signaling molecule-receptor complex acts as a transcription factor to regulate the transcription of specific genes. (**b**) Hydrophilic hormones, which are derived from amino acids, lipids, or polypeptides, cannot penetrate the plasma membrane and must therefore interact with specific receptors at the cell surface. The signaling molecule-receptor complex initiates the production of second messenger molecules inside the cell, which then triggers the cellular response. Hydrophilic signaling receptors are transmembrane proteins that undergo a conformational change upon binding to the signaling molecule. They include (**c**) the G protein-coupled receptors (GPCRs), and (**d**) receptor tyrosine kinases (RTKs).

c GPCR

d Receptor tyrosine kinase

---

element (HRE)—in the promoter region of specific genes to alter the rate of transcription to mRNA.

- **Nuclear receptors** are present in the nucleus already bound to DNA. These receptors alter the transcription of specific genes only when the appropriate signaling molecule diffuses to the nucleus and binds to them, allowing them to interact with additional proteins.

7.3.2 Hydrophilic Signaling Molecules and Their Receptors

Hydrophilic signaling molecules are water-soluble molecules that cannot diffuse through the hydrophobic core of cell membranes. Instead, these molecules bind to specific receptors at the cell surface, which triggers the activation (or inhibition) of signaling events downstream from the signaling molecule–receptor complex (▶ Fig. 7.3b). In general,

hydrophilic signaling molecules are small and are either derived from amino acids, obtained from lipid metabolism (e.g., epinephrine, acetylcholine), or exist as small polypeptides (e.g., glucagon, insulin). These signaling molecules share the following characteristics:

- Because they are water soluble, these signaling molecules do not require carrier proteins for transport in the bloodstream.
- They tend to have short half-lives (seconds to minutes).
- Their receptors are located at the cell surface.

Receptors for hydrophilic molecules are transmembrane proteins that undergo a conformational change upon binding to the signaling molecule. The resulting change in receptor activity triggers a cascade of signaling events that affect cellular processes. There are two important classes of receptors for hydrophilic signaling molecules (▶ Fig. 7.3c, d):

1. G protein–coupled receptors (GPCRs): Signaling via these seven α-helical transmembrane proteins is mediated by

trimeric G proteins, effector proteins, and second messengers.

2. Receptor tyrosine kinases: These single α-helical transmembrane proteins utilize their intrinsic enzymatic activity to initiate a cascade of signaling events mediated by monomeric G proteins and protein kinases.

Therapeutics
Lipophilic and hydrophobic medications

Oral contraceptives contain lipophilic signaling molecules (e.g., ethinyl estradiol—a derivative of estradiol) that have long half-lives (hours to days); hence they are often taken daily. On the other hand, hydrophilic molecules with short half-lives (seconds to minutes) are administered at the time that they are needed. For instance, epinephrine—contained within epinephrine autoinjectors—is taken to treat severe acute allergic reactions that may lead to anaphylactic shock.

Normal
Effects of glucagon, epinephrine, cortisol, and insulin on glucose metabolism

When glucose deficiency occurs (e.g., under starved conditions), the pancreas releases the peptide hormone glucagon. Glucagon then elevates blood glucose levels by promoting the breakdown of glycogen in the liver and inhibiting glycogen synthesis. Similarly, epinephrine stimulates the breakdown of glycogen by promoting glucagon secretion. If the glycogen stores have been depleted, then the steroid hormone cortisol stimulates gluconeogenesis by inducing the transcription of enzymes involved in this glucose-producing pathway. Conversely, under fed conditions, insulin serves to lower blood glucose levels by promoting the synthesis of glycogen (to store glucose), stimulating glycolysis (to catabolize glucose), and inhibiting the activity or synthesis of enzymes involved in gluconeogenesis. A deficiency in insulin production (type 1 diabetes) or insensitivity to insulin (type 2 diabetes) results in elevated blood glucose levels.

Therapeutics
Graves disease

Graves disease is an autoimmune disorder in which antibodies bind to and activate the thyroid-stimulating hormone (TSH) receptor, causing hyperthyroidism due to an increase in the production of thyroid hormones and an increase in the size of the thyroid gland (goiter). It is more common among women and usually presents by age 40. Weight loss, insomnia, and anxiety are common symptoms. About 50% of the affected patients exhibit bulging eyes (Graves ophthalmopathy). Serum TSH levels are low due to feedback inhibition. Treatment includes surgical resection of the thyroid gland, radioactive iodine to decrease the thyroid mass, or pharmacological intervention with antithyroid drugs, such as propylthiouracil and methimazole.

7.4 Signaling via G Protein–coupled Receptors

Structurally, GPCRs contain an extracellular domain that binds to a specific signaling molecule, a transmembrane domain composed of seven α-helices, and an intracellular domain that interacts with trimeric G proteins. Because signaling via GPCRs affects a variety of biological processes, numerous pharmacological agents have been developed to stimulate or inhibit their activities. Signaling via GPCRs involves the following common steps:

1. A signaling molecule (first messenger) binds to the extracellular domain of the receptor and causes a conformational change in the protein.
2. The intracellular domain activates its associated trimeric G protein by triggering the exchange of guanosine diphosphate (GDP) for guanosine triphosphate (GTP).
3. The activated GTP-bound G protein interacts with a membrane-bound effector protein, which is usually an enzyme that produces (or hydrolyzes) a second messenger.
4. Signaling is terminated by various mechanisms that include dissociation of the signaling molecule from the receptor, inactivation of the G protein, and reduction of cellular concentrations of second messengers.

7.4.1 Trimeric G Proteins, Effectors, and Second Messengers

Trimeric G Proteins

Trimeric G proteins are guanine nucleotide-binding proteins that contain three distinct subunits (α, β, and γ) and possess GTP hydrolyzing (GTPase) activity. They act as on–off molecular switches that are active when the α subunit is bound to GTP and inactive when it is bound to GDP (▶ Fig. 7.4). Different GPCRs interact with different types of G proteins, such as G_s, G_i, G_q, and G_t.

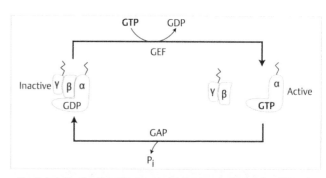

Fig. 7.4 Activation/inactivation cycle of trimeric G proteins. Trimeric G proteins contain three subunits (α, β, γ). An inactive G protein has guanosine diphosphate (GDP) bound to its α subunit, which is attached to the β and γ subunits. To become active, the G protein must exchange its GDP for guanosine triphosphate (GTP). This occurs via the action of a guanine nucleotide exchange factor (GEF). The active, GTP-bound α subunit separates from the β and γ subunits. To return to its inactive state, the intrinsic GTPase activity of the G protein hydrolyzes its bound GTP into GDP and phosphate (Pi). This action is accelerated by a GTPase-activating protein (GAP).

- Guanine nucleotide exchange factors (GEFs) are proteins that activate G proteins by promoting the exchange of GDP for GTP. For instance, a ligand-bound GPCR acts as a GEF for trimeric G proteins. Conversely, GTPase-activating proteins (GAPs) speed up the inactivation of G proteins by accelerating their intrinsic GTPase activity, which hydrolyzes GTP to GDP and phosphate (P_i).

Effector Proteins and Their Second Messengers

Once activated, the GTP-bound α subunit of a trimeric G protein interacts with an effector protein to activate or inhibit its activity. Typically, effector proteins are membrane-bound enzymes that catalyze reactions that produce a variety of second messengers—small molecules that affect the activity of enzymes that control critical biological processes. Examples of second messengers include cyclic adenosine monophosphate (cAMP), cyclic guanosine monophosphate (cGMP), diacylglycerol (DAG), inositol 1,4,5-triphosphate (IP_3), and Ca^{2+}. Some common GPCR signaling pathways and their corresponding G proteins, effector proteins, and second messengers are listed here:

1. **Signaling via G_s and G_i modulates adenylate cyclase activity and cAMP concentrations** (▶ Fig. 7.5a, b):
   - GPCR-mediated activation of the α subunit of G_s ($G_{s\alpha}$) activates the effector protein adenylate cyclase, an enzyme that converts ATP to cAMP. Conversely, activation of the α subunit of G_i ($G_{i\alpha}$) inhibits adenylate cyclase and prevents the production of cAMP.
   - The second messenger, cAMP, stimulates the activity of protein kinase A (PKA), an enzyme that alters the activity of various proteins via phosphorylation.
2. **Signaling via G_t activates cGMP phosphodiesterase and lowers the concentration of cGMP** (▶ Fig. 7.5c):
   - GPCR-mediated activation of the α subunit of G_t ($G_{t\alpha}$) activates the effector protein cGMP phosphodiesterase, an enzyme that hydrolyzes cGMP into the noncyclic 5′-GMP.
   - The reduced levels of cGMP cause hyperpolarization of visual cells, which is important for vision. The GPCR linked to G_t (transducin) is activated by light.

Foundations
Hydrolysis of cyclic nucleotides

Cellular levels of cyclic nucleotides are reduced by enzymes that hydrolyze their phosphodiester bonds to produce noncyclic nucleotides. For instance, cAMP is hydrolyzed into 5′-AMP by cAMP phosphodiesterase, and cGMP is hydrolyzed into 5′-GMP by cGMP phosphodiesterase. Several synthetic and natural compounds inhibit phosphodiesterases to prolong the effects of cyclic nucleotides on physiological processes. For instance, inhibitors of type 5 cGMP phosphodiesterase include sildenafil (Viagra, Pfizer, New York, NY), vardenafil (Levitra, Bayer, Pittsburgh, PA), and tadalafil (Cialis, Eli Lilly, Indianapolis, IN). Their action increases the concentration of cGMP, which leads to the relaxation of smooth muscles and vasodilation, resulting in an erection. Another inhibitor of phosphodiesterases is caffeine. Its consumption results in the accumulation of cAMP, which contributes to increased heart rate.

Foundations
Inhibition of G proteins by bacterial toxins

Cholera toxin prevents the inactivation of $G_{s\alpha}$, and pertussis toxin prevents the activation of $G_{i\alpha}$. These toxins do so by covalently modifying (via ADP ribosylation) the α subunits of G_s and G_i. ADP ribosylation of an arginine residue on $G_{s\alpha}$ decreases its intrinsic GTPase activity. As a result, it remains in the active GTP-bound form much longer, causing continued stimulation of adenylate cyclase and overproduction of cAMP. In intestinal cells, the elevated cAMP levels lead to the opening of chloride channels and a loss of electrolytes and water, which manifests as diarrhea. ADP ribosylation of a cysteine residue on $G_{i\alpha}$ prevents the activation and dissociation of this subunit from the trimeric G protein. The result is less inhibition of adenylate cyclase and once again an overproduction of cAMP. In airway epithelial cells, pertussis toxin causes loss of fluids and excessive mucus secretion, which presents as whooping cough.

Normal
Diversity of G protein–coupled receptor signaling

The same hormone in different cells may produce different physiological responses. For example, binding of epinephrine to the β-adrenergic receptors causes relaxation of bronchial and intestinal smooth muscle. However, binding of epinephrine to the β-adrenergic receptors on heart muscle causes it to contract. Even though epinephrine signaling produces the same second messenger, cAMP, in both cardiac and smooth muscle, the downstream signaling pathways diverge to allow different physiological effects in the two types of tissues. Thus, epinephrine can be used to relieve bronchospasms during an asthma attack and also to restore cardiac rhythms after shock or cardiac arrest.

Therapeutics
β-Agonists and their effects

The β-agonist albuterol is a hydrophilic molecule that binds to and activates β_2-adrenergic receptors. It is commonly administered directly to the lungs (via an inhaler or nebulizer) to treat airway-constricting conditions such as asthma, bronchitis, and COPD (chronic obstructive pulmonary disease). Additionally, patients who are unresponsive to albuterol treatment are often given epinephrine. These β-agonists relax bronchial smooth muscles and stimulate heart muscle contraction (through activation of β_1-adrenergic receptors). Therefore, one side effect of albuterol treatment is tachycardia (rapid heart rate).

3. **Signaling via G_q activates phospholipase C and elevates the concentrations of DAG, IP_3, and Ca^{2+}** (▶ Fig. 7.6):
   - GPCR-mediated activation of the α subunit of G_q ($G_{q\alpha}$) activates the effector protein phospholipase C (PLC), an enzyme that cleaves the membrane lipid phosphatidylinositol 4,5-bisphosphate (PIP_2) into DAG and inositol 1,4,5-triphosphate (IP_3).

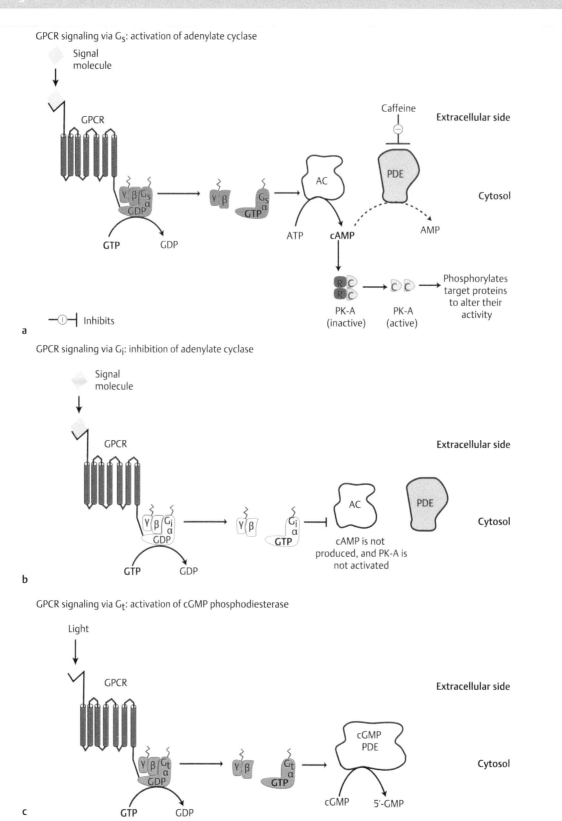

GPCR signaling via G_s: activation of adenylate cyclase

a

−①+ Inhibits

GPCR signaling via G_i: inhibition of adenylate cyclase

b

GPCR signaling via G_t: activation of cGMP phosphodiesterase

c

Fig. 7.5 G protein-coupled receptor (GPCR) signaling. Binding of a signaling molecule to a GPCR causes activation of G_s or Gi, which, in turn **(a)** stimulates or **(b)** inhibits adenylate cyclase (AC), respectively. Activated AC converts ATP to cAMP, a second messenger that regulates the activity of protein kinase A (PKA). Enzymatically inactive PKA exists as a tetrameric complex containing two regulatory subunits (R) and two catalytic subunits (C). Binding of cAMP to the regulatory subunits causes the complex to dissociate. The free, active catalytic subunits phosphorylate target proteins. cAMP is hydrolyzed into 5′-AMP by the action of phosphodiesterase (PDE), an enzyme that is inhibited by caffeine. **(c)** Light triggers the GPCR-mediated activation of G_t, which, in turn, stimulates the hydrolysis of cyclic guanosine mono-phosphate (cGMP) by cGMP PDE. GDP, guanosine diphosphate; GMP, guanosine monophosphate; GTP guanosine triphosphate.

II

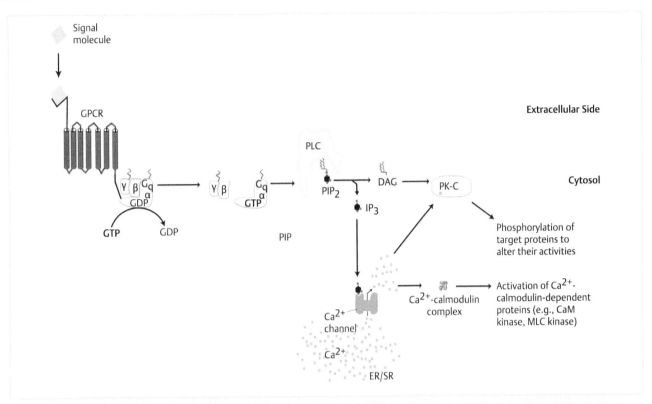

Fig. 7.6 G protein–coupled receptor (GPCR) signaling via G$_q$, phospholipase C (PLC) and protein kinase C (PKC). Binding of a signaling molecule to a GPCR triggers the activation of G$_q$, which stimulates the cleavage of phosphatidyl inositol 4,5-bisphosphate (PIP$_2$) by phospholipase C (PLC) to yield inositol 1,4,5-triphosphate (IP$_3$) and diacylglycerol (DAG). IP$_3$ causes the release of Ca^{2+} from the endoplasmic/ sarcoplasmic reticulum (ER/SR) into the cytosol. An increase in cytoplasmic Ca^{2+} causes the cytosolic enzyme protein kinase C (PKC) to translocate to the plasma membrane, where it is activated by DAG. Ca^{2+} also binds to the cytosolic protein calmodulin, forming a complex that activates Ca^{2+}-calmodulin-dependent proteins, which include Ca^{2+}-calmodulin-dependent protein kinase (CaM kinase) and myosin light-chain (MLC) kinase. Activated CaM kinase phosphorylates target proteins to alter their activities, whereas activated MLC kinase phosphorylates myosin light chains, causing smooth muscles to contract.

- The hydrophilic IP$_3$ translocates to the endoplasmic (or sarcoplasmic) reticulum, where it binds to and opens ligand-gated Ca^{2+} channels, allowing stored Ca^{2+} to be released into the cytoplasm.
- An increase in cytoplasmic Ca^{2+} causes the soluble enzyme protein kinase C (PKC) to translocate to the plasma membrane, where it is activated by the membrane-bound DAG, the other second messenger generated by PIP$_2$ hydrolysis. PKC phosphorylates the serine/threonine residues of protein targets, which has several consequences on cellular metabolism, growth, and differentiation.
- Ca^{2+} also binds to and forms a complex with the cytoplasmic protein calmodulin. This complex activates proteins such as the Ca^{2+}-calmodulin dependent protein kinases (CaM-kinases), phosphatases, ion channels, and cytoskeletal proteins.

Normal

Nitric oxide and smooth muscle relaxation

Nitric oxide (NO) is known as the endothelium-derived agent responsible for the relaxation of smooth muscle. It is generated from arginine in endothelial cells in a reaction promoted by Ca^{2+}-calmodulin. Released NO diffuses to neighboring smooth muscle and activates guanylate cyclase, leading to the production of cGMP. Cyclic GMP activates protein kinase G (PK-G), resulting in smooth muscle relaxation and vasodilation. This is the mechanism of the antianginal effect of nitroglycerin, which decomposes in the body to NO. Patients taking nitroglycerin should not take medications that inhibit cGMP phosphodiesterases—such as those used to treat erectile dysfunction (e.g., Viagra). Combining nitroglycerin and Viagra leads to extreme vasodilation and causes sometimes fatal drops in blood pressure.

Therapeutics

Antihistamines inhibit G protein–coupled receptor signaling

The symptoms of allergies—which include sneezing, runny nose, and itchy, watery eyes—are caused by histamine, a hydrophilic signaling molecule derived from the amino acid histidine. Histamine is a ligand that binds to the four histamine GPCRs (H1 to H4). Antihistamines are compounds that decrease allergic symptoms triggered by histamine by acting as the inverse agonists of the H1 and H2 GPCR. The antihistamines found in common allergy medications are cetirizine (Zyrtec, UCB Pharmaceuticals, Atlanta, GA), loratadine (Claritin, Merck, Whitehouse Station, NJ), and diphenhydramine hydrochloride (Benadryl, McNeil Consumer Healthcare, Fort Washington, PA). Other antihistamines that block the H1 receptors, such as meclozine and dimenhydrinate (Dramamine, McNeil Consumer Healthcare), can act as antiemetics and are used to inhibit symptoms of motion sickness.

The physiological effects of activating specific GPCRs are summarized in ▶ Table 7.2.

7.5 Signaling via Receptor Tyrosine Kinases

Structurally, receptor tyrosine kinases (RTKs) contain an extracellular signaling molecule-binding domain, a single α-helical transmembrane domain, and an intracellular domain that possesses tyrosine kinase activity (▶ Fig. 7.3d). The signaling molecules that bind to and activate RTKs include growth factors such as the epidermal growth factor (EGF), platelet-derived growth factor (PDGF), and nerve growth factor (NGF). Signaling via RTKs occurs through the following common steps:

1. A signaling molecule (or ligand) binds to the extracellular domain of the RTK. This induces a conformational change that causes receptor dimerization.
2. The dimerized receptor phosphorylates specific tyrosine residues on itself (autophosphorylation/ crossphosphorylation).
3. These phosphotyrosine residues are recognized and bound by adaptor and docking proteins, which activate downstream signaling pathways that are either dependent or independent of the small, monomeric G protein RAS.
4. RAS-dependent signaling is facilitated by members of the mitogen-activated protein kinase (MAPK) family, whereas RAS-independent signaling is facilitated by other types of kinases. Both signaling pathways trigger the phosphorylation of protein targets in the nucleus, plasma membrane, and cytoplasm, leading to alterations in gene transcription and protein activity.
5. Signaling via RTKs is terminated via multiple mechanisms that include degradation of the signaling molecules by extracellular proteases, ligand-induced endocytosis of the receptors followed by lysosomal degradation, accelerated RAS inactivation, and dephosphorylation of target proteins by phosphoprotein phosphatases.

Signaling via RTKs has both long-term and short-term effects on the target cell. The long-term effects (hours to days) include alterations in gene transcription. The short-term effects (seconds to minutes) include changes in the activity of proteins already present in the cell.

Monomeric G proteins such as RAS are similar to trimeric G proteins in that they both possess GTPase activity. They are inactive when bound to GDP and active when bound to GTP. RAS also cycles between the inactive and active states with the aid of GEFs and GAPs (▶ Fig. 7.7).

Table 7.2 Physiological effects of activating 6 protein-coupled receptors

Signal molecule, GPCR, and G protein	Physiological response
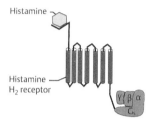 Epinephrine / β-adrenergic receptor	• Relaxation of bronchial and intestinal smooth muscle • Contraction of heart muscle • ↑ Breakdown of triacylglycerols in adipose tissue • ↑ Breakdown of glycogen in liver and muscle • ↑ Glycolysis in muscle
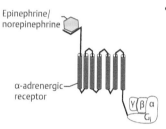 Histamine / Histamine H₂ receptor	• Bronchoconstriction and symptoms of allergic reactions (e.g., itchy, watery eyes)
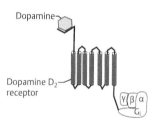 Epinephrine/ norepinephrine / α-adrenergic receptor	• Constriction of vascular smooth muscle
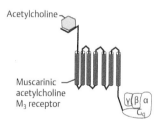 Dopamine / Dopamine D₂ receptor	• Increased heart rate
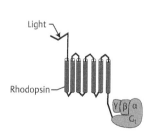 Acetylcholine / Muscarinic acetylcholine M₃ receptor	• Bronchoconstriction and stimulation of salivary glands
Light / Rhodopsin	• Vision

Normal

Receptors that possess enzymatic activity

Receptor tyrosine kinases are not the only single α-helical transmembrane receptors that catalyze enzymatic reactions. Others exhibit guanylate cyclase activity [e.g., atrial natriuretic peptide (ANP) receptor], serine/threonine kinase activity [e.g., transforming growth factor β (TGF-β) receptor], and protein tyrosine phosphatase activity (e.g., CD45).

Therapeutics

Receptor tyrosine kinases and cancer

RTKs are the targets of several pharmacological inhibitors because excessive signaling from mutated or overexpressed RTKs is associated with human cancer. For instance, the breast cancer drug herceptin targets HER2, which belongs to the family of EGF-binding RTKs.

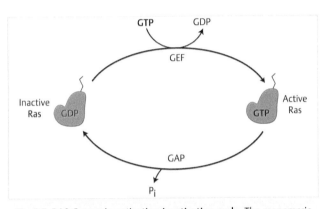

Fig. 7.7 RAS G protein activation-inactivation cycle. The monomeric G protein RAS is inactive when bound to guanosine diphosphate (GDP) and active when bound to guanosine triphosphate (GTP). A guanine nucleotide exchange factor (GEF) activates RAS by exchanging its bound GDP for GTP. A GTPase-activating protein (GAP) stimulates the intrinsic GTP hydrolyzing activity of RAS, returning it to an inactive GDP-bound state.

Therapeutics

RAS and cancer

Mutant forms of mammalian RAS or its GEFs and GAPs have been implicated in a wide range of human cancers. It is estimated that 30 to 50% of lung and colon cancers and nearly 90% of pancreatic cancers are associated with activating point mutations in *RAS*. Such mutations decrease the intrinsic GTPase activity of RAS and lock it for a much longer period in the active or GTP-bound state. Neurofibromatosis—a condition marked by the growth of tumors from nerve tissue—is caused by an inactivating mutation in the neurofibromin (*NF-1*) gene, which encodes a GTPase activating protein (GAP) for RAS. Thus, the absence of NF-1 allows RAS to excessively activate pathways that promote nerve tissue growth.

7.5.1 Insulin Signaling

Insulin is a hormone that binds to its cognate RTK to regulate the metabolism of the fuels glycogen and triacylglycerol through RAS-dependent and -independent signaling pathways (▶ Fig. 7.8).

RAS-dependent Insulin Signaling

1. Insulin binds to its RTK, which exists as a preformed dimer, causing autophosphorylation of the receptor's tyrosine residues.
2. The phosphotyrosine residues are recognized and bound by a docking protein called the insulin receptor substrate 1 (IRS-1).
3. IRS-1 is then phosphorylated on its tyrosine residues by the insulin receptor.
4. Phosphorylated IRS-1 is recognized and bound by the adaptor protein GRB-2, initiating the activation of RAS and the MAPK cascade. This results in the phosphorylation of nuclear proteins that increase the transcription of glucokinase—an enzyme that phosphorylates glucose in the first step of both glycolysis and glycogen synthesis.
5. Insulin receptor substrate 2 (IRS-2) is similar to IRS-1 in its function but has different specificity for adaptor proteins.

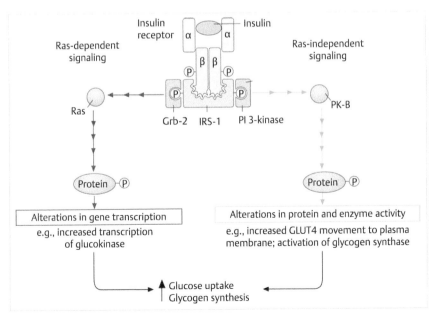

Fig. 7.8 RAS-dependent and -independent insulin signaling through receptor tyrosine kinase. Binding of insulin to its dimeric receptor causes autophos-phorylation of certain tyrosine residues in the cytosolic domain of the receptor. These phosphotyrosine motifs are recognized by docking proteins, such as insulin receptor substrate 1 (IRS-1). Binding of the adaptor protein GRB-2 to IRS-1 initiates the RAS-dependent signaling pathway that alters the transcription of specific genes. On the other hand, binding of phosphoinositide 3-kinase (PI 3-kinase) leads to the RAS-independent activation of protein kinase B (PKB). PKB mediates the positive effects of insulin on glucose uptake and storage. GLUT4, glucose transporter 4.

RAS-independent Insulin Signaling

The first three steps are identical to those in RAS-dependent insulin signaling.

1. Insulin binds to its RTK, which exists as a preformed dimer, causing autophosphorylation of the receptors' tyrosine residues.
2. The phosphotyrosine residues are recognized and bound by a docking protein called the insulin receptor substrate 1 (IRS-1).
3. IRS-1 is then phosphorylated on its tyrosine residues by the insulin receptor.
4. Phosphorylated IRS-1 recruits phosphoinositide 3-kinase (PI 3-kinase), an enzyme that phosphorylates phosphoinositides (a type of phospholipid) to generate phosphatidylinositol 3,4-bisphosphate and phosphatidylinositol 3,4,5-triphosphate (PIP_3).
5. These membrane-bound phosphoinositides act as second messengers that stimulate both the recruitment of protein kinase B (PKB) to the membrane and its activation via phosphorylation.
6. Active PKB (a serine/threonine kinase also known as Akt) phosphorylates and alters the activity of many intracellular proteins, which have stimulatory effects on glucose uptake and storage.
   - For instance, PKB plays a role in the insulin-induced movement of the glucose transporter 4 (GLUT4) from the cytoplasm to the plasma membranes of muscle and adipose cells.
   - PKB also promotes glycogen synthesis by phosphorylating and inhibiting glycogen synthase kinase-3 (GSK-3).

Foundations

Recognition domains

Adaptor proteins such as GRB-2 and IRS-1 have special domains known as SH2 domains or PTB domains that recognize and bind to motifs on the receptor that contain phosphorylated tyrosine residues.

Normal

Small G proteins

There are more than 150 members of the RAS superfamily of small G proteins (molecular weight of 20 to 25 kDa) that play an important role in the transduction of signals from plasma membrane receptors to the effector proteins such as soluble kinases. In contrast to the heterotrimeric G proteins associated with GPCR signaling, the small G proteins are monomeric in nature, consisting of a single polypeptide chain. They control such diverse processes as cell proliferation, intracellular vesicular traffic, survival and apoptosis, cell shape and polarity, and membrane transport and secretion. Small G proteins have intrinsic GTPase activity, and mutations that affect this activity can lead to cancer. Some of the subfamilies of small G proteins include RAS, RAB, RHO, ARF, and RAN.

Foundations

Insulin resistance

One of the critical aspects of insulin resistance leading to diabetes is a loss of insulin stimulation of glucose uptake by GLUT4 transporters in adipose and skeletal muscle. Several studies point to reduced activation of PKB by insulin in obese subjects. Although the site of impairment of the signaling pathway leading to this defect is not definitively established, probable early candidates are IRS-1 and IRS-2. It is known that, although tyrosine phosphorylation of IRS-1/2 is necessary for the recruitment of PI-3 kinase, serine/threonine phosphorylation appears to inactivate the IRSs and lead to their degradation. Multiple kinases may be involved in serine/threonine phosphorylation of IRS-1/2, which is stimulated by cytokines, free fatty acids, and hyperinsulinemia.

Review Questions: Membranes, Transport, and Signaling

1. Proteins found in membrane are identified by the manner in which they associate with the phospholipid bilayer. Some proteins are firmly embedded in the membrane and stabilized through hydrophobic interaction with membrane lipids. They span the entire lipid bilayer and interact with both internal and external environment. The membrane domain of these proteins embedded in the lipid bilayer is most likely composed of hydrophobic amino acids. Which of the following is an example of such transmembrane proteins?
   A) Monotopic
   B) Receptor
   C) Phospholipase
   D) G protein
   E) Protein kinase

2. Palytoxin (PTX, $C_{129}H_{227}N_3O_{52}$) is a water-soluble polyalcohol toxin produced by dinoflagellate algae of the genus *Ostreopsis*. Because of global warming, *Ostreopsis* has spread from tropical to temperate waters. It may now be found, for example, in algal blooms in the Mediterranean Sea, Sea of Japan, and the Gulf of Mexico during summer and may show up in seafood from these waters. PTX is particularly dangerous because it is not destroyed by cooking. Ingestion of contaminated food results in clupeotoxism marked by rhabdomyolysis, cramping, nausea, vomiting, diarrhea, paresthesia, exophthalmia, renal failure, cardiopulmonary arrest, and death within minutes to days. PTX binds to the extracellular domain of Na^+/K^+ ATPase, turning it into a permanently open ion channel. After poisoning with PTX, the sodium, potassium, and calcium concentrations in the cytosol would change as follows:
   A) Na^+ elevated, K^+ reduced, Ca^{2+} elevated

B) Na⁺ elevated, K⁺ reduced, Ca²⁺ reduced
C) Na⁺ elevated, K⁺ elevated, Ca²⁺ elevated
D) Na⁺ elevated, K⁺ elevated, Ca²⁺ reduced
E) Na⁺ reduced, K⁺ reduced, Ca²⁺ elevated

3. Thyroid hormone acts through intracellular receptors. Intracellular hormone receptors act by:
A) Activating adenylate cyclase
B) Stimulating the production of cyclic adenosine monophosphate (cAMP)
C) Stimulating feedback inhibition
D) Stimulating gene transcription
E) Stimulating the degradation of the hormone

4. A medical student attending to a woman with a high serum cortisol recalls that cortisol is a steroid hormone that regulates gene expression by binding to its receptor—the glucocorticoid receptor. The class of DNA-binding domain common to the steroid receptors is:
A) Beta sheet
B) Zinc finger
C) Alpha helical domain
D) Tyrosine kinase
E) Steroid response element

5. Identify the cell signaling pathway outlined below.

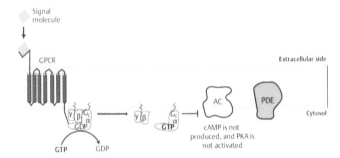

A) Epinephrine mediated α₂ adrenergic pathway.
B) Acetylcholine coupled M3 muscarinic pathway.
C) Insulin mediated receptor tyrosine kinase pathway.
D) Cytokine receptor coupled JAK STAT pathway.
E) Growth factor stimulation of the mitogen-activated protein kinase (MAPK) pathway.

6. Histamine H₂ receptors stimulate gastrointestinal motility and secretion of digestive juices. H₂ receptor antagonists such as cimetidine and ranitidine are used to treat peptic ulcers. They lead to
A) reduced hydrolysis of PIP₂ into IP₃ and DAG
B) increased hydrolysis of PIP₂ into IP₃ and DAG
C) decreased production of cAMP
D) increased production of cAMP
E) increased production of cyclic guanosine monophosphate (cGMP)

7. You are working with a disaster relief organization in an area where unusually heavy monsoon rainfalls caused widespread flooding in a shanty town. There is a lack of clean water, so people are forced to use floodwater for consumption, washing, and other needs. Your patients are suffering from severe rice-water-like diarrhea, resulting in dehydration and weakness. Which of the following describes the underlying pathomechanism?
A) ADP-ribosylation of elongation factor 2 (EF-2), so that protein synthesis is prevented
B) ADP-ribosylation of the α subunit of Gₛ by a bacterial toxin, so that this protein can no longer stimulate the production of cAMP by adenylate cyclase
C) ADP-ribosylation of the α subunit of Gᵢ by a bacterial toxin, so that this protein can no longer prevent the production of cAMP by adenylate cyclase
D) ADP-ribosylation of the α subunit of Gᵢ by a bacterial toxin, so that this protein constantly prevents the production of cAMP by adenylate cyclase
E) ADP-ribosylation of the α subunit of Gₛ by a bacterial toxin, so that this protein constantly stimulates the production of cAMP by adenylate cyclase

8. The mechanism of Insulin signaling involves the binding of the hormone to receptor tyrosine kinase causing autophosphorylation of receptor's tyrosine residues. The phosphotyrosine residues are recognized and bound by a docking protein called the insulin receptor substrate -1(IRS-1). The IRS-1 stimulate glucose uptake into cells by inducing translocation of the glucose transporter, GLUT4, from intracellular storage to the plasma membrane through which of the following signal transduction mechanism?
A) Phosphorylation and activation of protein kinase B through PI3 kinase.
B) Binding of GTP in exchange for GDP to rat sarcoma viral antigen (RAS) stimulated by a guanine nucleotide exchange factor (GEF)
C) Phosphorylation of mitogen/extracellular signal activated kinase (MEK) by protein kinase B (PKB)
D) Phosphorylation of GEF by insulin receptor substrate 1 (IRS-1)
E) Binding of GTP in exchange for GDP to phosphatide dependent kinase (PDK), stimulated by growth factor receptor bound protein 2 (GRB-2)

9. A 47-year-old man is delivered to the hospital for malaise, jaundice, edema, and ascites. On physical exam he had 2 cm hard hepatomegaly and 5 to 6 cm splenomegaly. His bloodwork revealed acanthocytosis (spur cells) and severe liver disease. Liver ultrasound showed nodular hepatomegaly, and biopsy showed advanced cirrhosis with iron accumulation. His bone marrow was hypercellular. While waiting for a liver transplant, the patient was treated with diuretics but progressed to grade IV hepatic encephalopathy and died. If you analyzed the lipid composition of the patient's red blood cells, you would find a relative increased concentration of
A) cholesterol
B) phosphatidylserine
C) phosphatidylcholine
D) phosphatidylethanolamine
E) plasmalogens

10. A 6-month-old female patient was scheduled for surgery to correct pulmonary stenosis and hypoplasia of the pulmonary arteries. Her weight was 16.3 lbs., the results of preoperative laboratory tests were as expected, and her

blood type was O Rh⁺. For the cardiopulmonary bypass, the priming solution consisted of 1 unit of packed erythrocytes, 1 unit of whole blood, and 200 mL of Ringer solution with appropriate medications. The patient was cooled to a core temperature of 84.2 °F for the operation. Five minutes after the bypass was started, the perfusionist realized that the machine prepared for the patient had been switched with that for another patient with blood group A Rh⁺, who was operated at the same time in a different theater. The patient was immediately infused with glucocorticoids, antihistamines, and diuretics. Urine was alkalized with bicarbonate. In addition, the patient received ultrafiltration to remove inflammatory cytokines and plasmapheresis with frozen plasma. Surgery was completed successfully, and the patient was transferred to an intensive care unit. During the following day, laboratory values indicated the formation of immune complexes and minor hemolysis but no change in liver and kidney function. Further recovery was uneventful. To remove isohemagglutinins in the patient's blood by plasmapheresis, plasma from a donor of which of the following blood groups should be used?

A) O

B) A

C) B

D) AB

E) Any blood type

11. A 54-year-old man smokes two packs of cigarettes a day and is on isosorbide dinitrate (Dilatrate, Sun Pharmaceutical, Mumbai, Maharashtra, India), a long-acting nitric oxide (NO) precursor for angina pectoris. His body mass index is 31. His managerial job leaves him little time for exercise, most of which consists of bowling. He was having problems in his marriage due to performance issues recently and has consulted his physician who put him on sildenafil (Viagra, Pfizer, New York, NY) tablet. One night, about 1 hour after taking this medication, he started to feel lightheaded; he also had the feeling of an irregular pulse. After near syncope, he reported to the emergency room of a nearby hospital. When he arrived there, his symptoms had largely resolved. His blood pressure was 15 mm Hg lower than usual, and there were isolated ventricular premature beats on his EKG. The patient was given fluids, a 24-hour Holter monitor, and referral to a cardiologist. The side effects this patient experienced originate from which of the following?

A) Increased cGMP levels due to the nitrate and increased 5′-GMP levels due to the effects of the inhibitor of type 5 cGMP phosphodiesterase

B) Attenuation of the effects of the nitrate by the inhibitor of type 5 cGMP phosphodiesterase, which blocks the ability of guanylate cyclase to produce cGMP.

C) Increased cGMP levels due to the nitrate and increased cGMP levels due to the effects of the inhibitor of type 5 phosphodiesterase

D) Exacerbation of the effects of the nitrate due to an increase in AMP levels triggered by the inhibitor of type 5 cGMP phosphodiesterase

E) An additive lowering of blood pressure because nitrates and sildenafil inhibit the same enzyme.

12. In an effort to create a mouse model for retinitis pigmentosa, Sakamoto and coworkers[1] induced mutations in the germ line of mice with ethyl nitrosourea and then screened the descendants. One line had a V685 M missense mutation in *PDE6A*, the mouse gene for the α subunit of phosphodiesterase 6. In homozygous mutant mice, phosphodiesterase activity was nondetectable, and photoreceptors were destroyed by day 14 after birth, even when the animals were reared in the dark. Heterozygous animals were not affected. How would you expect measurements of [cGMP] and [Ca²⁺] in cones of homozygous mutant mice to compare with those of normal mice? (Note: cGMP binds to the TRP-M1 ion channels and allows Na⁺ and Ca²⁺ to flow into the cell.) Assume normal ambient light.

A) Both are lowered.

B) Both are increased.

C) [cGMP] is elevated, and [Ca²⁺] is reduced.

D) [cGMP] is reduced, and [Ca²⁺] is elevated.

E) [cGMP] is elevated, and [Ca²⁺] is reduced.

13. The images in this set show normal (left) and apoptotic (right) cells. In the top row, the cells have intact plasma membranes. Thus, antibodies can bind only to substances in the outer leaflet of the membrane. In the bottom row, the cells were treated with digitonin, a substance that makes holes in the plasma membrane large enough for antibodies to enter the cell. Thus, antibodies against intracellular components can also bind their targets. All cells were stained with antibodies against the α subunit of G$_s$ (red color) and against a "mystery" membrane component (blue color). Purple color occurs where both labels are in close proximity. Which of the following is the "mystery" membrane component most likely to be?

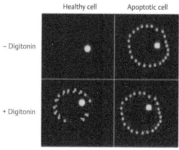

A) Phospholipase C

B) Phosphatidylserine

C) Cholesterol

D) The adenosine triphosphate (ATP)–binding site of Na⁺/K⁺- ATPase

E) Oligosaccharides on glycoproteins

14. Differential scanning calorimetry (DSC) is a technique to follow phase transitions (e.g., melting). Two chambers—one with buffer only, the other also containing the sample—are slowly heated in parallel, and the energy required for changing the temperature in both chambers is compared. As the sample approaches a phase transition temperature, it requires more energy to heat than the buffer ("excess heat," measured in J/mol·… °C). Once the temperature is high

enough for the transition to be complete, the excess heat drops to near 0 J/mol·... °C again. The experiment depicted below measures the "melting" ($L_\alpha \rightarrow L_{\beta'}$ transition) in two samples of phosphatidylcholine liposomes. The samples differ in the fatty acids that make up the phospholipid. What is the difference between the fatty acid chains of the samples?

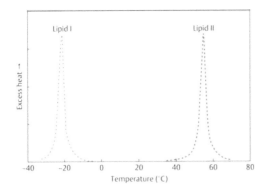

A) Lipid I contains stearic acid (C18:0), and lipid II contains oleic acid (C18:1).

B) Lipid I contains oleic acid (C18:1), and lipid II contains stearic acid (C18:0).

C) Lipid I contains stearic acid (C18:0), and lipid II contains palmitic acid (C16:0).

D) Lipid I contains palmitic acid (C16:0), and lipid II contains stearic acid (C18:0).

E) Lipid I contains oleic acid (C18:1), and lipid II contains palmitoleic acid (C16:1).

15. Growth factors bind to extracellular domain of receptor tyrosine kinases (RTK), thereby activating downstream signaling pathways that are dependent on the small, monomeric G protein, RAS. RAS is active when bound to:
A) H^+
B) GTP
C) Ca^{++}
D) ATP
E) c AMP

16. You may have already experienced the truth of the saying "Behind every successful doctor stands a whole lot of caffeine." Caffeine increases our ability to concentrate and makes us feel more awake. It also increases respiratory rate, blood pressure, and heart rate and stimulates metabolism (and therefore may have a protective effect against metabolic syndrome). Caffeine within cells inhibits the degradation of cAMP. Which of the following effects would be observed after ingestion of caffeine?
A) Decreased activity of protein kinase A.
B) Elevated cellular cAMP levels.
C) Increased cellular inositol 1,4,5-triphosphate (IP_3) levels.
D) Altered gene expression by binding to intracellular receptors.
E) Activation of phosphodiesterase.

17. The following experiments were performed with the peptide hormone "X":
• ^{125}I-labeled hormone "X" was injected into laboratory animals. The animals were sacrificed, and frozen sections

of various organs were placed on photographic film. The film darkened on liver sections whereas it stayed clear on skeletal muscle sections.
• The molecular mass of hormone "X" was determined by gel filtration to be approximately 3,500 Da.
• When the livers of animals treated with ^{125}I-labeled hormone "X" were homogenized and centrifuged at 3,000 g for 10 min, the radioactivity was found in the membrane fraction.
• The blood glucose levels in animals treated with hormone "X" increased; at the same time, the liver mass decreased.
• cAMP levels in cultured hepatocytes increased upon exposure to hormone "X."
   Hormone "X" is which of the following?
A) Cortisol
B) Glucagon
C) Epinephrine
D) Norepinephrine
E) Insulin

18. A 45-year-old woman with a body mass index (BMI) of 35 reports to you because of polydipsia, polyuria, and frequent nightly calls to the bathroom, which interfere with her sleep. Examination reveals a blood pressure of 150/90 mm Hg, pulse 90 beats/min, breathing 21/min. Urinalysis: glucose 2+, albumin and ketones negative. Blood: triglycerides 170 mg/dL, high-density lipoprotein (HDL) 30 mg/dL, random blood glucose 220 mg/dL, glycated hemoglobin (HbA1c) 9%. She is diagnosed as having insulin-resistant diabetes (diabetes mellitus type 2). Abnormal response of which of the following intracellular messaging pathways would be expected in the muscle tissue of this patient?
A) Altered transcription due to binding of a hormone-receptor complex to DNA
B) Na^+ and K^+ ion channel opening
C) Activation of protein kinase A
D) Activation of adenylate cyclase
E) Activation of mitogen-activated protein kinase (MAPK)

19. Membranes regulate the flow of biomolecules into and out of the cells. Some biomolecules diffuse directly through the membranes, whereas others require the assistance of proteins embedded within the membrane. Membrane carrier protein-assisted, energy dependent movement of molecules against their concentration gradient is
A) amino acid transport through the membrane
B) simple diffusion
C) facilitated diffusion
D) primary active transport
E) peptide transport through membrane

20. The energy -independent movement of molecules down their concentration gradient can occur unaided (simple diffusion) or with assistance (facilitated diffusion) of transmembrane proteins. Which of the following statements best describes the facilitated transport mechanism?
A) Transport through the membrane is an equilibration process
B) Transport can occur in only one direction
C) ATP is required as an energy source

D) It is not a significant process in eukaryotic cells

E) Solutes can only leave the cell by this process, not enter the cell

21. Lysergic acid diethylamide (LSD, "acid") was one of the favorite drugs of the hippie movement in the 1960s. In μg amounts it causes hallucinations, altered sense of time, synesthesia, and "spiritual" experiences. In Switzerland it is currently in clinical trial for the management of pain and end-of-life anxiety in patients with terminal cancer. LSD acts through $5HT_{2A}$ serotonergic receptors, which signal through G_q. Which of the following reactions is involved in the effects of LSD?

A) Stimulation of adenylate cyclase

B) Inhibition of adenylate cyclase

C) Binding of Ca^{2+} to calmodulin

D) Activation of phosphodiesterase

E) Closing of Ca^{2+} channels in the endoplasmic reticulum (ER)

22. In a well-fed state, modulation of metabolic activity by the predominant hormone binding to its receptor results in:

A) GPCR mediated activation of $G_{s\alpha}$.

B) Increased tyrosine phosphorylation.

C) Increased production of cyclic adenosine monophosphate (cAMP)

D) Increased protein kinase A activity.

E) increased production of cyclic guanosine monophosphate (cGMP).

23. Binding of a signaling molecule to G protein-coupled receptor (GPCR) triggers the activation of G_q. A GTP-bound $G_{q\alpha}$ subunit would initiate downstream signaling leading to increased second messengers, inositol 1,4,5-triphosphate (IP_3) and diacylglycerol (DAG). Increased DAG results in the activation of

A) a monomeric G protein.

B) phospholipase C activity.

C) adenylyl cyclase activity.

D) cAMP phosphodiesterase activity.

E) protein kinase C activity.

24. A student at the Metropolitan School of Nursing had a persistent cough, for which she visited her primary care doctor. She was given an inhaler to ease her symptoms, but she received no diagnosis or definitive treatment. Two weeks later, one of her lab instructors, a 48-year-old man without relevant previous history, also developed a runny nose and paroxysmal coughs ending in a noisy inspiratory stridor, with posttussive emesis. This got so bad that he sought help in the Metropolitan Mercy Hospital. Physical exam: temperature 37.4 °C, respiratory rate 45/min, pulse 150 beats/min, blood pressure 102/49 mm Hg, and an oxygen saturation rate of 90%. Studies: interstitial opacities with peribronchial wall thickening on chest X-ray, respiratory secretions positive for *Bordetella pertussis* in polymerase chain reaction (PCR). The patient was treated with inhaled epinephrine and albuterol plus a 5-day course of azithromycin. The school informed all students, faculty, and staff of their exposure to *Bordetella* and suspended clinical training activities until all involved had obtained prophylactic treatment according to the Centers for Disease Control and Prevention guidelines, supervised by the state's health authority. The production of which of the following second messengers would be higher than normal in the patient's lung epithelial cells?

A) cAMP

B) cGMP

C) Ca^{2+}

D) Diacylglycerol

E) IP_3

Answers and Explanations: Membranes, Transport, and Signaling

1. B Integral proteins that span the entire lipid bilayer and interact with both internal and external environment are referred to as transmembrane proteins. The transmembrane part of a protein is made up mostly of hydrophobic amino acids. Receptors whose functions regulate the flow of certain molecules into and out of the cells and receive and transmit extracellular signals to the intracellular environment is a transmembrane protein.

A Integral monotopic proteins do not span the lipid bilayer

C Phospholipases are peripheral proteins that are loosely bound to the membrane surface through electrostatic interaction with lipids or other proteins.

D Small G proteins (e.g., Ras) are lipid anchored proteins tethered to the membrane via a covalently attached lipid molecule.

E Lipid anchored protein

2. A The Na^+/K^+ ATPase is responsible for maintaining low intracellular concentrations of Na^+ and high intracellular concentrations of K^+ via the ATP-dependent movement of $2K^+$ in and $3Na^+$ out of a cell. The Na^+-Ca^{2+} exchanger maintains low levels of cytosolic Ca^{2+} by importing $3Na^+$ and exporting one

Ca^{2+} ion. Opening the ion channel of Na^+/K^+ ATPase leads to a breakdown of the ion gradient across the cell membrane, causing cytosolic levels of Na^+ to increase and K^+ to decrease. In addition, the breakdown of the Na^+ gradient would reduce the activity of the Na^+-Ca^{2+} exchanger, causing cytosolic Ca^{2+} levels to increase.

B Ca^{2+} is normally lower inside the cell than outside. A collapse of the ion gradients therefore would cause cytosolic Ca^{2+} to rise.

C K^+ is normally higher inside the cell than outside. A collapse of the ion gradients therefore would cause K^+ to decrease.

D Normally, K^+ is higher and Ca^{2+} is lower inside a cell than outside. A collapse of the ion gradient would therefore lower and increase, respectively, the intracellular concentration of these ions.

E Na^+ is normally lower inside a cell than outside. A collapse of the ion gradients would therefore increase cytosolic Na^+.

3. D Thyroid hormones are lipophilic substances that can freely cross the plasma membrane. In the cytosol, they bind to soluble receptors. The hormone/receptor-complex then migrates into the nucleus to affect gene expression via hormone response elements (HRE) in promoters and enhancers. They exhibit endocrine signaling. Long-distance signaling between different organs, where the signaling molecule is transported by the bloodstream, is called endocrine signaling.

A Adenylate cyclase is activated by the α subunit of G_s and inhibited by that of G_i. Activation of G proteins is the result of water-soluble hormones binding to the extracellular domain of G protein-coupled receptors (GPCRs). Steroids are fat soluble and cross the plasma membrane.

B. Cyclic AMP is produced by adenylate cyclase, an enzyme that is activated by some water-soluble hormones that bind to the extracellular domain of GPCRs.

C Principal mechanisms to regulate the concentration of the active enzymes in the tissue.

E Mechanism for signal termination.

4. B Zinc finger motifs are relatively small autonomously-folded domains that contain a nucleotide recognition signal. They are commonly found in the DNA binding domain of steroid hormone receptors.

A The Beta sheet is a common motif of regular secondary structure in proteins. The supramolecular association of β-sheets has been implicated in formation of the protein aggregates and fibrils observed in many human diseases, notably the amyloidosis such as Alzheimer disease.

C, D Structurally receptor tyrosine kinase (RTKs) contains an extracellular ligand binding domain, a single alpha helical transmembrane domain and an intracellular domain that possesses tyrosine kinase activity.

E Steroid hormones exert their effects by diffusing through the lipid bilayer and interacting with the intracellular receptor and then move into the nucleus and bind to its specific response element (HRE). Additionally, they activate other transcription factors to modulate gene expression of specific proteins.

5. A It is a G protein coupled receptor (GPCR) signaling pathway. Epinephrine binds to the α_2 adrenergic receptors and leads to the GPCR mediated activation of α subunit of G_i ($G_{i\alpha}$); inhibits adenylyl cyclase and prevents the production of cAMP. Conversely the GPCR mediated activation of α subunit of G_s ($G_{s\alpha}$); activates adenylyl cyclase, an enzyme that converts ATP into cAMP. The latter effect of adenylyl cyclase activation is achieved through binding of epinephrine to β-adrenergic receptor.

B Acetylcholine (ACh) binds to the M1 muscarinic receptor in brain results mainly in formation of diacylglycerol (DAG)/inositol 1,4,5-trisphosphate (IP3). Muscarinic ACh receptors act through second messengers. M_1 acts mostly via G_q, which stimulates phospholipase C. This enzyme hydrolyzes phosphatidylinositol-4,5-bisphosphate (PIP_2) into IP_3 and DAG. M_1 acts mainly through G_q, but in some tissues there may also be some activation of G_i, thus—if at all—and a reduction in cAMP synthesis. Muscarinic ACh receptors are metabotropic (i.e., they act through second messengers). Nicotinic receptors, on the other hand, are ionotropic (i.e., they form ion channels). The outlined pathway is a G protein coupled receptor (GPCR) signaling pathway mediated by epinephrine.

C Insulin binds to the receptor tyrosine kinase (RTK) and mediates RAS dependent and RAS independent signaling path-

way. The outlined pathway is a G protein coupled receptor (GPCR) signaling pathway mediated by epinephrine.

D Cytokines binding to a receptor protein complex leads to initiation of the Janus kinase (JAK) / signal transducer and activator of transcription (STAT) pathway. The outlined pathway is a G protein coupled receptor (GPCR) signaling pathway mediated by epinephrine.

E MAPK pathway is stimulated by growth factors and insulin. Growth factors coupled with tyrosine kinase receptor through active RAS protein mediate the mitogen-activated protein kinase (MAPK) pathway. The outlined pathway is a G protein coupled receptor (GPCR) signaling pathway mediated by epinephrine.

6. D H2 receptors act through G_s, which stimulates the production of cAMP. Antagonists of H2 receptors block this pathway and therefore decrease [cAMP].

A The hydrolysis of PIP_2 into IP_3 and DAG is a component of H1 receptor signaling facilitated by G_q. H1 receptor antagonists are used as antiallergic (Benadryl, McNeil Consumer Healthcare, Fort Washington, PA), sedative (doxylamine), and antiemetic (meclizine) drugs.

B The hydrolysis of PIP_2 into IP_3 and DAG is a component of H1 receptor signaling facilitated by G_q. H1 receptor antagonists would decrease, rather than increase, the production of these second messengers.

C Only H3 and H4, but not H2, receptors work through G_i. H3 receptors are found in the brain and are targets for experimental drugs against obesity. H4 receptors are found on white blood cells and regulate neutrophil release from the bone marrow and mast cell chemotaxis. They are targets for experimental allergy and asthma drugs.

E There are no known histamine receptors working with cGMP as a second messenger.

7. E The patients are suffering from cholera; the cholera toxin A1 subunit enters the cytosol and ADP-ribosylates the α subunit of G_s, preventing it from hydrolyzing bound GTP to GDP. Thus, G_s stays constantly active and stimulates the production of cAMP by adenylate cyclase. The cAMP turns on the cystic fibrosis transconductance regulator (CFTR), leading to the transport of chloride into the intestine. Water follows osmotically, leading to a "diarrhea on steroids" that helps the bacterium to spread.

A ADP-ribosylation of EF-2 occurs in diphtheria, not in cholera.

B ADP-ribosylation of the α subunit of G_s by cholera toxin turns the protein constitutively on, not off.

C ADP-ribosylation of the α subunit of G_i occurs in whooping cough, not in cholera.

D ADP-ribosylation of the α subunit of G_i occurs in whooping cough, not in cholera. In addition, it would turn G_i off so it can no longer prevent the synthesis of cAMP.

8. A Insulin stimulates glucose uptake into cells by inducing translocation of the glucose transporter, GLUT4, from intracellular storage to the plasma membrane. PI 3-kinase and AKT are known to play a role in GLUT4 translocation. AKT is also known as protein kinase B. Phosphorylated IRS-1 recruits PI 3-kinase that activates protein Kinase B. Active protein kinase B plays a role in insulin-induced movement of glucose transporter 4

(GLUT4) from the cytoplasm to the plasma membrane of muscle and adipose tissue.

B Active RAS (RAS-GTP) starts the mitogen-activated protein kinase (MAPK) pathway, which controls the expression of genes (slow effects of insulin).

C MEK is phosphorylated by receptor-associated factor (RAF) as part of the MAPK pathway, not by PKB. Phosphorylation by PKB regulates the fast (metabolic) effect of insulin.

D Guanine nucleotide exchange factor (GEF) [e.g., son of sevenless (SOS)] is not phosphorylated; rather, it is recruited to the insulin/insulin receptor/IRS-1/GRB-2 protein complex. Only then can it act as a GTP/GDP exchange factor for RAS, starting the MAPK pathway.

E PDK is regulated by PIP_3, not by GTP/GDP exchange. This is involved in the metabolic (fast) effects of insulin, not in gene regulation. GRB-2 is not a GTP/GDP exchange factor, but an adaptor protein, which recruits the exchange factor SOS to the insulin/insulin receptor/IRS-1 complex.

9. A In severe liver disease, "most frequently alcoholic liver cirrhosis," the erythrocyte membrane gets loaded with cholesterol and sphingomyelin. (This also happens if normal erythrocytes are incubated with the plasma of a patient with spur cell anemia.) Cholesterol and sphingomyelin reduce membrane fluidity and result in an irregular cell shape (remodeling by spleen). The high cholesterol content also leads to reduced repair of lipids after peroxidation, shortened lifetime of the erythrocyte, and anemia.

B The relative concentration of phosphatidylserine in spur cell membranes is decreased.

C The relative concentration of phosphatidylcholine in spur cell membranes is decreased.

D The relative concentration of phosphatidylethanolamine in spur cell membranes is decreased.

E The relative concentration of plasmalogens in spur cell membranes is decreased.

10. B Because plasma from a donor with blood group A does not contain any antibodies against the A antigen, it can be used to dilute out the antibodies present in the patient's blood. This reduces lysis of the foreign erythrocytes. Note that in the patient, the immune response against the A antigen had not fully formed, which may have contributed to the positive outcome. Transfusion of blood group-mismatched blood is reported to occur with a frequency of 2.5 to 253 per 100,000.

A Plasma from a donor with blood group O would contain antibodies against the A antigen and hence increase lysis of the foreign erythrocytes in the patient.

C Plasma from a donor with blood group B would contain antibodies against the A antigen and hence increase lysis of the foreign erythrocytes in the patient.

D Although plasma from an AB donor does not contain antibodies against the A antigen and therefore could be used to dilute the antibodies present in the patient against the foreign erythrocytes, the use of a donor of blood type A would avoid introducing another variable and would therefore be preferable.

E Using plasma from a random blood type would pose the risk of introducing antibodies against A antigen and increase the lysis of the foreign erythrocytes in the patient.

11. C NO stimulates the production of cGMP from GTP, whereas phosphodiesterase (PDE) inhibitors like sildenafil prevent the degradation of cGMP to 5′-GMP. Thus, both drugs increase the concentration of the same second messenger, leading to a synergistic (more than additive) lowering of blood pressure. The risk of unwanted effects is increased by excessive food intake and alcohol consumption, and also by an unfamiliar partner. Serious side effects (e.g., acute myocardial infarction) are apparently rare. Nevertheless, there should be a 24-hour interval between intake of nitrates and cGMP phosphodiesterase (PDE) inhibitors in either order.

A NO does lead to an increase in the production of cGMP, but cGMP PDE inhibitors like sildenafil prevent its degradation to 5′-GMP.

B Phosphodiesterases degrade cyclic nucleotide monophosphates; these are formed by nucleotide cyclases.

D Degradation of cGMP does not lead to AMP but to 5′-GMP.

E The NO produced by nitrates acts on guanylate cyclase, increasing the production of 5′-cGMP. Sildenafil acts on phosphodiesterase, preventing the breakdown of cGMP to 5′-GMP. Thus, both drugs act on different enzymes but conspire to increase the concentration of the same second messenger.

12. B Because there is no phosphodiesterase to bind and hydrolyze cGMP, the concentration of this second messenger will increase. Thus, more cGMP can bind to the ion channels, keeping them open and allowing Na^+ and Ca^{2+} to flow into the cell. This increases the current through the channel and also the concentrations of the ions in the cytosol. Indeed, it is speculated that the chronic increase of cytosolic Ca^{2+} stimulates destruction of photoreceptor cells by apoptosis.

A, C, D, E See explanation for B.

13. B The relocalization of phosphatidylserine from the inner sheet to the outer sheet of the plasma membrane's lipid bilayer serves to mark apoptotic cells for recognition by phagocytes. Thus, in normal cells, antibodies against both phosphatidylserine and G proteins cannot bind without permeabilization. In apoptotic cells, antibodies against phosphatidylserine, but not G proteins, can bind before the cells are permeabilized. (Note: Autoantibody production against phosphatidylserine is the cause of antiphospholipid syndrome, characterized by increased vascular thrombosis, about 10% of patients with recurrent arterial and venous thrombosis.)

A Phospholipase C is an enzyme that hydrolyzes the phospholipid, phosphatidylinositol 4,5-bisphosphate (PIP_2). It occurs on the cytoplasmic leaflet of both apoptotic and nonapoptotic cells. Thus, in both apoptotic and nonapoptotic cells, staining would require permeabilization.

C Cholesterol is present in the outer leaflet of both apoptotic and nonapoptotic cells. However, the images show no staining of the "mystery" component in the nonpermeabilized normal cells.

D Antibodies against the ATP-binding site of Na^+/K^+-ATPase would bind to an intracellular domain of the enzyme. Hence, its staining would require permeabilization in apoptotic and nonapoptotic cells.

E The sugar trees of glycosylated membrane proteins are always on the extracellular side. Hence, staining would be visible without permeabilization in both apoptotic and nonapoptotic cells.

14. B The melting point of lipid I is significantly lower than that of lipid II. The melting point of phospholipids containing the unsaturated oleic acid would be much lower than that of phospholipids containing the saturated stearic acid. Saturated fatty acids are straight molecules, whereas *cis*-unsaturated fatty acids have a 120-degree kink at the position of the double bond. This prevents tight packing of phospholipids in a membrane, making the membrane more fluid. Mammals have membranes with a melting temperature of 10 to 12 °C, well below body temperature. In thermophilic bacteria, the lipid melting temperature is higher than in mammals; in psychrophilic bacteria, it is lower.

A The melting point of phospholipids containing the saturated stearic acid would be higher than that of phospholipids containing the corresponding unsaturated oleic acid.

C The presence of the saturated stearic acid in phospholipids will make their melting point higher (not lower) than that of phospholipids containing the shorter palmitic acid.

D The longer-chain length in stearic acid compared to palmitic acid allows the former to have a slightly higher melting temperature (55 °C) than the latter (40 °C).

E The presence of the unsaturated oleic acid in phospholipids will cause their melting temperatures to be higher (not lower) than that of phospholipids containing the shorter, unsaturated palmitoleic acid.

15. B (C, D, E) Growth factor binds to the extracellular domain of the RTK. This induces a conformational change that causes receptor dimerization. The dimerized receptor phosphorylates specific tyrosine residues on itself. These phosphotyrosine residues are recognized and bound by adaptor and docking proteins, which activate downstream signaling pathways that are dependent on small, monomeric G protein RAS. RAS-dependent signaling is facilitated by members of the mitogen-activated protein kinase (MAPK) family. Monomeric G proteins RAS are similar to trimeric G proteins in that they both possess GTPase activity. They are inactive when bound to GDP and active when bound to GTP.

A Hydrophilic molecules and ions cannot easily traverse the hydrophobic interior of membranes without a special carrier or transport mechanism.

16. B Caffeine inhibits cAMP phosphodiesterase, thereby suppressing hydrolysis of 3′,5′-cAMP into 5′-AMP and thereby increases cAMP levels. It is perhaps pertinent that in clinical studies, caffeine consumption has inferior results on learning ability compared to a nap.

A E Caffeine inhibits 3′,5′-cAMP phosphodiesterase which inactivates cAMP to AMP. High cellular cAMP levels will increase the activity of protein kinase A.

C Caffeine does not stimulate G_q signaling which causes phospholipase C to cleave inositol 4, 5-bisphosphate (PIP_2) into IP_3 and diacylglycerol (DAG).

D Only hydrophobic hormones like steroids alter gene expression by binding to intracellular receptors.

17. B Glucagon binds to liver, but not skeletal muscle, as demonstrated by autoradiography. It is a peptide hormone, as demonstrated by its molecular mass (3485 Da) and the ability to be iodinated. It binds to receptors on the cell membrane, which can be separated from the cytosol by a brief centrifuga-

tion at moderate speed. Binding of glucagon to liver cells leads to the conversion of stored glycogen to glucose, which is released into the bloodstream. Glucagon receptors work via G_s, which stimulates adenylate cyclase.

A Cortisol is much smaller than 3,500 Da (362 Da, in fact) and is not a peptide. The cortisol-receptor complex does not act via adenylate cyclase. Cortisol has a slight insulin-like effect on the liver, stimulating the synthesis rather than the breakdown of glycogen.

C Epinephrine (adrenaline) is a small organic molecule (183 Da), not a peptide hormone like "X" although it can produce the same effects as "X." Epinephrine can also bind to the skeletal muscle.

D Norepinephrine (noradrenaline) is a small organic molecule with a molecular mass of 169 Da, not a peptide hormone like "X."

E Insulin would lower blood glucose by stimulating its uptake by muscle and adipose. Insulin would also lower the cAMP levels of hepatocytes.

18. E Insulin and growth factors act through autophosphorylation of their receptor, which stimulates the MAPK pathway. Therefore, the MAPK pathway will not respond normally in a patient with insulin-resistant diabetes (diabetes mellitus type 2).

A Only lipophilic hormones such as steroids can act through intracellular receptors to alter transcription. Insulin is a protein and cannot cross the plasma membrane.

B Insulin does not act through ion channels.

C Insulin does not act through a G protein-coupled receptor.

D Insulin does not act through a G protein-coupled receptor.

19. D Active transport—either primary (dependent on hydrolysis of energy-rich molecules, such as adenosine triphosphate [ATP]) or secondary (depending on cotransport of another solute, such as Na^+, down its concentration gradient)—always requires transmembrane proteins.

A Amino acids are taken up into cells via Na^+-coupled secondary active transport.

B Small gas molecules and hydrophobic substances can cross the plasma membrane by simple diffusion, which does not require any transmembrane proteins and hence is not subject to saturation.

C Facilitated diffusion down a concentration gradient is facilitated by membrane proteins.

E Peptide transport through membrane is by intestinal $H^+/$ peptide symport.

20. A Facilitated diffusion occurs downhill until the concentrations on both sides of the membrane are the same. It therefore requires no metabolic energy. However, because transport occurs through a transmembrane protein, the velocity as a function of concentration shows saturation.

B The facilitator simply increases the rate at which equilibrium is attained. The direction of transport is determined by the concentration gradient.

C ATP (or another energy-rich substrate) is required for primary active transport, not for diffusion (facilitated or not). Diffusion is down a concentration gradient; active transport is uphill (against the gradient) and thus requires energy.

D A significant process in eukaryotic cells that utilize facilitated diffusion is the uptake of glucose from the blood into cells.

E Facilitated diffusion allows for the uptake of solutes (e.g., glucose) from the blood as well as the release into the blood by the liver cell.

21. C $5HT_{2A}$ receptors act through G_q, which stimulates phospholipase C, resulting in the production of diacylglycerol (DAG) and inositol 1,4,5-triphosphate (IP_3). The latter opens Ca^{2+} channels in the ER, releasing Ca^{2+} into the cytosol, where it binds to CALcium-MODULated proteIN (calmodulin, CaM).

A $5HT_{2A}$ receptors act through G_q, not through G_s.

B $5HT_{2A}$ receptors act through G_q, not through G_i.

D $5HT_{2A}$ receptors act through G_q, not through G_t.

E $5HT_{2A}$ receptors act through G_q, which, via IP_3, actually opens Ca^{2+} channels in the ER.

22. B In the well-fed state, insulin is the predominant hormone. The insulin receptor belongs to the class of receptor tyrosine kinases, which autophosphorylate themselves upon hormone binding. This leads to further protein phosphorylation of downstream target proteins.

A, C, D Increased production of cAMP occurs after binding of hormones whose receptors are coupled to G_s. Increased production of cAMP activates protein kinase A. Glucagon mediates GPCR $G_{s\alpha}$ activation, increasing intracellular cAMP. In the well-fed state, insulin is the predominant hormone. Insulin receptors are not coupled to G_s.

E Production of cGMP is caused by either membrane-bound (e.g., for atrial natriuretic factor) or cytosolic receptors (e.g., for nitric oxide). In the well-fed state, insulin is the predominant hormone. Insulin does not signal via either of these receptors.

23. E G protein-coupled receptor (GPCR) signaling via G_q, phospholipase C yields two second messengers, IP_3 and DAG. IP_3 causes the release of cytosolic Ca^{2+} which then translocates cytosolic protein kinase C to the plasma membrane where it is activated by DAG.

A IP3 causes the release of cytosolic Ca^{2+} which then translocates cytosolic protein kinase C (not monomeric G protein) to the plasma membrane where it is activated by DAG.

B Phospholipase C yields messengers IP_3 and DAG. IP3 causes the release of cytosolic Ca^{2+} which then translocates cytosolic protein kinase C (not Phospholipase C) to the plasma membrane where it is activated by DAG.

C After fasting, glucagon is the predominant hormone. Its receptors signal via the trimeric G_s triggers the activation of adenylate cyclase.

D cAMP phosphodiesterase (hydrolysis of 3′, 5′-cAMP into 5′-AMP), is not stimulated by G_q pathway.

24. A Pertussis toxin adenosine diphosphate (ADP) ribosylates $G_{i\alpha}$, preventing GDP/GTP exchange and thus inhibition of adenylate cyclase. *Bordetella* infections claim the lives of some 400,000 children worldwide each year; without mandatory immunization, this would be much worse. Weakening protection from childhood immunization creates a reservoir of susceptible adults; these may spread the infection to infants and elderly, in whom it is particularly dangerous. Presentation of these infections in adults may be unusual.

B cGMP is involved in transducin signaling (G_t) in vision, smell, and the taste of sweet, bitter, and savory. It is also produced by receptors with guanylate cyclase domains (e.g., nitric oxide, atrial natriuretic peptide) that do not require G proteins for coupling.

C Ca^{2+} is increased by G_q signaling.

D Diacylglycerol is increased by G_q signaling.

E IP_3 is increased by G_q signaling.

Reference

[1] Sakamoto K, McCluskey M, Wensel TG, Naggert JK, Nishina PM. New mouse models for recessive retinitis pigmentosa caused by mutations in the Pde6a gene. Human Mol Gen. 2009; 18:178–192

Part III

Cellular Respiration

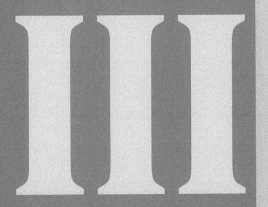

III

8 Principles of Cellular Respiration

8.1 Overview

Cellular respiration is the process by which the energy contained within the bonds of carbohydrates, proteins, and lipids is harvested and converted into adenosine triphosphate (ATP). The energy stored in ATP is then released upon hydrolysis and used to perform mechanical work (e.g., muscle contraction) or chemical work (e.g., biomolecule synthesis). Cellular respiration depends on the integration of several metabolic pathways that link the breakdown of nutrients to oxidation-reduction (redox) reactions that culminate in the transfer of electrons to O_2 and

the phosphorylation of adenosine diphosphate (ADP) into ATP. A summary of the pathways involved follows (▶ Fig. 8.1):

1. **Glycolysis:** This cytosolic pathway splits glucose (a six-carbon carbohydrate) into two molecules of pyruvate (a three-carbon compound). In doing so, ATP and a reduced form of nicotinamide adenine dinucleotide (NADH) are produced. (The starting material, glucose, is obtained from the catabolism of carbohydrates or from de novo synthesis via gluconeogenesis.)
2. **Decarboxylation of pyruvate:** Under aerobic conditions, pyruvate is transported into the mitochondria, where it is

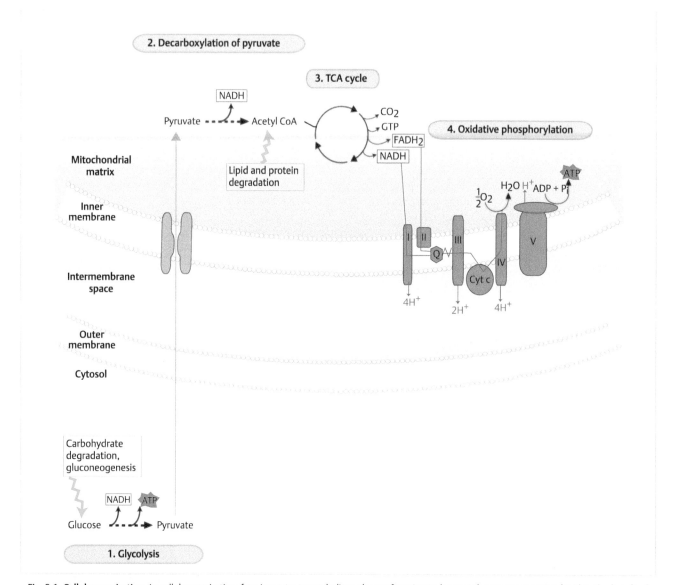

Fig. 8.1 Cellular respiration. In cellular respiration, four important metabolic pathways function to harvest the energy contained within the bonds of carbohydrates, proteins, and lipids and convert it to adenosine triphosphate (ATP). Those metabolic pathways are (1) glycolysis, (2) decarboxylation of pyruvate, (3) tricarboxylic acid (TCA) cycle, and (4) oxidative phosphorylation. The degradation of carbohydrates and the de novo synthesis of glucose (gluconeogenesis) supply the glucose. The degradation of lipids and proteins, as well as the metabolism of glucose, supply acetyl coenzyme A (CoA). ADP, adenosine diphosphate; FADH$_2$, reduced flavin adenine dinucleotide; GTP, guanosine triphosphate; NADH, reduced nicotinamide adenine dinucleotide.

converted (via oxidative decarboxylation) to acetyl coenzyme A (CoA) in a reaction that produces NADH.

3. **Tricarboxylic acid (TCA) cycle:** In the mitochondria, the reactions of the TCA cycle oxidize acetyl CoA into CO_2 and generate NADH, a reduced form of flavin adenine dinucleotide ($FADH_2$), and guanosine triphosphate (GTP). (The starting substrate, acetyl CoA, is obtained from the breakdown of glucose as well as the catabolism of proteins and lipids.)

4. **Oxidative phosphorylation:** This pathway is performed by a collection of inner mitochondrial membrane protein complexes (I, II, III, IV) that facilitate the transfer of electrons from NADH and $FADH_2$ to O_2 and establish a proton gradient across the inner membrane. This gradient provides the energy needed for an enzyme complex called ATP synthase (also known as complex V) to phosphorylate ADP into ATP.

8.2 ATP

8.2.1 Structure

ATP—the fundamental energy currency of the cell—is a ribonucleotide made up of adenine, ribose, and three phosphate groups in the following arrangement (▶ Fig. 8.2):

- The adenine (a double-ringed purine nitrogenous base) is attached to carbon-1 of ribose (a 5-carbon cyclic sugar) via an N-glycosidic bond.
- The first phosphate group (α) is attached to carbon-5 of ribose via a phosphoric acid ester bond. The second phosphate group (β) is attached to the α-phosphate group via a phosphoric acid anhydride bond. The third phosphate

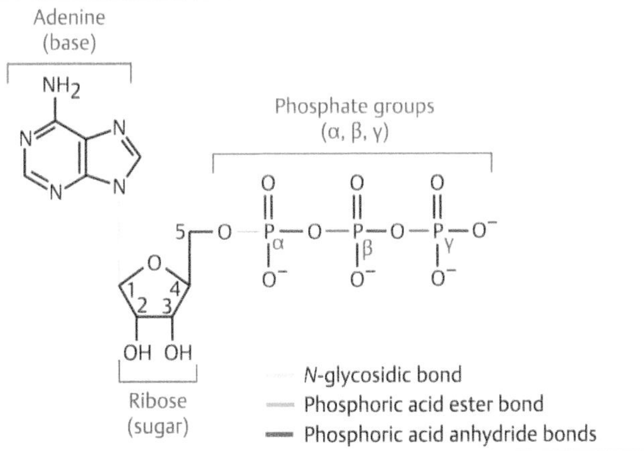

Fig. 8.2 Structure of adenosine triphosphate. ATP is a ribonucleotide formed from the purine base adenine, the sugar ribose, and three phosphate groups. Adenine is attached to carbon-1 of ribose via an N-glycosidic bond (blue). The α-phosphate group is attached to carbon-5 of ribose via a phosphoric acid ester bond (green). The β-phosphate group is attached to the α-phosphate group via a phosphoric acid anhydride bond (red). The terminal γ-phosphate group is attached to the β-phosphate group via another phosphoric acid anhydride bond (red).

group (γ) is attached to the β-phosphate group via another phosphoric acid anhydride bond.

III

Foundations

Nucleosides versus nucleotides

Nucleosides (e.g., adenosine) are composed of a nitrogenous base (e.g., adenine) attached to carbon-1 of ribose (or deoxyribose) via an N-glycosidic bond. When one or more phosphate groups are attached to the nucleoside, the resulting compound is referred to as a nucleotide.

8.2.2 ATP Hydrolysis

In the presence of water, the high-energy phosphoric acid anhydride bonds of ATP are cleaved (hydrolyzed), and a large amount of standard free energy ($\Delta G^{\circ\prime}$) is released (▶ Fig. 8.3a), as follows:

- The hydrolysis of the terminal phosphoric acid anhydride bond of the γ-phosphate group generates ADP and inorganic phosphate (PO_4^{3-}; P_i) and is associated with a $\Delta G^{\circ\prime}$ value of −7.3 kcal/mol (−30.5 kJ/mol).
- The hydrolysis of the phosphoric acid anhydride bond between the α- and β-phosphate groups of ATP generates adenosine monophosphate (AMP) and pyrophosphate ($P_2O_7^{4-}$; PP_i) and is associated with a $\Delta G^{\circ\prime}$ value of −10.9 kcal/mol (−45.6 kJ/mol).
- The spontaneous hydrolysis of pyrophosphate (PP_i) into two P_i is associated with a $\Delta G^{\circ\prime}$ value of −4.0 kcal/mol (−19.2 kJ/mol).

Reaction coupling. As indicated by its negative $\Delta G^{\circ\prime}$, the hydrolysis of ATP is an exergonic (energy-releasing) reaction that proceeds to the right as written and is said to be spontaneous. It is often coupled with endergonic (energy-consuming) reactions where $\Delta G^{\circ\prime} > 0$. As such, these reactions will proceed to the left as written and are said to be nonspontaneous. A commonly used example of the coupling of ATP hydrolysis to a thermodynamically unfavorable reaction is the first step in glycolysis in which the enzyme hexokinase (or glucokinase) phosphorylates glucose into glucose 6-phosphate to trap it inside a cell (▶ Fig. 8.3b).

Foundations

High-energy phosphoric acid anhydride and thioester bonds

Similar to ATP, other triphosphate nucleotides such as guanosine triphosphate (GTP), cytidine triphosphate (CTP), uridine triphosphate (UTP), and thymidine triphosphate (TTP) store energy within their high-energy phosphoric acid anhydride bonds. Energy is also stored in the thioester bond formed between the thiol group of coenzyme A and carboxylic acids. The energy released upon hydrolysis of this thioester bond is equivalent to that of ATP hydrolysis of the terminal phosphoric acid anhydride bond of ATP.

Hydrolysis energies

ATP $\longrightarrow$ ADP + P$_i$ ($\Delta G^{\circ\prime}$ = − 7.3 kcal/mol)

ATP $\longrightarrow$ AMP + PP$_i$ ($\Delta G^{\circ\prime}$ = − 10.9 kcal/mol)

PP$_i$ $\longrightarrow$ P$_i$ + P$_i$ ($\Delta G^{\circ\prime}$ = − 4.0 kcal/mol)

a

Coupled reaction

Reaction 1: Glucose + P$_i$ $\longrightarrow$ glucose 6-phosphate + H$_2$O $\Delta G^{\circ\prime}$ = + 3.3 kcal/mol

Reaction 2: ATP + H$_2$O $\longrightarrow$ ADP + P$_i$ $\Delta G^{\circ\prime}$ = − 7.3 kcal/mol

Coupled
b reaction: Glucose + ATP $\longrightarrow$ glucose 6-phosphate + ADP $\Delta G^{\circ\prime}$ = − 4.3 kcal/mol

Fig. 8.3 Energetics of adenosine triphosphate (ATP) hydrolysis and coupled reactions. (a) The hydrolysis of ATP into adenosine diphosphate (ADP) and phosphate (P$_i$) is associated with a standard free energy ($\Delta G^{\circ\prime}$) of −7.3 kcal/ mol. The hydrolysis of ATP into adenosine monophosphate (AMP) and pyrophosphate (PPi) is associated with $\Delta G^{\circ\prime}$ of −10.9 kcal/mol. Pyrophosphate is spontaneously hydrolyzed into two phosphates, with a $\Delta G^{\circ\prime}$ of −4.0 kcal/mol of free energy. **(b)** The $\Delta G^{\circ\prime}$ for the transfer of a phosphate group to carbon-6 of glucose (the first step in glycolysis) is + 3.3 kcal/mol. When coupled to ATP hydrolysis, the resulting $\Delta G^{\circ\prime}$ is −4.3 kcal/mol for the phosphorylation of glucose, which allows the reaction to proceed spontaneously and to the right as written. This reaction is catalyzed by hexokinase (glucokinase).

Normal

Energy storage in ion gradients

Energy is stored within the electrochemical gradients formed across membranes by ions such as Na$^+$ and H$^+$. The movement of these ions across membranes, down their gradients, to an area of lower concentration provides the energy to do work. For instance, by moving Na$^+$ into a cell, the sodium-glucose transporter 1 (SGLT1) harnesses the energy contained within the Na$^+$ gradient to drive the transport of glucose into the cell. (The Na$^+$ concentration is higher outside relative to inside the cell.) Likewise, by moving H$^+$ into the mitochondrial matrix from the intermembrane space, ATP synthase harnesses the energy contained within the H$^+$ gradient to power the phosphorylation of ADP to ATP. (The H$^+$ concentration is higher in the mitochondrial intermembrane space relative to the matrix during active electron transport.)

Foundations

Gibbs free energy change

Gibbs free energy (G) describes the energy available to do useful work. The change in free energy (ΔG) refers to the difference in G between the product(s) and the reactant(s) of a chemical reaction. The rate at which the reaction proceeds does not depend on the magnitude of ΔG but on the enzyme that catalyzes the reaction. The standard free energy change ($\Delta G^{\circ\prime}$) refers to the free energy change under standard conditions where the initial concentration of reactants and products is 1 M, the temperature is 298 K (25 °C), the pressure is 1 atm, and the pH is 7.0.

8.2.3 ATP Production: Substrate-Level versus Oxidative Phosphorylation

Substrate-level phosphorylation and oxidative phosphorylation are two ways in which cells generate ATP. They are similar in that they do so via the transfer of a phosphate group onto ADP. They differ, however, in the following ways:

- In substrate-level phosphorylation, the transfer of the phosphate group to ADP is catalyzed by kinases using PO$_4^{3-}$ groups obtained from metabolic intermediates that possess high-energy phosphate bonds (▶ Fig. 8.4).
- In oxidative phosphorylation, the transfer of the phosphate group to ADP is catalyzed by the mitochondrial ATP synthase using phosphate groups obtained from H$_2$PO$_4^-$ and HPO$_4^{2-}$ found in the mitochondrial matrix. ATP synthase harnesses the energy contained within the proton gradient across the inner mitochondrial membrane to synthesize ATP.

Foundations

GTP production via substrate-level phosphorylation

Guanosine triphosphate (GTP) is an essential molecule that is required for metabolic reactions (e.g., nucleotide synthesis) and for the activation of proteins (e.g., G proteins). Substrate-level phosphorylation is the mechanism by which GTP is generated from GDP and a phosphate group. In the tricarboxylic acid cycle, the enzyme succinate thiokinase concomitantly catalyzes the conversion of succinyl CoA into succinate and the phosphorylation of GDP to GTP (see Fig. 10.3). The energy released from the conversion of succinyl CoA into succinate is used to generate a high-energy phosphohistidine intermediate on the enzyme. The phosphate group is then transferred to GDP to form GTP.

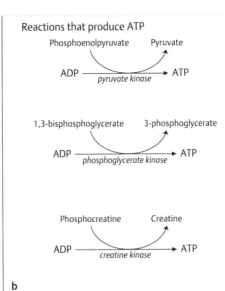

Donors of phosphate groups
Phosphoenolpyruvate
($\Delta G°'$ of hydrolysis = –14.8 kcal/mol)

1, 3-bisphosphoglycerate
($\Delta G°'$ of hydrolysis = –11.9 kcal/mol)

Phosphocreatine
($\Delta G°'$ of hydrolysis = –10.3 kcal/mol)

a

Reactions that produce ATP

Phosphoenolpyruvate → Pyruvate

ADP —— pyruvate kinase —→ ATP

1,3-bisphosphoglycerate → 3-phosphoglycerate

ADP —— phosphoglycerate kinase —→ ATP

Phosphocreatine → Creatine

ADP —— creatine kinase —→ ATP

b

Fig. 8.4 Phosphate donors in substrate-level phosphorylation. (a, b) In substrate-level phosphorylation, the transfer of the phosphate group to ADP is catalyzed by protein kinases (e.g., pyruvate kinase, phosphoglycerate kinase, creatine kinase) using PO_4^{3-} groups obtained from compounds (e.g., phosphoenolpyruvate, 1,3-bisphosphoglycerate, phosphocreatine) that possess high-energy phosphate bonds. The substrate-level phosphorylations carried out by pyruvate kinase and phosphoglycerate kinase are found in the glycolytic pathway.

Therapeutics

Creatine kinase: a marker for myocardial infarction

Using a phosphate group derived from ATP, creatine kinases phosphorylate creatine to generate the high-energy compound, phosphocreatine, which serves as an energy storage reserve in resting muscle. When needed, phosphocreatine rapidly (2 to 7 seconds) donates its phosphate group for the phosphorylation of ADP into ATP. This helps to maintain adequate energy levels to support muscle contractions. The form of creatine kinase that is normally found in muscle and brain tissue (CK-MB or CK2) is used as a marker for the diagnosis of myocardial infarctions (MIs) because damage to heart muscle cells results in abnormally high levels of serum CK-MB within the first 4 to 8 hours after an MI. Peak levels are seen 12 to 24 hours after an MI, and levels return to normal in 3 to 4 days. It should be noted that CK levels in serum may also go up if there is damage to skeletal muscle in the absence of any damage to the cardiac muscle (although the isoform in this case is CK-MM or CK3). Therefore, confirmation of the diagnosis of MI requires other cardiac markers such as troponin T/I and glycogen phosphorylase BB.

Normal serum creatine kinase level is 25 to 90 U/L for males and 10 to 70 U/L for females.

9 Glycolysis and the Fate of Pyruvate

9.1 Glucose Uptake

Before glucose can be metabolized, it needs to be taken up from the blood plasma into the cell. The normal concentration of glucose in the plasma is between 4 and 8 mM (70 to 140 mg/dL), although it may be as much as 20 mM in portal blood after a meal.

To accomplish the transfer of glucose, the cell uses glucose transporters. They facilitate the transport of glucose and other sugars (e.g., galactose, fructose) in and out of cells along the concentration gradient of the sugar. There are 14 glucose transporters, 4 of which are important in the current context:

1. **GLUT1** (*glucose transporter, isoform 1*) is a ubiquitous transporter found especially in red blood cells, the cornea, the placenta, the brain, tissue cultures, and transformed (cancerous) cells. It facilitates the transport of glucose in an unregulated manner. GLUT1 has a high affinity for glucose with a $K_m = 1$ mM. K_m is defined as the substrate concentration at which the reaction velocity is half-maximal. Maximal reaction velocity occurs at a substrate concentration of approximately 10 times the K_m. Because GLUT1 has a K_m of 1 mM, and the [glucose] in the plasma is between 4 and 8 mM, GLUT1 is almost saturated at all times. There is some evidence that GLUT1 expression may be downregulated by fasting and free fatty acids and upregulated by insulin and hypoxia. Cancer cells have increased expression of GLUT1 and small molecule inhibitors of GLUT1 (e.g., fasentin) are being explored as possible chemotherapeutic agents.

2. **GLUT2** is the main glucose transporter found in the liver, basolateral surface of intestinal cells and in kidney proximal tubules. This transporter allows glucose uptake/release independent of insulin. This is a high-capacity, low affinity ($K_m = \sim 10$ mM) transporter with no regulation. The high capacity coupled with low affinity allows GLUT2 to let glucose and galactose into the liver extremely quickly from portal blood (e.g., after a meal) to minimize hyperglycemia and galactosemia. GLUT2 also allows glucose to be released from the liver during gluconeogenesis (i.e., when blood glucose levels fall). GLUT2 is also present in the β cells of the pancreas. These cells sense blood glucose levels through GLUT2 and release insulin accordingly.

3. **GLUT3** is the major glucose transporter in neurons. Like GLUT1, GLUT3 acts by facilitated transport in an insulin-independent manner, with high affinity ($K_m = 1$ mM). GLUT3 can also be considered to be saturated, which is necessary because the brain depends on glucose for its energy (*only* metabolizes glucose), except in very extreme starvation conditions, at which time it will use ketone bodies.

4. **GLUT4** is important for glucose transport in the skeletal muscle, adipose tissue, and heart. Surface expression of this transporter is dependent on insulin. GLUT4 is normally sequestered in microvesicles in the cytosol (▶ Fig. 9.1). Insulin binds to the plasma membrane, generating a signaling cascade that allows surface expression of GLUT4. When expressed, this transporter has a K_m of 5 mM and is therefore normally ~ 50% saturated. The end result of insulin

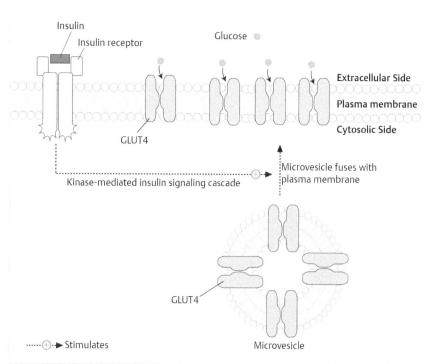

Fig. 9.1 Regulation of cell surface expression of glucose transporter 4 (GLUT4) by insulin. GLUT4 transporters in muscle and in adipose tissue are normally sequestered in microvesicles in the cytoplasm. Insulin signaling causes the microvesicles to fuse with the plasma membrane, thus enabling the expression of GLUT4 to facilitate glucose uptake.

Insulin

Insulin receptor

Glucose

Extracellular Side

Plasma membrane

GLUT4

Cytosolic Side

Microvesicle fuses with plasma membrane

Kinase-mediated insulin signaling cascade

GLUT4

Microvesicle

⊕▶ Stimulates

III

release from the pancreas is a decrease in the concentration of glucose in the plasma.

Therapeutics

Fanconi-Bickel syndrome

Fanconi-Bickel syndrome results from an inherited deficiency of GLUT2 glucose transporters in the liver, pancreatic β cells, and proximal renal tubules. Children and infants with this disorder exhibit stunted growth, hepatomegaly, and bouts of hypoglycemia between meals but hyperglycemia (and hypergalactosemia) after a meal. Due to the deficiency of GLUT2 in the liver, glucose and galactose are not rapidly cleared from circulation after feeding. Also, glucose generated via gluconeogenesis is not released from the liver during the fasting state. Insulin secretion remains low because the pancreatic β cells fail to sense an increase in blood glucose levels. Hepatomegaly is the result of glycogen accumulation in the liver. Dwarfism is the result of vitamin D–dependent hypophosphatemic rickets due to proximal tubular nephropathy. Treatment consists of ingesting frequent small meals to ensure adequate calorie intake and avoidance of galactose in the diet. Electrolytes are replaced, and vitamin D and phosphate supplements are given.

9.2 Overview of Glycolysis

Glycolysis is a series of cytoplasmic reactions employed by all human cell types to harness the chemical energy contained within glucose. In these reactions, adenosine triphosphate (ATP) and the reduced form of nicotinamide adenine dinucleotide

(NADH) are generated when glucose is degraded into pyruvate in the presence of oxygen (aerobic glycolysis) or into lactate when the oxygen supply is limited (anaerobic glycolysis).

Aerobic glycolysis and beyond. As summarized in ▶ Fig. 9.2a, aerobic glycolysis involves the breakdown of one molecule of glucose into two molecules of pyruvate, with a net production of two molecules each of ATP and the electron carrier NADH. When oxygen is available, pyruvate is transported into the mitochondrial matrix where it is completely oxidized into CO_2 concomitant with the generation of an additional 34 to 36 molecules of ATP.

Anaerobic glycolysis and beyond. As summarized in ▶ Fig. 9.2b, anaerobic glycolysis also involves the breakdown of one molecule of glucose into two molecules of pyruvate concomitant with the production of two ATP and two NADH molecules. When the oxygen supply is deficient, however, pyruvate is reduced to lactate in a reaction that oxidizes the NADH back to NAD^+.

- Anaerobic glycolysis serves as a critical source of ATP for those cells that lack mitochondria (e.g., red blood cells), are poorly vascularized (e.g., cornea), or are deprived of oxygen (e.g., cells of overworked skeletal muscles or infarcted heart muscles).

Glucose supply. The supply of glucose used in the glycolytic pathway comes from dietary glucose, fructose, and galactose and the breakdown of glycogen (the stored form of glucose). Alternatively, glucose may be supplied by gluconeogenesis (see Chapter 12, section "Gluconeogensis: De novo Synthesis of Glucose), a pathway in which noncarbohydrate precursors such as glycerol, lactate, glucogenic amino acids, and tricarboxylic acid (TCA) cycle intermediates are used to synthesize glucose de novo via a series of reactions that are similar to those of glycolysis in reverse.

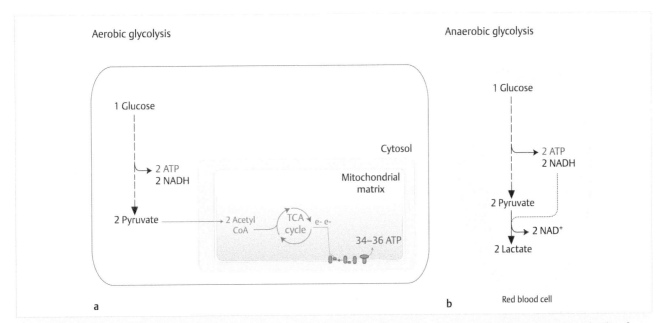

Fig. 9.2 Aerobic and anaerobic glycolysis. (a) Aerobic glycolysis is a series of cytoplasmic reactions that oxidize glucose into two molecules of pyruvate and generates two molecules each of adenosine tri-phosphate (ATP) and the reduced form of nicotinamide adenine dinucleotide (NADH). Pyruvate is then completely oxidized to CO_2 in mitochondria, generating an additional 34 to 36 molecules of ATP. (b) Anaerobic glycolysis also involves the breakdown of glucose into two molecules each of pyruvate, ATP, and NADH, but the pyruvate is then reduced to lactate, oxidizing the NADHs to generate two NAD^+ molecules. CoA, coenzyme A; TCA, tricarboxylic acid.

III

Therapeutics

Hypoxemia

Hypoxemia refers to a low partial pressure of O_2 in arterial blood (PaO_2). It may be caused by hypoventilation, low inspired O_2, diffusion impairment, ventilation/perfusion (V/Q) mismatch, or right-to-left-shunt. Clinical signs include pallor and cyanosis.

Normal

O_2 content of blood

The O_2 content of blood is defined as the volume of oxygen (both free and bound to hemoglobin) that is carried in 100 mL of blood and normally ranges from 95 to 100% of full saturation. It is calculated using values that represent the concentration of hemoglobin (Hb) in g per 100 mL of blood (Normal range: Men, 13.8–17.2; Women, 12.1–15.1), the percentage of saturation of arterial hemoglobin with O_2 SaO_2, the partial pressure of O_2 in the plasma of arterial blood PaO_2, and Hüfner's constant (1.34), in the following equation:

$$O_2 \text{ content of blood} = (1.34 \times [Hb] \times SaO_2) + (PaO_2)$$

Peripheral O_2 saturation (SpO_2) can be measured with a pulse oximeter. SpO_2 values 90% or lower are indicative of hypoxemia and imminent respiratory failure. It should be noted that oxygen saturation does not directly reflect tissue oxygenation. In the newborn, whose blood contains predominantly fetal hemoglobin with higher affinity for oxygen, SpO_2 levels lower than 94 to 95% may be indicative of hypoxemia.

Normal

Red blood cells and glycolysis

Red blood cells (RBCs) lack mitochondria; hence glycolysis serves as their only mechanism for producing ATP. Therefore, a disruption in the glycolytic pathway of RBCs inactivates the ATP-dependent ion pumps, which are essential for the maintenance of intracellular-extracellular ion gradients and thus cell viability. The resulting effect is the lysis of RBCs, which manifests as hemolytic anemia. The normal range for RBC (erythrocyte) count for men is 4.3 to 5.9 million/mm³ (4.3 to 5.9×10^{12}/L), and 3.5 to 5.5 million/mm³ (3.5 to 5.5×10^{12}/L) for women.

9.3 Glycolytic Reaction Steps

The glycolytic pathway consists of a series of enzyme-catalyzed, cytoplasmic reactions, of which three are irreversible. Grouping of these reactions into three phases allows for a helpful summary of the role of each reaction in glycolysis (▶ Fig. 9.3).

1. **Investment phase (steps 1–3):** This phase is defined by the first three reactions of glycolysis (two of which are irreversible under physiological conditions). The first reaction consumes one ATP for the purpose of trapping glucose inside the cell via its phosphorylation into glucose 6-phosphate. After the latter has been isomerized to fructose 6-phosphate, an additional molecule of ATP is consumed to convert it into fructose 1,6-bisphosphate.

- The two ATP-dependent, irreversible glycolytic reactions in this investment phase are catalyzed by hexokinase/glucokinase and phosphofructokinase-1. These enzymes are known regulators of the glycolytic pathway. Phosphofructokinase-1, which catalyzes the slowest of the glycolytic reactions, is rate limiting.

2. **Splitting phase (steps 4 and 5):** This phase is defined by the reaction catalyzed by aldolase A in which it splits the 6-carbon molecule—fructose 1,6-bisphosphate—into two three-carbon molecules: glyceraldehyde 3-phosphate (G3P) and dihydroxyacetone phosphate (DHAP).

- G3P and DHAP are isomers of each other and are reversibly interconverted by the enzyme triose phosphate isomerase. Two molecules of G3P are utilized in subsequent glycolytic reactions. When conditions favor the DHAP isomer (such as when the NAD^+ supply is depleted), it is converted to glycerol 3-phosphate—a precursor used for the synthesis of triacylglycerols (fats).

3. **Recoup phase (steps 6–10):** This phase is defined by the next five reactions (only one of which is irreversible) that convert G3P into pyruvate while generating NADH and ATP molecules. The most noteworthy reactions of this phase are catalyzed by the following:

- Glyceraldehyde 3-phosphate dehydrogenase, an enzyme that reduces NAD^+ into NADH during the conversion of G3P into the high-energy compound 1,3-bisphosphoglycerate
- Phosphoglycerate kinase, an enzyme that catalyzes the substrate-level phosphorylation of adenosine diphosphate (ADP) into ATP in a reaction that also converts 1,3-bisphosphoglycerate into 3-phosphoglycerate
- Pyruvate kinase, an enzyme that catalyzes the next substrate-level phosphorylation of ADP to form ATP in an irreversible reaction that converts the high-energy phosphoenolpyruvate into pyruvate

Regeneration of NAD^+. The amount of NAD^+ in the cytosol is limiting and must be regenerated in order for glycolysis to continue. Thus, under aerobic conditions, cytosolic NADH is oxidized to NAD^+ by either the malate-aspartate shuttle or the glycerophosphate shuttle (see Chapter 11). However, under anaerobic conditions or in cells lacking mitochondria, NADH is oxidized to NAD^+ when pyruvate is reduced to lactate by lactate dehydrogenase (step 11).

Foundations

Glycolysis versus gluconeogenesis

Although the cytoplasmic glycolytic reactions function to degrade glucose, the cytoplasmic and mitochondrial reactions of gluconeogenesis serve to synthesize glucose de novo—particularly when blood glucose levels are low. The steps of gluconeogenesis are a reversal of the steps of glycolysis with three exceptions:

1. In glycolysis, glucose is phosphorylated into glucose 6-phosphate by hexokinase/glucokinase. The reverse of this (i.e., the dephosphorylation of glucose 6-phosphate) is catalyzed by glucose 6-phosphatase in gluconeogenesis.
2. In glycolysis, fructose 6-phosphate is phosphorylated into fructose 1,6-bisphosphate by phosphofructokinase-1. The

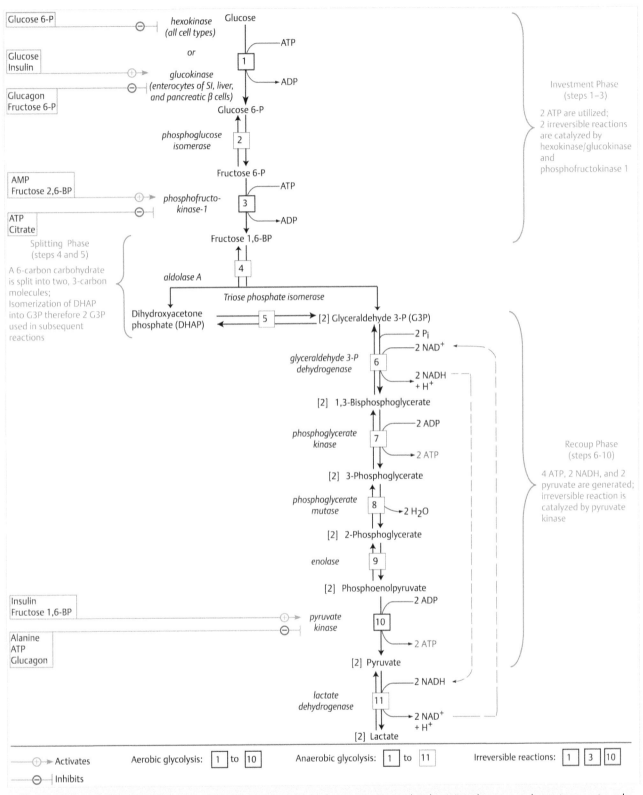

Fig. 9.3 Reaction steps of glycolysis. Glycolysis consists of a series of cytoplasmic, enzyme-catalyzed reactions that convert glucose to pyruvate under aerobic conditions or lactate under anaerobic conditions. The pathway is regulated by the three enzymes that catalyze the irreversible reactions of steps 1, 3, and 10. Key glycolytic reactions are summarized in ▶ Table 9.1. ADP, adenosine diphosphate; ATP, adenosine triphosphate; BP, bisphosphate; NAD, nicotinamide adenine dinucleotide; NADH, reduced form of nicotinamide adenine dinucleotide.

Table 9.1 Enzymes that catalyze ATP-consuming/producing reactions and produce NADH/NAD$^+$

Step	Enzyme	ATP consuming reaction	ATP use
1	Hexokinase/glucokinase (in liver)	Glucose → glucose 6-P	1 ATP
3	Phosphofructokinase-1	Fructose 6-P → fructose 1,6-BP	1 ATP
		ATP-producing reaction	**ATP yield**
7	Phosphoglycerate kinase	1,3-Bisphosphoglycerate → 3-phosphoglycerate	2 ATP
10	Pyruvate kinase	Phosphoenolpyruvate → pyruvate	2 ATP
		NADH-producing reaction	**Yield**
6	Glyceraldehyde 3-P dehydrogenase	Glyceraldehyde 3-P → 1,3-bisphosphoglycerate	2 NADH

Abbreviations: ATP, adenosine triphosphate; NAD, nicotinamide adenine dinucleotide; NADH, reduced form of nicotinamide adenine dinucleotide. Net ATP yield from glycolysis is two ATP/glucose.
NAD$^+$ must be regenerated for glycolysis to continue; therefore, reducing equivalents from NADH are shuttled into the electron transport chain via glycerol-phosphate shuttle, or malate-aspartate shuttle or NADH is oxidized by lactate dehydrogenase.

reverse (i.e., the de-phosphorylation of fructose 1,6-bisphosphate) is catalyzed by fructose 1,6-bisphosphatase in gluconeogenesis.

3. In glycolysis, phosphoenolpyruvate (PEP) is converted to pyruvate by pyruvate kinase. The reverse of this (i.e., the conversion of pyruvate into PEP) is performed in two steps by the enzymes pyruvate carboxylase (located in the mitochondria) and PEP carboxykinase.

Therapeutics
Hypoxia

Hypoxia is described as low oxygen concentration in body tissues. It may occur in local tissue sites as a consequence of vascular occlusion (infarction). Hypoxia occurs in the whole body at high altitude, when ventilation is impaired, or when cardiac output is decreased. To compensate for the low levels of O$_2$, cells switch to anaerobic metabolism of glucose, which leads to the buildup of lactate, causing lactic acidosis.

Normal
The brain and glucose

Brain cells are exceptionally dependent on glucose for energy because it is the predominant fuel molecule that can cross the blood–brain barrier. Consequently, during periods of starvation, brain cells obtain their supply of glucose from that which is generated via gluconeogenesis in the liver. Under prolonged conditions of starvation, the brain can utilize ketone bodies as fuel.

Normal
Carbohydrate metabolism in fed versus fasting states

In the fed state, abundant glucose is available, leading to increases in uptake, trapping within the cells, rates of glycolysis and glycogen synthesis, and a decrease in gluconeogenesis. Fasting state leads to a reversal of these effects, leading to decreases in uptake, catabolism, and storage and an increase in the rate of gluconeogenesis by the liver. The metabolic effects in fed versus fasting states are orchestrated by the relative amounts of insulin versus glucagon in circulation.

9.4 Regulation and Integration of Glycolysis and Associated Disorders

9.4.1 Regulation

The glycolytic pathway is regulated by hexokinase/glucokinase, phosphofructokinase-1, and pyruvate kinase. These kinases catalyze the three irreversible phosphorylation reactions that either consume ATP or generate it. The activity of these enzymes is modulated by fluctuations in the concentrations of molecules such as ATP, adenosine monophosphate (AMP), glucose, insulin, and glucagon. In general, glycolysis is

- promoted after a meal when blood glucose and insulin levels are high but that of glucagon is low;
- inhibited during periods of fasting when blood glucose and insulin levels are low but that of glucagon is high;
- stimulated by signals of a low-energy charge, such as elevated AMP levels; and
- inhibited by signals of a high-energy charge, such as elevated ATP levels.

Hexokinase/Glucokinase

Hexokinase is present in most tissues, whereas its isozyme, glucokinase (hexokinase IV), is found mainly in liver cells and pancreatic β cells. Although both enzymes catalyze the ATP-dependent phosphorylation of glucose into glucose 6-phosphate, which traps it in the cell's cytosol, they differ in their affinity for glucose and their sensitivity to changes in the levels of glycolytic intermediates, as follows:

- Hexokinase has a low K_m (0.1 mM) and therefore a high affinity for glucose (▶ Fig. 9.4a). This allows it to catalyze its reaction even when blood glucose levels are low. Hexokinase is inhibited by its product, glucose 6-phosphate (see ▶ Fig. 9.3) and is therefore most active when this product is being used up rapidly.
- Glucokinase, in contrast, does not exhibit Michaelis-Menten kinetics with respect to glucose and has low affinity for glucose (▶ Fig. 9.4a). It is half-saturated ($S_{0.5}$) at 8 mm glucose and is only weakly inhibited by the product, glucose 6-phosphate. These characteristics make

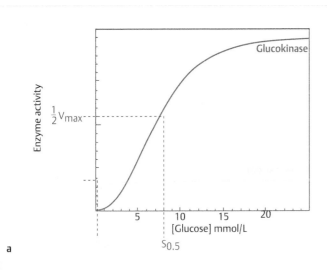

Fig. 9.4 Hexokinase, glucokinase, and serum glucose ranges. (a) Enzyme kinetics: hexokinase versus glucokinase: Hexokinase (blue) has a low K_m (0.1 mmol/L) and therefore a high affinity for glucose. Glucokinase (red) has a high $S_{0.5}$ (8 mmol/L) and therefore a low affinity for glucose and exhibits a sigmoidal saturation curve for glucose. **(b)** Glycemic status based on serum glucose concentrations: The normal range for serum glucose concentrations after a period of fasting (e.g., after sleeping) is 5.6 mmol/L, or 2 hours after a meal (postprandial) is < 7.8 mmol/L. A person is considered hypoglycemic when the random blood glucose level falls below 2.78 mmol/L. For diabetics, the fasting serum glucose level is ≥ 7.0 mmol/L, and 2 hours postprandial it is > 11.1 mmol/L.

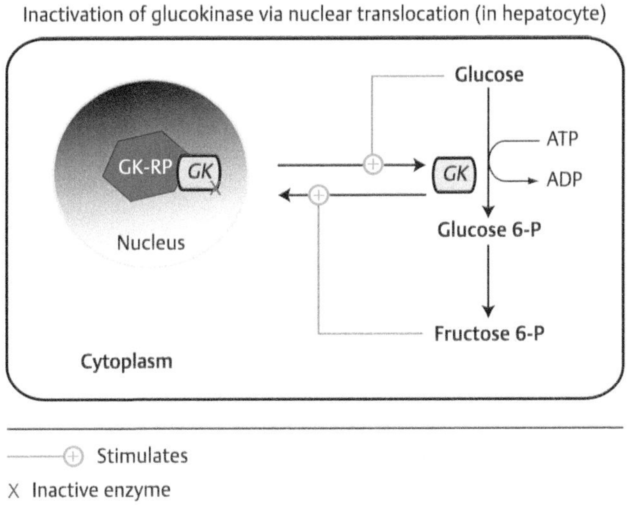

	Hypoglycemic	Normal		Diabetic	
		Fasting	*2 h postprandial*	*Fasting*	*2 h postprandial*
Serum [glucose]	< 2.78 mmol/L (< 50 mg/dL)	5.6 mmol/L (100 mg/dL)	< 7.8 mmol/L (< 140 mg/dL)	≥ 7.0 mmol/L (≥ 126 mg/dL)	≥ 11.1 mmol/L (≥ 200 mg/dL)

b

Inactivation of glucokinase via nuclear translocation (in hepatocyte)

Fig. 9.5 Regulation of glucokinase. Fructose 6-phosphate stimulates the translocation of glucokinase (GK) to the nucleus, where it binds to and thus is inhibited by the glucokinase regulatory protein (GK-RP) located in the nucleus. GK is inactive when bound to GK-RP in the nucleus. High levels of blood glucose, however, promote the dissociation of GK from GK-RP and its subsequent translocation back to the cytosol, where it is active. ADP, adenosine diphosphate; ATP, adenosine triphosphate; P, phosphate.

glucokinase most active when blood glucose levels are high. It is indirectly inhibited by fructose 6-phosphate, which promotes the translocation of glucokinase to the nucleus, where it binds to, and is thus sequestered by, a nuclear protein called glucokinase regulatory protein (GK-RP) (▶ Fig. 9.5). When glucose levels are high, glucokinase dissociates from GK-RP and is released back into the cytosol, where it becomes active.

Hormonal modulation of glucokinase. Elevated levels of insulin induce the synthesis of glucokinase, whereas elevated levels of glucagon decrease it.

Normal

Glucokinase as a glucose sensor and blood glucose buffer

Glucokinase (GK) is a monomeric protein of 50 kDa mass with a $S_{0.5}$ of 8 mM for glucose. Cellular expression of GK is governed by a single gene with two promoters, one of which is regulated by insulin. The insulin-sensitive promoter controls hepatic expression of GK, whereas the constitutive promoter is important in pancreatic β cells. Hormone-producing α and β cells of pancreas are present in regions known as islets of Langerhans. The α cells produce glucagon, whereas the β cells secrete insulin in response to blood glucose levels. GK, together with the ATP-sensitive K channel (K_{ATP} channel) and voltage-sensitive L-type Ca channels, serves as the glucose sensor to determine the threshold for glucose-stimulated insulin release. When blood glucose levels rise above 5 mM, such as after a meal, glucose enters pancreatic β cells via the constitutive glucose transporter 2 (GLUT2). GK controls the glycolytic and oxidative production of ATP, which closes the K_{ATP} channel and depolarizes the β cell membrane. As a result, the L-type Ca channel opens, allowing calcium influx. Calcium triggers insulin release via several signaling pathways that involve cAMP, inositol 3-phosphate, and protein kinase C.

The concentration of glucose in portal blood can reach as high as 20 mM after a meal. GK, with its low affinity and high capacity for glucose, is ideally suited to process the increased load and maintain blood glucose homeostasis. When glucose levels are low, hepatic GK is sequestered in the nucleus in complex with an inhibitory 68 kDa protein (GK-RP). High glucose and fructose 1-phosphate promote dissociation of the GK/GK-RP complex, allowing GK to translocate to cytosol. GK in the liver regulates glycolysis, the pentose phosphate shunt, and ATP production.

Phosphofructokinase-1

Phosphofructokinase-1 (PFK-1), the rate-limiting enzyme of glycolysis, catalyzes the ATP-dependent phosphorylation of fructose 6-phosphate into fructose 1,6-bisphosphate. It is activated by high concentrations of AMP and fructose 2,6-bisphosphate (F26BP) but inhibited by high concentrations of ATP and citrate (▶ Fig. 9.3).
- F26BP is formed by the bifunctional enzyme phosphofructo-kinase-2/fructose-bisphosphatase-2 (PFK-2/FBPase-2), which functions as a kinase in the dephosphorylated state and as a phosphatase in the phosphorylated state.
- Citrate is the first intermediate formed in the TCA cycle.

Hormonal modulation of PFK-1. Elevated levels of insulin stimulate PFK-1 activity, whereas elevated levels of glucagon reduce it via the mechanisms listed here (▶ Fig. 9.6). When PFK-1 activity is reduced, glycolysis is inhibited, but gluconeogenesis is favored.
- The activity of PFK-1 is simulated via the insulin-induced activation of protein phosphatases, which dephosphorylate PFK-2/FBPase-2, triggering its kinase activity. Consequently, F26BP levels increase, and PFK-1 activity is stimulated.
- The activity of PFK-1 is reduced via the glucagon-induced increase in cyclic AMP (cAMP) levels, which activate protein kinase A (PKA)—an enzyme that phosphorylates PFK-2/FBPase-2 and triggers its phosphatase activity. Consequently, F26BP levels decrease and cause a reduction in PFK-1 activity.

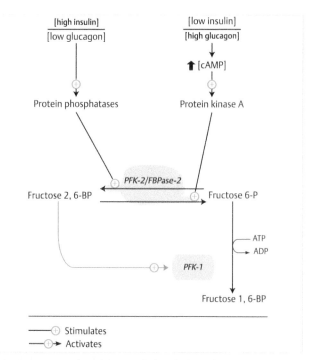

Fig. 9.6 Hormonal modulation of phosphofructokinase-1 and -2 activities
Fructose 2,6-bisphosphate, which is formed by phosphofructokinase-2/ fructose-bisphosphatase-2 (PFK-2/FBPase-2), activates phosphofructo-kinase-1 (PFK-1). PFK-2/FBPase-2 is a bifunctional enzyme that functions as a kinase in its unphosphorylated form or as a phosphatase in its phosphorylated form. In the fed state (when blood glucose levels are high), elevated levels of insulin activate protein phosphatases, which dephosphorylate PFK-2 in the liver. As a result, PFK-2 functions as a kinase to increase the concentrations of fructose 2,6-bisphosphate (BP), which stimulates PFK-1 activity. In the fasting state, however, elevated levels of glucagon increase cyclic adenosine monophosphate (cAMP) levels, which activate protein kinase A (PKA), an enzyme that phosphorylates PFK-2 in the liver. As a result, PFK-2 functions as a phosphatase to decrease the concentrations of fructose 2,6-bisphosphate, which decreases PFK-1 activity. ADP, adenosine diphosphate; ATP, adenosine triphosphate; P, phosphate.

Normal

Regulation of PFK-2 in heart muscle

Cardiac muscle contains a different isoenzyme of the bifunctional enzyme that interconverts fructose 6-phosphate/ fructose 2,6-bisphosphate. Epinephrine acts on the β-adrenergic receptor in the heart as in the liver and increases the intracellular levels of cAMP and consequently activated PKA. However, phosphorylation of bifunctional enzyme by PKA in the cardiac muscle increases fructose 2,6-bisphosphate levels rather than decreasing them. This differential effect is due to the fact that while PKA phosphorylates serine 32 on the bifunctional enzyme in the liver, it modifies serine 466 in the heart. As a result, epinephrine increases the rate of glycolysis in the heart while lowering it in the liver. The isoform of PFK-2 found in the skeletal muscle lacks serine 32 and is therefore insensitive to epinephrine.

Pyruvate Kinase

Pyruvate kinase irreversibly converts phosphoenolpyruvate into pyruvate with the production of ATP. It is activated by fructose 1,6-bisphosphate (the product of PFK-1 activity) but inhibited by elevated levels of ATP and alanine—a molecule that pyruvate can be converted into (▶ Fig. 9.3).

Hormonal modulation of pyruvate kinase activity. Elevated levels of insulin trigger an increase in pyruvate kinase activity, whereas elevated levels of glucagon decrease it via the mechanisms listed here (▶ Fig. 9.7). When pyruvate kinase activity is reduced, glycolysis is inhibited, and phosphoenolpyruvate enters the gluconeogenesis pathway to create glucose instead.

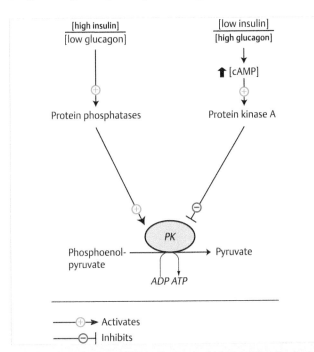

Fig. 9.7 Hormonal modulation of pyruvate kinase activity. Elevated levels of insulin activate protein phosphatases, which dephosphorylate and activate pyruvate kinase (PK). In contrast, elevated levels of glucagon activate protein kinase A (via cyclic adenosine monophosphate), which phosphorylates and inactivates PK.

- Insulin stimulates a protein phosphatase that dephosphorylates and activates pyruvate kinase.
- Glucagon causes cAMP-mediated activation of PKA—an enzyme that phosphorylates and inhibits pyruvate kinase.

9.4.2 Integration

Several intermediates in the glycolytic pathway are utilized by other pathways and systems, as summarized in ▶ Table 9.2.

9.4.3 Glycolysis-associated Disorders

Several human disorders are attributed to deficiencies in glycolytic pathway enzymes. Approximately 95% of glycolysis-related disorders that manifest as hemolytic anemia (i.e., anemia caused by the destruction of red blood cells) may be attributed to defects in pyruvate kinase, and 4% is attributed to defects in phosphoglucose isomerase. ▶ Table 9.3 summarizes the defects in some glycolytic enzymes and the resulting disorders, as well as the enzymes which are inhibited by arsenate and fluoride.

Therapeutics

Diabetes mellitus

Diabetes mellitus is a group of diseases characterized by hyperglycemia. The two major forms are type 1 and type 2. Type 1 diabetes results from a loss of pancreatic β cell mass (likely due to immune destruction) leading to severe insulin deficiency. Type 2 diabetes is initially caused by insulin resistance and slowly progresses to a loss of function of β cells. Other types of diabetes may be caused by genetic or physiological factors. Mutations in glucokinase and mitochondrial tRNA$_{leu}$ genes are associated with diabetes. Some cases of aberrant conversion of proinsulin to mature insulin as well as defective insulin receptor have also been described. Pancreatitis, trauma, infection, cystic fibrosis, hemochromatosis and pancreatic carcinoma may cause diabetes. Gestational diabetes refers to impaired glucose tolerance during pregnancy.

Table 9.2 Glycolytic intermediates and the pathways and systems in which they are used

Glycolytic intermediate	Use in other pathways or systems
Glucose 6-phosphate	Precursor for • pentose phosphate pathway Converted to glucose 1-phosphate, which is used in • galactose metabolism • glycogen synthesis (i.e., glucose storage) • uronic acid pathway (for the synthesis of glucuronic and iduronic acids, which are found in glycosaminoglycans)
Fructose 6-phosphate	Precursor for the synthesis of • mannose (involved in the glycosylation of proteins) • amino sugars (e.g., galactosamine and glucosamine, which are also found in glycosaminoglycans and glycoproteins)
Dihydroxyacetone phosphate	Converted to glycerol 3-phosphate for • triacylglycerol synthesis in liver cells • glycerophosphate shuttle
1,3-bisphospho-glycerate	Converted to 2,3-bisphosphoglycerate, which is an allosteric effector that reduces the affinity of hemoglobin for O_2 (i.e., right shifts Hb-O_2 binding curve) by binding to and stabilizing deoxyhemoglobin, which effectively triggers the release of O_2 for use by local tissues

Table 9.3 Glycolytic enzymes that may be defective and their clinical presentations

Enzyme	Defect	Disorder
Glucokinase	Autosomal dominant mutations	Inactivating mutation in one allele causes maturity onset diabetes of the young (MODY-2) Inactivating mutation in both alleles causes neonatal diabetes Activating mutation causes hyperinsulinemic hypoglycemia that can cause life-threatening seizures
Phosphoglucose isomerase	Autosomal recessive mutations	Mutations affect the protein's folding and activity and lead to nonspherocytic hemolytic anemia and neurologic impairment
Aldolase A	Deletion	Hemolytic anemia
Triose phosphate isomerase	Autosomal recessive mutations	Mutations cause intermediate enzyme deficiency and are associated with neonatal onset hemolytic anemia and neurologic dysfunction
Pyruvate kinase	Mutation in erythrocytes	Hemolytic anemia

Normal fasting blood glucose levels are defined as < 100 mg/dL (< 5.6 mM). Values of 100 to 125 mg/dL are considered as prediabetic, and values > 125 mg/dL are provisionally classified as diabetic. Another method of diagnosis is the glucose tolerance test in which patients are orally administered glucose solution (1.75 g/kg body weight), and blood glucose levels are measured 2 hours later. Values of 140 to 199 mg/dL suggest a prediabetic condition, and values > 200 mg/dL give a provisional diagnosis of diabetes. A combination of diabetic values under both of the foregoing criteria together with common symptoms of diabetes such as a random blood glucose value of > 200 mg/dL, polydipsia (increased thirst), polyuria (increased urination), and unexplained weight loss confirm the diagnosis of diabetes.

Therapeutics
Warburg effect
Warburg effect refers to the phenomenon that rapidly growing malignant tumors have rates of glycolysis that are up to 200 times greater than normal tissues under aerobic conditions. It has been speculated that the Warburg effect could be the result of mitochondrial damage in cancer and the fact that glycolysis provides the building blocks for cell replication. Unlike normal cells that contain the tetrameric form of pyruvate kinase, tumor cells appear to contain the dimeric form of the enzyme (M2-PK). The dimeric form has lower affinity for phosphoenolpyruvate, causing the glycolytic intermediates to accumulate. These intermediates could serve as the building blocks for the synthesis of nucleotides, phospholipids, and amino acids required by the rapidly dividing tumor cells. Tumor hypoxia leads to the expression of hypoxia inducible factor-1 (HIF-1) which stimulates the production of GLUT1 and glycolytic enzymes such as hexokinase, G3P dehydrogenase and enolase and contributes to the Warburg effect.

Therapeutics
Hemolytic anemia
Hemolytic anemia results from premature destruction of erythrocytes. The causes of chronic hemolytic anemia could be due to inherited defects in red blood cell membranes (spherocytosis, elliptocytosis), to its metabolism (nonspherocytic anemia due to a deficiency of glycolytic enzymes or of glucose 6-phosphate dehydrogenase), or to hemoglobinopathies (thalassemias, sickle cell disease). Nutritional deficiencies in iron, folate, and vitamin B_{12} contribute to hemolytic anemia, as do viral, bacterial, and protozoal infections. Clinical markers of hemolytic anemia include elevated lactate dehydrogenase and unconjugated bilirubin (which is a product of hemoglobin catabolism).

Deficiencies of glycolytic enzymes (phosphoglucose isomerase, triose-phosphate isomerase, and, in particular, pyruvate kinase) may be inherited in either autosomal recessive or dominant fashion. The consequence of enzyme deficiency is a decrease in energy stores of erythrocytes because they depend solely on glycolysis for their energy production. The lack of ATP leads to aberrant function of ATP-dependent ion pumps, leading to an accumulation of Na^+ and attendant swelling and hemolysis.

Therapeutics
Maturity onset diabetes of the young
Maturity onset diabetes of the young (MODY) is characterized by nonketotic diabetes mellitus due to pancreatic β cell dysfunction, with an onset in adolescence (usually before the age of 25 years). MODY can result from mutations inherited in an autosomal dominant fashion in at least six separate genes expressed in β cells. They include hepatocyte nuclear factor HNF-4α (MODY-1), glucokinase (MODY-2), HNF-1α (MODY-3), insulin promoter factor 1 (MODY-4), HNF-1β (MODY-5), and neurogenic differentiation factor 1 (MODY-6). The patients, who are nonobese, usually present with a mild, asymptomatic hyperglycemia and have a strong family history of diabetes in successive generations. It is estimated that MODY may account for up to 5% of all cases of diabetes in the United States. The mutations in MODY, with the exception of glucokinase, affect transcription factors that modulate the transcription of the insulin gene. Inactivating mutations in glucokinase, on the other hand, lead to defective secretion of insulin.

Therapeutics
Hyperinsulinemia

Hyperinsulinemia is a heterogeneous disorder that results in mild to severe hypoglycemia. Persistent hyperinsulinemia in infants is a cause for concern due to the risk of seizures, coma, and neurologic sequelae. Environmental factors for transient hyperinsulinemia include maternal diabetes, poor fetal growth, and birth asphyxia, all of which lead to excessive insulin release. Uncontrolled maternal diabetes exposes the fetus to high glucose levels and causes fetal β cell hyperplasia and increased insulin secretion. The resultant postnatal hypoglycemia is treated with glucose infusion and usually resolves within 1 to 2 days. Genetic causes of persistent congenital hyperinsulinemia include activating mutations in the genes that encode subunits of the ATP-sensitive potassium channel, glutamate dehydrogenase-1, and glucokinase. In addition to glucose administration, treatment may include administration of diazoxide, which is an activator of potassium channel. Another cause of hyperinsulinemia, particularly among women, are insulinomas which are usually benign tumors of the pancreas.

9.5 Pyruvate

Pyruvate, the end product of aerobic glycolysis, is considered to be the most central molecule in cellular respiration because it serves as a substrate for the following biological processes:
1. Generation of ATP
2. Gluconeogenesis (see Chapter 12, Section 2)
3. Protein synthesis (see Chapter 19, Section 2)
4. Fatty acid synthesis (see Chapter 13)

9.5.1 Pyruvate Supply

In addition to being generated by the glycolytic reactions described in the previous sections, pyruvate is produced from the degradation of amino acids via reactions that transfer (transaminate) or remove (deaminate) the amino group bound to the α-carbon. For instance, the six amino acids serine, cysteine, alanine, glycine, threonine, and tryptophan (abbreviated SCAGTT) are converted to pyruvate, as summarized in ▶ Fig. 9.8 and described further in Chapter 10.

9.5.2 Pyruvate's Fates

Pyruvate's contribution, making biological processes that generate energy (in the presence or absence of oxygen) or synthesize glucose de novo (gluconeogenesis) or biomolecules (proteins and fatty acids), is dependent on whether pyruvate is converted to acetyl CoA, alanine, oxaloacetate, or lactate. The different fates of pyruvate are driven by certain conditions, as follows (▶ Fig. 9.8):
1. Aerobic fed conditions: pyruvate → acetyl CoA or alanine
   - Pyruvate is transported into the mitochondrial matrix, where it is decarboxylated by the pyruvate dehydrogenase complex to form acetyl CoA (see Chapter 10). This is important for the synthesis of fatty acids and the function

of the TCA cycle to break down acetyl CoA into CO_2, H_2O, and energy (in the form of ATP).
   - An amino group can also be transferred from glutamate to pyruvate by alanine aminotransferase (ALT) to form alanine. ALT requires pyridoxal phosphate as a cofactor, and its action contributes to the synthesis of proteins.
2. Aerobic fasting conditions: pyruvate → oxaloacetate
   - Pyruvate is carboxylated to oxaloacetate by pyruvate carboxylase, an enzyme that requires biotin as a cofactor, and is allosterically activated by acetyl CoA. Oxaloacetate then enters the gluconeogenesis pathway to generate glucose.
3. Anaerobic conditions: pyruvate → lactate
   - Pyruvate is reduced to lactate by lactate dehydrogenase. Lactate is then used by the Cori cycle (lactic acid cycle) (see **Fig. 12.6**), in which it is first expelled into the bloodstream and then taken up by the liver, where it is converted into glucose via gluconeogenesis. This newly formed glucose is then sent to the bloodstream, where it is taken up by exercising muscles (and red blood cells) and used to generate more ATP via anaerobic glycolysis.
   - Pyruvate is also converted to alanine by ALT in oxygen deprived muscle and exported to the liver (alanine cycle). In the liver alanine is used for gluconeogenesis (via transamination to pyruvate) and the nitrogen is disposed of in the urea cycle (via glutamate).

Foundations
Glucogenic versus ketogenic amino acids

Glucogenic amino acids are those that can be degraded into pyruvate or intermediates of the TCA cycle and can be converted to glucose via gluconeogenesis. Ketogenic amino acids, however, are those that can be broken down into acetyl CoA or acetoacetyl CoA only and cannot be converted into glucose. Some amino acids exhibit both glucogenic and ketogenic properties (see Chapter 15, Fig. 15.6).

Foundations
Amino acid versus oxoacid

An amino acid is a carboxylic acid with an amino group attached to its α-carbon. Removal of the amino group generates an oxoacid. For instance, pyruvate is the oxoacid of alanine.

Therapeutics
Lactate dehydrogenase and myocardial infarction

Lactate dehydrogenase (LDH) is a tetrameric enzyme. Each of the subunits occurs as one of the two isozymes, a heart form (H) and a muscle form (M). Therefore, LDH can have five tetrameric structures HHHH (LDH1), HHHM (LDH2), HHMM (LDH3), HMMM (LDH4), and MMMM (LDH5). LDH1 and LDH2 are predominantly localized to heart muscle and to erythrocytes, LDH3 to lung and brain and LDH4 to pancreas, kidney and placenta, whereas liver and skeletal muscle express LDH5. When the cardiac muscle is damaged after myocardial infarction (MI), the levels of LDH1 and LDH2 increase in the

Suppliers of pyruvate: glucose and amino acids (SCAGTT)

Fates of pyruvate

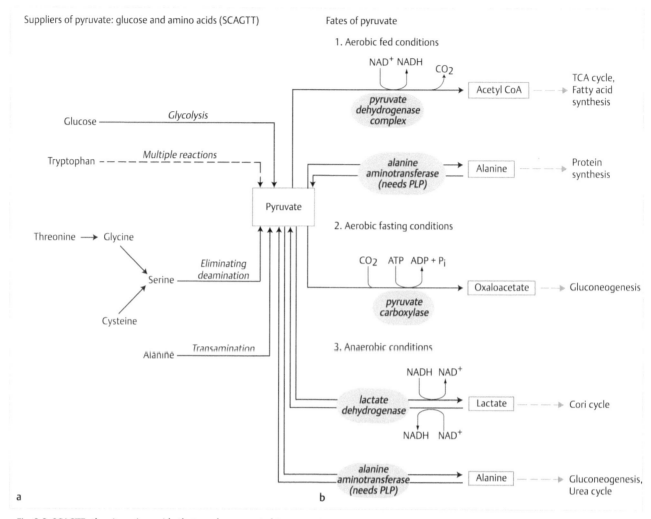

Fig. 9.8 SCAGTT, the six amino acids that can be converted to pyruvate
(a) Suppliers of pyruvate: glucose and amino acids (SCAGTT): The paths to generating pyruvate from glucose and the amino acids serine, cysteine, alanine, glycine, threonine, and tryptophan (SCAGTT). (b) Fates of pyruvate: (1) Under aerobic fed conditions, pyruvate is converted to acetyl coenzyme A (CoA) (by pyruvate dehydrogenase complex) and alanine (by the pyridoxal phosphate-dependent alanine aminotransferase). (2) Under aerobic fasting conditions, pyruvate is converted to oxaloacetate (by the biotin-dependent pyruvate carboxylase). (3) Under anaerobic conditions, pyruvate is converted to lactate (by the enzyme lactate dehydrogenase). In oxygen-deprived muscle, alanine aminotransferase converts pyruvate to alanine. ADP, adenosine diphosphate; ATP, adenosine triphosphate; NAD, nicotinamide adenine dinucleotide; NADH, reduced form of nicotinamide adenine dinucleotide; PLP, pyridoxal phosphate; TCA, tricarboxylic acid.

blood and peak 24 to 48 hours after the MI. Interestingly, although initially the level of LDH2 is higher than that of LDH1, the pattern switches after the first 24 hours, with LDH1 being higher than LDH2. On the other hand, creatine phosphokinase isozyme 2 (CK-MB/CK2) level in the blood increases rapidly after an MI, reaching the peak 20 to 28 hours after the event and returning to baseline by 48 to 60 hours. The combination of elevated CK-MB together with the LDH isozyme switch is a reliable diagnostic for an MI.

Therapeutics
Lactic acidosis
Lactic acidosis is a type of metabolic acidosis and is caused by a buildup of D-lactate (> 5 mM) in blood and tissues. The

patients present with rapid breathing, vomiting, and abdominal pain. Because lactate is the end product of glycolysis under anaerobic conditions, its accumulation usually signifies hypoxia. Some medications (e.g., antidiabetics, antiretrovirals) and poisons (e.g., arsenic) can cause lactic acidosis. Alternatively, neonatal lactic acidosis can be caused by an inborn error of metabolism. Mutations in mitochondrial DNA leading to mitochondrial encephalopathy, lactic acidosis, and stroke (MELAS) and deficiencies of pyruvate dehydrogenase (PDH) and pyruvate carboxylase are examples of genetic causes underlying lactic acidosis. The most common form of PDH complex deficiency involves mutations in the X-linked gene for the α subunit affecting the activity of the E1 enzyme that uses thiamine pyrophosphate (vitamin B_1) as a cofactor. In some cases, administration of vitamin B_1 sufficiently improves E1 activity to correct the acidosis. A deficiency of pyruvate carboxylase not only causes a buildup of lactate via pyruvate but also leads to hypoglycemia due to the disruption of the gluconeogenic pathway. Alcoholics are prone to lactic acidosis due to the fact that ethanol metabolism consumes available NAD^+ in hepatic cells, leading to increased conversion of pyruvate to lactate as the means of regenerating the NAD^+. Alcoholics are also usually deficient in vitamin B_1, thus limiting oxidation of pyruvate via PDH.

Therapeutics

Fatty liver disease in alcoholics

Excessive alcohol consumption (≥ 60 g/d) causes fatty liver. Ethanol is metabolized in the liver by alcohol dehydrogenase to acetate via acetaldehyde. Increased $NADH/NAD^+$ ratio due to alcohol and aldehyde dehydrogenases causes hepatic accumulation of glycerol 3-phosphate, which serves as the backbone for excessive triglyceride synthesis. Acetate also serves as the substrate for increased fatty acid synthesis. Lastly, ethanol inhibits fatty acid catabolism via β-oxidation and also very low-density lipoprotein (VLDL) secretion by the liver. These factors combine to significantly elevate liver triglyceride content (alcoholic steatosis).

Normal

Fermentation: pyruvate fate in yeast and microorganisms

Regeneration of NAD^+ is essential for the continued operation of glycolytic pathway. In higher organisms, pyruvate is metabolized to lactate (homolactic fermentation) under anaerobic conditions and undergoes oxidative decarboxylation under aerobic conditions. In brewer's yeast, pyruvate undergoes anaerobic alcoholic fermentation to generate ethanol. This process is made use of in the preparation of beer and wine. Microorganisms such as lactobacilli and streptococci employ homolactic fermentation, whereas propionibacteria and bifidobacteria can process pyruvate via oxaloacetate to propionic acid.

III

10 Tricarboxylic Acid Cycle

10.1 Overview

The tricarboxylic acid (TCA) cycle, also known as the citric acid cycle or Krebs cycle, metabolizes carbon skeletons obtained from the catabolism of energy nutrients into CO_2 to generate guanosine triphosphate (GTP) and the electron carriers $FADH_2$ (the reduced form of flavin adenine dinucleotide) and NADH (the reduced form of nicotinamide adenine dinucleotide). It takes place in mitochondria and functions only under aerobic conditions. The TCA cycle is an amphibolic pathway because it carries out both the breakdown (catabolism) and the synthesis (anabolism) of biomolecules, as follows:

Catabolism: The two-carbon skeleton of acetyl coenzyme A (CoA) is oxidized into CO_2.

Anabolism: Several TCA cycle intermediates serve as precursors for the synthesis of glucose, amino acids, and lipids, as well as other important biomolecules.

10.2 Acetyl CoA Supply

Acetyl coenzyme A (CoA) is the "activated" form of acetate, one of the simplest carboxylic acids. It is composed of acetate bound to CoA via a high-energy thioester bond. Acetyl CoA is obtained from the degradation of the three energy nutrients—carbohydrates, lipids, and proteins—as follows (▶ Fig. 10.1):

1. **Carbohydrates** are degraded into glucose, which gets oxidized into pyruvate via glycolysis. Pyruvate is then decarboxylated by the pyruvate dehydrogenase enzyme complex to generate acetyl CoA. This reaction is a critical step that links glycolysis to oxidative phosphorylation and, as such, is discussed in further detail in Section "Pyruvate dehydrogenase complex regulation."
2. **Lipids,** such as the fat stored as triacylglycerols in adipose tissue, are degraded into fatty acids, which are broken down into acetyl CoA units via β-oxidation.
3. **Proteins** are broken down into various amino acids, seven of which undergo a variety of reactions to be converted into acetyl CoA.

These seven ketogenic amino acids are phenylalanine, isoleucine, threonine, tryptophan, tyrosine, lysine, and leucine (PITTTLL).

Normal
Coenzyme A

Coenzyme A is a complex molecule that serves as an activator of acyl groups. It is synthesized from pantothenic acid (vitamin B_5), adenosine tri-phosphate (ATP), and cysteine. It forms a high-energy thioester linkage with acyl groups such as acetate or fatty acids. The thioester linkage in acetyl CoA has a slightly greater negative standard free energy of hydrolysis ($\Delta G°´ = -7.5$ kcal/mol) than the γ-phosphate ester bond in ATP ($\Delta G°´ = -7.3$ kcal/mol). Formation of acetyl CoA from acetate and coenzyme A by the action of CoA acetylase therefore requires the energy of hydrolysis of the β-phosphate ester linkage of ATP ($\Delta G°´ = -10.9$ kcal/mol). Activation of acyl groups with CoA facilitates transacylation, condensation, and oxidation-reduction reactions.

III

Foundations
Energy from glucose versus fatty acids

Fats are more energy dense than either carbohydrates or proteins (9 kcal/g vs 4 kcal/g). Complete oxidation of a molecule of glucose to CO_2 and H_2O via glycolysis and TCA cycle, followed by oxidative phosphorylation, can yield a maximum of 36 to 38 molecules of ATP. In comparison, complete oxidation of a molecule of palmitic acid, a 16-carbon, saturated fatty acid, can yield up to 129 ATP molecules (see Chapter 13, Section 4.2).

Foundations
Glucogenic and ketogenic amino acids

Although the nitrogen in amino acids is catabolized through the urea cycle (see **Fig 15.14**), the carbon skeletons are processed to yield either the intermediates of glycolysis and the TCA cycle or acetyl CoA. Amino acids that are metabolized to pyruvate or a TCA cycle intermediate can be utilized as substrates for synthesis of glucose and are hence classified as gluconeogenic. Two amino acids, leucine and lysine, can only be metabolized to acetyl CoA and are classified as purely ketogenic. Acetyl CoA is completely oxidized by the TCA cycle and as a result cannot serve as a substrate for gluconeogenesis. On the other hand, it is the precursor for ketone bodies (see Chapter 13, Section "Ketone Bodies"). Five amino acids can be broken down to both a gluconeogenic precursor and acetyl CoA. Phenylalanine, isoleucine, threonine, tryptophan, and tyrosine (PITTT) are therefore both glucogenic and ketogenic.

Foundations
Acetyl CoA in other metabolic pathways

In addition to serving as a substrate for the TCA cycle, acetyl CoA serves as the sole building block for the synthesis of lipids such as fatty acids and isoprenoids (including sterols and steroid hormones). Thus, acetyl CoA sits at the junction of catabolic and anabolic pathways. Under conditions of severe fasting or diabetes, much acetyl CoA is generated due to fatty acid breakdown. However, it cannot be oxidized through the TCA cycle due to the fact that the other substrate, oxaloacetate, is committed to gluconeogenesis. The liver therefore converts acetyl CoA into ketone bodies (acetoacetate and β-hydroxybutyrate), which can serve as an alternative energy source for muscle and brain.

10.3 Decarboxylation of Pyruvate

To link aerobic glycolysis to oxidative phosphorylation, pyruvate must enter the mitochondria with the help of mitochondrial pyruvate carrier (MPC), where the pyruvate dehydrogenase complex (PDC) catalyzes the oxidative decarboxylation of pyruvate into CO_2 and acetyl CoA with the production of

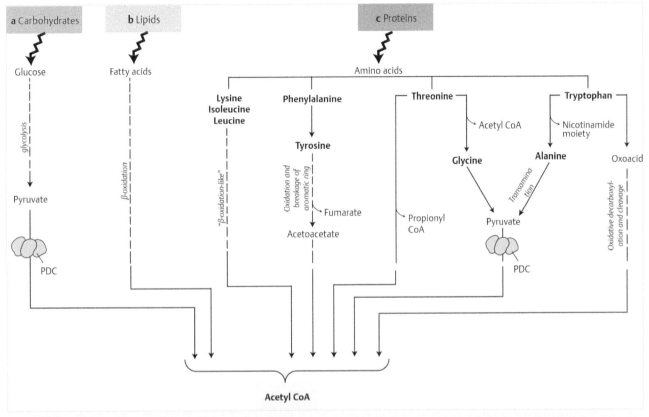

Fig. 10.1 Sources of acetyl coenzyme A. Acetyl CoA is obtained from the degradation of the three energy nutrients—(a) carbohydrates, (b) lipids, and (c) proteins. The amino acids that can be converted into acetyl CoA are phenylalanine, isoleucine, threonine, tryptophan, tyrosine, lysine and leucine (PITTTLL). Note that the oxidation of one molecule of glucose generates two molecules of acetyl CoA. PDC, pyruvate dehydrogenase complex.

NADH (▶ Fig. 10.2a). The PDC is composed of three enzymes and five coenzymes with the following features (▶ Fig. 10.2b):

- The three enzymes are E1 (pyruvate decarboxylase), E2 (dihydrolipoyl transacetylase), and E3 (dihydrolipoyl dehydrogenase).
- The five coenzymes are thiamine pyrophosphate (TPP), lipoic acid, flavin adenine dinucleotide (FAD), CoA, and nicotinamide adenine dinucleotide (NAD+). The first three are prosthetic groups that are permanently bound to the PDC, and the latter two, CoA and NAD+, are cosubstrates that associate with PDC temporarily. All of the coenzymes, except lipoic acid, are derived from various types of B vitamins (▶ Table 10.1).

Pyruvate dehydrogenase complex regulation. Tightly bound to PDC are two enzymes—pyruvate dehydrogenase phosphatase (PDP) and pyruvate dehydrogenase kinase (PDK)—which respectively catalyze the activating dephosphorylation and inactivating phosphorylation of PDC (on E1). Consequently, certain molecules alter PDC's activity either directly or via modulation of the activities of PDP and PDK (▶ Table 10.2b), as follows:

- PDC is activated by its substrates and low-energy signals (e.g., elevated [NAD+] and [ADP]). Activation is favored under conditions in which the concentration of insulin is high (e.g., after a meal).
- PDC is inhibited by its end-products and high-energy signals (e.g., elevated [NADH] and [ATP]). Inhibition is favored under fasting conditions where levels of acetyl CoA and NADH are high due to the oxidation of fatty acids.

Normal

PDC in tissues

PDC plays an important role in the energy metabolism of both skeletal and cardiac muscle as well as in adipose tissue. Calcium released during muscle contraction stimulates PDC activity by directly binding to PDP. In cardiac muscle, Ca^{2+} may also inhibit PDK, leading to further activation of PDC. PDP is a Mg^{2+}-dependent enzyme, and in adipose tissue insulin may activate the enzyme by lowering the K_m for Mg^{2+}. The mediators of insulin stimulation of PDP are yet to be identified. In heart, the stimulation of PDC by catecholamines such as epinephrine appears to be mediated by Ca^{2+}.

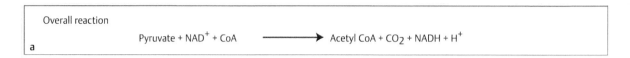

Overall reaction

a

$$\text{Pyruvate} + \text{NAD}^+ + \text{CoA} \longrightarrow \text{Acetyl CoA} + \text{CO}_2 + \text{NADH} + \text{H}^+$$

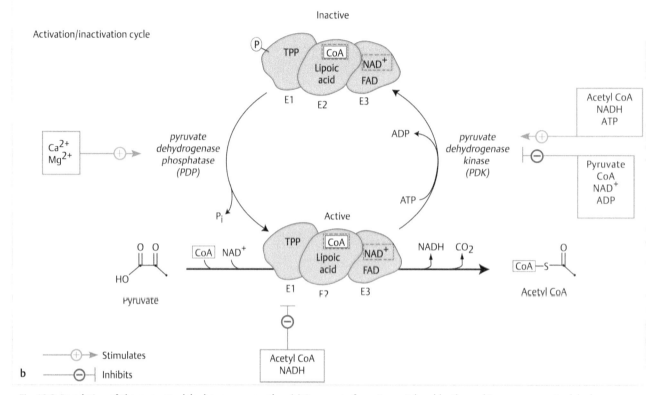

b

Fig. 10.2 Regulation of the pyruvate dehydrogenase complex. (a) Summary of reaction catalyzed by the multienzyme pyruvate dehydrogenase complex (PDC). **(b)** PDC consists of three enzymes (E1, E2, E3), which catalyze the decarboxylation of pyruvate into acetyl CoA. Tightly bound to PDC are two enzymes—pyruvate dehydrogenase phosphatase (PDP) and pyruvate dehydrogenase kinase (PDK)—which respectively catalyze the activating dephosphorylation and inactivating phosphorylation of PDC (on E1). Thus, PDC is active when PDP is activated or PDK is inhibited. Conversely, PDC is inactive when PDP is inhibited and PDK is activated. ADP, adenosine diphosphate; ATP, adenosine triphosphate; CoA, coenzyme A; FAD, flavin adenine dinucleotide; NAD, nicotinamide adenine dinucleotide; NADH, reduced form of nicotinamide adenine dinucleotide; TPP, thiamine pyrophosphate.

Table 10.1 Pyruvate dehydrogenase complex coenzymes and vitamins from which they are derived

Coenzyme	Vitamin
Thiamine pyrophosphate (TPP)	B$_1$ (thiamine)
Coenzyme A (CoA)	B$_5$ (pantothenic acid)
Lipoic acid	None
Flavin adenine dinucleotide (FAD)	B$_2$ (riboflavin)
Nicotinamide adenine dinucleotide (NAD$^+$)	B$_3$ (niacin)

Table 10.2 Modulators of pyruvate dehydrogenase complex (PDC) activity

Activators	Inhibitors
Ca^{2+}, Mg^{2+} (via allosteric activation of PDP)	Acetyl CoA, NADH (via allosteric activation of PDK)
ADP, CoA, NAD$^+$, pyruvate (via inhibition of PDK)	Acetyl CoA, ATP (via PDK activation), NADH
Insulin in adipose tissue, catecholamines in cardiac muscle (via increased Ca^{2+} and activation of PDP)	Arsenite (via inhibition of PDC by binding to lipoic acid in E2)

Abbreviations: ADP, adenosine diphosphate; ATP, adenosine triphosphate; CoA, coenzyme A; NAD, nicotinamide adenine dinucleotide; NADH, reduced form of nicotinamide adenine dinucleotide; PDK, pyruvate dehydrogenase kinase; PDP, pyruvate dehydrogenase phosphatase.

Therapeutics

Beriberi and Wernicke-Korsakoff syndrome

Beriberi is a nutritional deficiency condition in which the body does not have sufficient thiamine (vitamin B$_1$). Symptoms include weight loss, shortness of breath, difficulty walking, mental confusion and speech difficulties, lack of coordination, pain, and involuntary eye movements. There are two main types of beriberi: dry beriberi and Wernicke-Korsakoff syndrome, both of which involve peripheral neuropathy. Dry beriberi affects cardiovascular function. These conditions are diagnosed by measuring blood levels of thiamine. Treatment usually involves thiamine supplementation together with other water-soluble vitamins. In the Western world, these conditions are rare due to vitamin fortification of all essential foods. Thiamine deficiency is commonly seen in alcoholics due to their poor nutrition and because ethanol tends to inhibit the absorption of thiamine. Thiamine deficiency in chronic alcoholics is termed Wernicke-Korsakoff syndrome. Thiamine deficiency leads to increased blood levels of pyruvate and α-ketoglutarate due to impaired action of PDC and α-ketoglutarate dehydrogenase, which require thiamine pyrophosphate as an essential cofactor.

Therapeutics

Arsenite and lipoic acid

The lipoic acid subunit (E2) of PDC is modified by arsenite (derivative of arsenic) which links to lipoic acid's two sulfhydryl (SH) groups. It is a suicide inhibitor that binds to thiol groups irreversibly and limits the availability of lipoic acid. This will have an effect not only on PDC but on all the enzymes that use lipoic acid coenzyme (including α-ketoglutarate dehydrogenase and branched chain α-keto acid dehydrogenase). Arsenic is a slow poison because it takes time for it to affect enough enzymes to become lethal. It builds up in the body and can be detected in the hair.

Normal

Pyruvate dehydrogenase deficiency (neonatal lactic acidosis)

Some instances of neonatal lactic acidosis in male infants appear to be due to defects in PDC, particularly in E1. The gene for E1 is located on the X chromosome. Affected infants demonstrate high serum pyruvate and lactate, though the ratio of pyruvate to lactate is normal. Lactate levels may be normalized by the combined administration of vitamin B_1 (thiamine pyrophosphate), lipoic acid, and biotin. Vitamin B_1 serves as a cofactor of E1. Lipoic acid may help stimulate the overall activity of PDC. Biotin serves to metabolize pyruvate by an alternate enzyme, pyruvate carboxylase. Treatment may also include dichloroacetate, which is an inhibitor of PDK and serves to activate PDC. A ketogenic diet, to minimize pyruvate formation and to generate acetyl CoA bypassing the PDC, is also used.

10.4 Tricarboxylic Acid (TCA) Cycle

In the TCA cycle, the oxidation of the two-carbon skeleton of acetyl CoA into CO_2 occurs via eight enzyme-catalyzed reactions (▶ Fig. 10.3). Because these reactions form a closed loop, the substrate—oxaloacetate—used in the first reaction is regenerated in the last. The TCA cycle functions mainly in the mitochondrial matrix. One of its enzymes (succinate dehydrogenase) is found in the inner mitochondrial membrane, whereas the remaining seven soluble enzymes are found in the mitochondrial matrix. Each turn of the TCA cycle produces the following molecules:

1 Oxaloacetate, 2 CO₂, 3 NADH, 1 FADH₂, 1 GTP

Although ATP is not directly produced by the TCA cycle, the energy equivalent of 3, 2, and 1 molecules of ATP is ultimately generated from each NADH, $FADH_2$, and GTP molecule, respectively. Therefore, the oxidation of one molecule of acetyl CoA

produces the equivalent of 12 ATPs, as summarized in the following calculations:

$$3NADH \frac{3ATP}{1NADH} = 9ATP$$

$$1FADH_2 \frac{2ATP}{1FADH_2} = 2ATP$$

$$1GTP \frac{1ATP}{1GTP} = 1ATP$$

Sum = 12 ATP/acetyl CoA (or 24 ATP/glucose)

10.4.1 Reactions and Regulation of the TCA cycle

The eight enzymes of the TCA cycle catalyze a variety of reactions that involve condensation, isomerization, oxidation, decarboxylation, cleavage, and phosphorylation of substrates (▶ Fig. 10.3). Regulation of the cycle is controlled by the three enzymes (citrate synthase, isocitrate dehydrogenase, and α-ketoglutarate dehydrogenase), which catalyze the irreversible reactions. A summary of key characteristics of groups TCA cycle reactions follows:

Steps 1 and 2: Condensation and Isomerization to Generate Isocitrate

The TCA cycle begins with the condensation of acetyl CoA with oxaloacetate to generate citrate (tricarboxylic acid) via an irreversible reaction catalyzed by citrate synthase. Citrate is then isomerized to isocitrate by the enzyme aconitase. Citrate synthase is subject to regulation by insulin, substrates, cycle intermediates, and high-energy signals, and aconitase is inhibited by fluorocitrate, as summarized in ▶ Table 10.3.

Steps 3 and 4: Irreversible Oxidations and Decarboxylations to Generate NADH, CO_2, and Succinyl CoA

Isocitrate is oxidized and decarboxylated into α-ketoglutarate via a reaction catalyzed by isocitrate dehydrogenase, the rate-limiting enzyme of the TCA cycle. This is followed by another oxidation and decarboxylation reaction, which, catalyzed by α-ketoglutarate dehydrogenase, converts α-ketoglutarate into succinyl CoA. α-Ketoglutarate dehydrogenase requires the same five coenzymes as the pyruvate dehydrogenase complex to function. They are NAD⁺, FAD, thiamine pyrophosphate, lipoic acid, and CoA.
- The irreversible reactions catalyzed by isocitrate dehydrogenase and α-ketoglutarate dehydrogenase each generate 1 NADH and 1 CO_2 molecule. The activities of these enzymes are subject to regulation, as summarized in ▶ Table 10.4.

Normal

Differential effects of citrate on rate-limiting enzymes

High concentrations of citrate in a cell are indicative of an ATP-rich state. Consistent with this notion, citrate serves as an allosteric inhibitor of PFK-1, the rate-limiting enzyme of

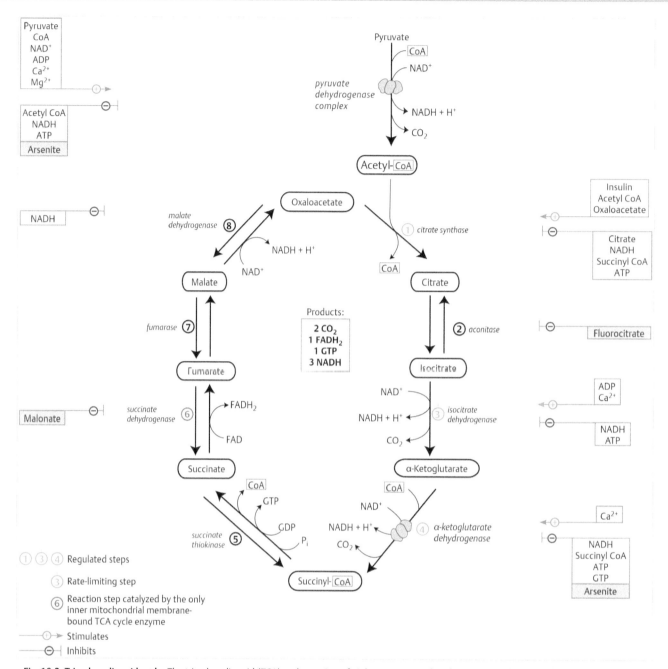

Fig. 10.3 Tricarboxylic acid cycle. The tricarboxylic acid (TCA) cycle consists of eight enzyme-catalyzed reactions in the mitochondria. These produce the reduced coenzymes NADH and FADH₂, which shuttle electrons to the electron transport chain for oxidative phosphorylation. Regulation of the TCA cycle occurs at three enzymes (citrate synthase, isocitrate dehydrogenase, and α-ketoglutarate dehydrogenase), which catalyze the irreversible reactions of the cycle. Inhibitory compounds include arsenite, fluorocitrate, and malonate (gray boxes). ADP, adenosine diphosphate; ATP, adenosine triphosphate; CoA, coenzyme A; FAD, flavin adenine dinucleotide; FADH₂, reduced form of flavin adenine dinucleotide; GDP, guanosine diphosphate; GTP, guanosine triphosphate; NAD, nicotinamide adenine dinucleotide; NADH, reduced form of nicotinamide adenine dinucleotide.

glycolysis, to limit further catabolism of glucose. Citrate is also an allosteric activator of acetyl CoA carboxylase, which converts acetyl CoA to malonyl CoA in the rate-limiting first step of fatty acid biosynthesis. Thus, citrate promotes the storage of excess energy as fat. By preventing further production of ATP and by promoting its utilization for fatty acid synthesis, citrate helps maintain the energy charge of cells in the desired range.

Because both the pyruvate dehydrogenase complex and α-keto-glutarate dehydrogenase require the five coenzymes thiamine pyrophosphate, FAD, NAD⁺, CoA, and lipoic acid for their function, a deficiency in their precursor vitamins (except for lipoic acid which is not a vitamin) disrupts the function of the TCA cycle and causes a dramatic decrease in ATP production. Some of the disorders that are linked to these vitamin deficiencies are summarized in ▶ Table 10.5.

Table 10.3 Modulators of citrate synthase and aconitase activities

Enzyme	Activators	Inhibitors
Citrate synthase	Acetyl CoA, insulin, oxaloacetate	ATP, citrate, NADH, succinyl CoA
Aconitase	-	Fluorocitrate (a metabolic product of the rat poison fluoroacetate)

Abbreviations: ATP, adenosine triphosphate; CoA, coenzyme A; NADH, reduced form of nicotinamide adenine dinucleotide.

Table 10.4 Modulators of isocitrate dehydrogenase and α-ketoglutarate dehydrogenase activities

Enzyme	Activators	Inhibitors
Isocitrate dehydrogenase	ADP (allosterically), Ca^{2+}	ATP, NADH
α-Ketoglutarate dehydrogenase	Ca^{2+}	ATP, arsenite, GTP, NADH, succinyl CoA

Abbreviations: ADP, adenosine diphosphate; ATP, adenosine triphosphate; CoA, coenzyme A; GTP, guanosine triphosphate; NADH, reduced form of nicotinamide adenine dinucleotide.

Table 10.5 Disorders associated with vitamin deficiencies that affect pyruvate dehydrogenase complex and α-ketoglutarate dehydrogenase activities

Vitamin deficiency disorder	Precursor vitamin	Coenzyme
Beriberi, polyneuritis, Wernicke-Korsakoff syndrome	B_1 (thiamine)	Thiamine pyrophosphate (TPP)
Fatigue, sleep disturbances, impaired coordination, alopecia, dermatitis, enteritis, adrenal insufficiency	B_5 (pantothenic acid)	Coenzyme A (CoA)
Neonatal-onset epilepsy, muscular hypotonia	None	Lipoic acid
Cheilosis (angular stomatitis), dermatitis	B_2 (riboflavin)	Flavin adenine dinucleotide (FAD)
Pellagra with diarrhea, dermatitis, and dementia	B_3 (niacin)	Nicotinamide adenine dinucleotide (NAD^+)

Table 10.6 Genetic defects associated with partial loss of TCA cycle enzymes (TCA cycle enzymopathies)

Enzyme defect	Consequences
Aconitase	Mitochondrial iron-sulfur protein deficiency in Friedreich ataxia
α-Ketoglutarate dehydrogenase	Severe encephalopathy, hypotonia, psychotic behavior, pyramidal symptoms
Succinate dehydrogenase	Leigh-like syndrome, paraganglioma and pheochromocytoma, early-onset encephalomyopathies
Succinyl CoA synthase	Encephalomyopathy and mtDNA depletion
Fumarase	Early encephalomyopathy, seizures, dystonia, uterine leiomyomas, papillary renal cell cancer

Abbreviation: mtDNA, mitochondrial DNA.

Step 5: Cleavage of Succinyl CoA and Phosphorylation to Generate Succinate and GTP

The high-energy thioester bond of succinyl CoA is cleaved to form succinate in a reaction that is coupled to the substrate-level phosphorylation of guanosine diphosphate (GDP) into GTP. This step is catalyzed by succinyl thiokinase (also known as succinyl CoA synthetase).

Steps 6 to 8: Reversible Oxidations to Produce FADH₂ and NADH and Regenerate Oxaloacetate

Succinate is oxidized to fumarate with the production of $FADH_2$ via a reaction catalyzed by succinate dehydrogenase. Fumarate is then converted to malate via the enzyme fumarase. In the

final step, malate is converted to oxaloacetate, with the production of NADH via the action of malate dehydrogenase. Some noteworthy characteristics of succinate dehydrogenase, as well as inhibitors of the latter and malate dehydrogenase's activities, are as follows:

- Succinate dehydrogenase is the only TCA cycle enzyme that is bound to the inner mitochondrial membrane and the only one that generates $FADH_2$. It is also called Complex II because it is a component of the electron transport chain, where it serves to transfer electrons from $FADH_2$ to coenzyme Q.
- Succinate dehydrogenase is inhibited by malonate (a competitive inhibitor).
- Malate dehydrogenase is inhibited by NADH.

Some of the disorders associated with genetic defects in TCA cycle enzymes are summarized in ▶ Table 10.6.

Foundations

ATP:ADP and NADH:NAD⁺ ratios

The anabolic and catabolic pathways of a cell are broadly regulated by the energy status of the cell. The energy charge of a cell may be defined as the ratio of [ATP] to [ADP], or more precisely as follows:

$$\frac{[ATP] + \frac{1}{2}[ADP]}{[ATP] + [ADP] + [AMP]}$$

The [ATP]:[ADP] ratio is high in energy-rich cells and low in cells that are energy poor. In actuality, the energy charge of a cell is strictly regulated in a very narrow range (0.8 to 0.95). The reducing power in a cell, denoted predominantly by the [NADH]:[NAD⁺] ratio, represents the potential energy and varies inversely with the [ATP]:[ADP] ratio. Thus, when cellular ATP levels are low, the activity of the TCA cycle is increased to provide more NADH to serve as a substrate for oxidative phosphorylation to generate ATP. Conversely, when cellular ATP levels are high, the production of NADH via the TCA cycle and its oxidation via the mitochondrial electron transport chain are inhibited.

III

Normal
Succinyl CoA in heme synthesis

The amphibolic pathway of the TCA cycle serves not only to oxidize acetyl CoA but to generate precursors for the synthesis of important biomolecules. An example is the condensation of succinyl CoA and the amino acid glycine, with decarboxylation, to generate δ-aminolevulinic acid (δ-ALA) as the first step in heme biosynthesis (see Chapter 16). This reaction is catalyzed by ALA synthase, the rate-limiting enzyme of heme biosynthesis, and requires pyridoxal phosphate (vitamin B_6) as a cofactor.

Normal
Dehydrogenases that require the same five coenzymes as PDC

Pyruvate (the product of glycolysis), δ-ketoglutarate (an intermediate of the TCA cycle) and branched-chain keto acids (generated by transamination of valine, isoleucine, and leucine) all represent α-keto acids that are oxidatively decarboxylated by similarly organized mitochondrial multi-enzyme complexes. Like the PDC, α-ketoglutarate dehydrogenase and branched-chain keto acid dehydrogenase complexes are made of similar E1 and E2 enzymes and an identical E3 enzyme. All three complexes utilize the same five vitamin-derived coenzymes (TPP, lipoic acid, CoA, FAD+, and NAD+). Thus, deficiencies of the precursor vitamins would simultaneously affect all three multienzyme complexes.

Therapeutics
Rat poison inhibits the TCA cycle

Fluoroacetate is a rat poison that inhibits the TCA cycle. Fluoroacetate reacts with CoA to form fluoroacetyl CoA, which (instead of acetyl CoA) condenses with oxaloacetate to produce fluorocitrate. Fluorocitrate is an analogue of citrate and is a competitive inhibitor of aconitase, a TCA cycle enzyme that catalyzes the isomerization of citrate to isocitrate. Thus, inhibition of aconitase leads to the accumulation of citrate, which inhibits citrate synthase, the enzyme that catalyzes the first step of the TCA cycle. Fluorocitrate, like citrate, is also an allosteric inhibitor of PFK-1 and acts to inhibit glycolysis.

Therapeutics
Competitive inhibitors of succinate dehydrogenase

Compounds that are structurally similar to succinate inhibit the TCA cycle by competing with succinate for binding to succinate dehydrogenase, the only TCA cycle enzyme that generates

$FADH_2$. Such inhibitory molecules include the TCA cycle intermediates malate and oxaloacetate, as well as the chemical malonate. Malonate, a dicarboxylic acid, is a structural analogue of succinate and is a strong competitive inhibitor of succinate dehydrogenase. Malonate was used in studies to map the active site of succinate dehydrogenase. Malonate may be generated from malonyl CoA, an important intermediate in fatty acid synthesis (Chapter 13).

10.5 Anaplerotic Reactions and Anabolic Functions of the TCA Cycle

10.5.1 Anaplerotic Reactions

In order for the TCA cycle to continue functioning, it must constantly replenish its intermediates because they are also consumed by anabolic pathways. Reactions that replenish TCA cycle intermediates are called anaplerotic reactions. The two major types of anaplerotic reactions are the degradation of amino acids and the carboxylation of pyruvate (▶ Fig. 10.4):

1. **Degradation of amino acids** replenishes oxaloacetate, α-ketoglutarate, succinyl CoA, and fumarate. This occurs via transaminations (transfer of amino groups), deaminations (removal of amino groups), or oxidation of aromatic rings.
2. **Carboxylation of pyruvate** replenishes oxaloacetate. This ATP-consuming reaction is catalyzed by pyruvate carboxylase—an enzyme that requires biotin for its activity and is stimulated by acetyl CoA. This reaction preferentially occurs under glucose-deprived conditions (e.g., fasting) in which the acetyl CoA supply is high, and the resulting oxaloacetate will be used to synthesize glucose via gluconeogenesis.
   - It is important to note that lipids (e.g., fatty acids with even number of carbons) are degraded exclusively to acetyl CoA (which loses both carbons during the TCA cycle as CO_2) and therefore do not have anaplerotic activity.
   - Expression of pyruvate carboxylase in the liver is suppressed by insulin.

Therapeutics
Pyruvate carboxylase deficiency

Mutations in the pyruvate carboxylase gene that alter the amount or activity of this enzyme lead to a condition called pyruvate carboxylase deficiency. A disruption in pyruvate carboxylase activity causes more pyruvate to be converted to lactic acid than oxaloacetate, the former of which accumulates in the blood. The symptoms of this condition appear shortly after birth and include seizures, muscle weakness (hypotonia), and uncontrolled muscle movement (ataxia). Although the incidence is 1 in 250,000 births in general, it appears more prevalent among Algonkian Indian tribes in eastern Canada. This genetic defect is inherited in an autosomal recessive pattern.

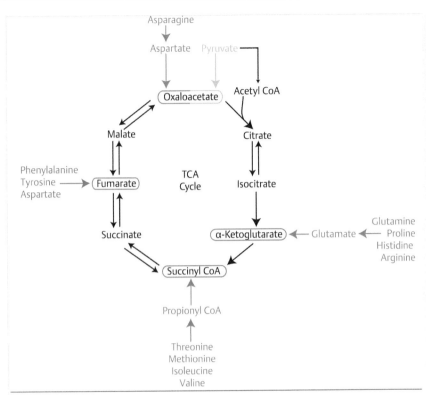

Fig. 10.4 Anaplerotic reactions of the tricarboxylic acid (TCA) cycle. Reactions that replenish TCA cycle intermediates are called anaplerotic reactions, of which there are two major types. The first and most important is the degradation of amino acids into oxaloacetate, α-ketoglutarate, succinyl coenzyme A (CoA), and fumarate. The second is the carboxylation of pyruvate into oxaloacetate, which occurs when blood glucose levels are low. (When blood glucose is high, pyruvate is converted to acetyl CoA by pyruvate dehydrogenase complex for the TCA cycle and fatty acid synthesis.)

■ Amino acid degradations that replenish α-ketoglutarate, succinyl CoA, and fumarate

■ Pyruvate carboxylation which, replenishes oxaloacetate

10.5.2 Anabolic Functions

Several TCA cycle intermediates serve as precursors for anabolic pathways that synthesize biomolecules such as glucose, lipids, and amino acids, as follows:

Oxaloacetate contributes to the synthesis of glucose (▶ Fig. 10.5a): Under glucose-deprived conditions (e.g., fasting), oxaloacetate is preferentially used to synthesize glucose de novo via the cytoplasmic pathway, gluconeogenesis (see **Fig. 12.7**).

• For this to occur, oxaloacetate is reduced to malate in mitochondria, transported to the cytoplasm, and oxidized back into oxaloacetate. The latter then becomes committed to the gluconeogenesis pathway through its phosphorylation and decarboxylation into phosphoenolpyruvate (PEP) by the enzyme PEP carboxykinase.

Citrate contributes to the synthesis of lipids (▶ Fig. 10.5a): In the fed state, citrate is used to generate acetyl CoA, the building block for the synthesis of all lipids in the cytosol (see **Fig. 13.3**).

• For this to occur, citrate must be transported into the cytoplasm, where it is cleaved into acetyl CoA and oxaloacetate. (The latter is reduced to malate, and then to pyruvate, which reenters mitochondria.)

Oxaloacetate and α-ketoglutarate contribute to amino acid synthesis (▶ Fig. 10.5b): Addition of an amino group to the α-carbon of oxaloacetate and α-ketoglutarate produces the amino acids aspartate and glutamate, respectively.

• Aspartate is converted into asparagine, whereas glutamate is converted into glutamine, proline, and arginine.

Oxaloacetate and citrate's respective paths to glucose synthesis (green) and lipid synthesis (orange)

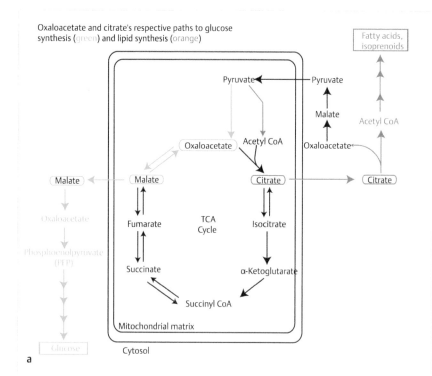

a

Oxaloacetate and α-ketoglutarate's paths to the synthesis of amino acids

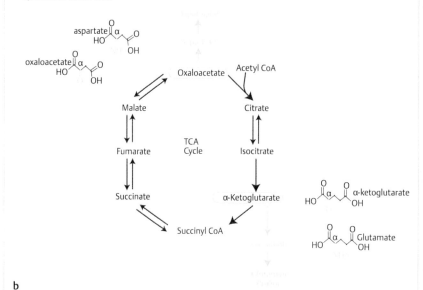

b

Fig. 10.5 Tricarboxylic acid (TCA) cycle intermediates used to synthesize (a) glucose, lipids, and (b) amino acids. (a) Synthesis of glucose via gluconeogenesis (green): Oxaloacetate, produced from the carboxylation of pyruvate, is reduced to malate. Malate is transported from the mitochondrial matrix into the cytoplasm, where it is oxidized back to oxaloacetate, which is carboxylated to phosphoenolpyruvate (PEP). PEP is then converted to glucose via a series of reactions. Synthesis of lipids (orange): Citrate, produced from the condensation of acetyl coenzyme A (CoA) with oxaloacetate, is transported into the cytoplasm and cleaved to form acetyl CoA and oxaloacetate. Acetyl CoA is used to synthesize lipids such as fatty acids and isoprenoids, whereas oxaloacetate is reduced to malate and then to pyruvate, which reenters mitochondria. **(b)** Oxaloacetate and α-ketoglutarate belong to a family of compounds called α-keto acids. These compounds contain a carbonyl group (C=O) at the α-carbon position (first carbon attached to a functional group). Addition of an amino group (via transamination) to the α-carbon of oxaloacetate and α-ketoglutarate produces the amino acids aspartate and glutamate, respectively, which serve as precursors for additional amino acids such as asparagine, glutamine, proline, and arginine.

11 Oxidative Phosphorylation and Mitochondria

11.1 Overview

Oxidative phosphorylation is the most important means by which adenosine triphosphate (ATP) is produced under aerobic conditions. It involves the integration of several metabolic pathways that link the breakdown of nutrients to oxidation-reduction (redox) reactions that culminate in the transfer of electrons to O_2, and the phosphorylation of adenosine diphosphate (ADP) to ATP. Two important characteristics of oxidative phosphorylation are its location and its protein/lipid mediators.

Location: Oxidative phosphorylation takes place in mitochondria (▶ Fig. 11.1a). These cellular organelles are composed of a central mitochondrial matrix enclosed by an inner membrane that is bent into folds called cristae. The inner membrane is surrounded by an outer membrane, and the space separating the two membranes is called the intermembrane space. Mitochondria are found in large numbers per cell, and several metabolic processes occur in specific regions of this organelle due to its structural organization, as follows (▶ Fig. 11.1b):

- The *mitochondrial matrix* has a pH that is higher than that of the intermembrane space and serves as the site for the β-oxidation of fatty acids, pyruvate dehydrogenase activity, the tricarboxylic acid (TCA) cycle, ketone body synthesis, some

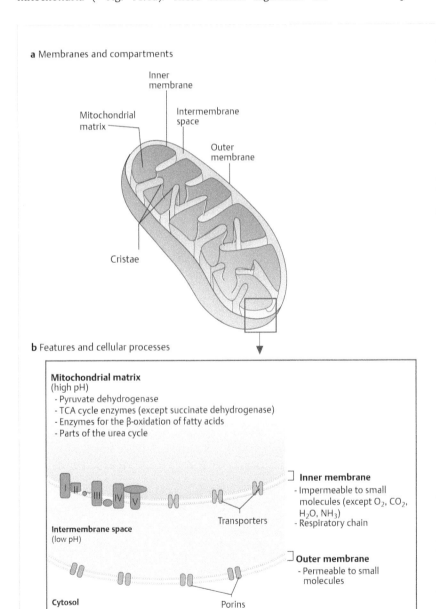

a Membranes and compartments

Inner membrane

Mitochondrial matrix

Intermembrane space

Outer membrane

Cristae

b Features and cellular processes

Mitochondrial matrix
(high pH)
- Pyruvate dehydrogenase
- TCA cycle enzymes (except succinate dehydrogenase)
- Enzymes for the β-oxidation of fatty acids
- Parts of the urea cycle

I II III IV V

Transporters

Inner membrane
- Impermeable to small molecules (except O_2, CO_2, H_2O, NH_3)
- Respiratory chain

Intermembrane space
(low pH)

Outer membrane
- Permeable to small molecules

Cytosol

Porins

Fig. 11.1 Mitochondrion. (a) Mitochondria are cellular organelles composed of a central mitochondrial matrix enclosed by an inner membrane that is bent into folds (called cristae). The inner membrane is surrounded by an outer membrane, and the space separating both membranes is called the intermembrane space. **(b)** Mitochondria are the major site of cellular respiration. The mitochondrial matrix is the site of β-oxidation of fatty acids, the tricarboxylic acid (TCA) cycle, parts of the urea cycle, activity of pyruvate dehydrogenase, parts of heme synthesis, and storage of Ca^{2+} ions. The inner mitochondrial membrane harbors the protein complexes of the respiratory chain. The intermembrane space contains nucleoside and creatine kinases.

reactions of the urea cycle and heme biosynthesis, and as a reservoir for Ca^{2+}.

- *The inner mitochondrial membrane* has a large surface area as a result of its cristae. It is only permeable to ammonia (NH_3), O_2, and CO_2. It harbors all the necessary protein complexes and mobile electron carriers that facilitate oxidative phosphorylation, as well as the transporters (integral proteins) that move other molecules across the membrane's lipid bilayer.
- *The intermembrane space* contains a high concentration of protons (and thus has a lower pH than the matrix), which is essential for oxidative phosphorylation.
- *The outer mitochondrial membrane* is permeable to small molecules (< 10 kDa) due to the presence of protein channels called porins.

Protein and lipid mediators: Oxidative phosphorylation is mediated by the respiratory chain—a collection of inner mitochondrial membrane proteins called complexes I, II, III, IV, and V and cytochrome-c, as well as a lipophilic molecule called coenzyme Q (ubiquinone). ▸ Table 11.1 contains a summary of the structural and functional details of each component of the respiratory chain (▸ Fig. 11.2).

Foundations

Cytochrome-c and apoptosis

Cytochrome-c is a protein that functions as a mobile carrier of electrons between complexes III and IV of the mitochondrial electron transport chain. *Apoptosis* refers to programmed cell death, which occurs for many different reasons, such as normal development, DNA damage, and growth factor deprivation. Many apoptotic stimuli (e.g., reactive oxygen species [ROS], stress, DNA damage) initiate the process by opening the mitochondrial permeability transition pore complex, causing a release of cytochrome-c. Cytochrome-c, in turn, induces a cascade of biochemical reactions that result in the activation of a subfamily of cysteine proteases called caspases. Caspases serve as the executors of apoptosis, leading to cell death. The release of cytochrome-c into the cytosol can therefore serves as a biochemical marker for cells undergoing apoptosis. The assay for released cytochrome-c involves fractionation of cell lysates by differential centrifugation to isolate mitochondria and postmitochondrial supernatant fractions followed by detection of cytochrome-c in each fraction by Western blotting using anticytochrome-c antibodies.

Table 11.1 Components of the respiratory chain

Protein/Lipid mediators	Structural details	Function/Action
Complex I (NADH dehydrogenase)	• Transmembrane protein • e^- transfers are facilitated by tightly bound FMN and Fe-S clusters	• Accepts $2e^-$ from NADH and donates them to coenzyme Q • Pumps $4 H^+$ from the matrix into the intermembrane space
Complex II (succinate dehydrogenase)*	• Protein bound to the matrix side of the inner mitochondrial membrane • e^- transfers are facilitated by tightly bound FAD and Fe-S clusters	• Transfers $2e^-$ from $FADH_2$ to coenzyme Q
Coenzyme Q (ubiquinone)	• Lipophilic molecule composed of an aromatic six-membered ring and a long hydrophobic side chain • Mobile; it moves freely within the lipid bilayer of the inner mitochondrial membrane • Converted to ubiquinol upon acceptance of $2e^-$	• Accepts $2e^-$ from either Complex I or Complex II and transfers them to Complex III
Complex III (cytochrome-c reductase)	• Transmembrane protein • e^- transfers are facilitated by Fe-S clusters and cytochromes-b and -c_1, which harbor iron-containing heme-b and -c molecules	• Accepts $2e^-$ from ubiquinol and donates them to cytochrome-c • Pumps $4 H^+$ from the matrix into the intermembrane space
Cytochrome-c	• Small protein bound to the intermembrane space side of the inner mitochondrial membrane • Mobile; it is held to the membrane via electrostatic forces • e^- transfers are facilitated by an iron-containing heme c group	• Accepts electrons from Complex III and donates them to Complex IV
Complex IV (cytochrome-c oxidase)	• Transmembrane protein • e^- transfers are facilitated by Cu centers and cytochromes-a and -a_3, which harbor iron-containing heme-a molecules	• Accepts electrons from cytochrome-c and transfers them to O_2, which forms water • Pumps $2 H^+$ from the matrix into the intermembrane space
Complex V (ATP synthase)	• Multisubunit transmembrane protein • Proton movement is facilitated by its membrane spanning F_0 domain, and ATP synthesis is facilitated by its F_1 domain, which protrudes into the matrix	• Moves protons from the intermembrane space into the matrix to obtain the energy needed to synthesize ATP from ADP and P_i

* Succinate dehydrogenase is also a TCA cycle enzyme.

Abbreviations: ADP, adenosine diphosphate; ATP, adenosine triphosphate; FAD, flavin adenine dinucleotide; Fe-S, iron-sulfur; FMN, flavin mononucleotide; NADH, reduced form of nicotinamide adenine dinucleotide.

a Organization

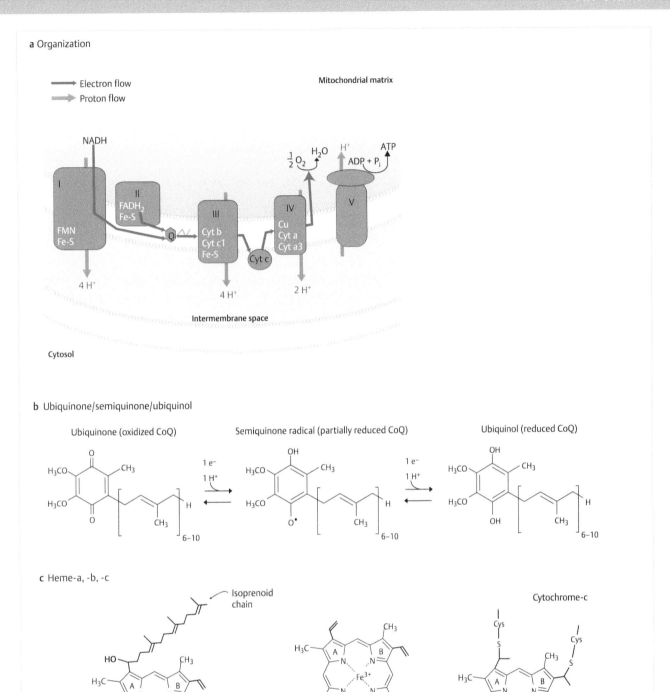

Fig. 11.2 Respiratory chain. (**a**) Organization: Components of the respiratory chain. (**b**) Ubiquinone/semiquinone/ubiquinol: Oxidized and reduced states of ubiquinone. (**c**) Heme-a, -b, -c: Heme-a in cytochromes-a and -a₃ is isoprenylated and harbors a formyl group. Heme-b in cytochrome-b is akin to heme in hemoglobin. Heme-c in cytochrome-c is covalently bound to this protein. ADP, adenosine diphosphate; ATP, adenosine triphosphate; CoQ, conenzyme Q; FADH₂, reduced form of flavin adenine dinucleotide; FMN, flavin mononucleotide.

11.1.1 Redox Reactions

Redox reactions involve the transfer of electrons from a donor (reductant) to an acceptor (oxidant). There are two types of such reactions.

1. **In the electron-only transfer** (▶ Fig. 11.3a), electrons are transferred between two metal ions. For example, Cu^+ can reduce Fe^{3+} to Fe^{2+}. Cu^+ gets oxidized to Cu^{2+} in the process because the former gives one of its electrons to Fe^{3+}.
   • The reactant that gets oxidized is the reductant (Cu^+). The reactant that gets reduced is the oxidant (Fe^{3+}).
   • This process can be split into two half reactions: the oxidation half reaction and the reduction half reaction. The rule of thumb is that the oxidant is always on the side of the reaction with the electrons. Cu^{2+} and Cu^+ are a redox pair, and Fe^{3+} and Fe^{2+} are the other redox pair. These reactions are reversible.
2. **Reducing-equivalent transfer** (▶ Fig. 11.3b) involves transfer of a proton plus an electron. An example is the reduction of pyruvate (the oxidant that gets reduced) by $NADH + H^+$ (the reductant that gets oxidized) to lactate and nicotinamide adenine dinucleotide (NAD^+) (catalyzed by lactate dehydrogenase).
   • This reaction can also be split into two half reactions, namely, the oxidation half reaction and the reduction half reaction. $NADH/NAD^+$ and pyruvate/lactate are the redox pairs.

Normal

Ferredoxins

Ferredoxins are small proteins that serve as carriers of electrons in mitochondrial cytochrome P-450 systems. They contain clusters of iron and sulfur (e.g., Fe_2-S_2, Fe_4-S_4, and Fe_3-S_4). Reduction and oxidation of iron between Fe^{3+} and Fe^{2+} states allow transfer of electrons between members of the ferredoxin family. Adrenodoxin, which is an Fe_2-S_2 ferredoxin (FDX1), is known to participate in the biosynthesis of steroid hormones in

adrenal glands and also functions in the metabolism of vitamin D and bile acids. Another ferredoxin (FDX2) appears to be necessary for the biogenesis of heme-a (found in cytochrome oxidase), as well as of iron-sulfur proteins (e.g., aconitase). Ferredoxins also play important roles in bacterial metabolism and photosynthesis in plant chloroplasts.

11.1.2 Standard Redox Potential

The standard redox potential (E_0') is a measure of the affinity of a redox pair for electrons. Its units are in volts (V), and it is measured in reference to the standard half reaction, $H^+ + e^- \rightarrow \frac{1}{2}H_2$. The standard half reaction takes place in a hydrogen cell containing 1 M H^+ (pH = 0).
• A redox pair in the test cell (at pH = 7) that donates electrons to the hydrogen cell would have a negative E_0', whereas a redox pair that accepts electrons from the hydrogen cell would have a positive E_0'.
• A redox pair with a lower E_0' has a lower affinity for electrons and thus gives them up easily to a redox pair with a higher E_0', which has a higher affinity for electrons.
• The molecule with the lower E_0' is described as the reducing agent, whereas that with the higher E_0' is known as an oxidizing agent (▶ Fig. 11.4).

11.2 Mechanism of Oxidative Phosphorylation

The success of oxidative phosphorylation depends on the respiratory chain's ability to accomplish three key goals:
1. Transfer electrons from NADH and the reduced form of flavin adenine dinucleotide ($FADH_2$) to O_2
2. Establish a proton gradient across the inner mitochondrial membrane
3. Synthesize ATP

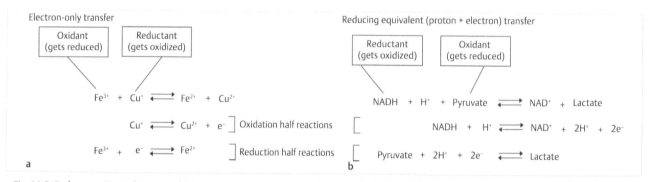

Fig. 11.3 Redox reactions: Electron-only transfer and reducing equivalent transfer. Redox reactions involve the transfer of electrons from a donor (reductant) to an acceptor (oxidant). **(a)** In the electron-only transfer, electrons are transferred between two metal ions. For example, Cu^+ can reduce Fe^{3+} to Fe^{2+}. Cu^+ gets oxidized to Cu^{2+} in the process (as it gives one of its electrons to Fe^{3+}). **(b)** Reducing-equivalent transfer involves transfer of a proton plus an electron. An example is the reduction of pyruvate by $NADH + H^+$ to lactate and NAD^+. In the half reactions, the oxidant is always on the side of the reaction with the electrons.

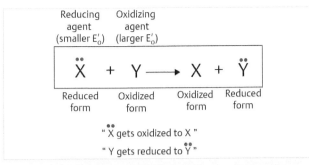

Fig. 11.4 Reducing and oxidizing agents. In the reaction depicted here, com pound $\ddot{X}$ donates a pair of electrons to compound Y. X/$\ddot{X}$ and Y/$\dot{y}$ are known as redox pairs. $\ddot{X}$, which has a small E'_0, is the reducing agent (reductant) that gets oxidized in the reaction, and Y, which has the larger E_0, is the oxidizing agent (oxidant) that gets reduced.

Table 11.2 Standard redox potential of redox pairs/Couples of oxidative phosphorylation

Redox pair or couple (oxidized form/reduced form)	E_0' (V)
NAD^+/NADH	-0.32
FMN/$FMNH_2$	-0.22
FAD/$FADH_2$	-0.22
Ubiquinone/ubiquinol	+0.10
Cytochrome-b (Fe^{3+}/Fe^{2+})	+0.12
Cytochrome-c (Fe^{3+}/Fe^{2+})	+0.22
Cytochrome-a (Fe^{3+}/Fe^{2+})	+0.29
½ O_2/H_2O	+0.82

Abbreviations: FAD, flavin adenine dinucleotide; $FADH_2$, reduced form of flavin adenine dinucleotide; FMN, flavin mononucleotide; FMNH, reduced form of flavin mononucleotide; NAD^+, nicotinamide adenine dinucleotide; NADH, reduced form of nicotinamide adenine dinucleotide.

11.2.1 (1.) Transfer of Electrons from NADH and FADH₂ to O₂

The components of the electron transport chain are arranged in a manner that allows electrons to flow from the molecules with the lowest E_0' (e.g., NADH = -0.32 V; $FADH_2$ = -0.22 V) to that with highest E_0' (O_2 = +0.82 V). Additional characteristics of electron transfer reactions of the electron transport chain are as follows:

- Electrons are transferred along the electron transport chain in various forms, such as electrons (e^-), hydride ion (:H^-), and hydrogen atoms (·H).
- Electron transfers are facilitated by pairs of molecules that serve as oxidizing and reducing agents (redox pairs), such as NAD^+/NADH, FAD/$FADH_2$, ubiqinone/ubiquinol, and the flavin mononucleotides (FMN/$FMNH_2$).
- Electron transfers are also facilitated by redox couples, which are the oxidized and reduced forms of an element, such as Fe^{3+}/Fe^{2+} and Cu^{2+}/Cu^+.

The difference in redox potential between acceptor and donor molecules ($\Delta E_0' = E_0'^{\text{acceptor}} - E_0'^{\text{donor}}$) is associated with a free energy change ($\Delta G°'$). $\Delta G°'$ can be calculated using the following equation, where n is the number of electrons transferred, and $\mathscr{F}$ (Faraday constant) is 96.5 kJ/volt·mol (23.06 kcal/volt·mol).

$$\Delta G°' = -n\mathscr{F}\Delta E_0'$$

As the foregoing equation implies, $\Delta G°'$ and $\Delta E_0'$ are directly related but are opposite in magnitude. Thus, the greater the $\Delta E_0'$, the more negative is the $\Delta G°'$. The $\Delta E_0'$ associated with the transfer of electrons along the electron transport chain complexes results in a negative $\Delta G°'$ that is used to pump protons (H^+) from the mitochondrial matrix into the intermembrane space, leading to a pH and electrical gradient across the inner membrane. The potential energy associated with this gradient (known as the proton motive force) is later utilized to synthesize ATP by Complex V. The standard redox potentials of molecules involved in oxidative phosphorylation are summarized in ▶ Table 11.2.

Inhibition of electron transport. Oxidative phosphorylation is disrupted when the transfer of electrons along the electron transport chain is inhibited. The resulting effect is a decrease in the pumping of protons across the inner membrane, a decrease in the proton gradient, and inhibition of ATP synthesis. Blockage of electron transfer occurs at the following complexes (▶ Fig. 11.5):

- Inhibition of Complex I by amytal (amobarbital), rotenone, myxothiazol, and piericidin A
- Inhibition of Complex II by malonate and thenoyltrifluoroacetone (TTFA)
- Inhibition of Complex III by antimycin A
- Inhibition of Complex IV by carbon monoxide, cyanide, and hydrogen sulfide

Mutations in mitochondrial DNA that lead to the production of defective electron transport chain components are associated with disorders summarized in ▶ Table 11.3.

11.2.2 (2.) Establishment of a Proton Gradient across the Inner Mitochondrial Membrane

The carefully controlled electron transfers are linked to the pumping of protons across the inner membrane from the mitochondrial matrix into the intermembrane space. This generates a pH gradient ($\Delta pH = pH_{\text{matrix}} - pH_{\text{intermembrane space}}$) in which the mitochondrial intermembrane space is more acidic than the matrix, which results in the following:

- The more positively charged outer surface of the inner mitochondrial membrane (relative to the inner surface) gives rise to a membrane potential ($\Delta\Psi$) – (i.e., the voltage difference between the two surfaces of the inner mitochondrial membrane).
- The amount of energy stored within the H^+ gradient is represented by the proton motive force (pmf), a value that reflects contributions from the membrane potential ($\Delta\Psi$) and pH gradient (ΔpH), as seen in the Nernst equation below, where R is the gas constant (1.987×10^{-3} kcal/mol·K), T is temperature in kelvins, and $\mathscr{F}$ is Faraday's constant (23.06 kcal/V).

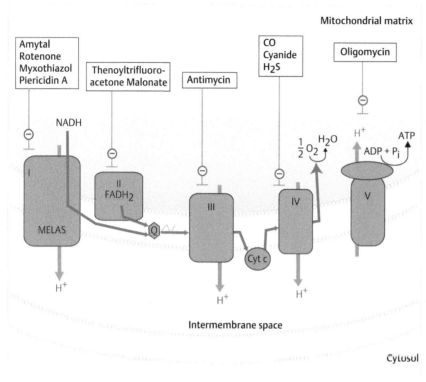

Fig. 11.5 Compounds that inhibit oxidative phosphorylation. Several compounds block electron transfer along the electron transport chain by targeting specific complexes. Complex I is inhibited by amytal, rotenone, myxothiazol, and piericidin A. Complex II is inhibited by malonate. Complex III is inhibited by antimycin A. Complex IV is inhibited by carbon monoxide (CO), cyanide, and hydrogen sulfide (H_2S). Complex V, which does not participate in the transport of electrons, is inhibited by oligomycin. All of these compounds inhibit ATP synthesis. ADP, adenosine diphosphate; ATP, adenosine triphosphate; $FADH_2$, reduced form of flavin adenine dinucleotide; NADH, reduced form of nicotinamide adenine dinucleotide.

→ Electron flow
⇒ Proton flow ——⊝⊣ Inhibits complex

Table 11.3 Disorders associated with mutations in mitochondrial genes

Disorder	Affected mitochondrial gene	Affected ETC complexes	Signs, symptoms, onset
Mitochondrial encephalopathy, lactic acidosis, and stroke (MELAS)	tRNA^{Leu}	Complex I, IV	Muscle weakness and pain, accumulation of lactic acid, vomiting, loss of appetite, seizures, strokelike episodes. Onset: Infancy to early childhood
Kearns-Sayre syndrome	Single large deletion of 1.1–10 kb of mtDNA affecting multiple genes	All	Eye pain, ophthalmoplegia, ptosis, pigmentary retinopathy, defects in cardiac conduction, ragged red fibers. Onset: before age 20
Leber hereditary optic neuropathy (LHON)	ND1, ND4, Cyt b	Complex I, III	Degenerated optic nerve, continued loss of central vision. Onset: early adulthood
Leigh syndrome	ND5, cytochrome-c oxidase	Complex I, IV	Difficulty swallowing, weak motor skills, vomiting, lesions in basal ganglia and brainstem. Onset: first year of life
Myoclonic epilepsy and ragged-red fiber disease (MERRF)	tRNA^{Lys}	Complex I, IV	Muscle spasms, hearing loss, dementia
Hypertrophic cardiomyopathy (exercise intolerance)	Cyt b, cytochrome-c oxidase	Complex III, IV	Enlargement and degeneration of cardiac muscle. Onset: birth to young adulthood
Pearson syndrome	Single large deletion of 4977 bp of leukocyte mtDNA	All	Sideroblastic anemia, exocrine pancreas dysfunction
Hypertension and hypercholesterolemia	tRNA^{Ileu}, tRNA^{Met}, tRNA^{Lys}	Complex I, IV	BP > 140/90 mm Hg, total serum cholesterol > 200 mg/ dL, hypomagnesemia (< 1.7 mg/dL)
Diabetes with deafness	tRNA^{Leu}(UUR)	Complex I, IV	Maternal inheritance, defective ATP production and insulin release in pancreatic β cells (different from glucokinase mutation seen in MODY2), lack of insulin resistance, impaired hearing; may respond to ubiquinone supplements

Abbreviations: ATP, adenosine triphosphate; ETC, electron transport chain; MODY, maturity onset diabetes of the young; ND1 and ND4, NADH dehydrogenase genes.

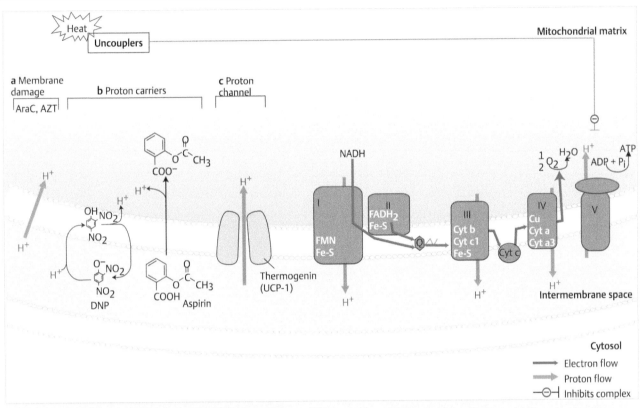

Fig. 11.6 Uncouplers generate heat and inhibit ATP synthase. The inner mitochondrial membrane is normally impermeable to protons; however, uncoupling agents and proteins support the movement of protons across the inner mitochondrial membrane by **(a)** damaging the membrane, **(b)** binding to and transporting protons across the membrane, and **(c)** serving as a channel that allows protons to pass through the inner membrane. The effect of uncouplers includes the generation of heat and inhibition of adenosine triphosphate (ATP) synthase (Complex V). ADP, adenosine diphosphate; AraC, cytosine arabinoside; AZT, azidothymidine; DNP, 2,4-dinitro-phenol; FADH$_2$, reduced form of flavin adenine dinucleotide; NADH, reduced form of nicotinamide adenine dinucleotide.

$$pmf = \Delta\psi \frac{2.3RT}{\mathscr{F}} \bullet \Delta pH$$

Uncoupling—disruption of the proton gradient. In oxidative phosphorylation, the formation of the proton gradient couples the transfer of electrons (from NADH and FADH$_2$ to O$_2$) to the phosphorylation of ADP to ATP. This coupling is called chemiosmosis. As such, if the proton gradient is disrupted, then phosphorylation of ADP becomes uncoupled from the transfer of electrons. Uncouplers are defined as those chemicals and proteins that allow protons to reenter the mitochondrial matrix from the intermembrane space independent of the proton-channeling function of ATP synthase. The resulting reduction in the proton gradient leads to the following:

- Acceleration of both the TCA cycle and electron transfer to O$_2$
- Inhibition of ATP synthase
- Generation of heat due to the flow of protons into the matrix

Uncouplers are categorized as membrane-damaging agents, mobile proton carriers, or proton channels (▶ Fig. 11.6), as follows:

- **Membrane-damaging agents:** Oxidative phosphorylation cannot occur efficiently in mitochondria with damaged inner mitochondrial membranes because this will render them permeable to protons. Some agents that break down the structural integrity of mitochondrial membranes are

nucleoside analogues such as cytosine arabinoside (AraC) and azidothymidine (AZT) (▶ Fig. 11.6a).
  ○ AraC and AZT are drugs used in the treatment of cancer and human immunodeficiency virus (HIV), respectively. Metabolism of these compounds to their 5′-triphosphate form makes them potent inhibitors of DNA synthesis, including that of the mitochondria.

- **Mobile proton carriers:** Certain lipid-soluble substances bind to and transport protons through the inner membrane. They include compounds such as 2,4-dinitrophenol (DNP) and aspirin (▶ Fig. 11.6b).

- **Proton channels:** Certain ion channels (known as uncoupling proteins) transport protons across the inner mitochondrial membrane in a controlled manner (▶ Fig. 11.6c). One such proton channel is thermogenin (also known as UCP-1), a naturally occurring uncoupler in humans and hibernating animals. It is found in the brown fat tissue of newborns to serve exclusively for generating heat.

11.2.3 (3.) Synthesis of ATP

Synthesis of ATP is catalyzed by a large membrane-bound protein complex called ATP synthase (Complex V). It harnesses the energy contained within the proton motive force (pmf) by passing protons through its proton channel, down their concentration gradient, and into the matrix. In doing so, ATP synthase

III

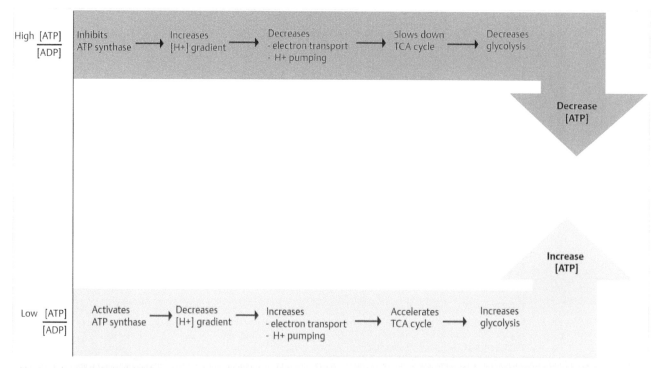

Fig. 11.7 Respiratory control. Respiratory control allows the body to regulate the production of ATP by oxidative phosphorylation in order to meet the changing energy requirements of the body. A high ATP:ADP ratio (pink) slows down oxidative phosphorylation by reducing ATP synthase (Complex V) activity, disrupting the [H⁺] gradient, inhibiting electron transport and thus proton pumping, inhibiting the TCA cycle, and decreasing the rate of glycolysis and the conversion of pyruvate to acetyl CoA. A low ATP:ADP ratio (green) speeds up oxidative phosphorylation by having opposing effects on the aforementioned processes. ADP, adenosine diphosphate; ATP, adenosine triphosphate; CoA, coenzyme A; TCA, tricarboxylic acid.

obtains the necessary power (– 7.3 kcal/mol) to form ATP from ADP and inorganic phosphate (PO_4^{3-}).

The consensus based on thermodynamic considerations is that the synthesis of each ATP molecule by ATP synthase requires the passage of at least three protons from the intermembrane space into the matrix. In addition, the electrogenic exchange of ATP and ADP across the inner mitochondrial membrane by the adenine nucleotide translocator uses another proton.

Inhibition of ATP synthase. The uncouplers mentioned earlier inhibit ATP synthase via disruption of the proton gradient. ATP synthase is also the target of several pharmacological compounds, including oligomycin. This antibiotic is produced by various types of *Streptomyces* and exerts its effect by disrupting ATP synthase's ability to transport protons through its channel. As a result, the proton gradient increases to a level that triggers the cessation of electron transport.

11.2.4 Regulation

Oxidative phosphorylation generates most of the ATP produced by the body. To meet changing energy requirements, the body relies on respiratory control to regulate the production of ATP by oxidative phosphorylation. Respiratory control is sensitive to O_2 and the ATP:ADP ratio, as follows:

• **O_2:** Oxidative phosphorylation will not occur if O_2 is absent.

• **ATP:ADP ratio:** The rate of oxidative phosphorylation is dependent on the energy demand of the cell, as marked by fluctuations in the ATP:ADP ratio.
  ○ When energy is needed, the ATP:ADP ratio is low. This signal speeds up the rate of oxidative phosphorylation to produce ATP by first stimulating the activity of ATP synthase, which then stimulates all upstream processes, as summarized in ▶ Fig. 11.7.
  ○ When energy is more than sufficient, the ATP:ADP ratio is high. This signal slows down the rate of oxidative phosphorylation and thus the production of ATP by first inhibiting ATP synthase, which then attenuates all upstream processes, as summarized in ▶ Fig. 11.7.

Foundations

Respiratory chain components encoded by mtDNA

Human mitochondrial DNA is a circular, double-stranded molecule of 16,569 bp and is present in most cells at 100 to 10,000 copies/cell and replicates independently of chromosomal DNA. It codes for 2 rRNAs, 22 tRNAs, and 13 proteins that function in the respiratory chain and ATP synthesis. These proteins include 7 of the more than 43 subunits of Complex I (NADH dehydrogenase), 1 of the 11 subunits of Complex III (cytochrome-c reductase), 3 of the 13 subunits of Complex IV (cytochrome-c oxidase), and 2 of the 8 subunits of Complex V (ATP synthase). None of the four subunits of Complex II (succinate dehydrogenase) are encoded by the mitochondrial genome. Defects in mitochondrially encoded components of the respiratory chain do lead to defects in oxidative phosphorylation. However, the severity of symptoms is variable due to heteroplasmy. Mitochondrial density varies from tissue to tissue, and also mitochondria contain multiple copies of the genome. Defects in respiratory chain component proteins are also associated with a high incidence of certain types of cancer (e.g., midgut carcinoid tumors) due to an increased production of reactive oxygen species (ROS) by defective mitochondria. Production of ROS can lead to damage of nuclear proto-oncogenes (see Chapter 20) and cause unregulated cell division.

Therapeutics
Rotenone
Rotenone is a naturally occurring pesticide and has been used as fish poison for many centuries. It can be obtained from the roots of *Lonchocarpus* or *Derris* plant species. It is moderately toxic in humans, with an LD_{50} of 150 to 300 mg/kg. Its rapid photodecomposition in sunlight prevents it from becoming a groundwater contaminant. Rotenone is a potent inhibitor of NADH dehydrogenase (Complex I) of the mitochondrial electron transport chain. It appears to prevent the electron transfer from the Fe-S centers to ubiquinone. The inhibition by rotenone may be overcome by menadione (vitamin K_3), which allows the electrons to bypass the site of rotenone blockade. In case of acute rotenone poisoning, treatment includes washing of contaminated skin and eyes, gastric lavage, intravenous administration of glucose and menadione, and maintaining adequate hydration. Chronic rotenone poisoning has, in some cases, been linked to Parkinson disease.

Therapeutics
Amytal (amobarbital)
Amytal (amobarbital), also known as truth serum, is a barbiturate. Its sedative effects are mediated through an activation of gamma-aminobutyric acid type A ($GABA_A$) receptors in the central nervous system. It is more potent than phenobarbital and barbital but less potent than pentobarbital and secobarbital. Amytal is used in the treatment of anxiety, insomnia, and epilepsy. It is a reversible inhibitor of NADH dehydrogenase (Complex I) of the respiratory chain. Blockade of electron transport chain with amytal has been shown to protect cardiac muscle during ischemia-reperfusion by limiting the production of ROS.

Therapeutics
Cyanide poisoning
Cyanide (CN) binds to the oxidized or ferric (Fe^{3+}) form of iron in the heme of the cytochrome-a_3 component of Complex IV of the mitochondrial respiratory chain and prevents O_2 reduction (terminal step of electron transport). Mitochondrial respiration

and ATP production cease, leading to rapid cell death. Death occurs from tissue asphyxia, especially in the central nervous system. If caught early, nitrites can convert Fe^{2+} in hemoglobin into Fe^{3+}, resulting in the formation of methemoglobin, which scavenges CN to protect Complex IV. Subsequent administration of thiosulfate allows enzymatic conversion of CN to thiocyanate, which is nontoxic. Another treatment for suspected cyanide poisoning is intravenous administration of hydoxocobalamin (Cyanokit®, Meridian Medical Technologies). Cynide reacts with hydroxocobalamin to form nontoxic cyanocobalamin which is excreted. Azide (N_3^-), another respiratory chain inhibitor, also binds to Fe^{3+} in Complex IV.

Therapeutics
Cyanide versus carbon monoxide action
Both carbon monoxide (CO) and nitric oxide (NO) compete with O_2 for binding to reduced heme-a_3 (Fe^{2+}) in Complex IV, whereas CN, N_3^-, and hydrogen sulfide (H_2S) bind to the oxidized form of heme-a_3 (Fe^{3+}). Thus, CO acts as a competitive inhibitor (raises the K_m). whereas CN and H_2S act as noncompetitive inhibitors (decrease V_{max}). The kinetics of NO inhibition are a bit more complex because NO can be metabolized to NO_2^- by oxidized heme-a_3.

Therapeutics
Ragged red fibers and abnormal mitochondria
Myoclonic epilepsy and ragged-red fiber disease (MERRF) is the result of a mutation in the tRNA^{Lys} gene of the mitochondrial genome. The mutation affects the synthesis of several proteins that require mitochondrial lysyl-tRNA. This is a rare disease with an incidence of 1 in 400,000 (in Europe), and the severity of the disease varies due to heteroplasmy. Skeletal muscle biopsy stained with modified Gomori trichrome shows aggregates of abnormal mitochondria in red-staining irregularly shaped fibers in the subsarcolemmal and intermyofibrillar regions. Associated clinical symptoms include ptosis, extraocular muscle weakness, ataxia, deafness, heart conduction defects, and raised cerebrospinal fluid (CSF) protein. There is no cure, and symptomatic treatment in some cases includes high doses of coenzyme Q_{10} and L-carnitine.

Thermogenesis in Brown Adipose Tissue

Brown adipose tissue is an important source of heat production during cold adaptation for hibernating mammals and newborn humans. Unlike white adipose, it is rich in mitochondria and has a high expression of UCP-1 (uncoupling protein-1, thermogenin) in the inner mitochondrial membranes. UCP is present in different isoforms in different tissues. UCP-1 uncouples the electron transport from ATP synthase by providing a pathway for protons to leak across the inner mitochondrial membrane back into the matrix. The energy stored in the proton gradient is dissipated as heat rather than used for the production of ATP. When the brain senses cold, it sends sympathetic stimulation to the brown adipose tissue. Norepinephrine is released by postganglionic sympathetic nerves to activate β-adrenergic

III

receptors on the surface of brown adipose cells. As a result, a cytosolic lipase is stimulated to break down triglycerides into fatty acids. The fatty acids activate UCP-1 and stimulate H^+ transport to release heat. It is thought that a long-chain fatty acid anion binds to UCP-1 in a non-dissociable fashion and helps in the symport of a proton into the matrix. Chronic norepinephrine signaling also upregulates gene expression of UCP-1, leading to increased mitochondrial biogenesis.

Foundations

P:O ratio

The P:O ratio is a measure of the efficiency of oxidative phosphorylation, which couples ATP synthesis to cell respiration and is defined as molecules of ATP generated from ADP and inorganic phosphate per atom of oxygen consumed. The theoretical maximum P:O ratio for the oxidation of NAD-linked substrates (e.g., pyruvate) is 3 and for that of FAD-linked substrates (e.g., succinate) is 2. In laboratory studies with freshly isolated mitochondria, nonintegral P:O ratios (~ 2.5 for pyruvate and ~ 1.5 for succinate) are commonly observed. Such nonintegral P:O ratios are explained as the result of several competing processes that are coupled to proton translocation, such as transport of inorganic cations, anionic metabolites, and nicotinamide nucleotide transhydrogenase reaction.

Foundations

Sources of NADH and FADH₂

The NADH that serves as the substrate of Complex I of the respiratory chain is derived mainly from the TCA cycle (isocitrate dehydrogenase, α-ketoglutarate dehydrogenase, and malate dehydrogenase), from oxidative decarboxylation of pyruvate (pyruvate dehydrogenase), and from the oxidation of ketone bodies (β-hydroxybutyrate dehydrogenase). NADH generated by cytosolic reactions such as glyceraldehyde phosphate dehydrogenase cannot enter the mitochondrial matrix. However, the electrons from cytosolic NADH can be transferred to mitochondrial NAD^+ or FAD by malate-aspartate or glycerol phosphate shuttles, respectively. $FADH_2$ that provides electrons to ubiquinone can also come from multiple sources, such as succinate dehydrogenase (Complex II), glycerol phosphate shuttle and fatty acyl CoA dehydrogenase.

Normal

Ubiquinone radical

The partially reduced ubiquinone radical (Q^-) is an intermediate in the transfer of electrons from Complex I to ubiquinone, as well as in the transfer from reduced ubiquinone to Complex III. The Q^- can pass an electron to O_2 to generate the free radical superoxide ($\cdot O_2^-$) anion. Superoxide, along with hydrogen peroxide (H_2O_2) and the hydroxyl radical ($\cdot OH$), constitute the reactive oxygen species (ROS) capable of damaging proteins, membrane lipids, and nucleic acids. The enzyme superoxide dismutase can catalyze the conversion of superoxide to H_2O_2, and the H_2O_2 can be detoxified to water by the action of glutathione peroxidase.

Foundations

Other electron transport systems

The cytochrome P-450 superfamily (CYP) of enzymes is another example of an electron transfer system that is of high biological relevance. CYP enzymes are localized mainly to the endoplasmic reticulum but also occur in the mitochondria (e.g., desmolase or cholesterol side-chain cleavage complex, P-450_{scc}). These enzymes are active in the metabolism of many hydrophobic compounds, such as steroid hormones, eicosanoids, and vitamin D, as well as xenobiotics, such as drugs and toxins. CYP enzymes are hemoproteins that act as mono-oxidases by utilizing a pair of electrons from NADPH to incorporate one atom of molecular oxygen into a substrate while reducing the second oxygen atom to water, as shown here:

$$NADPH + H^+ + O_2 + R\text{-}H \rightarrow NADP^+ + H_2O + R\text{-}OH$$

Electron transfer from NADPH to the heme in mitochondrial CYP involves a flavoprotein (adrenodoxin reductase) and an Fe-S protein (adrenodoxin). In the microsomal CYP system, cytochrome-b_5 serves as the intermediate in the electron transfer.

Foundations

Daily ATP production

The normal daily caloric intake of an adult weighing 70 kg (154 lb) is ~ 2000 kcal (8360 kJ). The free energy ($\Delta G°'$) of ATP synthesis from ADP and Pi is 7.3 kcal/mol (30.5 kJ/mol) under standard conditions. However, under physiological conditions, assuming a temperature of 37 °C and concentrations of ATP, ADP, and Pi to be 3.5 mM, 1.5 mM, and 5 mM, respectively, the actual ΔG can be calculated to be 11 kcal/mol (46 kJ/mol). Assuming that the efficiency of conversion of food energy into ATP is 40%, the amount of ATP synthesized per day would be 72.7 mol. Given the molecular weight of ATP as 503, this figure translates into 36.6 kg of ATP or ~ 52% of typical body weight!

Therapeutics

Nucleoside analog treatments and fatigue

Many of the side effects of nucleoside analogs such as azidothymidine (AZT), cytosine arabinoside (AraC), and 2'-3'-dideoxycytidine (ddC) used in antiretroviral therapy may be traced to their mitochondrial toxicity. These prodrugs are activated by phosphorylation to nucleotides by the mitochondrial isoform of thymidine kinase (TK2). The activated drugs inhibit mitochondrial DNA polymerase γ and deplete mitochondrial DNA. As a result, the synthesis of locally produced components of the respiratory chain, particularly in Complex I, is inhibited, leading to a loss of ATP production. The decrease in Complex I activity causes overutilization of Complex II, resulting in elevated levels of ROS and further damage to other cellular systems. The symptoms of antiretroviral toxicity mimic mitochondrial genetic diseases and include fatigue, lactic acidosis, skeletal myopathy, cardiac dysfunction, and hepatic failure.

III

Therapeutics

Aspirin overdose

Aspirin (acetyl salicylate) is used frequently as an antipyretic drug to lower elevated body temperatures. However, acute aspirin poisoning at doses above 150 mg/kg paradoxically causes hyperthermia. At high concentrations, salicylate uncouples oxidative phosphorylation by disrupting the proton gradient across the inner mitochondrial membrane and causes the dissipation of energy as heat. It also stimulates the respiratory center in the brain and causes hyperventilation. Treatment for aspirin overdose includes gastric lavage and hemodialysis. The classical uncoupling agent, dinitrophenol, also causes hyperthermia when ingested.

Therapeutics

Hypoxia and ATP preservation

Hypoxic conditions that follow myocardial infarction or stroke cause a decrease in the activity of the respiratory chain and in the proton motive force. Oxygen starvation also causes the cell to depend on glycolysis for energy production, leading to lactic acidosis. Lowered pH in the mitochondrial matrix causes dimerization and activation of a small inhibitory protein (IF_1) that binds to ATP synthase and prevents it from acting in reverse to hydrolyze ATP. Thus, ATP levels are preserved.

11.3 Mitochondrial Transport Systems

Most of the molecules generated or used in metabolic processes that take place in the mitochondria can cross the outer mitochondrial membrane through protein pores called porins. However, to cross the inner mitochondrial membrane, these molecules/ions require assistance from specific transport or shuttle systems, some of which harness the energy contained within the proton gradient or membrane potential to transport molecules in the following manner:

- **Uniport:** One molecule/ion is transported alone.
- **Symport:** More than one molecule/ion are transported simultaneously in the same direction.
- **Antiport**: More than one molecule/ion are transported simultaneously but in opposite directions.

11.3.1 Malate-Aspartate and Glycerophosphate Shuttles

One of the end-products of the cytosolic reactions of glycolysis is the reduced coenzyme NADH, which cannot cross into the mitochondrial matrix to transfer its electrons to components of the electron transport chain (ETC) to generate ATP via oxidative phosphorylation. As such, two shuttle systems have been identified that function to transfer the reducing equivalents of NADH from the cytosol to the mitochondrial matrix via a set of redox and transamination reactions.

1. **Malate-aspartate shuttle** (▶ Fig. 11.8a)**:** operates in the heart, liver, and kidneys.
   - Its action generates NADH (in the mitochondrial matrix), which then enters the ETC at complex I (NADH dehydrogenase).
2. **Glycerophosphate shuttle** (▶ Fig. 11.8b)**:** operates in skeletal muscle and brain.
   - Its action generates $FADH_2$ (in the inner mitochondrial membrane), which donates its electrons to the ETC at co-enzyme Q.

Mechanism. Both shuttles carry out a series of redox reactions that transfer electrons from cytosolic NADH (which was generated from the conversion of glyceraldehyde 3-phosphate into 1,3-bisphosphglycerate). Because NADH enters the respiratory chain at a lower redox potential than $FADH_2$, NADH generates 3 molecules of ATP versus the 2 generated per $FADH_2$. As such, depending on the shuttle system used, the complete oxidation of glucose into CO_2 and water may generate 36 or 38 molecules of ATP (including the 2 ATP molecules generated during glycolysis).

11.3.2 Antiporters for Phosphate/OH⁻ and Phosphate/ Malate Exchange

The concentration of phosphate in the mitochondrial matrix is low due to its consumption by the ATP synthase. Phosphate is imported into the mitochondrial matrix via antiport mechanisms that simultaneously import phosphate in the form of $H_2PO_4^-$ and HPO_4^{2-} and export a hydroxide ion (OH^-) or a molecule of malate (▶ Fig. 11.9). The energy for the antiport of phosphate and OH^- is obtained from the proton gradient (ΔpH).

11.3.3 Antiporter for ADP/ATP Exchange

The ATP/ADP translocase facilitates the antiport of ATP and ADP such that when one molecule of ATP is transported out to the intermembrane space, one molecule of ADP is moved into the matrix (▶ Fig. 11.9). This process is driven by the low concentration of ATP in the intermembrane space. The energy for this exchange is provided by both the proton gradient (ΔpH) and the membrane potential ($\Delta \Psi$).

- Because ADP has three negative charges and ATP has four, their exchanges are energetically favored by the proton gradient across the inner mitochondrial membrane.

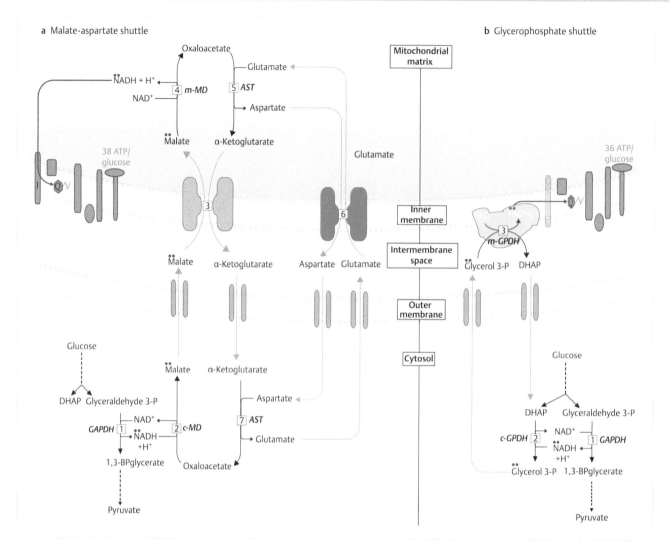

Fig. 11.8 Malate-aspartate and glycerophosphate shuttles. (a) The malate-aspartate shuttle transfers the reducing equivalents (electrons, *red dots*) of the reduced form of nicotinamide adenine dinucleotide (NADH) in the cytosol to NADH in the mitochondrial matrix via the following steps: (1) The conversion of glyceraldehyde 3-P to 1,3-bisphosphoglycer-ate (1,3-BPglycerate) by glyceraldehyde 3-P dehydrogenase (GAPDH) generates NADH, which is used by cytosolic malate dehydrogenase (c-MD) (2) to reduce oxaloacetate to malate. Malate crosses the mitochondrion's outer membrane and is transported (3) into the matrix simultaneously as one α-ketoglutarate is transported out through the same transporter. The oxidation (4) of malate (in the matrix) to oxaloacetate (by mitochondrial malate dehydrogenase (m-MD) regenerates NADH, which enters the electron transport chain at Complex I (NADH dehydrogenase). (5) Oxaloacetate reacts with glutamate in a transamination reaction catalyzed by aspartate aminotransferase (AST) that generates α-ketoglutarate and aspartate (Asp). α-Ketoglutarate is then transported to the cytoplasm (3) simultaneously as one malate is imported into the matrix. In the cytoplasm, α-ketoglutarate (7) reacts with Asp in a transamination reaction that generates oxaloacetate and glutamate. Glutamate is simultaneously imported into the matrix with the export of one Asp via the same antiporter (6). (**b**) The glycerophosphate shuttle transfers the reducing equivalents of NADH in the cytoplasm to $FADH_2$ in the mitochondrial matrix via the following steps: (1) Dihydroxyacetone phosphate (DHAP) and glyceraldehyde 3-phosphate are generated via glycolysis. The conversion of glyceraldehyde 3-phosphate to 1,3-bisphosphoglycerate by GAPDH generates NADH, which is used by cytosolic glycerol 3-P dehydrogenase (c-GPDH) to reduce DHAP to glycerol 3-P (2). (3) Glycerol 3-P enters the intermembrane space, where mitochondrial glycerol 3-P dehydrogenase (m-GPDH)—bound to the inner mitochondrial membrane—simultaneously oxidizes glycerol 3-P to DHAP (3) and reduces FAD to $FADH_2$. $FADH_2$ then donates its electrons to the electron transport chain at coenzyme Q (CoQ), and DHAP reenters the cytosol. ATP, adenosine triphosphate; NAD^+, nicotinamide adenine dinucleotide.

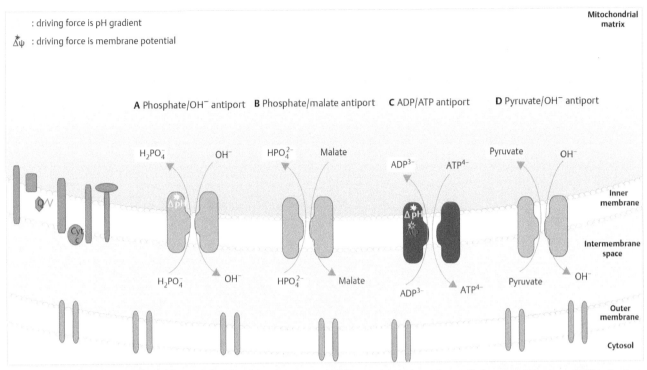

: driving force is pH gradient

$\Delta\Psi$: driving force is membrane potential

Mitochondrial matrix

A Phosphate/OH⁻ antiport **B** Phosphate/malate antiport **C** ADP/ATP antiport **D** Pyruvate/OH⁻ antiport

$H_2PO_4^-$ OH⁻ HPO_4^{2-} Malate ADP³⁻ ATP⁴⁻ Pyruvate OH⁻

Inner membrane

ΔpH ΔpH $\Delta\Psi$

Intermembrane space

$H_2PO_4^-$ OH⁻ HPO_4^{2-} Malate ADP³⁻ ATP⁴⁻ Pyruvate OH⁻

Outer membrane

Cytosol

Fig. 11.9 Mitochondrial transport. (a-d) Molecules are moved across the inner mitochondrial membrane. Their transport is powered either by the normal membrane potential ($\Delta\Psi$) or the proton gradient (ΔpH). ADP, adenosine diphosphate; ATP, adenosine triphosphate.

Review Questions: Cellular Respiration

1. Erythrocytes are red blood cells that make up about 50% of the blood volume. As an erythrocyte matures in the bone marrow, it extrudes its nucleus and most of its other organelles. Which of the following cellular processes will be active in an erythrocyte?
   A) Tricarboxylic acid cycle
   B) β Oxidation
   C) Oxidative phosphorylation
   D) Anaerobic Glycolysis
   E) Gluconeogenesis

2. In mitochondria treated with the uncoupler dinitrophenol (DNP), which among the following is the possible outcome?
   A) The proton gradient generated from the oxidation of NADH and FADH₂ is increased.
   B) The protons flow back from the intermembrane space into the matrix after passing through the ATP synthase.
   C) The energy conserved in the proton gradient is used to generate ATP.
   D) Electron transport chain is inhibited by DNP binding to Complex IV.
   E) Permeability of inner mitochondrial membrane to protons is increased.

3. The transfer of electrons in the electron transport chain (ETC) is essential for oxidative phosphorylation to occur. Which of the following statements is correct regarding the flow of electrons through the electron transport chain?
   A) Coenzyme Q is the final electron acceptor.
   B) Complex II transfers electrons from NADH to ubiquinone (CoQ).

   C) Complex IV accepts electrons from oxygen.
   D) Complex I transfers electrons from FADH2 to CoQ.
   E) Complex III accepts electrons from reduced coenzyme Q (CoQH2).

4. How many high-energy phosphates are generated through the complete metabolism of one acetyl CoA molecule to CO_2 and H_2O?
   A) 1
   B) 3
   C) 6
   D) 11
   E) 12

5. A 25-year-old marathon runner presents to the hospital with complaints of muscle pain, troubled breathing, feeling tired, dizzy and light-headed immediately after the run. Serum lactate was elevated. Further urine analysis, blood gas analysis and serum enzyme studies are ordered to confirm the underlying cause. An increase in which of the following in the muscle may best explain lactate accumulation in this patient?
   A) ATP
   B) NAD+
   C) NADH
   D) Oxygen
   E) NADPH

6. Tracy, a 15-year-old female, arrived at the clinic with an emaciated look and at a height of 5 ft 3 in (1.6 m) and a weight of 75 lbs (34 kg). She was accompanied by her

brother who informed the physician that Tracy was a good student and active in extracurricular activities. However, a year ago she stopped participating in any school activities, and at about the same time, her grades deteriorated drastically. Her brother also reported that Tracy had restricted her food intake but with no binging and purging. The physician advised immediate admission for Tracy. The primary treatment plan was to replenish macronutrients to her body to provide an energy source. After macronutrient replenishment, which among the following will be the immediate driving force that powers the phosphorylation of ADP to ATP by ATP synthase in her body?
A) High [ADP] in the mitochondrion
B) High [NADH] in the cytoplasm
C) Gradient of ATP across the inner mitochondrial membrane
D) Gradient of glucose across the plasma membrane
E) Gradient of H^+ across the inner mitochondrial membrane

7. The term **oxidative phosphorylation** refers to a process in which
A) ATP energy is used to drive protons across the inner mitochondrial membrane
B) A proton gradient provides power for electron transfer from substrate to oxygen
C) ATP energy supplies power for the transfer of electrons from substrate to oxygen
D) Electron transfer creates a proton gradient needed for ATP synthesis
E) phosphorylation of ADP creates a pH gradient across the inner mitochondrial membrane

8. A neonate is admitted to the ICU and is a known case of inherited defect in the E1 subunit of pyruvate dehydrogenase complex (PDC). The infant demonstrates elevated serum pyruvate and lactate. Which vitamin may help manage this enzyme defect?
A) Thiamine (vitamin B_1)
B) Biotin (vitamin B_7)
C) Pyridoxine (vitamin B_6)
D) Folate (vitamin B_9)
E) Cobalamin (vitamin B_{12})

9. Pyruvate dehydrogenase, α-ketoglutarate dehydrogenase, and branched-chain α-keto acid dehydrogenase share one common protein, the E3 subunit. Which molecule is used as a prosthetic group by this subunit?
A) NAD^+
B) FAD
C) Lipoamide
D) CoA
E) Thiamine pyrophosphate

10. The activities of phosphofructokinase 1 (PFK-1), pyruvate dehydrogenase, and citrate synthase will be reduced in the presence of high
A) ATP
B) AMP
C) Ca^{2+}

D) NADPH
E) Insulin

11. According to a 2006 report by the US Department of Health and Human Services, cyanide produces toxic effects at levels ≥ 0.05 mg/dL of blood, and deaths have occurred at levels ≥ 0.3 mg/dL. The report also found that 1 hour of exposure to air containing 110 ppm of hydrogen cyanide gas can be life threatening, whereas 10 minutes of exposure at 546 ppm can be deadly. At the molecular level, cyanide's effect on the cell leads to an impaired conversion of:
A) NADPH to NADP
B) Pyruvate to lactate
C) ATP to ADP
D) Acetyl Co A to CO_2 and H_2O
E) Reduced glutathione to oxidized glutathione

12. The protein and lipid members of the electron transport chain harbor molecules that facilitate the transfer of electrons. Which of the following electron-carrying molecules is harbored in the protein that transfers electrons directly to oxygen?
A) $NADH + H^+$
B) Heme-a_3
C) Heme-b
D) Heme-c
E) $CoQH_2$

13. The presence of an electrochemical gradient of protons across the inner mitochondrial membrane is required for the production of which metabolite?
A) ATP
B) H_2O_2
C) $FADH_2$
D) O_2
E) $NADH + H^+$

14. A medical student attending to a 65-year-old female at the health clinic noticed cheilosis and angular stomatitis on careful oral examination. The student recalled that riboflavin deficiency symptoms are nonspecific and have a similar presentation. Which of the following enzyme activities may be affected in this individual?
A) Succinate dehydrogenase
B) Isocitrate dehydrogenase
C) Pyruvate Carboxylase
D) Lactate dehydrogenase
E) Malate dehydrogenase

15. The reaction catalyzed by which of the following enzymes is an oxidation-reduction (redox) reaction allosterically activated by ADP and inhibited by ATP?
A) Succinate dehydrogenase
B) Malate dehydrogenase
C) Isocitrate dehydrogenase
D) Lactate dehydrogenase
E) Citrate synthase

16. A 32-year-old female is brought to the emergency in a coma. The husband informed the attending physician that within one hour after ingestion of her last meal, she

experienced nausea, vomiting and abdominal pain. Later her condition deteriorated with confusion followed by agitation, seizures and coma. Toxicological analysis was positive for acute fluoroacetate poisoning with significant hypocalcemia. Acute poisoning with fluoroacetate may inhibit cellular metabolic enzyme:
A) Succinate dehydrogenase
B) Branched chain keto acid dehydrogenase
C) α-Ketoglutarate dehydrogenase
D) Aconitase
E) Pyruvate dehydrogenase

17. Cellular respiration depends on the integration of several metabolic pathways that link the breakdown of nutrients to oxidation reduction (redox) reactions that culminate in the transfer of electrons to O_2, the final acceptor of electrons in the electron transport chain. Electrons produced directly from pyruvate enter the mitochondrial electron transport chain as
A) Coenzyme Q
B) NADH + H^+
C) $FADH_2$
D) Acetyl CoA
E) Tetrahydrobiopterin

18. Mitochondrial inner membrane is impermeable to NADH and $FADH_2$. The glycerophosphate shuttle system functions to transfer:
A) the reducing equivalents of NADH in the cytoplasm to FAD in the mitochondrial matrix.
B) the reducing equivalents of NADH in the cytoplasm to NAD in the mitochondrial matrix
C) the reducing equivalents of $FADH_2$ in the cytoplasm to NAD in the mitochondrial matrix.
D) the reducing equivalents of NADH in the cytoplasm to NADP in the mitochondrial matrix.
E) the reducing equivalents of $FADH_2$ in the cytoplasm to NADP in the mitochondrial matrix.

19. In glycolysis, most enzymatic reactions are reversible and can also be used for gluconeogenesis. However, there are three glycolytic reactions that are irreversible, and different enzymes are required to bypass them in gluconeogenesis. Which of the following enzymes catalyzes such an irreversible step in glycolysis?
A) Phosphoglucose isomerase
B) Phosphofructokinase 1
C) Aldolase A
D) Glyceraldehyde-3-phosphate dehydrogenase
E) Phosphoglycerate kinase

20. In a national training center, an athlete runs 800 m. Afterward, a blood sample is taken and analyzed. Which of the following was most likely increased in his serum at the end of his jog?
A) Glucose
B) Lactate
C) Free fatty acids
D) Acetoacetate
E) β-Hydroxybutyrate

21. Identify the bond marked by arrow 4 in the image below:

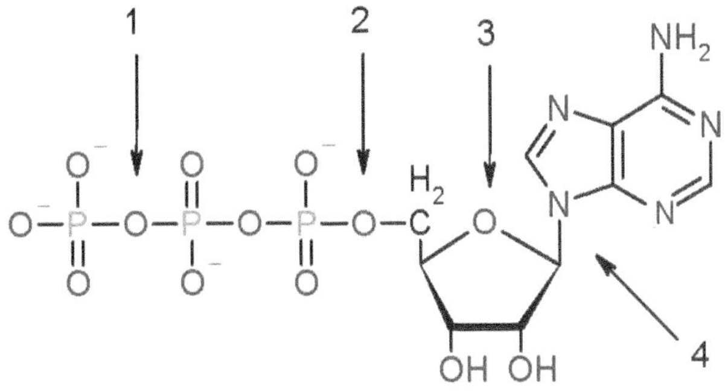

Adenosine triphosphate

A) Anhydride
B) Ester
C) Glycosidic
D) Hemiacetal
E) Amide

22. Consider the following reactions:
1. Glutamate + NH_3 ⇆ Glutamine + H_2O ($\Delta G^{0'}_1$ = + 3.4 Kcal/mol)
2. ATP + H_2O ⇆ ADP + Phosphate ($\Delta G^{0'}_2$ = -7.3 Kcal/mol)
3. Coupled: Glutamate + NH_3 + ATP ⇆ Glutamine + ADP + Phosphate

In which direction would reactions 1 and 2 and the coupled reaction proceed spontaneously?

	Reaction 1	Reaction 2	Coupled reaction
A.	Right	Right	Right
B.	Right	Left	Right
C.	Right	Left	Left
D.	Left	Right	Right
E.	Left	Right	Left

A) Row A
B) Row B
C) Row C
D) Row D
E) Row E

23. Which of the following rows pairs the correct electron transport chain complex with its inhibitor?

	Cyanide	Oligomycin	Antimycin A
A.	V	II	I
B.	I	III	V
C.	II	IV	IV
D.	IV	V	III
E.	IV	I	II

A) Row A
B) Row B
C) Row C

D) Row D
E) Row E

24. A 15-year-old girl with known seizure disorders and on phenobarbital (barbiturates) was rushed to the emergency room due to barbiturate overdose. The resident at the emergency room immediately started her on activated charcoal via nasogastric tube because barbiturates are toxic and inhibit oxidative phosphorylation by binding to:
A) Complex I (NADH dehydrogenase)
B) Complex II (succinate dehydrogenase)
C) Complex III (cytochrome-c reductase)
D) Complex IV (cytochrome-c oxidase)
E) Complex V (ATP synthase)

25. A 35-year-old man was rushed to the emergency room because he was unconscious. He was an experienced runner and had participated in a marathon race (42 km/26.1 miles). It was a cloudy day, and the organizers had provided service stations at regular intervals on the track where isotonic drinks were served. Celebrating his fifth place in the race with his friends, the patient was drinking his third glass of champagne when he suddenly collapsed. Which immediate intervention could save the life of this patient?
A) Ringer/lactate, intravenous (IV)
B) Insulin IV
C) Glucose IV
D) Blood clot dissolvers
E) Oxygen mask

26. A newly-developed laboratory method to isolate mitochondrial matrix as well as inner and outer mitochondrial membranes needs to be evaluated. Enzyme assays are commonly used in cell biology after separations to test cellular fractions for contamination with extraneous material. Which of the following enzymes could be used to test the matrix fraction for contamination with inner membrane and vice versa?

	To assess purity of matrix	To assess purity of inner membrane
A.	Pyruvate dehydrogenase	Cytochrome-c oxidase
B.	Pyruvate kinase	Glycerol 3-phosphate dehydrogenase (FAD-dependent)
C.	Thermogenin	Succinate dehydrogenase
D.	NADH dehydrogenase	α-Ketoglutarate dehydrogenase
E.	Glycerol 3-phosphate dehydrogenase (NADH-dependent)	Cytochrome-c reductase

A) Row A
B) Row B
C) Row C
D) Row D
E) Row E

27. A newborn girl is transferred to the neonatal intensive care unit for severe nonspherocytic hemolytic anemia and jaundice. She was born by cesarean section at week 32 as the third child to a first-cousin couple; none of her older siblings had survived. She was given two exchange transfusions on her first day and phototherapy for 8 days. She was maintained with monthly red blood cell transfusions until a splenectomy was performed at age 3. From then on, transfusions were required only rarely, usually after infections. Her mental development was normal, physical development was delayed. She is now 13 years old. Investigating the metabolite concentrations in the erythrocytes of this patient (before the first transfusion) resulted in the following: high levels of glucose-6-phosphate, 1,3-bisphosphoglycerate, 3-phosphoglycerate, phosphoenolpyruvate, ADP, and AMP and low levels of ATP, pyruvate, and lactate. Which of the following glycolytic enzymes is most likely defective?[1,2]
A) Hexokinase
B) Glyceraldehyde-3-phosphate dehydrogenase
C) Phosphoglycerate kinase
D) Enolase
E) Pyruvate kinase

28. A 10-week-old boy was presented to the metabolic unit of a pediatric hospital for irregularities in brain development. He was born by vaginal delivery after 38 weeks gestation with a birth weight of 2.7 kg (5.95 lb) to a 33-year-old woman of Hispanic descent. From week 10 of gestation ultrasonography had shown progressive enlargement of ventricles, absence of corpora callosa, and hypoplasia of the brainstem and cerebellum. After birth he had been in respiratory distress, showed hypotonia, was feeding poorly, and had frequent seizures. Laboratory: blood pH 7.2, serum pyruvate, lactate, and alanine elevated, citrate reduced. Imaging: [1]H-MRI at 1.5 T confirmed the ultrasonographic findings, 2D chemical shift spectroscopy demonstrated a doublet at 1.33 ppm and a singlet at 2.37 ppm—attributed to lactate and pyruvate, respectively—in the cerebrospinal fluid. The best treatment plan in this case be:
A) a low galactose diet
B) coenzyme Q and carnitine
C) uncooked corn starch meals in the evening
D) allopurinol
E) dichloroacetate, thiamine, and citrate

29. Sodium 2-fluoroacetate (compound 1080) is used as a rodenticide. It is activated inside cells to fluoroacetyl CoA by acetyl CoA synthetase (acetate thiokinase), which is then converted to (-)-*erythro*-2-fluorocitrate by citrate synthase. The latter compound acts as a suicide substrate for aconitase, forming 4-OH- *trans*-aconitate inside the enzyme and directly reducing the synthesis of:
A) Acetyl CoA
B) Oxaloacetate
C) Isocitrate
D) Pyruvate
E) 1–3, bisphosphoglycerate

30. A 48-year-old man is admitted to the emergency room complaining of nausea, malaise, and palpitations. A physical exam reveals flushed, sweaty skin, tachycardia, rapid respiration, and a body temperature of 105.8 °F. Upon questioning, he admits taking a "purely natural" weight

reduction supplement obtained from an Internet source. The active ingredient of that supplement is most likely
A) 2,4-Dinitrophenol
B) Cyanide
C) Rotenone
D) Oligomycin
E) Antimycin A

31. A 64-year-old woman from Botswana (in southern Africa) visits her primary care physician because of weakness, weight loss, and diarrhea. Medical history: several years of alcohol abuse, strangulated hernia repair by bowel resection. Physical exam: erythematous, hyperpigmented, nonpruritic (nonitchy), scaling rash of face, neck, and arms (Casal necklace), glossitis (inflamed, swollen tongue with abnormal color), diminished sense of touch and pain on all extremities. She is apathic (without sensation or feeling), confused, and disoriented. As far as can be gleaned from her, she eats corn-based staple foods but little meat and few fresh vegetables, which she cannot afford. The patient requires supplementation with a vitamin that will increase the amounts of a coenzyme required for the activity of which of the following enzymes?[3]
A) Pyruvate carboxylase
B) Alanine aminotransferase
C) Pyruvate dehydrogenase
D) Hexokinase
E) Succinate dehydrogenase

32. Fowler solution, named after the English physician who invented it in 1786, was a tonic that was prescribed in the United States until the 1950s against malaria, syphilis, chorea, asthma, and other diseases not tractable at the time. It is a 1% solution of potassium arsenite (liquor kali arseniatum). Many patients who took this solution for a long time suffered from chronic arsenite poisoning (which made them take more of the tonic). Much of the toxicity of arsenite is due to its forming chemical bonds with SH groups, especially when two of them are close together. Which of the following mitochondrial enzymes uses a cofactor susceptible to arsenite poisoning?
A) α-ketoglutarate dehydrogenase
B) Citrate synthase
C) Aconitase
D) Isocitrate dehydrogenase
E) Succinyl CoA synthase

33. About 15% of the world's population currently is overweight, and 4% is obese. According to World Health Organization predictions, these numbers are expected to double by 2025, with a commensurate increase in cardiovascular disease, cancer, and Alzheimer disease. Because therapies based on reduction of energy intake have proven largely unsuccessful in stemming this tide, one current focus of research includes therapies that increase energy expenditure. One obvious target is thermogenin (UCP1). How does UCP1 increase energy expenditure?
A) It binds a proton on the outer side of the inner mitochondrial membrane and then facilitates its release into the matrix.

B) It forms a pore through the inner mitochondrial membrane through which NADH can move from the intermembrane space into the matrix.
C) It is an ATPase, which transports protons against the gradient from the intermembrane space into the matrix.
D) Protons flow through this protein together with glucose (symport), which is then burned by the mitochondria.
E) UCP1 allosterically activates the NADH dehydrogenase (complex I), and this is controlled by β-adrenergic receptors.

34. Impila (*Callilepsis laureola de Candolle*, Asteraceae, aka ox-eye daisy) is a plant used for medicinal purposes in southern Africa; the name actually means "good health" in Zulu. It is used to treat tapeworm infections, stomach problems, impotency in males, infertility in females, and to induce labor. In the ritual administered by shamans, dilute aqueous extracts of the plant are ingested by the patient and immediately removed again by induction of vomiting. This procedure is known as *phalaza* and is supposed to cleanse the patient from the influence of evil spirits. Lately, impila has made it into esoteric "health" shops, and parents, without the supervision of shamans, have given the extracts to their children as enemas. The children were brought to local hospitals suffering from nausea, vomiting, epigastric pain (upper abdominal pain), diarrhea, anxiety, and convulsions. Laboratory investigations revealed hypoglycemia, proteinuria, glucosuria, ketonuria, and high concentrations of potassium in urine. Needle biopsies showed destruction of kidney tubules and liver parenchyma by apoptosis. The toxic agent was identified as atractyloside by liquid chromatography coupled mass spectrometry. This substance is known to interfere with ATP synthesis by inhibition of which of the following mitochondrial proteins? [4,5,6]
A) ATP/ADP exchanger
B) Cytochrome-c
C) ATP synthase
D) Succinate dehydrogenase
E) Cytochrome-c reductase

35. One of the purported mechanisms of action of the hypoglycemic drug metformin is to inhibit NADH dehydrogenase (complex I) and thereby increase the concentration of AMP in the cytosol, which activates AMP-dependent protein kinase (AMPK). One of the effects is increased transport and expression of glucose transporter at the plasma membrane of muscle. At the same time, expression of hexokinase is also increased. Both these effects have which of the following possible outcome on glucose utilization in the cell? [7,8]
A) GLUT4 will transport extracellular glucose into the cell together with Na^+ (symport); hexokinase II will prepare the glucose for entry into glycolysis.
B) GLUT4 utilizes the energy of ATP hydrolysis to actively transport glucose into the cells; hexokinase II prepares glucose for conversion into glycogen.
C) GLUT4 allows for passive diffusion of glucose into the cell; hexokinase prevents it from slipping back out.

III

D) GLUT2 will transport extracellular glucose into the cell together with Na⁺ (symport); hexokinase will prepare the glucose for entry into glycolysis.

E) GLUT2 utilizes the energy of ATP hydrolysis to actively transport glucose into the cells; hexokinase prepares glucose for conversion into glycogen.

36. Tumor cells survive on anaerobic glycolysis in the cytoplasm rather than aerobic tricarboxylic acid (TCA) cycle/oxidative phosphorylation in mitochondria (Warburg effect). This is an adaption to the oxygen-poor microenvironment inside a tumor, and it also reduces apoptotic signals from mitochondria. Dichloroacetate is a simple molecule that inhibits PDK and thereby stimulates mitochondrial metabolism, making the tumor cell more sensitive to apoptosis. A similar effect can be achieved by an inhibitor of which of the following enzymes?[9]
A) Phosphofructokinase
B) Pyruvate kinase
C) Lactate dehydrogenase
D) Citrate synthase
E) NADH dehydrogenase

37. In Tarui disease (glycogen storage disease VII), the muscle isoform of phosphofructokinase 1 is defective. This enzyme is subject to allosteric control; it is activated by some and inhibited by other modulators. To make a definitive diagnosis of Tarui disease, the activity of this enzyme in muscle biopsies needs to be measured. Because the amount of tissue in a biopsy is very small, the assay needs to be as sensitive as possible (i.e., all activating), but none of the inhibiting modulators should be present. Which among the following should be left out of the assay mixture?
A) ADP
B) AMP
C) Citrate
D) Fructose-6-phosphate
E) Fructose -2,6-bisphosphate

38. A 12-year-old girl was brought to the emergency room after attempting suicide with an overdose of *N*-acetyl- *para*-aminophenol (acetaminophen). At admission (1 hour after ingestion) she was lethargic. Complete blood count (CBC) and tests for liver and renal function were normal. A Foley catheter and nasogastric tube were placed, and oral activated charcoal and intravenous *N*-acetylcysteine were given. Oxygen was applied as needed to maintain saturation above 90%. During the next 3 hours she developed encephalopathy, hypotension, tachycardia, and mild respiratory distress. *N*-Acetyl-p-benzoquinone imine (NAPQI) was detected in her serum. Venous blood gas analysis was pH 7.22, P CO_2 34 mm Hg, P O_2 71 mm Hg, HCO_3^- 14 mEq/L, base excess -13 mEq/L. Transaminase levels increased but started to decline again after day 6. She could be transferred to the psychiatric ward on day 12. Accumulation of which among the following contributed to acidosis in this case?[10,11]
A) Fatty acids
B) Formic acid
C) Lactic acid
D) Acetoacetic acid
E) β-Hydroxybutyric acid

39. In 1860 the explorers Burke, Gray, King, and Wills started on an expedition to cross Australia for the first time in a south–north direction (Melbourne to the Gulf of Carpentaria). On their return journey they ran short of food and had to supplement their diet with local freshwater mussels *Velesunio ambiguous* Philippi,) and sporocarps of an aquatic fern known as nardoo (*Marsilea drummondii* A. Braun). After a few weeks on this diet they fell ill, suffering from a weakness that made it difficult and painful to get up or walk, tachycardia, confusion, convulsions, vomiting, and emaciation. Gray, Burke, and Wills died; the only survivor, King, never recovered from peripheral neuropathy. Like many mussels and sea food, *Velesunio ambiguus* contains thiaminase, which destroys the vitamin B_1 (thiamine) in the diet. The major pathway inhibited in these explorers would be
A) Glycolysis
B) Fatty acid synthesis
C) TCA cycle
D) Oxidative phosphorylation
E) β-Oxidation

40. Some people have a P446 L mutation in the glucokinase regulatory protein (GK-RP), which reduces binding of fructose-6-phosphate to this protein. How would this mutation affect glucokinase activity and the fasting plasma levels of glucose and triglycerides?

	Glucokinase	Fasting glucose	Fasting triglycerides
A.	Higher	Higher	Lower
B.	Higher	Lower	Higher
C.	Lower	Higher	Lower
D.	Lower	Lower	Higher
E.	Lower	Lower	Lower

A) Row A
B) Row B
C) Row C
D) Row D
E) Row E

41. Mutations in succinate dehydrogenase subunit A (SDHA), a mitochondrial enzyme whose gene is found on chromosome 5, result in encephalocardiomyopathy with leukodystrophy, dementia, myoclonic seizures, retinopathy, ataxia, cardiac conduction defects, short stature, generalized muscle weakness and wasting with easy fatigability. Muscle biopsies show ragged red fibers and excessive lipid droplets. Because two copies of the *SDH* gene must be mutated in order for the disease to manifest, what is the inheritance of the disease?
A) Autosomal dominant
B) Autosomal recessive
C) X-linked dominant
D) X-linked recessive
E) Mitochondrial

42. The cause of death of a couple found dead in a closed tent with the camping lantern burning inside the tent was carbon monoxide poisoning. Carbon monoxide poisoning

may have which of the following effects on mitochondrial oxidative phosphorylation?
A) Increased ATP synthesis and increased oxygen consumption.
B) Increased ATP synthesis and decreased oxygen consumption.
C) Decreased ATP synthesis and increased oxygen consumption.
D) Decreased ATP synthesis and decreased oxygen consumption.
E) Unchanged ATP synthesis and Decreased oxygen consumption.

43. The rate of mitochondrial respiratory chain function is dependent on the energy demand of the cell and is stimulated in the presence of increased intracellular:
A) ATP
B) ADP
C) Rotenone
D) NADPH
E) Antimycin

44. Which among the following is a "low-energy" compound?
A) Cytidine triphosphate (CTP)
B) ATP
C) Acetyl CoA
D) Glucose 6-phosphate
E) Phosphoenolpyruvate

45. If you wanted to develop an assay for pyruvate dehydrogenase activity, use of which substrate or production of which product would yield an easily measurable signal, with routine laboratory equipment, and high sensitivity?
A) Oxidized nicotinamide adenine dinucleotide (NAD$^+$)
B) ATP
C) Flavin adenine dinucleotide (FAD)
D) Thiamine pyrophosphate (TPP)
E) Inorganic phosphate (P$_i$)

46. If the standard free energy change ($\Delta G°'$) for a reaction A + B → C + D$_{(gas)}$ is positive, then which of the following best describes this reaction under standard condition?
A) It is exergonic.
B) It is spontaneous.
C) It is at equilibrium.
D) A change from standard conditions will drive the reaction towards the right or left.
E) K$_{eq}$ > 1 for this reaction.

47. Copper (Cu), one of the most abundant microelements in the human body serves as a cofactor for the activity of many enzymes and is a component of complex IV of the electron transport chain with:
A) Reduced form of nicotinamide adenine dinucleotide (NADH) + H$^+$)
B) Cytochrome-a$_3$
C) Cytochrome-b
D) Flavin mononucleotide (FMN)
E) Coenzyme Q

48. A 40-year-old male presents to the clinic with ankle edema, exertional dyspnea, and is diagnosed with beriberi on

further evaluation. An enzyme of the TCA cycle that has a mechanism and cofactor requirement very similar to those of pyruvate dehydrogenase and may also be affected in this individual is:
A) Succinate dehydrogenase
B) Malate dehydrogenase
C) Isocitrate dehydrogenase
D) α-Ketoglutarate dehydrogenase
E) Aconitase

49. In aerobic metabolism, most of the high-energy phosphate is generated by
A) glycolysis acting on glucose generating lactate.
B) glycolysis acting on glucose generating pyruvate.
C) pyruvate dehydrogenase reaction.
D) TCA cycle.
E) oxidative phosphorylation.

50. In the TCA cycle, four reactions produce reducing equivalents. The word that characterizes the name of the enzyme in all four cases is
A) oxidase.
B) reductase.
C) dehydrogenase.
D) isomerase.
E) synthetase.

51. The reaction catalyzed by which enzyme of the TCA cycle generates a high energy compound that is used for synthesis of ATP by substrate-level phosphorylation?
A) Succinate dehydrogenase
B) Succinate thiokinase
C) Fumarase
D) Malate Dehydrogenase
E) α-Ketoglutarate dehydrogenase

52. Which among the following events is directly responsible for the synthesis of ATP in the mitochondria?
A) transfer of electrons from NADH to Co Q.
B) transfer of electrons from FADH2 to Co Q.
C) movement of protons across the inner membrane.
D) transfer of electrons from cytosolic NADH to mitochondrial NAD +
E) protons passing through the Fo–F1 complex.

53. Which of the following electron carriers is an integral component of Complex I of the mitochondrial electron transport chain?
A) NAD$^+$
B) NADP$^+$
C) FMN
D) FAD
E) Cu center

54. The standard redox potential of NADH is -320 mV, the most negative of all components of the electron transport chain. Therefore, under standard conditions,
A) NADH readily accepts electrons from all other components.
B) NADH's oxidation is not coupled with ATP synthesis.
C) NADH provides a high $^-\Delta G$ when oxidized.
D) NADH can donate electrons to α-ketoglutarate.

55. Cytochrome-c oxidase (complex IV)
    A) is inhibited by rotenone.
    B) is the terminal enzyme of the mitochondrial electron transport chain.
    C) binds oxygen, resulting in the formation of hydrogen peroxide
    D) contains two atoms of zinc/heme-a.
    E) can be reduced by cytochrome-b

56. What is the effect of an "uncoupler" on metabolism?
    A) The formation of ATP continues, but oxidation of TCA cycle intermediates ceases.
    B) ATP formation ceases because TCA cycle activity is inhibited.
    C) Mitochondrial metabolism is blocked.
    D) The movement of ATP and ADP across mitochondrial membranes is impaired.
    E) ATP formation ceases, but O_2 consumption increases.

57. Pyruvate dehydrogenase controls the rate with which pyruvate (a product of sugar and amino acid metabolism) can be broken down by the TCA cycle. Which of the following intermediates of the TCA cycle is a feedback inhibitor of pyruvate dehydrogenase?
    A) Citrate
    B) Isocitrate
    C) α-Ketoglutarate
    D) NADH
    E) $FADH_2$

58. *SLC25A13* is a gene that encodes the mitochondrial aspartate/glutamate antiporter known as citrin. Mutations in this gene result in a defective aspartate/glutamate antiporter which can manifest as adult-onset-type II citrullinemia. Patients with this disorder suffer with recurrent hyperammonemia, neuropsychotic symptoms, aberrant behaviors (e.g., aggression, hyperactivity and irritability). They may have a fatty liver and have an aversion to carbohydrate-rich foods (e.g., sweets), and an overwhelming preference for foods rich in proteins and/or lipids. You have generated a *SLC25A13*-knockout mouse model. What metabolic change would you expect to find in the livers of homozygous *SLC25A13*(–/–) knockout animals?
    A) Increased use of cytosolic aspartate to generate oxaloacetate and glutamate from α-ketoglutarate.
    B) Decreased activity of malate-aspartate shuttle.
    C) Increased transfer of reducing equivalents (electrons) from NADH to complex I of the electron transport chain (ETC).
    D) Decreased transfer of reducing equivalents (electrons) from $FADH_2$ to complex I of the ETC.
    E) Increased production of urea.

59. A 2-year-old girl is evaluated in an emergency room for seizures. Her older brother, father, a paternal aunt (with two normal daughters), and her paternal grandfather had all been diagnosed with persistent hyperinsulinemic hypoglycemia. Their disease could be controlled with dietary modification and/or diazoxide (a drug that reduces insulin secretion). Age of onset and disease severity showed anticipation in this family. Lab results: serum insulin, C peptide, growth hormone, cortisol, and ammonia increased;

free fatty acids, ketone bodies, and glucose (29 mg/dL) decreased; lactate, carnitine, triiodothyronine (T_3), thyroxine (T_4), and thyroid-stimulating hormone (TSH) were normal. Glucose tolerance test result was within normal limits. Pancreas ultrasound, computed tomography (CT) and magnetic resonance imaging (MRI) were also normal. Activating mutations in which enzyme would explain this clinical picture?[12]
    A) Hexokinase
    B) Pyruvate kinase
    C) Lactate dehydrogenase
    D) Glucokinase
    E) Enolase

60. A 3-year-old boy was brought to the emergency room by his parents after they found him in his bed stiff and unresponsive, with rolling eyes and clenched teeth. Four days earlier, the patient had developed lethargy, reduced appetite, and a dry cough; the family doctor had prescribed 300 mg acetylsalicylate (aspirin) 3 times a day. Physical exam revealed dehydration, tachypnea, a ketotic breath, body temperature of 38 °C, and unresponsiveness to nonpainful stimuli. Lab results: lymphocytosis, metabolic acidosis, and increased prothrombin time. Glucose, ammonia, and liver enzymes were normal. Salicylate was present in toxic concentrations. The boy was treated with gastric washout, intravenous bicarbonate, glucose, potassium, and diuretics. Twenty-four hours after admission, he had deteriorated, with dilated pupils, raised blood pressure, papilledema (swelling of the optic disk secondary to elevated intracranial pressure), and crepitations (crackles) on both lung bases. His temperature had risen to 39 °C, and he had to be intubated because of cyanosis, but ventilation was stopped after 48 hours. The boy recovered and was discharged on day 13. What is the most likely cause for fever, tachypnea, and cyanosis in this patient?[13]
    A) Hospital-acquired viral infection
    B) Hospital-acquired bacterial infection
    C) Reye syndrome
    D) Uncoupling of oxidative phosphorylation
    E) Anaphylaxis due to drug incompatibility

61. An athlete has been jogging on a treadmill in a national training center for Olympic athletes for 10 min wearing a spirometer mask. He is consuming 15 L/min of air and producing 3 L/min of carbon dioxide. Which among the following substrates is he burning, assuming that the air oxygen is consumed completely?
    A) Carbohydrate
    B) Protein
    C) Saturated fatty acids
    D) Monounsaturated fatty acids
    E) Polyunsaturated fatty acids

62. The most likely presentation of an individual with a glycolytic enzyme deficiency would be
    A) Hyperglycemia
    B) Decreased glucose absorption
    C) Hemolytic anemia
    D) Cataract
    E) Lactic acidosis

63. Which of the following pairs of electron carriers are components of Complex III of the mitochondrial electron transport chain?
A) Ubiquinone and Cytochrome-a_3
B) Ubiquinone and Fe-S cluster
C) Ubiquinone and Cytochrome-c
D) Fe-S cluster and Cytochrome-a_3
E) Fe-S cluster and Cytochrome-b

64. Which of the following is an example of an oxidation-reduction (redox) reaction?
A) Malate + NAD^+ → oxaloacetate + NADH + H^+
B) Succinyl CoA + GDP + P_i → succinate + GTP
C) Acetyl CoA + oxaloacetate → citrate + CoA
D) Fumarate + H_2O → malate
E) ATP + H_2O → ADP + P_i

65. The TCA cycle is an amphibolic pathway. It has a role in catabolism and its intermediates serve as precursors of anabolic pathways. Which among the following do you think is the primary role of TCA cycle in the body?
A) Be part of the pathway that converts carbons of glucose to the carbon skeleton of glutamate
B) Metabolize the carbon skeleton of aspartate to CO_2
C) Be part of the pathway that converts the carbon skeleton of glutamate to glucose
D) Contribute to metabolizing a majority of the carbons of glucose to CO_2
E) Provide part of the pathway for net synthesis of glucose from fatty acids with an even number of carbons

66. TCA cycle is a common pathway for oxidation of all metabolic fuels. It also provides intermediates that can be used in other pathways.
Which of the following statements regarding this pathway is correct?
A) Two carbons enter the cycle as oxaloacetate.
B) Glucose is metabolized to lactate through the pathway.
C) One of the intermediate of the pathway, oxaloacetate, crosses from the mitochondria to the cytosol as malate.
D) The high ratio of NADH /NAD^+ in the body activates the pathway.
E) It is an essential energy producing pathway in the erythrocytes.

67. A component of the electron transport chain that can accept electrons from more than one donor is:
A) cytochrome-c.
B) cytochrome-b.
C) cytochrome-c_1.
D) cytochrome-a_3.
E) ubiquinone.

68. Which of the following components of the electron transport chain is inhibited by malonate?
A) Complex I (NADH dehydrogenase)
B) Complex II (succinate dehydrogenase)
C) Complex III (cytochrome-c reductase)
D) Complex IV (cytochrome-c oxidase)
E) Complex V (ATP synthase)

69. Creatinine is an anhydride of creatine and
A) requires creatine kinase for its synthesis.

B) is a component of the urea cycle.
C) is excreted by the lungs.
D) is an important hormone.
E) is a marker of renal function.

70. The image below shows the structures of succinate and malonate, substrate and inhibitor, respectively, of succinate dehydrogenase. Given the most likely mechanism of inhibition, what will be the consequences of the presence of malonate on the apparent K_m and V_{max} of succinate dehydrogenase for succinate?

	K_m	V_{max}
A.	Increased	Increased
B.	Increased	unchanged
C.	Increased	Decreased
D.	Decreased	Increased
E.	Decreased	Unchanged

A) Row A
B) Row B
C) Row C
D) Row D
E) Row E

71. Mitochondrial encephalopathy, lactic acidosis and stroke (MELAS) is characterized by muscle weakness and pain, accumulation of lactic acid, vomiting, loss of appetite, seizures and stroke-like episodes. MELAS is associated with mutations in mitochondrial genes encoding subunits of Complex I of the electron transport chain (ETC) and may have the following effect on ETC function:

Succinate   Malonate

A) No effect on electron transport chain.
B) Allow electron transport to proceed without ATP synthesis.
C) Inhibits respiration without impairment of ATP synthesis.
D) Prevents the binding and oxidation of $CoQH_2$ (ubiquinol).
E) Prevent NAD^+-requiring reactions.

72. In tightly-coupled mitochondria, the rate of oxidative phosphorylation is limited mainly by the concentration of which of the following?
A) NADH
B) ATP
C) ADP
D) Citric acid
E) Pyruvate

73. A 6-day-old infant girl was transferred to a tertiary care hospital with severe hepatic failure, dehydration, axial

(truncal) hypotonia, and lactic and ketoacidosis. A diagnosis of pyruvate carboxylase deficiency was made. In pyruvate carboxylase deficiency, cells lack the major source of compounds that replenish the TCA cycle (anaplerotic reaction), specifically, the generation of
A) acetyl CoA from pyruvate.
B) oxaloacetate from pyruvate.
C) pyruvate from phosphoenolpyruvate.
D) lactate from pyruvate.
E) phosphoenolpyruvate from phosphoglycerate.

74. Arsenate (AsO_4^{3-}, the pentavalent form of arsenic) can mimic inorganic phosphate. However, in an aqueous environment, acyl arsenates spontaneously hydrolyze much faster than the corresponding phosphates. Which intermediate of glycolysis will occur as an unstable compound in the presence of arsenate?
A) Glucose-6-phosphate
B) Fructose-6-phosphate
C) Fructose-1,6-bisphosphate
D) Glyceraldehyde-3-phosphate (GAP)
E) 1,3-Bisphosphoglycerate (1,3-BPG)

75. A 47-year-old woman was brought to the emergency room unconscious after ingesting about 25 mg/kg rotenone with intent to self-harm. She was reported by her family to have vomited profusely. Her blood pressure was 93/52 mm Hg with normal heart rate and electrocardiogram. Respiration was rapid. Blood analysis revealed elevated liver enzymes, normal kidney function, and severe metabolic acidosis. She was intubated, continuous venovenous hemodialysis was started, and she was put on intravenous bicarbonate and adrenaline. Acetylcysteine, multivitamins, zinc, and iron (substances shown in cell culture to reduce damage by rotenone) were also given. However, she died after 48 hours from multiorgan failure. Her acidosis was most likely caused by which of the following?[14]
A) Pyruvate
B) Lactate
C) Fumarate
D) Succinate
E) Malate

76. A 23-year-old woman reports to her doctor because of polydipsia, polyuria, and nightly calls to the bathroom. Physical exam reveals the following: height 1.70 m (67 in.), normal weight of 60 kg (132 lb). Urinalysis: glucose

2 + (which could be normalized by low-dose sulfonylurea); albumin, ketones, and erythrocytes negative; pH 4.6. Blood: random glucose 10 mM, erythrocytes $3.5 \times 10^6/mm^3$, white blood cells (WBC) 8000/mm^3, hematocrit (HCT) 35%, human chorionic gonadotropin (hCG) negative. Family history: mother has diabetes.
If this patient is found to suffer from a single gene disorder, a mutation iin which of the following genes could explain her presentation?
A) Pyruvate kinase
B) Malate dehydrogenase
C) Glucokinase
D) α-Ketoglutarate dehydrogenase
E) Enolase

77. A 41-year-old woman was treated in a hyperbaric chamber for carbon monoxide (CO) poisoning due to a defective water heater in her home. After 6 days, she was released from the hospital in good health. After about 1 month, she started to have neurologic and psychiatric problems (forgetfulness, nervousness, and disordered speech). Her situation worsened to depression, kleptomania (addiction to stealing regardless of economic need), and paranoia until she was hospitalized for evaluation 10 months after her accident. Blood and urine analysis results were unremarkable; electroencephalogram (EEG) and neurologic exams were also normal. Magnetic resonance imaging (MRI) revealed ischemic and necrotic lesions in the cortex, subcortical white matter, and globus pallidus. She was put on quetiapine and, once stabilized, followed as an outpatient. The damage was caused mainly by binding of CO to which of the following?[15]
A) Cytochrome-c
B) Enolase
C) Hemoglobin
D) Pyruvate dehydrogenase
E) Glyceraldehydes-3-phosphate dehydrogenase

78. A 1-week-old boy is diagnosed with an inborn deficiency of the pyruvate dehydrogenase E1 subunit. Which among the following can be safely supplemented in his diet?
A) Alanine
B) Glycine
C) Serine
D) Tryptophan
E) Leucine

Answers and Explanations: Cellular Respiration

1. D Glycolysis, also called Embden-Meyerhof-Parnas pathway, occurs in the cytosol. Erythrocytes lack mitochondria and rely on anaerobic glycolysis for energy.

A The tricarboxylic acid (TCA) cycle, also known as the citric acid or Krebs cycle, occurs in the mitochondrial matrix. In the TCA cycle, one molecule of acetyl coenzyme A (CoA) is broken down to two molecules of CO_2; the hydrogens are saved in the form of three molecules of NADH + H^+ and one molecule of FADH$_2$. These are oxidized to water during oxidative phosphorylation. Erythrocytes lack mitochondria.

B During β oxidation, fatty acids are broken down to acetyl CoA; this reaction occurs in the mitochondrial matrix. Erythrocytes lack mitochondria.

C Oxidative phosphorylation occurs on the inner mitochondrial membrane. During this reaction sequence, metabolic hydrogen (in the form of NADH + H^+ and FADH$_2$) is safely oxidized to water. The chemical energy of that reaction is used to convert ADP and P$_i$ into ATP. Erythrocytes lack mitochondria.

E Gluconeogenesis is formation of glucose from noncarbohydrate substrates. The cytosolic and mitochondrial reactions of gluconeogenesis serves to synthesize glucose. Erythrocytes lack mitochondria.

2. E In an uncoupled system, increased transport of H + across membrane abolishes the electrochemical proton gradient.

A In an uncoupled system, the proton gradient generated from the oxidation of NADH and $FADH_2$ is dissipated.

B In an uncoupled system, the proton gradient is short circuited allowing protons to flow back from the intermembrane space into the matrix without passing through the ATP synthase.

C In an uncoupled system, the energy conserved in the proton gradient is converted to heat, rather than being used to generate ATP.

D Carbon monooxide (CO) binds to the reduced or ferrous (Fe2 +) form of iron in the heme component of cytochrome -a3 component of Complex IV of the mitochondrial respiratory chain and prevents O2 reduction (terminal step of electron transport).

3. E Complex III contains heme-b, which is part of cytochrome-b, accepts electrons from the mobile carrier coenzyme Q (ubiquinone), and transfers them to another mobile carrier cytochrome-c.

A Coenzyme Q is a lipid-soluble molecule in the ETC. Complex III accepts electrons from reduced coenzyme Q ($CoQH_2$) and transfers them to cytochrome-c (the mobile protein of the ETC). Oxygen and not coenzyme Q, is the final electron acceptor in the ETC.

B $FADH_2$ is a prosthetic group for succinate dehydrogenase (complex II), a non-proton-pumping member of the ETC. Complex II transfers electrons from $FADH_2$ to ubiquinone (a lipid-soluble molecule in the ETC), but not to cytochrome-c (the mobile protein of the ETC).

C Heme-a is a prosthetic group found within cytochrome-c oxidase (complex IV). Complex IV accepts electrons from cytochrome-c (the mobile protein member in the ETC) and transfers them to the final electron acceptor, oxygen.

D FMN is a prosthetic group found within NADH dehydrogenase (complex I), the first proton-pumping member of the ETC. However, complex I transfers electrons from NADH to CoQ (the lipid-soluble molecule in the ETC).

4. E According to conventional wisdom, 9 ATP originate from oxidation of 3 NADH + H+, 2 from the single $FADH_2$, and 1 at the substrate level from the succinyl CoA synthetase reaction (actually GTP, but the equilibrium constant of GTP + ADP ⇆ GDP + ATP is near 1).

A, B, C, D See explanation for **E**.

5. C An anaerobic episode may underlie the above clinical presentation. The amount of NAD+ in the cytosol is limiting and must be regenerated in order for glycolysis to continue. Thus under aerobic condition, cytosolic NADH is oxidized to NAD+ by either malate aspartate shuttle or glycerophosphate shuttle. Lack of oxygen in the muscle may lead to increase in NADH and lactate accumulation.

A An anaerobic episode may underlie the above clinical presentation. Under aerobic condition, cytosolic NADH is oxidized to NAD+ by either malate aspartate shuttle or glycerophosphate shuttle producing ATP.

B Lack of oxygen in the muscle may lead to increase in NADH and lactate accumulation.

D An anaerobic episode may underlie the above clinical presentation with lack of oxygen to the muscles.

E Lack of oxygen in the muscle may lead to increase in NADH (not NADPH) and lactate accumulation.

6. E Macronutrients through TCA cycle are oxidized to two molecules of CO_2; the hydrogens are saved in the form of three molecules of NADH + H+ and one molecule of $FADH_2$. The driving force for phosphorylation is the electrochemical energy in the H+ gradient produced by oxidation of metabolic hydrogen (NADH and $FADH_2$).

A Although [ADP] controls the rate of oxidative phosphorylation, it does not provide the driving force for it.

B NADH in the cytoplasm cannot enter the mitochondria directly; its reducing equivalents have to be transported in by either the malate-aspartate or glycerophosphate shuttle. Inside the mitochondria, NADH is oxidized to NAD+ and water, and the energy of that process generates a proton gradient, which drives ATP synthesis.

C Because ATP is produced inside but consumed outside the mitochondria, a concentration gradient across the mitochondrial membrane must exist. But this gradient does not drive ATP formation.

D Glucose is used in cells as fuel; hence [glucose] is lower inside the cell than in the plasma. However, the gradient drives only transport of glucose into the cell; ATP production is driven by oxidation of glucose to CO_2 and H_2O.

7. D The sequence of events is the oxidation of NADH and $FADH_2$ with delivery of the electrons to the electron transport chain, electron transfer to O_2 with production of a pH and electrical gradient across the inner mitochondrial membrane, reentry of protons through ATP synthase (complex V) with phosphorylation of ADP to ATP.

A Although it is possible for the ATP synthase (complex V) to use the energy of ATP hydrolysis to generate a proton gradient, under physiological conditions, the reaction happens the other way around: oxidation of NADH and $FADH_2$ produces a proton gradient that is then used by the ATP synthase to convert ADP to ATP.

B Electron transfer from substrates (NADH and $FADH_2$) to oxygen releases energy that is conserved as a proton gradient across the inner mitochondrial membrane. This proton gradient is then used to drive the ATP synthase, which phosphorylates ADP to ATP.

C Electron transfer from substrates (NADH and $FADH_2$) to oxygen releases energy that is conserved as a proton gradient across the inner mitochondrial membrane. This proton gradient is then used to drive the ATP synthase, which phosphorylates ADP to ATP.

E Although it is possible for the ATP synthase (complex V) to use the energy of ATP hydrolysis to generate a proton gradient, under physiological conditions, the reaction happens the other way around: oxidation of NADH and $FADH_2$ produces a proton gradient that is then used by the ATP synthase to convert ADP to ATP.

8. A Milder form of the above deficiency is due to a defect wherein the enzyme has a low affinity for the cofactor. The PDC requires thiamine pyrophosphate as a cofactor.

B Biotin is required by carboxylases and is not used by pyruvate dehydrogenase.

C Pyridoxine is required mainly for transaminases and for the aromatic amino acid decarboxylases.

D Folate carries one-carbon groups from amino acid breakdown to nucleotide synthesis.

E Cobalamin is required for two reactions in the human body: the conversion of homocysteine to methionine and the conversion of methylmalonyl CoA to succinyl CoA.

9. B The E3 subunit oxidizes dihydrolipoamide on the E2 subunit to lipoamide, forming a disulphide bond. The hydrogens on the SH groups of dihydrolipoamide are transferred to the prosthetic group FAD, and then from $FADH_2$ to the cosubstrate NAD^+.

A The E3 subunit does transfer hydrogens from the dihydrolipoamide in the E2 subunit to NAD^+, forming NADH. However, NAD^+ is a cosubstrate, not a prosthetic group. Prosthetic groups stay in the enzyme throughout its life, whereas cosubstrates bind, are modified, and then dissociate again.

C Lipoamide is a prosthetic group of the E2 subunits of pyruvate dehydrogenase, α ketoglutarate dehydrogenase, and branched-chain α-keto acid dehydrogenase, not the E3 subunit.

D CoA is a cosubstrate of pyruvate dehydrogenase, α-ketoglutarate dehydrogenase, and branched-chain α-keto acid dehydrogenase, not a prosthetic group. Prosthetic groups stay in the enzyme throughout its life, whereas cosubstrates bind, are modified, and then dissociate again. CoA also takes the acetyl group from S-acetyl-dihydrolipoamide in the E2, not the E3, subunit.

E Thiamine pyrophosphate (TPP) is a prosthetic group of the E1, not the E3, subunit of pyruvate dehydrogenase, α-ketoglutarate dehydrogenase, and branched-chain α-keto acid dehydrogenase.

10. A Elevated levels of molecules such as ATP and NADH are indicative of a state of high energy charge. This means that the cell has plenty of energy, so the pathways that lead to the production of more energy (glycolysis, tricarboxylic acid cycle) are inhibited by allosteric regulation of their key enzymes. For instance, PFK-1 (the rate-limiting enzyme of glycolysis) is inhibited by ATP; pyruvate dehydrogenase (the enzyme that links glycolysis to the TCA cycle) is inhibited by both ATP and NADH; citrate synthase (the enzyme that catalyzes the first step of the TCA cycle) is inhibited by ATP and NADH.

B Elevated levels of molecules such as ATP and NADH are indicative of a state of high-energy charge. This means that the cell has plenty of energy, so the pathways that lead to the production of more energy (glycolysis, tricarboxylic acid cycle) are inhibited by allosteric regulation of their key enzymes.

C Ca^{2+} is an activator isocitrate dehydrogenase and alpha ketoglutarate dehydrogenase.

D Pyruvate dehydrogenase (the enzyme that links glycolysis to the TCA cycle) is inhibited by both ATP and NADH; citrate synthase (the enzyme that catalyzes the first step of the TCA cycle) is inhibited by ATP and NADH and not NADPH.

E Insulin is a well-fed state hormone. The pathways that lead to the production of more energy (glycolysis, tricarboxylic acid

cycle) are activated by covalent modification (dephosphorylation) of their key enzymes (PDH, PFK-2).

11. D The TCA cycle breaks down acetyl CoA into CO_2 and reducing energy in the form of NADH and $FADH_2$. Oxidation of these hydrogens—that is, transport of electrons from hydrogen ([H] → $H^+ + e^-$) to oxygen ($O_2 + 4 e^- → 2 O^{2-}$) in a stepwise, safe fashion—provides most of the ATP produced by the catabolism of food. Cyanide blocks electron transport at the level of cytochrome-c oxidase (complex IV) and stops the generation of the H^+ gradient that drives the ATP synthase (complex V). At the same time, NADH will no longer be oxidized to NAD^+ and hence the TCA cycle will stop for lack of NAD^+ as well as due to the feedback inhibition of key enzymes of TCA cycle by NADH.

A Cyanide blocks electron transport at the level of cytochrome-c oxidase (complex IV) and stops the generation of the H^+ gradient that drives the ATP synthase (complex V). At the same time, NADH will no longer be converted back to NAD^+ not NADPH to $NADP^+$

B Cyanide blocks electron transport at the level of cytochrome-c oxidase (complex IV) and stops the generation of the H^+ gradient that drives the ATP synthase (complex V). At the same time, NADH will no longer be oxidized to NAD^+ Pyruvate to lactate conversion will be enhanced as the cell becomes dependent on anaerobic respiration.

C Electron transport is required to generate the proton gradient that drives ATP formation. Cyanide decreases both electron transport and ATP formation. In the absence of new ATP production, there would be increased hydrolysis of ATP to ADP.

E Cyanide blocks electron transport at the level of cytochrome-c oxidase (complex IV) and stops the generation of the H^+ gradient that drives the ATP synthase (complex V). At the same time, NADH will no longer be converted back to NAD^+. Cyanide has no direct effect on glutathione peroxidase.

12. B Cytochrome-c oxidase (complex IV), which contains heme-a, -a_3, and Cu, transfers electrons directly to oxygen.

A NADH dehydrogenase (complex I), which contains FMN and Fe-S centers, transfers electrons and H^+ from NADH + H^+ onto CoQ, not oxygen.

C, D Cytochrome-c reductase (complex III), which harbors heme-b, heme-c, and Fe-S centers, transfers electrons to cytochrome-c, not oxygen.

E $CoQH_2$ transfers electrons to cytochrome-c reductase (complex III), not oxygen.

13. A Phosphorylation of ADP to ATP requires energy derived from the potential energy of the proton gradient when protons pass back through ATP synthase.

B Hydrogen peroxide (H_2O_2) is produced by most flavoproteins according to $FADH_2 + O_2 → FAD + H_2O_2$. These enzymes are located in the peroxisome, which also contains catalase to deal with the toxic (disinfectant!) H_2O_2. Mitochondrial flavoproteins like succinate dehydrogenase have evolved to transfer most (> 98%) of the hydrogen onto coenzyme Q (CoQ) instead of oxygen. Only if the electron transport chain is interrupted—for example, by poisons such as antimycin A—is H_2O_2 production significant. Even then, however, it does not require a proton gradient.

C $FADH_2$ is consumed, not produced, in the electron transport chain.

D O_2 is consumed, not produced, in the electron transport chain.

E NADH is consumed, not produced, in the electron transport chain.

14. A Succinate dehydrogenase as it is the only enzyme in the list that uses FAD as a cosubstrate. FAD is a cofactor derived from Vitamin B_2 (riboflavin).

B Isocitrate dehydrogenase uses NAD^+ as a cosubstrate, not FAD.

C Pyruvate carboxylase uses biotin as a cosubstrate, not FAD.

D Lactate dehydrogenase uses NAD^+ as a cosubstrate, not FAD.

E Malate dehydrogenase uses NAD^+ as a cosubstrate, not FAD.

15. C Isocitrate dehydrogenase is one of the control points of the TCA cycle and is activated by ADP but inhibited by ATP.

A Succinate dehydrogenase performs a redox reaction, but it is not controlled by [ATP] or [ADP]. Instead, it is competitively inhibited by the substrate analogue malonate.

B Malate dehydrogenase performs a redox reaction, but it is not controlled by [ATP] or [ADP]. Instead, it is inhibited by NADH.

D Lactate dehydrogenase performs a redox reaction, but it is not controlled by [ATP] or [ADP].

E Isocitrate dehydrogenase is one of the control points of the TCA cycle and is activated by ADP but inhibited by ATP. So is citrate synthase, but that is not an oxidation-reduction reaction.

16. D Sodium 2-fluoroacetate (compound 1080) is used as a rodenticide. Fluoroacetate is absorbed from gastrointestinal tract after ingestion. It is activated inside cells to fluoroacetyl CoA by acetyl CoA synthetase (acetate thiokinase), and is then converted to (-)-erythro-2-fluorocitrate by citrate synthase. The latter compound acts as a suicide substrate for aconitase, forming 4-OH- trans-aconitate inside the enzyme.

A Malonate, a dicarboxylic acid, is a structural analog of succinate and is a strong competitive inhibitor of succinate dehydrogenase.

B, C, E Enzymes which use a lipoic acid derivative as a cofactor, such as branched-chain ketoacid dehydrogenase, α-ketoglutarate dehydrogenase and pyruvate dehydrogenase are inhibited by arsenite (derivative os arsenic). Arsenite links to lipoic acid's two sulfhydryl (SH) groups. It is a suicide inhibitor that binds to thiol groups irreversibly and limits the availability of lipoic acid.

17. B Pyruvate dehydrogenase forms acetyl CoA, CO_2, and $NADH + H^+$ from pyruvate. NADH then enters the mitochondrial ETC at complex I.

A Coenzyme Q is not produced from pyruvate. It is a lipid molecule that transfers electrons from complexes I and II to III in the ETC.

C $FADH_2$ is generated by succinate dehydrogenase (a TCA cycle and ETC enzyme), not directly from pyruvate.

D Although acetyl CoA is generated from the decarboxylation of pyruvate, acetyl CoA itself does not carry electrons to the ETC in this form. Instead, acetyl CoA is oxidized in the TCA cycle to generate $NADH + H^+$ and $FADH_2$, which then enter the ETC.

E Tetrahydrobiopterin is a carrier of reducing equivalents in the metabolism of amino acids, not the ETC.

18. A Glycerophosphate shuttle is one of two ways that reducing equivalents from NADH can cross the mitochondrial membrane. The glycerophosphate shuttle operates mainly in muscle and brain. The cytosolic NADH is used by glycerol-3 phosphate dehydrogenase to reduce DHAP to glycerol-3-phosphate. The glycerol-3-phosphate formed in the cytosol is reduced by a dehydrogenase located on the outer face of the inner mitochondrial membrane, which produces $FADH_2$ and dihydroxyacetone phosphate. $FADH_2$ then reduces coenzyme Q (ubiquinone) to ubiquinol.

B Malate-aspartate shuttle is one of the ways that reducing equivalents from NADH can cross the mitochondrial membrane. The malate-aspartate shuttle operates mainly in the heart, liver and kidneys. The cytosolic NADH is used by the malate dehydrogenase in the cytosol to reduce oxaloacetate to malate. The malate-formed in the cytosol crosses the mitochondrial outer membrane and is transported into the matrix. The oxidation of malate in the matrix to oxaloacetate generates NADH which enters electron transport chain I (NADH dehydrogenase).

C, E The glycerophosphate shuttle system is one of two ways that reducing equivalents from NADH can cross the mitochondrial membrane and not from $FADH_2$.

D The glycerophosphate shuttle system is one of two ways that reducing equivalents from NADH can cross the mitochondrial membrane, and does not involve NADPH.

19. B The reaction Fru-6-P + ATP → Fru-1,6-BP + ADP, catalyzed by PFK-1, is irreversible. For gluconeogenesis, Fru-1,6-bisphosphatase hydrolyzes Fru-1,6-BP to Fru-6-P and P_i (BP, bisphosphate).

A The conversion of Glc-6-P into Fru-6-P by phosphoglucose isomerase (also known as glucose-6-phosphate isomerase) is readily reversible.

C Splitting Fru-1,6-BP into glyceraldehyde-3-P and dihydroxyacetone phosphate by aldolase A is readily reversible, even though a C-C bond is split.

D The reaction glyceraldehyde-3-P + P_i + NAD^+ ⇄ 1,3-BPG + NADH + H^+, catalyzed by glyceraldehyde-3-phosphate dehydrogenase, is readily reversible. The free energy of substrate oxidation is almost completely preserved by formation of a high-energy phosphate (BPG, bisphosphoglycerate).

E The reaction 1,3-BPG + ADP ⇄ 3-PG + ATP, catalyzed by phosphoglycerate kinase, is readily reversible, even though an ATP is formed. 1,3-BPG is an energy-rich compound (PG, phosphoglycerate).

20. B In a sprint, the first 2 to 4 seconds are fueled by ATP stored in the muscle, then creatine phosphate takes over for up to ~ 20 seconds. From then on, anaerobic glycolysis is used to provide energy to white muscle fibers, using glucose and producing lactate. After ~ 2 minutes, tissue becomes too acidic, and red muscle fibers take over, using aerobic glycolysis of glucose. In endurance sports, the glycogen stores of muscle and liver are eventually depleted (in a marathon race after ~ 30 km), then fatty acids become the main fuel source of muscular activity (with glycerol fueling gluconeogenesis).

A In a sprint, the first 2 to 4 seconds are fueled by ATP stored in the muscle, then creatine phosphate takes over for up to ~ 20 seconds. From then on, anaerobic glycolysis is used to provide energy to white muscle fibers, decreasing glucose as it is used to produce lactate. After ~ 2 minutes tissue becomes too acidic, and red muscle fibers take over, using aerobic glycolysis of glucose. In endurance sports, the glycogen stores of muscle and liver are eventually depleted (in a marathon race after ~ 30 km), then fatty acids become the main fuel source of muscular activity (with glycerol fueling gluconeogenesis).

C Fatty acids become the main fuel source of muscular activity (with glycerol fueling gluconeogenesis) during endurance sports, where the glycogen stores of muscle and liver are eventually depleted (e.g., after ~ 30 km of a marathon race). During an 800 m race, however, the first 2 to 4 seconds are fueled by ATP stored in the muscle, then creatine phosphate takes over for up to ~ 20 seconds. From then on, anaerobic glycolysis is used to provide energy to white muscle fibers, using glucose and producing lactate. After ~ 2 minutes tissue becomes too acidic, and red muscle fibers take over, using aerobic glycolysis of glucose.

D Acetoacetate is a ketone body that is generated in the liver from elevated levels of acetyl CoA, the product of fatty acid breakdown. Glycogen stores of muscle and liver are eventually depleted, and fatty acids become the main fuel source of muscular activity during endurance sports (e.g., after ~ 30 km of a marathon race), not an 800 m race.

E β-Hydroxybutyrate is a ketone body that is generated in the liver from elevated levels of acetyl CoA, the product of fatty acid breakdown. Glycogen stores of muscle and liver are eventually depleted, and fatty acids become the main fuel source of muscular activity during endurance sports (e.g., after ~ 30 km of a marathon race), not an 800 m race.

21. C The N-glycosidic bond marked by arrow 4 is formed between a C1 of ribose and N9 of adenine.

A An anhydride is a bond between two acids; marked by arrow 1 and is between two phosphoric acid molecules. The N-glycosidic bond is formed between ribose and adenine.

B Esters are formed between an alcohol and an acid, marked by arrow 2, and it is between a phosphoric acid and the alcoholic OH group on C5 of ribose. The N-glycosidic bond is formed between ribose and adenine.

D Hemiacetal marked by arrow 3. The N-glycosidic bond is formed between ribose and adenine.

E Amides are formed between an acid and an amine. The N-glycosidic bond is formed between ribose and adenine.

22. D (A, B, C, E) The first reaction has, as written, a positive $\Delta G^{0\prime}$. It will therefore proceed to the left unless free energy is provided to make it go to the right. The second reaction has a negative $\Delta G^{0\prime}$; thus, free energy is released when the reaction proceeds to the right, and it will do so spontaneously. The coupled reaction has a free energy of $\Delta G = \Delta G^{\circ\prime}1 + \Delta G^{0\prime}2 = +3.4$ Kcal/mol + (- 7.3 Kcal/mol) = - 3.9 Kcal/mol. Thus, the coupled reaction will proceed spontaneously to the right.

23. D (A, B, C, E) Cyanide inhibits cytochrome-c oxidase (complex IV), oligomycin binds to and inhibits the transmembrane (F_o) part of ATP synthase (complex V), and antimycin A inhibits cytochrome-c reductase (complex III).

24. A Barbiturates bind to the CoQ-binding site of complex I and prevent electron transfer from internal Fe-S centers to coenzyme Q (CoQ). Note that CoQ can still be reduced by succinate dehydrogenase, electron-transferring flavoprotein (ETF, β-oxidation), and glycerol-3-phosphate:CoQ oxidoreductase (cytosolic NADH via glycerol phosphate shuttle). Hence barbiturates are somewhat less toxic than compounds acting on complexes III and IV, which block oxidative phosphorylation altogether (e.g., cyanide).

B Barbiturates do not inhibit complex II.

C Barbiturates do not inhibit complex III.

D Barbiturates do not inhibit complex IV.

E Barbiturates do not inhibit complex V.

25. C After ~ 30 km (18.6 miles) into a marathon race, even well-trained athletes have used up their glycogen stores. They continue to run on fatty acids and ketone bodies. The reduced rate of ATP production is experienced as "hitting the wall." Blood glucose levels in this situation are maintained by gluconeogenesis. This is required given that brain, erythrocytes, and kidneys absolutely depend on glucose for fuel. When the patient drank alcohol after this strenuous exercise, he blocked gluconeogenesis and hence his only remaining source of blood glucose, resulting in a (life-threatening) hypoglycemic coma.

A Ringer/lactate, often used to treat hypoglycemia, would not work in this patient. With gluconeogenesis blocked, he can no longer convert lactate into glucose.

B The patient is suffering from a hypoglycemic coma; injecting insulin would only accelerate his demise.

D The patient is suffering from a hypoglycemic coma, not a stroke.

E The patient is suffering from a hypoglycemic coma, not a lung problem.

26. D NADH dehydrogenase is also known as complex I of oxidative phosphorylation. This enzyme is located in the inner mitochondrial membrane; thus, it can translocate 4 H^+ ions across the inner membrane for each NADH + H^+ oxidized. This enzyme is therefore suitable to check a preparation of mitochondrial matrix for contamination with inner membranes. α-Ketoglutarate dehydrogenase is a soluble enzyme of the tricarboxylic acid (TCA) cycle and therefore occurs in the mitochondrial matrix. Absence of this enzyme in a preparation of inner membranes would exclude contamination with matrix proteins.

A Pyruvate dehydrogenase is a soluble enzyme of the citric acid cycle and therefore supposed to be in preparations of mitochondrial matrix. On the other hand, cytochrome-c oxidase is also known as complex IV of oxidative phosphorylation. It is located in the inner mitochondrial membrane and translocates 2 H^+ ions across the membrane for each cytochrome-c oxidized. Its presence in a preparation of inner mitochondrial membrane is therefore expected and would not exclude contamination with mitochondrial matrix enzymes.

B Pyruvate kinase is an enzyme of glycolysis and located in the cytosol. Its presence in a preparation of mitochondrial matrix would therefore indicate contamination with cytosol, not inner membranes. The FAD-dependent glycerol-3-phosphate dehydrogenase (G3PDH isoform 2) is located on the outside of the inner mitochondrial membrane, facing the intermembrane space. It functions as part of a shuttle system that transports hydrogen from cytosolic NADH + H⁺ into oxidative phosphorylation, together with the cytosolic G3PDH isoform 1, which is NADH-dependent. Presence of FAD-dependent G3PDH in preparations of mitochondrial inner membranes is therefore to be expected and not an indication of contamination with matrix enzymes.

C Thermogenin is a proton channel in the inner mitochondrial membrane of brown adipose tissue that short-circuits the H⁺ gradient across the membrane to produce heat, especially in newborns and in hibernating animals. This protein would be a suitable marker to check preparations of mitochondrial matrix for contamination with inner membranes only if the mitochondria used were from brown adipose tissue. Succinate dehydrogenase is the only enzyme of the TCA cycle that occurs in the inner mitochondrial membrane. Its presence in preparations of these membranes is therefore to be expected and not an indication of contamination with matrix enzymes.

E The NADH-dependent glycerol-3-phosphate dehydrogenase (G3PDH isoform 1) is located in the cytosol. Its main function is to help shuttle reducing equivalents from cytosolic NADH + H⁺ into oxidative phosphorylation. Its presence in preparations of mitochondrial matrix would therefore indicate contamination with cytosol, not mitochondrial inner membranes. CoQH₂: cytochrome-c oxidoreductase is also known as complex III of oxidative phosphorylation. Its presence in mitochondrial inner membrane preparations is therefore to be expected and not an indication of contamination with mitochondrial matrix.

27. E Enzymopathies are almost always recessive and result in disease due to either substrate accumulation and/or product deficiency. Pyruvate is low; thus, the defect has to be in pyruvate kinase, the enzyme that catalyzes the conversion of phosphoenolpyruvate and ADP to pyruvate and ATP in glycolysis. The concentrations of the substrates of this enzyme are elevated, the product concentrations reduced. In addition, lactate concentrations are reduced because lactate is produced from pyruvate. AMP is elevated due to conversion of 2 ADP into ATP and AMP by adenylate kinase. Concentrations of glycolytic metabolites before the inhibited step are also elevated, as one would expect. Pyruvate kinase deficiency is the most frequent cause of nonspherocytic hemolytic anemia.

A If hexokinase were defective, one would expect reduced rather than elevated concentrations of glucose-6-phosphate.

B If glyceraldehyde-3-phosphate dehydrogenase were defective, one would expect reduced rather than elevated concentrations of 1,3-bisphosphoglycerate.

C If phosphoglycerate kinase were defective, one would expect reduced rather than elevated concentrations of 3-phosphoglycerate.

D If enolase were defective, one would expect reduced rather than elevated concentrations of phosphoenolpyruvate.

28. E Low citrate and high pyruvate are indicative of pyruvate dehydrogenase deficiency, which also explains the secondary increased lactate and alanine. Dichloroacetate inhibits pyruvate dehydrogenase kinase; thiamine is a cofactor of pyruvate dehydrogenase; citrate treats acidemia.

A A low galactose diet would be appropriate for a patient suffering from galactosemia, a defect in one of the three enzymes required to metabolize galactose. Signs of galactosemia are cataracts, jaundice, hepatomegaly, galactosuria, aminoaciduria, albuminuria, hypoglycemia, hyperbilirubinuria (both direct and indirect), and elevated liver enzymes.

B Carnitine is used to treat certain deficiencies in fatty acid metabolism, either to ease fatty acid transport into the mitochondria (primary carnitine deficiency, carnitine-acylcarnitine translocase deficiency, carnitine palmitoyltransferase II deficiency) or to remove toxic intermediates that accumulate (acyl CoA dehydrogenase deficiencies, *mut*-type methylmalonic aciduria). Coenzyme Q can be helpful in deficiencies of oxidative phosphorylation.

C Uncooked cornstarch is used in the glycogen storage diseases affecting the liver, mainly in von Gierke disease. Because it is broken down in the intestine only very slowly, it can supply the patient with a constant trickle of glucose during an overnight fast, given that their liver is unable to do so. This prevents the fasting hypoglycemia that could cause severe brain damage.

D Allopurinol inactivates xanthine oxidase and hence prevents the formation of uric acid. In a child, hyperuricemia would probably be primary, and gout would be a presenting problem.

29. C The TCA cycle begins with the condensation of acetyl CoA with oxaloacetate to generate citrate via an irreversible reaction catalyzed by citrate synthase. Citrate is then isomerized to isocitrate by the enzyme aconitase. Fluorocitrate acts as a suicide substrate for aconitase thereby reducing the synthesis of isocitrate.

A Synthesis of acetyl CoA requires pyruvate dehydrogenase complex. Hence its synthesis will not be reduced by fluorocitrate.

B. Synthesis of oxaloacetate from pyruvate requires pyruvate carboxylase. Hence its synthesis will not be reduced by fluorocitrate.

D. Synthesis of pyruvate requires pyruvate kinase. Hence its synthesis will not be reduced by fluorocitrate.

E. Synthesis of 1,3- bisphosphoglycerate requires glycerladehyde-3-phosphate dehydroghenase. Hence its synthesis will not be reduced by fluorocitrate.

30. A The signs and symptoms are typical for an uncoupler, a substance that shuttles protons down the concentration gradient across the inner mitochondrial membrane. The energy contained in that gradient is converted into heat. The body temperature of the patient needs to be kept below the fatal 107.6 °F by ice packs. At the same time, fluids and electrolytes lost with sweat should be replaced. Oxygen may be given as needed. There is a considerable black market for dinitrophenol as a weight-loss aid, which turns body fat into heat. Although this sounds like an easy way out, it is not without considerable risk, which is why dinitrophenol is not a licensed drug.

B Cyanide inhibits cytochrome-c oxidase, that is, complex IV of oxidative phosphorylation. This results in a complete failure of ATP production from oxidative phosphorylation. Initial signs include weakness, headache, confusion, and the feeling of suffocation. This progresses rapidly (seconds to minutes) into unconsciousness, seizures, and cardiac arrest. Places that work with cyanide (laboratories, electroplating) usually have accident kits nearby, which contain amyl nitrite to convert hemoglobin into methemoglobin (Fe^{2+} to Fe^{3+}), which acts as a binding site for cyanide. Then thiosulphate is injected to convert cyanomethemoglobin into thiocyanate, which is excreted by the kidney. An alternative method of treatment is hydroxycobalamin (vitamin B_{12}), which binds cyanide to form cyanocobalamin.

C The insecticide, acaricide, and piscicide rotenone (banned in most countries other than the United States) is the poison of the Mexican jicama vine *Pachyrhizus erosus* (L.), Fabaceae). The roots of this plant are edible and usually consumed raw but may also be cooked into soups or stews. All other parts of the plant are toxic. Rotenone also occurs in several other tropical plant species. Indigenous people release the juice of these plants into rivers to catch fish; the fish can be eaten because rotenone is poorly absorbed by our intestine. Its use as an insecticide is now strictly regulated because it is nonspecific and also kills useful insects like bees. Rotenone acts by inhibiting the interaction of complex I (NADH oxidase) with coenzyme Q (CoQ). The gills and trachea of insects and fish absorb rotenone much better than does the human intestine, which is why this substance is so toxic to them. In addition, ingestion of rotenone causes vomiting. However, long-term occupational exposure to rotenone is suspected to cause Parkinson disease.

D Oligomycin binds to the transmembrane part of the ATP synthase, which is hence called F_o for oligomycin binding (as opposed to the F_1 head, where ATP synthesis occurs). Binding blocks the proton channel and hence ATP synthesis. It is a 26-membered macrolide produced by *Streptomyces* and used in small amounts in laboratories only. In rats, oligomycin injection leads to lactic acidemia and reduced oxygen consumption. Its effects on humans are unknown but probably similar.

E The fungicide, insecticide, and piscicide antimycin A (Fintrol, produced by strains of *Streptomyces*) blocks oxidative phosphorylation by binding to the CoQ site of complex III (cytochrome-c reductase). This leads not only to a reduction of both oxygen consumption and ATP production but also to production of massive amounts of reactive oxygen species. It is probably these that are lethal.

31. C Pyruvate dehydrogenase requires the niacin (vitamin B_3)–derived coenzyme NAD^+ for its activity. This patient is suffering from pellagra, a disease characterized by the "4Ds": diarrhea, dermatitis, dementia, and death. Intestinal surgery, alcohol abuse, and corn-based nutrition make her more sensitive to this disease, which, if left untreated, would kill her. Recall that corn does contain considerable amounts of niacin, however, in a chemically bound form not available to human nutrition unless the corn is nixtamalized (cooked with an alkali-like lime water ($Ca(OH)_2$) or potash (K_2CO_3)). Pellagra used to be a big problem in the Mediterranean and in the southern United States, but fortification and a more variable diet have largely eliminated it there. However, in parts of India and southern Africa pellagra in people relying on corn is still endemic. Females are more sensitive than males because estrogen prevents niacin synthesis from tryptophan.

A Pyruvate carboxylase requires biotin for its activity and not niacin.

B Alanine aminotransferase requires the vitamin B_6–derived cofactor pyridoxal phosphate for its activity. Patients suffering from pellagra are deficient in vitamin B_3 (niacin).

D Hexokinase does not require a niacin-derived coenzyme for its activity.

E The activity of succinate dehydrogenase requires the tightly bound cofactor FAD. It is derived from riboflavin (vitamin B_2), not from niacin.

32. A α-Ketoglutarate dehydrogenase, like other thiamine-dependent oxidative decarboxylases, utilizes lipoamide to transfer the decarboxylated product onto coenzyme A. Lipoamide is converted to dihydrolipoamide in the process, which has two closely spaced SH groups sensitive to arsenite.

B Citrate synthase does not need a cofactor; it relies on acid/base synthesis with several histidine and aspartate residues acting as proton donors/acceptors.

C Aconitase relies on a 4Fe-4S cluster to accomplish its task, which is not sensitive to arsenite.

D Isocitrate dehydrogenase utilizes NAD^+ as a cosubstrate and manganese in the active center. Neither is sensitive to arsenite poisoning.

E Succinyl CoA synthase (succinyl thiokinase) uses a phosphate group to split succinyl CoA into CoA and succinyl phosphate. The "high-energy" phosphate is then transferred onto a His residue of the enzyme, releasing succinate. In a third step, the phosphate is transferred from His to GDP, making GTP. None of these compounds avidly react with arsenite.

33 A During oxidative phosphorylation, protons are pumped from the matrix into the intermembrane space by complexes I through IV, except for complex II. In most cells this gradient is used to drive ATP synthesis in complex V (ATP synthase). Brown adipose tissue is special in that its mitochondria express UCP1 in the inner mitochondrial membrane. A long-chain fatty acid anion bound to UCP-1 acts as a proton carrier, which allows protons to move down the concentration gradient back into the mitochondrial matrix. This in effect creates a short-circuit; the energy of the proton gradient is converted into heat. Brown adipose tissue is essential for newborn mammals, where it maintains body temperature until enough heat can be generated by muscular and metabolic activity. It is also used by hibernating mammals. Even adult humans have brown adipose tissue (mostly between the shoulder blades); it is only lost after intensive dieting.

B NADH cannot pass through the mitochondrial inner membrane.

C During oxidative phosphorylation, protons are pumped from the matrix into the intermembrane space by complexes I through IV. Thus, the flow of protons from the intermembrane space into the matrix is downhill (not against its gradient) and does not require energy (i.e., ATP hydrolysis).

D Glucose does not enter the mitochondria, it is converted into pyruvate in the cytosol. Pyruvate then enters the mitochondria through a membrane protein. Because pyruvate is produced in the cytosol and consumed in mitochondria, this transport is downhill and does not require cotransport.

E There is no direct interaction between UCP1 and the complexes of oxidative phosphorylation.

34. A Atractyloside is a toxic agent in plants that inhibits the mitochondrial ADP/ATP exchanger. It should be noted that herbal remedies are active not by magic but because of the chemical compounds they contain, as is the case for industrially produced pharmaceuticals. This is true both for clinically intended effects and for side effects. Contrary to popular belief, herbal drugs are neither inherently safe nor free of side effects (remember that many chemotherapeutic drugs used against cancer are of herbal or fungal origin). The risks increase when these drugs are used outside their cultural contexts.

B Atractyloside does not interact with cytochrome-c.

C Atractyloside does not interact with the ATP synthase.

D Atractyloside does not interact with succinate dehydrogenase (complex II).

E Atractyloside does not interact with cytochrome-c reductase (complex III).

35. C GLUT4 facilitates the transport of glucose down a concentration gradient from the extracellular fluid into the cell (or vice versa). It therefore needs no energy source like a Na^+-gradient or ATP. Once inside the cell, the glucose is phosphorylated by hexokinase, the negative charge of the phosphate group prevents the Glc-6-phosphate from leaving the cell again. This latter reaction causes the concentration gradient of Glc across the plasma membrane. AMPK is activated by high [AMP], that is, when the energy charge of the cell is low (e.g., in a contracting muscle). It therefore activates glycolysis.

A The Na^+/glucose symporter (SGLT1) occurs in the enterocytes of the small intestine and allows the concentration of glucose to be some 30,000 times higher inside the enterocyte than in the intestinal lumen. Muscle cells, however, are bathed in an extracellular fluid that contains a high concentration of glucose.

B Primary active transport of glucose occurs only in bacteria, not in mammals. Bacteria may have to take up this nutrient from very dilute solutions; transport is often fueled by phosphoenolpyruvate rather than ATP. Glucose uptake into muscle is down the concentration gradient and does not require metabolic energy. AMPK is activated by high [AMP], that is, when the energy charge of the cell is low (e.g., in a contracting muscle). It therefore activates glycolysis rather than glycogen synthesis.

D GLUT2 is expressed in kidney, liver, small intestine, and pancreatic β-cells, all of which require "bidirectional" flow of sugar and can also handle fructose and galactose. The Na^+/glucose symporter (SGLT1) occurs in the enterocytes of the small intestine and allows the concentration of glucose to be some 30,000 times higher inside the enterocyte than in the intestinal lumen. Muscle cells, however, are bathed in an extracellular fluid that contains a high concentration of glucose, and they express GLUT4, which, like GLUT2, allows for passive diffusion of glucose down a concentration gradient.

E Primary active transport of glucose occurs only in bacteria, not in mammals. Bacteria may have to take up this nutrient from very dilute solutions, and transport is often fueled by phosphoenolpyruvate rather than ATP. GLUT2 is expressed in kidney, liver, and pancreatic β-cells, all of which require "bidirectional" flow of sugar and can also handle fructose and galactose. Glucose uptake into muscle is by GLUT4, down the concentration gradient, and does not require metabolic energy. AMPK is activated by high [AMP], that is, when the energy charge of the cell is low (e.g., in a contracting muscle). It therefore activates glycolysis rather than glycogen synthesis.

36. C Inhibition of lactate dehydrogenase would prevent the recycling of cytoplasmic NADH to NAD^+ and hence stop anaero-bic glycolysis. The cell would have to rely on aerobic metabolism.

A Inhibitors of phosphofructokinase would block a key step in both aerobic and anaerobic sugar metabolism. This would starve not only cancer cells but also normal tissue.

B Inhibitors of pyruvate kinase would block a key step in both aerobic and anaerobic sugar metabolism. This would starve not only cancer cells but also normal tissue.

D Citrate synthase is part of the TCA cycle, which we want to stimulate, not inhibit.

E NADH dehydrogenase (complex I) is part of oxidative phosphorylation, which we want to stimulate, not inhibit.

37. C The enzyme defective in Tarui disease is phosphofructokinase 1, the rate-limiting enzyme of glycolysis. This enzyme is allosterically inhibited by markers of high cellular energy charge (ATP, phosphoenolpyruvate, citrate) and activated by markers of low energy charge (ADP, AMP and phosphate). In addition, it is potently activated by fructose 2,6-bisphosphate. Citrate is produced from acetyl CoA in the mitochondria and exported into the cytosol for fatty acid synthesis. It is therefore a marker of high energy charge; glycolysis is downregulated by citrate. ADP, AMP, and phosphate are markers of low energy.

A High cellular ADP concentration is an indication of low energy charge; it activates glycolysis, including the PFK-1 that is defective in Tarui disease.

B High cellular AMP concentration is an indication of low energy charge; it activates glycolysis, including the PFK-1 that is defective in Tarui disease. AMP is produced from ADP by adenylate kinase.

D Fructose-6-phosphate is a substrate of PFK-1, which is defective in Tarui disease. It also allosterically stimulates the enzyme as a homotropic allosteric modulator.

E Fructose -2,6-bisphosphate is the product of bifunctional enzyme phosphofructokinase 2/fructose -bisphosphatase -2(PFK-2/FBPase-2) and allosterically stimulates the enzyme PFK-1.

38. C Lactic acid is produced by muscle during anaerobic exercise and is converted back to glucose by the liver. This is called the Cori cycle. This patient had mild hypoxia and hence increased lactate production, and at the same time liver damage (marked by increased transaminase levels), that prevented gluconeogenesis from lactate. The resulting hypoglycemia may also raise ketone bodies, but the major acid present is lactic acid. Acetaminophen poisoning occurs relatively frequently (56,000 emergency room visits per year in the United States), and in lactic acidemia of unknown origin acetaminophen poisoning should be on the differential diagnosis. Alcohol can amplify the toxic effect of acetaminophen. In part, overdosing happens by accident (60% of cases) when people in pain take too much of an over-the-counter analgesic: "It's non-prescription, so it must be harmless." In 40% of cases, acetaminophen overdose is taken with intent to self-harm because of its easy availability. Part of the ingested acetaminophen is converted by CYP450 into *N*-acetyl-*p*-benzoquinone imine (NAPQI); this intermediately reacts with SH groups. If enough glutathione is available, NAPQI is converted into a mercapturic acid by conjugation to glutathione (phase II detoxification). If NAPQI production exceeds the available glutathione, protein SH-groups are modified instead, leading to liver toxicity and necrosis. *N*-acetylcysteine (NAC) can be given to such patients to restore glutathione levels.

A Long-chain free fatty acids are not soluble enough to markedly affect plasma pH.

B Methanol is metabolized to formic acid in the body and its accumulation is not contributing to acidosis in her case.

D Acetoacetic acid is a ketone body; these are produced from fatty acids by the liver. In this patient, failure to complete the Cori cycle led to lactic acidosis. The resulting hypoglycemia may raise ketones somewhat, but this is not the major cause of her acidosis.

E β-Hydroxybutyric acid is a ketone body; these are produced from fatty acids by the liver. In this patient, failure to complete the Cori cycle led to lactic acidosis. The resulting hypoglycemia may raise ketones somewhat, but this is not the major cause of her acidosis. β-Hydroxybutyric acid is produced in lieu of acetoacetic acid when the NADH:NAD⁺ratio in the liver is high, especially during diabetic ketoacidosis. This is clinically important because β-hydroxybutyrate, unlike acetoacetate, does not react with the nitroprusside-sodium present in urine test sticks. Therefore, one can obtain a false-negative urine test for ketone bodies, and that is about the only situation where measuring ketone bodies makes clinical sense.

39. C Thiamine is required as a cofactor by pyruvate dehydrogenase and α-ketoglutarate dehydrogenase in the TCA cycle, and also by the branched chain α-keto acid dehydrogenase in the breakdown of Leu, Ile, and Val. These enzymes perform oxidative decarboxylations of their substrates and transfer the product onto coenzyme A. Thiamine is required for the first step of these reactions. Thiamine is also required for transketolase, which occurs in the pentose phosphate shunt. Transketolase measurement in erythrocytes before and after addition of thiamine can be used to assess the thiamine status of a patient: if addition of thiamine increases the activity, the patient is deficient.

A Thiamine is not required for glycolysis. Glycolysis requires NAD⁺ and hence niacin.

B Thiamine is not required for fatty acid synthesis; this reaction requires pantothenic acid to make the acyl-carrier protein (ACP).

D Thiamine is not required for oxidative phosphorylation, which regenerates NAD⁺ and FAD. Thus, oxidative phosphorylation involves niacin and riboflavin in addition to Fe and Cu.

E Thiamine is not required for β-oxidation, which produces FADH$_2$ and NADH. This pathway therefore requires niacin and riboflavin.

40. B (A, C, D, E) GK-RP binding to glucokinase (hexokinase IV) in the liver is regulated by glucose, insulin, Fru-1-phosphate, and Fru-6-P (and possibly other factors). If the glucose concentration is low (fasting state), GK-RP binds to glucokinase, and the complex moves into the nucleus, where it is stored until glucose concentrations rise again after the next meal. Without GK-RP, glucokinase would be degraded, and reaction to rising glucose-concentration would be more sluggish. Binding of Fru-6-P to GK-RP increases its binding to glucokinase. Note that Fru-1-P has opposite effects from Fru-6-P, which makes sense because Fru-1-P is produced from dietary fructose and hence signals a postprandial state; Fru-6-P accumulates during glycogenolysis and gluconeogenesis, both of which occur during the fasting state. A mutation that reduces Fru-6-P binding therefore reduces GK-RP-glucokinase interactions, and glucokinase

remains active at higher product concentrations. Therefore, fasting plasma glucose is reduced. On the other hand, because more glucose will be converted to fat, fasting plasma triglycerides will rise.

41. B Most mitochondrial (Mt) enzymes are encoded in the nucleus; mutations therefore usually have an autosomal recessive inheritance. Mt DNA contains only 37 genes: the genes for 13 subunits of enzymes involved in oxidative phosphorylation, 2 rRNAs and 22 tRNAs

A Although SDHA is, like most mitochondrial proteins, encoded in the nucleus, inheritance is autosomal recessive, not dominant. Dominant inheritance requires either a gain of function (which is much rarer than loss of function), or a dominant negative effect. The latter occurs in homo-oligomeric proteins, when a single defective subunit renders the entire protein nonfunctional. Overall, dominant inheritance is much rarer than recessive.

C There are only seven diseases with X-linked dominant inheritance, none of which involve mitochondrial proteins.

D Of the 26 known X-linked recessive diseases, only three involve the mitochondria: Barth syndrome, ornithine transcarbamoylase deficiency, and sideroblastic anemia.

E Most mitochondrial enzymes (including SDHA) are encoded in the nucleus; mutations therefore usually have an autosomal recessive inheritance. MtDNA contains only 37 genes: the genes for 13 subunits of enzymes involved in oxidative phosphorylation, 2 rRNAs, and 22 tRNAs. SDHA happens to be encoded on chromosome 5.

42. D Carbon monoxide (CO) binds to the reduced or ferrous (Fe2+) form of iron in the cytochrome-a3 component of Complex IV of the mitochondrial respiratory chain and prevents O2 reduction (terminal step of electron transport). Hence oxygen consumption is decraesed, mitochondrial respiration and ATP production ceases, leading to rapid cell death.

A,B Carbon monoxide is an inhibitor of electron transport chain function and in its presence, ATP synthesis is decraesed, not increased.

C Uncouplers like dinitrophenol short-circuit the proton gradient across the inner mitochondrial membrane and thereby remove the driving force for adenosine triphosphate (ATP) generation. However, all processes that move protons out of the matrix into the intermembrane space (complexes I to IV) not only continue to work, but can work even faster, as they do not have to act against a proton gradient. In addition, the increased [ADP] and reduced [ATP] upregulate glycolysis and the tricarboxylic acid (TCA) cycle. Thus, oxygen consumption increases, and the chemical energy contained in the food is converted to heat.

E Carbon monoxide is an inhibitor of electron transport chain function and in its presence, ATP synthesis is decreased, not unchanged.

43. B When energy is needed, the ATP/ADP ratio is low. This signals to speed up the rate of oxidative phosphorylation to produce ATP by first stimulating ATP synthase.

A When energy is more than sufficient, the ATP/ADP ratio is high. This signals to slow the rate of oxidative phosphorylation and thus the production of ATP by first inhibiting ATP synthase.

C Rotenone is a naturally occurring pesticide and has been used as fish poison for many centuries. Rotenone is a potent inhibitor of NADH dehydrogenase (Complex I) of the mitochondrial electron transport chain function.

D ATP/ADP ratio regulates the rate of oxidative phosphorylation and not NADPH/NADP$^+$.

E Antimycin is a potent inhibitor of cytochrome-c reductase (Complex III) of the mitochondrial electron transport chain function.

44. D Glucose 6-phosphate cannot transfer its phosphate group to ADP. The hexokinase reaction, which generates glucose 6-phsophate, is not reversible. Therefore, liver has glucose-6-phosphatase to remove the phosphate group so that the freed glucose can be exported to the bloodstream.

A, B Nucleoside triphosphates are all "high-energy" compounds.

C The thioester bond in acetyl CoA preserves the energy contained in a C-C bond split during β-oxidation of fatty acids and by thiamine-dependent dehydrogenases.

E Phosphoenolpyruvate is a "super energy-rich" compound. The phosphate group cannot only be transferred to ADP (making ATP), but there is considerable excess free energy in that reaction to make it irreversible. Therefore, during gluconeogenesis, the pyruvate kinase reaction has to be circumvented by pyruvate carboxylase, malate dehydrogenase, and phosphoenolpyruvate carboxykinase (PEPCK). In effect, two molecules of ATP are used to convert one molecule of pyruvate into phosphoenolpyruvate.

45. A Reduction of NAD$^+$ to the NADH + H$^+$ increases its absorbance at 340 nm; this can be used to measure the rate of conversion in a photometer using Lambert-Beer's law. This type of assay was invented by Otto Warburg and is named for him.

B ATP is neither a substrate nor a product of the reaction catalyzed by pyruvate dehydrogenase.

C FAD is a coenzyme of pyruvate dehydrogenase and is not used up in this reaction.

D TPP is a coenzyme of pyruvate dehydrogenase and is not used up in this reaction.

E P$_i$ is neither a substrate nor a product of the reaction catalyzed by pyruvate dehydrogenase.

46. D The $\Delta G^{\circ\prime}$ predicts the position of the equilibrium under standard conditions. If the conditions are changed, the equilibrium will shift so as to counteract the change (Le Chatelier principle); like an increase of [A] would shift the equilibrium toward the right. To proceed toward the right (positive $\Delta G^{\circ\prime}$), the system would require energy, and lowering the temperature would therefore shift the equilibrium to the left. Because D is a gas, sealing the vessel would increase the pressure. To counteract this effect, the equilibrium would shift to the left.

A, B The $\Delta G^{\circ\prime}$ predicts the position of the equilibrium under standard conditions. When $\Delta G^{\circ\prime} > 0$, the reaction cannot occur spontaneously and is endergonic.

C When $\Delta G^{\circ\prime} = 0$, the reaction is at equilibrium and no useful energy is produced. The $\Delta G^{\circ\prime} > 0$ for this reaction.

E When $K_{eq} > 1$, then $\Delta G^{\circ\prime} < 0$, which means that reaction is spontaneous. The $\Delta G^{\circ\prime} > 0$ for this reaction.

47. B Cytochrome-a$_3$ and two copper centers (CuA and CuB) are in complex IV (cytochrome c oxidase).

A NADH + H$^+$ are substrates of complex I (NADH dehydrogenase).

C Complex III (cytochrome-c reductase) contains cytochromes-b and -c$_1$.

D FMN occurs in complex I (NADH dehydrogenase).

E Coenzyme Q is a lipid-soluble mobile molecule in the ETC.

48. D Poor nutrition and excess alcohol intake may lead to thiamine deficiency known as beriberi. Thiamine deficiency involving cardiovascular system is known as cardiac or wet beriberi. Both pyruvate dehydrogenase and α-ketoglutarate dehydrogenase decarboxylate their substrate concomitant with the reduction of NAD$^+$ to NADH + H$^+$ and the transfer of the remaining acid onto CoA. They both use thiamine (vitamin B$_1$), lipoamide and FAD as cofactors.

A Succinate dehydrogenase reduces FAD to FADH$_2$, not NAD$^+$ to NADH, like pyruvate dehydrogenase. In addition, the reaction mechanism and cofactor requirements of these two enzymes are quite different.

B Although both malate dehydrogenase and pyruvate dehydrogenase reduce NAD$^+$ to NADH, their reaction mechanism and cofactor requirements are quite different.

C Although both isocitrate dehydrogenase and pyruvate dehydrogenase reduce NAD$^+$ to NADH, their reaction mechanism and cofactor requirements are quite different.

E Aconitase catalyzes the molecular rearrangement of citrate to isocitrate via aconitate, not an oxidative decarboxylation like pyruvate dehydrogenase.

49. E By far, the most ATP is made by oxidative phosphorylation in which electron transport generates a pH gradient that in turn drives the F$_0$-$\prime$F^1 AT Pase. The protons pass through the F$_0$-F^1 complex down their concentration gradient into the matrix, and, in doing so, ATP synthase obtains the necessary power to form ATP from ADP and inorganic phosphate. Glycolysis and the TCA cycle contribute only two ATP and two guanosine triphosphates (GTPs), respectively, per glucose.

A Lactate is produced in anaerobic, not aerobic, glycolysis. The former also produces only two molecules of ATP per molecule of glucose. Most of the chemical energy contained in the glucose molecule is still in the two lactate molecules produced, which are therefore used for gluconeogenesis as soon as the oxygen supply improves.

B Conversion of one molecule of glucose into two molecules of pyruvate during aerobic glycolysis produces only two molecules of ATP.

C The pyruvate dehydrogenase reaction produces acetyl CoA and no high-energy phosphates. The thioester bond in acetyl CoA, however, has a high standard energy of hydrolysis.

D During the TCA cycle, each molecule of acetyl CoA produces only one molecule of GTP, that is, two per molecule of glucose.

50. C In the TCA cycle, acetyl CoA is broken down into two molecules of CO$_2$, and the hydrogens of acetyl CoA are transferred to NADH and FADH$_2$, respectively. Transfer of hydrogens is catalyzed by dehydrogenases, a subset of oxidoreductases.

A Although the removal of hydrogens from the substrates in these reactions is an oxidation, these hydrogens from acetyl CoA are transferred onto NAD$^+$ or FAD via reduction reactions. Oxidases transfer hydrogen or electrons onto oxygen, which none of the four enzymes of the TCA cycle in question do. Do not confuse oxidases with oxygenases, which introduce oxygen into an organic substrate.

B The term *reductase* is used unsystematically for enzymes that reduce a metabolite, where the source of reducing equivalents is ignored. The four TCA cycle reactions that produce reducing equivalents are catalyzed by enzymes that transfer hydrogen onto (or reduce) NAD^+ or FAD, as they remove these hydrogens from (i.e., oxidize) their respective substrates.

D Isomerases catalyze the intramolecular transfer of functional groups.

E Synthetases are enzymes that convert a substrate into a product using the hydrolysis of ATP as the energy source.

51. B Succinate thiokinase utilizes the energy of the thioester bond in succinyl CoA to synthesize GTP. GTP is the high energy compound that is used for synthesis of ATP by nucleoside diphosphate kinase. This process of ATP generation is known as substrate level phosphorylation.

A Succinate dehydrogenase does not catalyze the reaction in the TCA cycle that results in a high energy compound that is used for synthesis of ATP by substrate-level phosphorylation.

C Fumarase does not catalyze the reaction in the TCA cycle that results in a high energy compound that is used for synthesis of ATP by substrate-level phosphorylation.

D Malate dehydrogenase does not catalyze the reaction in the TCA cycle that results in a high energy compound that is used for synthesis of ATP by substrate-level phosphorylation.

E α-Ketoglutarate dehydrogenase decarboxylates α-ketoglutarate and uses the chemical energy of the C-C bond to form a thioester bond between the resulting succinate and CoA.

52. E ATP is made by ATP synthase (complex V, F_0–F^1 ATPase) which harnesses the energy of protons flowing down their concentration gradient into the matrix.

A B The success of oxidative phosphorylation depends on the respiratory chain's ability to transfer electrons from NADH and $FADH_2$ to O_2, but it is not the mechanism to explain ATP synthesis.

C Uncouplers also increase permeability of inner mitochondrial membrane to protons without generating any ATP.

D NADH in the cytoplasm cannot enter the mitochondria directly; its reducing equivalents have to be transported in by the malate shuttle. Inside the mitochondria, NADH is oxidized to NAD^+ and water, and the energy of that process generates a proton gradient, which drives ATP synthesis.

53. C FMN occurs in NADH dehydrogenase (complex I). Electron transfers are facilitated by tightly bound FMN nad Fe-S centers.

A NAD^+ is converted to NADH by PDH and three enzymes in the TCA cycle. The NADH is then oxidized back to NAD^+ by complex I of the ETC. NAD^+ and NADH are dissociable components of complex I.

B Nicotinamide adenine dinucleotide phosphate ($NADP^+$) is the product of biosynthetic (anabolic) reactions that use the reduced form of nicotinamide adenine dinucleotide phosphate (NADPH) as a donor of reducing equivalents. $NADP^+$/NADPH are not components of complex I.

D FAD is a component of complex II and accepts reducing equivalents from succinate (TCA cycle), glycerol-3-phosphate (NADH from glycolysis), and electron-transferring flavoprotein (ETF, β-oxidation). All these reducing equivalents are then transferred to coenzyme Q (CoQ) in the inner membrane.

E Cu centers occur in complexes IV of the ETC. Electron transfers are facilitated by Cu centers and cytochromes -a and -a_3.

54. C The bigger the difference in standard redox potential between an oxidizing and a reducing species, the higher the free energy of the redox reaction.

A Because of its very negative standard redox potential, NADH donates electrons to all other components of the electron transport chain. Electrons go from negative (lower) to positive (higher) redox potential.

B The P:O ratio is the measure of oxidative phosphorylation, which couples ATP synthesis to cellular respiration. The theoretical P:O ratio of NAD + linked substrate is 3.

D α-Ketoglutarate is part of the TCA cycle, not the electron transport chain. NAD^+ accepts electrons and hydrogens from α-ketoglutarate to become NADH. As one would expect, the standard redox potential for α-ketoglutarate is somewhat more negative (-380 mV) than that of NADH.

55. B In the electron transport chain, protons and electrons (in effect, but not mechanistically) from different sources are first collected on CoQ, then separated in complex III (cytochrome-c reductase). The protons are released into the intermembrane space. The electrons are transferred via cytochrome-c onto complex IV, where molecular oxygen, four electrons and four protons (from the mitochondrial matrix) form two molecules of water.

A The insecticide/acaricide/piscicide (used to kill insects, ticks and mites, and fish) rotenone binds to the CoQ site of complex I (NADH dehydrogenase).

C Most reactive (incompletely reduced) oxygen species are formed by flavoproteins (enzymes using $FAD/FADH_2$). Such enzymes are located in the peroxisome, where catalase destroys the resulting H_2O_2. One of the things evolution has achieved in the electron transport chain of the mitochondria is to minimize incomplete reduction of oxygen, even by the flavoproteins involved. Instead, electrons and protons are transferred to CoQ and from there to the complexes III (cytochrome-c reductase) and IV (cytochrome-c oxidase). The latter is remarkably effective in completely reducing molecular oxygen to water. Organisms without an efficient transport chain can only grow where oxygen is absent (e.g., *Clostridia* deep inside wounds).

D Complex IV (cytochrome-c oxidase) contains copper, heme-a, and heme-a_3 as centers. Zinc cannot serve in redox reactions, as all its compounds contain Zn^{2+}. Copper, however, can occur as Cu^+ and Cu^{2+}, and iron occurs as Fe^{2+} and Fe^{3+}. Both can participate effectively in electron transfer (redox) reactions.

E Heme-b occurs in complex III. There is no direct interaction between complexes III and IV.

56. E Uncouplers "short-circuit" the proton gradient across the inner mitochondrial membrane and thereby deprive the ATP synthase (complex V) of its energy source. Examples include dinitrophenol, pentachlorophenol, certain drugs such as aspirin or zidovudine (AZT), and metabolites such as bilirubin. Thermogenin (UCP1) is a protein that forms a proton channel in the mitochondria of brown adipose tissue. The high [ADP] and low [ATP] in the presence of uncouplers lead to increased glycolysis, TCA cycle and complex I to IV activity, and hence oxygen consumption.

A Because the TCA cycle produces the reducing equivalents used by the electron transport chain to produce ATP, ATP production cannot increase while TCA cycle ceases.

B Uncouplers do not inhibit the TCA cycle, but "short-circuit" the proton gradient formed by the electron transport chain and thus deprive the ATP synthase of its energy source. The TCA cycle, like glycolysis and electron transport chain, will actually be stimulated by the high [ADP]/[ATP] ratio.

C The activity of pathways like the TCA cycle and electron transport chain will even increase in the presence of an uncoupler.

D Inhibition of the ADP/ATP exchanger, and thus movement of ATP and ADP across mitochondrial membranes, is the mechanism of action of atractyloside, not of uncouplers.

57. D High ratios of NADH/NAD$^+$and acetyl CoA/CoA drive the reactions of both the E2 and E3 component of pyruvate dehydrogenase backward. As a result, the E1 subunit cannot transfer the hydroxyethyl intermediate onto E2, and the pyruvate dehydrogenase reaction ceases. The acetylated E2 will also stimulate pyruvate dehydrogenase kinase, which inactivates E1. Both NADH and acetyl CoA can be produced from fatty acid breakdown. Thus, fatty acids will be used for energy production in favor of sugars and amino acids.

A Citrate serves as a "high-energy" state signal in the cytosol, not the mitochondria.

B Isocitrate has no significant effect on pyruvate dehydrogenase activity.

C α-Ketoglutarate has no significant effect on pyruvate dehydrogenase activity.

E FAD acts as a prosthetic group in dehydrogenases and therefore cannot signal its redox status to other enzymes.

58. B Absence of the aspartate/glutamate antiporter disrupts the functioning of the malate-aspartate shuttle due to a reduction in the availability of aspartate.

A A deficiency in the aspartate/glutamate antiporter reduces the availability of cytosolic aspartate. As a result, there will be a decrease in its use for the cytosolic reaction that generates oxaloacetate and glutamate from α-ketoglutarate.

C A defect in the aspartate/glutamate antiporter would reduce (not increase) the transfer of reducing equivalents from NADH to complex I of the ETC.

D Reducing equivalents from FADH$_2$ are transferred to complex II (not complex I) of the ETC.

E Reduced cytosolic activity of aspartate would decrease the activity of urea cycle and lead to hyperammonemia.

59. D Glucokinase is expressed mainly in liver and pancreas. It has a lower affinity (higher K_m) for glucose than hexokinase. In the liver it serves to rapidly phosphorylate glucose for glycogenesis and lipogenesis, thereby removing glucose from the bloodstream after a meal. In pancreatic β-cells, glucokinase serves as a glucose sensor. In the family described, a V455M mutation resulted in a K_m some 60% lower than normal (increased affinity). Thus, glucokinase does not switch off when plasma glucose becomes low, and insulin secretion by pancreas and glucose storage by liver continue inappropriately. The result is hyperinsulinemic hypoglycemia. Because this is a gain-of-function mutation, inheritance is autosomal dominant. Note that apart from this activating mutation, there are also inactivating mutations of glucokinase, which result in maturity onset diabetes of the young (MODY).

A Hexokinase is a housekeeping enzyme that is expressed in most tissues and not controlled by hormones or glucose concentration. It simply provides glucose 6-phosphate for the catabolic needs of each individual cell.

B, C, E Genetic causes of persistent congenital hyperinsulinemia include activating mutations in the genes that encode subunits of the ATP-sensitive potassium channel, glutamate dehydrogenase-1, and glucokinase, not pyruvate kinase, enolase or lactate dehydrogenase.

60. D Aspirin toxicity involves respiratory stimulation, inhibition of the TCA cycle, uncoupling of oxidative phosphorylation, inhibition of aminotransferases, and increased breakdown of glycogen and fatty acids in the liver. This results in a brief respiratory alkalosis that within a few hours is followed by metabolic acidosis (lactate, pyruvate, ketones, amino acids). Treatment is by limiting absorption (activated charcoal and/or gastric lavage) and urine alkalization with bicarbonate, while maintaining electrolyte balance and preventing acute renal failure. Hemodialysis may be considered in severe cases.

A, B A hospital-acquired infection, whether bacterial or viral, needs time to develop and would be preceded by an asymptomatic period of several days.

C The features of Reye syndrome (which develop in children who have a viral illness and are given aspirin) are rash, persistent vomiting, encephalopathy, and enlarged, fatty liver; these were not present in this case. This case occurred before physicians became aware of the association of aspirin use and Reye syndrome in children. Today prescribing aspirin to pediatric patients with a possible viral illness would be considered a mistake.

E The features of anaphylaxis include a rapid drop of blood pressure, hives and flushing, angioedema, wheezing, and stridor. It usually develops quickly, not in a protracted manner, as in this patient.

61. A (B, C, D, E) There are two ways to answer this question: (1) 15 L of air (20% oxygen) are equivalent to 3 L pure oxygen; thus, the respiratory quotient (RQ = CO$_2$ eliminated/O$_2$consumed) is 1.0. This corresponds to carbohydrates. The empirical RQ for protein is 0.9, and for fatty acids it is 0.7. (2) After running for 10 min, the athlete will have used up his ATP/phosphocreatine stores and his capacity for anaerobic glycolysis. He will be using aerobic metabolism of glycogen. Only during prolonged exercise will glycogen stores become depleted and oxidation of fatty acids becomes the major energy source (e.g., after about 30 km [~18 miles] during a marathon).

62. C (A, B, D, E) Red blood cells (RBCs) lack mitochondria; hence, glycolysis serves as their only mechanism for producing ATP. Therefore a disruption in the glycolytic pathway may inactivate the ATP-dependent ion pumps, which are essential for the maintenance of intracellular-extracellular ion gradients and thus cell viability. The resultant effect is the destruction of RBCs, which manifests as hemolytic anemia.

63. E Fe-S clusters occur in complex I, II and III of the electron transport chain. Cytochrome-b occurs in complex III of the electron transport chain. Therefore, the pair can be found in complex III.

A, B, C, D Ubiquinone (Coenzyme Q) and cytochrome-c are mobile electron carriers not permanently associated with any of the ETC complexes. Cytochrome-a_3 is a component of complex IV, which contains several subunits. Subunit I binds heme-a and the heme-a_3/Cu_B binuclear center, which transfers electrons onto oxygen. This is the last reaction of the electron transport chain. Subunit II contains the Cu_A center that accepts electrons from cytochrome-c and passes them on to heme-a in subunit I. The remaining subunits of complex IV are not directly involved in the enzymatic reaction. Ubiquinone (coenzyme Q, CoQ) collects reducing equivalents from NADH dehydrogenase (complex I), succinate dehydrogenase (complex II), glycerol-3-phosphate dehydrogenase (cytosolic NADH), and electron-transferring flavoprotein (ETF, β-oxidation) and transfers them to complex III.

64. A The removal of electrons from an organic molecule is an oxidation reaction; addition is a reduction.

B In this reaction, succinyl CoA is hydrolyzed to succinate and CoA, and GDP (guanosine diphosphate) is phosphorylated to GTP (guanosine triphosphate).

C The total number of electrons "owned" by C atoms is not changed in this reaction, even though some are redistributed. There is no removal of hydrogen atoms (but, again, redistribution) and no introduction of electronegative elements. Hence, this is not a redox reaction.

D In this reaction, water is added to a double bond. This is a lyase reaction.

E The hydrolysis of ATP (adenosine triphosphate) to ADP (adenosine diphosphate) and P_i does not change the oxidation status of the reactants.

65. D In glycolysis, the six-carbon molecule glucose is broken down to 2 three-carbon molecules, pyruvate. The first carbon of pyruvate is lost in the pyruvate dehydrogenase reaction, forming acetyl CoA. This enters the TCA cycle, where both carbons are lost as CO_2. Thus, four out of six carbons from glucose are lost in the TCA cycle which generates NADH, $FADH_2$ and GTP.

A Glutamate can be made by transamination of the TCA cycle intermediate, α-ketoglutarate. Of the three carbon atoms in pyruvate, two are lost on the way to α-ketoglutarate, but the remaining carbon would become part of glutamate. This is not the primary function of TCA cycle in the body.

B Aspartate is converted into oxaloacetate by transamination; this enters the TCA cycle. Note that the enzyme responsible for this reaction, glutamate:oxaloacetate aminotransferase (GOT), also known as aspartate transaminase (AST), is clinically important to diagnose cell damage in the heart, skeletal muscle, and liver. This is not the primary function of TCA cycle in the body.

C Glutamate can be transaminated or deaminated to α-ketoglutarate, which is converted to malate by the TCA cycle. Malate is a precursor for gluconeogenesis. This is not the primary function of TCA cycle in the body.

E Mammalian cells cannot do net synthesis of glucose from even-chain fatty acids because both carbons of acetyl CoA are lost (as CO_2) in passing through the TCA cycle. The glycerol in fat can be converted to glucose, but this does not require the TCA cycle. However, fatty acids with odd number of carbons yield propionyl CoA at the end of β-oxidation, which can be converted to succinyl CoA and eventually to glucose.

66. C Oxaloacetate crosses from the mitochondria to the cytosol as malate for gluconeogenesis. The intermediates of the TCA cycle neither accumulate nor are used up during each turn of the cycle; two carbon atoms enter as acetyl CoA, and two come out as CO_2. Only when TCA cycle intermediates are used up for gluconeogenesis do they have to be replaced by anaplerotic (TCA cycle intermediate generating) reactions.

A Two carbon atoms enter the pathway as acetyl CoA.

B It is a common pathway for all the metabolic fuel for complete oxidation to CO_2 and H_2O.

D The high ratio of NADH /NAD+ reflects "high energy" in the body and slows the pathway.

E TCA is a mitochondrial pathway and erythrocytes lack mitochondria.

67. E Ubiquinone collects reducing equivalents from NADH dehydrogenase (complex I), succinate dehydrogenase (complex II), glycerol-3-phosphate dehydrogenase (cytosolic NADH), and ETF (β-oxidation) and transfers them to complex III.

A Cytochrome-c accepts electrons from complex III and delivers them to complex IV.

B Cytochrome-b, found in complex III, accepts electrons from ubiquinone and delivers them to cytochrome-c_1 of complex III.

C Cytochrome-c_1, found in complex III, accepts electrons from cytochrome-b and delivers them to an Fe-S center.

D Cytochrome-a_3 (complex IV or cytochrome-c oxidase) accepts electrons from cytochrome-c and passes them to O_2.

68. B Malonate inhibits complex II. It is a competitive inhibitor of succinate dehydrogenase.

A Malonate does not inhibit complex I. Rotenone and amytal are examples of poisons that inhibit complex I.

C Malonate does not inhibit complex III. Antimycin A inhibits complex III.

D Malonate does not inhibit complex IV. Cyanide binds very tightly to cytochrome-c oxidase and prevents the transfer of electrons to oxygen.

E Malonate does not inhibit complex V. Oligomycin, Aurovertin and dicyclohexylcarbodiimide (DCCD) are examples of poisons that inhibit complex V.

69. E Creatine phosphate does not leave the cell because it is charged. Only a breakdown product, creatinine, does so and is transported by blood to the kidneys, where it is excreted. Because creatinine is neither actively transported into the urine nor reabsorbed from it, we can use the concentrations of creatinine in plasma and urine, and the urine production rate, to calculate the volume of plasma filtered per unit time. This is useful to assess the function of Bowman's capsule (glomerular capsule).

A The phosphorylated form of creatine is a source of high-energy phosphate for ATP formation in muscle. The creatine phosphate in muscle acts as a high-energy phosphate donor to ADP during the first 10 to 20 seconds of muscle activity to help maintain ATP levels for continued contractions. This allows a "flight or fight" response without delay. Creatine phosphate requires creatine kinase for its synthesis and not creatinine.

B Neither creatine nor creatine phosphate participates in the urea cycle.

C Creatine phosphate does not leave the cell because it is charged. Only a breakdown product, creatinine, does so and is transported by blood to the kidneys, where it is excreted.

D Neither creatine nor creatine phosphate is a hormone.

70. B (A, C, D, E) Malonate resembles succinate structurally; the only difference is the number of methylene groups between the two carboxyl groups. Thus, the most likely mechanism of inhibition is competitive. In competitive inhibition, the V_{max} stays constant, as whatever the inhibitor's concentration is, it could be displaced from the binding site by substrate. However, more substrate is required to reach a given velocity; therefore, the apparent K_m (substrate concentration required for V_{max}) increases.

71. E Complex I accepts e$^-$ from NADH and donates them to coenzyme Q. Mutations in mitochondrial genes encoding subunits of complex I will prevent regeneration of NAD+ and therefore prevent NAD$^+$- requiring reactions in the mitochondrion.

A, C Mitochondria cannot synthesize ATP if respiration is inhibited. Mutations in mitochondrial genes encoding subunits of complex I inhibit ATP synthesis by interfering with respiration.

B The electron transport chain produces an H$^+$ gradient across the inner mitochondrial membrane that drives ATP synthesis. An uncoupler short-circuits that gradient, so that the energy contained is converted to heat rather than being used for ATP synthesis. The electron transport chain itself is not inhibited by uncouplers. Mutations in mitochondrial genes encoding subunits of Complex I inhibit ATP synthesis by interfering with respiration.

D Mutations in mitochondrial genes encoding subunits of complex I do not interfere with this ETC function. However, antimycin A binds to cytochrome-b in complex III of oxidative phosphorylation and prevents the binding and oxidation of CoQH$_2$(ubiquinol), thus disrupting electron transport.

72. C If there is not enough ADP to utilize the proton gradient, oxidation of NADH and the reduced form of flavin adenine dinucleotide (FADH$_2$) will cease. This also will inhibit the TCA cycle.

A Some oxidative phosphorylation can occur even if complex I (NADH dehydrogenase) is inhibited by rotenone or amytal.

B Although the ATP concentration influences the rate of glycolysis, it does not directly control the rate of oxidative phosphorylation.

D Although the citrate concentration influences the rate of glycolysis, it does not directly control the rate of oxidative phosphorylation.

E Although the pyruvate concentration influences the rate of glycolysis, it does not directly control the rate of oxidative phosphorylation.

73. B (D) In pyruvate carboxylase deficiency, cells lack the major source of compounds that replenish the TCA cycle (anaplerotic reaction), specifically, the generation of oxaloacetate from pyruvate. Mutation in the pyruvate carboxylase gene that alter the amount or activity of this enzyme lead to a condition called pyruvate carboxylase deficiency. A disruption in pyru-

vate carboxylase activity causes more pyruvate to be converted into lactate than oxaloacetate.

A Generation of acetyl CoA from pyruvate requires pyruvate dehydrogenase complex. Acetyl CoA (which loses both carbons during TCA cycle as CO$_2$) does not have anaplerotic activity.

C Generation of pyruvate from phosphoenolpyruvate requires pyruvate kinase is not an anaplerotic reaction.

E. Generation of phosphoenolpyruvate from phosphoglycerate requires enolase and is not anaplerotic reaction.

74. E 1,3-BPG is formed by glyceraldehyde-3-phosphate dehydrogenase: $(GAP + P_i + NAD^+ \leftrightarrows 1,3\text{-}BPG + NADH + H^+)$. In the presence of arsenate, 1-arseno-3-phosphoglycerate is formed and hydrolyzed—once released from the enzyme—to 3-phosphoglycerate. Therefore, one of the two ATP formed during the pay-off phase of glycolysis does not get made, making net ATP synthesis of glycolysis zero.

A Glucose-6-phosphate is formed using ATP, not inorganic phosphate. The reaction would not be affected by the presence of arsenate.

B Fructose-6-phosphate is formed from glucose-6-phosphate. The reaction would not be affected by the presence of arsenate.

C Fructose-1,6-bisphosphate is formed from Fru-6-P and ATP. The reaction would not be affected by the presence of arsenate.

D Glyceraldehyde-3-phosphate is formed by the breakdown of fructose-1,6-bisphosphate. The reaction would not be affected by the presence of arsenate

75. B The insecticide/acaricide/piscicide rotenone is an inhibitor of complex I (NADH dehydrogenase) of the electron transport chain, as it prevents the binding of CoQ to complex I. As a result, aerobic catabolism is no longer possible, and cells will switch to anaerobic metabolism, forming lactate. In addition, reactive oxygen species are formed, which are thought to be the actual cause of death. Rotenone poisoning is very rare, in part because this substance is poorly absorbed in the intestines and through skin (unlike gills and trachea). However, no effective treatment is known. Antioxidants and potassium channel openers are somewhat effective in cell culture studies, but no animal studies are available. There is also no established analytical routine for rotenone determination in patient's serum.

A Rotenone causes failure of aerobic metabolism; cells have to switch to anaerobic metabolism. This requires the conversion of pyruvate to lactate to maintain cytosolic NAD$^+$.

C, D, E Rotenone blocks complex I (NADH dehydrogenase) of the electron transport chain. Thus NADH is not recycled, and the TCA cycle fails for lack of NAD$^+$. Therefore, fumarate cannot be produced in significant amounts.

76. C (A, B, D, E) Diabetes types I and II are not single gene disorders. Negative hCG excludes pregnancy and therefore gestational diabetes. Family history makes mature onset diabetes of the young (MODY) the most likely diagnosis.

MODY is characterized by non ketotic diabetes mellitus due to pancreatic β cell dysfunction with onset in adolescence. MODY can result from mutations inherited in an autosomal dominant fashion in at least six separate genes expressed in β-cells. They include hepatocyte nuclear factor (HNF) 4α (MODY -1), glucokinase (MODY -2), HNF-1α (MODY-3), insulin promotor factor 1 (MODY-4), HNF-1β (MODY-5) and neurogenic differentiation factor 1 (MODY -6). About 35% of cases of MODY exhibit inactivating mutations in glucokinase which affect the ability of pancreas to secrete insulin appropriately.

77. C CO binds to hemoglobin with a 230-fold higher affinity than oxygen, forming carboxyhemoglobin. CO blocks the ability of hemoglobin to bind oxygen as well as to release any bound oxygen. Treatment is with oxygen; higher oxygen concentrations work faster: While at a partial pressure of 200 mbar (air), the half-life of CO is 320 min; it is 80 min at 1 bar (pure oxygen) and 23 min at 3 bar (hyperbaric chamber). However, even after successful treatment, about 10% of patients develop neurologic or psychiatric problems after an asymptomatic phase of about 1 month (delayed encephalopathy). This is reversible in most cases after about 1 year. CO poisoning is quite frequent; 15,600 cases occur every year in the United States, resulting in some 120 deaths.

A CO binds to and inhibits cytochrome-c oxidase (complex IV), not cytochrome-c.

B Enolase is the target of fluoride.

D Pyruvate dehydrogenase and other lipoic acid-containing enzymes are the target of arsenite (As^{III}).

E Glyceraldehyde-3-phosphate dehydrogenase is the target of arsenate (As^{V}).

78. E The breakdown of leucine starts with transamination followed by oxidative decarboxylation; the result is acetyl CoA and derivatives.

A The breakdown of alanine starts with transamination; the result is pyruvate, which the patient cannot metabolize to acetyl CoA, but can metabolize to lactate, leading to lactic acidosis.

B, C, D Glycine, serine and tryptophan are metabolized to pyruvate, which the patient cannot metabolize to acetyl Co A.

References

[1] Diez A, Gilsanz F, Martinez J, Pérez-Benavente S, Meza NW, Bautista JM. Life-threatening nonspherocytic hemolytic anemia in a patient with a null mutation in the PKLR gene and no compensatory PKM gene expression. Blood. 2005; 106(5):1851–1856

[2] Schröter, et al. Monatsschr Kinderheilkd. 1977; 125(7):713–9

[3] Ashourian N, Mousdicas N. N Engl J Med. 2006; 354:1614

[4] Watson AR, Coovadia HM, Bhoola KD. The clinical syndrome of Impila (Callilepis laureola) poisoning in children. S Afr Med J. 1979; 55(8):290–292

[5] Popat A, Shear NH, Malkiewicz I, et al. The toxicity of Callilepis laureola, a South African traditional herbal medicine. Clin Biochem. 2001; 34(3):229–236

[6] Stewart MJ, Steenkamp V. The biochemistry and toxicity of atractyloside: a review. Ther Drug Monit. 2000; 22(6):641–649

[7] Del Prato S, Penno G, Miccoli R. Changing the treatment paradigm for type 2 diabetes. Diabetes Care. 2009; 32 Suppl 2:S217–S222

[8] Miller RA, Birnbaum MJ. An energetic tale of AMPK-independent effects of metformin. J Clin Invest. 2010; 120(7):2267–2270

[9] Michelakis ED, Webster L, Mackey JR. Dichloroacetate (DCA) as a potential metabolic-targeting therapy for cancer. Br J Cancer. 2008; 99(7):989–994

[10] Shah AD, Wood DM, Dargan PI. Understanding lactic acidosis in paracetamol (acetaminophen) poisoning. Br J Clin Pharmacol. 2011; 71(1):20–28

[11] Wang GS, Monte A, Bagdure D, Heard K. Hepatic failure despite early acetylcysteine following large acetaminophen-diphenhydramine overdose. Pediatrics. 2011; 127(4):e1077–e1080

[12] Glaser B, Kesavan P, Heyman M, et al. Familial hyperinsulinism caused by an activating glucokinase mutation. N Engl J Med. 1998; 338(4):226–230

[13] Brown DC, Savage JM. Therapeutic aspirin overdose in a three-year-old boy. Ulster Med J. 1987; 56(1):63–65

[14] Wood DM, Alsahaf H, Streete P, Dargan PI, Jones AL. Fatality after deliberate ingestion of the pesticide rotenone: a case report. Crit Care. 2005; 9(3): R280–R284

[15] Yüksel EG, Taskin EO, Ovali GY. Türk Psikiyatri Dergisi. 2007; 18(1):80–8–6

Part IV

Metabolism

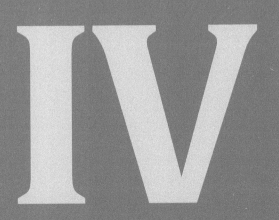

12 Carbohydrate Metabolism

12.1 Carbohydrates

Carbohydrates are a class of nutrients that serve as a major energy source for humans. They contain 4.1 kcal/g of energy, a value equivalent to that of proteins, but half of the energy contained in lipids. Carbohydrates have the general formula $C_n(H_2O)_n$ and are classified as monosaccharides, disaccharides, oligosaccharides, and polysaccharides based on the number of simple sugar units they contain (▶ Table 12.1).

12.1.1 Carbohydrate Digestion and Absorption

In the oral cavity and small intestine, polysaccharides and oligosaccharides are digested into disaccharides by α-amylases. Subsequent digestion of disaccharides by intestinal enzymes (e.g., maltase, lactase, sucrase) generates monosaccharides, which are rapidly absorbed by the small intestine. The movement of monosaccharides into and out of cells is facilitated by members of a family of glucose transporters (GLUTs), which have the following characteristics:

- Each GLUT functions in the cells of specific tissues (▶ Fig. 12.1) and binds to Glc, Gal, or Fru on one side of the plasma membrane, then undergoes a conformational change to transport and deposit them on the other side of the plasma membrane. In this manner, simple sugars are transported down their concentration gradient from an area of high concentration to one of low concentration.
  - Fanconi-Bickel syndrome is a disorder caused by a mutation in GLUT2 (See Therapeutics Box). This impairs the transport of Glc, Gal, and Fru in cells that express GLUT2.

- The sodium-glucose transporter 1 (SGLT1), however, cotransports two ions of Na^+ with each Glc or Gal into cells via secondary active transport. SGLT1 harnesses the energy supplied by the movement of Na^+ down its concentration gradient, to power the transport of Glc or Gal against their concentration gradient. SGLT1 is found on only the apical surfaces of both enterocytes (absorptive cells that line the walls of the small intestine) and epithelial cells of the S3 segment of kidney proximal tubules (▶ Fig. 12.2). In the S1 segment of proximal tubules, a similar cotransporter, SGLT2, functions in the reab-sorption of glucose from the glomerular filtrate.
  - Mutations in SGLT1 result in malabsorption of glucose and galactose, whereas mutations in SGLT2 lead to familial renal glycosuria.

Normal
GLUT2 in glucose sensing

Pancreatic β cells are one of the principal locations of GLUT2 transporters. GLUT2 allows for the bidirectional transport of glucose depending on the glucose concentration on either side of the plasma membrane. This process is made highly efficient due to its high capacity but low affinity for glucose. GLUT2 maintains intracellular levels of glucose equal to extracellular levels and as such is considered to be a "glucose sensor." If extracellular glucose levels rise, then so too do intracellular levels, stimulating pancreatic β cells to produce more insulin to maintain blood glucose homeostasis. A fall in extracellular glucose has the opposite effect. Glucose binds to a GLUT2 transporter located in the plasma membrane of pancreatic β cells and enters the cell by facilitated diffusion. Once inside, it is rapidly metabolized, generating adenosine triphosphate (ATP). This rise in ATP levels causes K^+ channels to close, resulting in depolarization of the β cell. Depolarization opens voltage-gated Ca^{2+} channels, and the subsequent Ca^{2+} influx stimulates the release of insulin from stores (rapid release). This influx of Ca^{2+} also activates calmodulin and Ca^{2+}/calmodulin-dependent protein kinase (CamK). This activation increases insulin synthesis (and allows a slow second phase of insulin release).

Table 12.1 Classification of carbohydrates

Class	Examples	Composition and relevant information
Monosaccharides (1 sugar unit)	Glucose (Glc)	$C_6H_{12}O_6$; most abundant simple sugar
	Galactose (Gal)	$C_6H_{12}O_6$; obtained from mammalian milk
	Fructose (Fru)	$C_6H_{12}O_6$; obtained from fruit and honey
	Ribose/deoxyribose	$C_5H_{10}O_5$/$C_5H_{10}O_4$; components of ribonucleic/deoxyribonucleic acids
Disaccharides (2 sugar units)	Maltose	Glc + Glc; found in malt sugars and hydrolyzed by maltase
	Lactose	Glc + Gal; found in mammalian milk and hydrolyzed by lactase
	Sucrose	Glc + Fru; found in table sugar, fruits, and honey and hydrolyzed by sucrase
Oligosaccharides (3–10 sugar units)	Polymers composed of a mixture of sugar units	Found attached to lipids (glycolipids) and proteins (glycoproteins)
Polysaccharides (>10 sugar units)	Cellulose	Polymer of Glc units: found in plants but indigestible by humans
	Starch	Polymer of Glc units: the stored form of glucose in plants
	Glycogen	Polymer of Glc units; the stored form of glucose in animals
	Glycosaminoglycans	Polymers of disaccharides; components of proteoglycans

IV

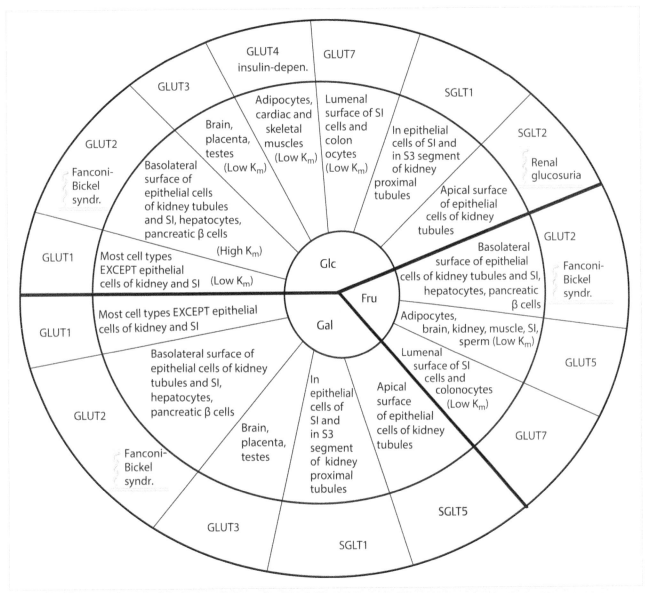

Fig. 12.1 Features of glucose transporters. Members of the family of glucose transporters (GLUTs) function in the cells of specific tissues to transport glucose (Glc), galactose (Gal), or fructose (Fru) across cellular membranes. ER, endoplasmic reticulum; SGLT, sodium-glucose transporter; SI, small intestine.

Therapeutics

Fanconi-Bickel syndrome

This rare autosomal recessive condition is caused by a mutation in the GLUT2 transporter located in hepatocytes, pancreatic β cells, enterocytes, and renal tubular cells. This leads to impaired transport of glucose, galactose, and fructose in these cells. Signs and symptoms of this syndrome include failure to thrive, hepatomegaly (secondary to glycogen accumulation), severe tubular nephropathy, abdominal bloating, and resistant rickets (phosphate is "lost" into urine due to tubular nephropathy). The patient will show fasting ketotic hypoglycemia and postprandial hyperglycemia due to the low hepatic uptake of glucose. Treatment involves restricrtion of galactose intake, supplementation with electrolytes, vitamin D and phosphate and ingestion of uncooked corn starch, which provides a sustained (~ 7 hours) release of glucose.

12.1.2 Carbohydrate Metabolism

The metabolism of carbohydrates involves their breakdown (catabolism) and synthesis (anabolism) via various mechanisms that serve either to generate energy, to store energy, or to produce compounds essential for the synthesis of other biomolecules. Some of these mechanisms include the following:

- **Cellular respiration:** In cellular respiration, the energy contained within the bonds of carbohydrate molecules is harnessed via the breakdown of glucose by glycolysis alone, or in combination with the tricarboxylic acid (TCA) cycle and oxidative phosphorylation (see Part III).
- **Gluconeogenesis:** In gluconeogenesis, glucose is synthesized *de novo* from carbon compounds derived from carbohydrate and noncarbohydrate sources.
- **Glycogen metabolism (glycogenesis and glycogenolysis):** Glygogenesis is the pathway by which glycogen is

IV

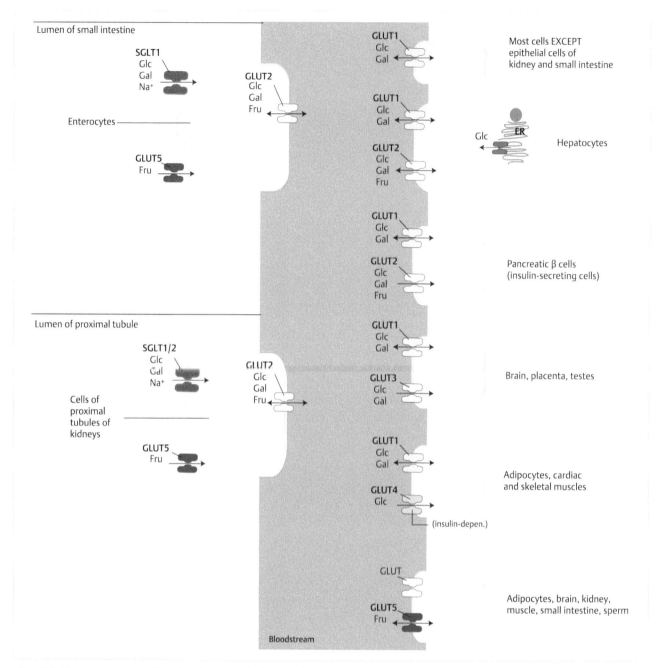

Fig. 12.2 Glucose transporters in action. Tissue-specific location of glucose transporters (GLUTs) and the monosaccharides they transport. ER, endoplasmic reticulum; Fru, fructose; Gal, galactose; Glc, glucose; SGLT, sodium-glucose transporter.

synthesized to store excess amounts of glucose in the liver or muscle. On the other hand, glycogenolysis is the pathway by which glycogen is degraded one glucose unit at a time

- **Fructose and galactose metabolism:** The breakdown of these two monosaccharides generates intermediates that— depending on the needs of the cell—can be utilized for glycolysis or gluconeogenesis. Moreover, galactose provides intermediates for the synthesis of lactose and glycogen and compounds for attachment to proteins and lipids.

- **Pentose phosphate pathway:** This pathway metabolizes the phosphorylated form of glucose (glucose 6-phosphate) to generate the reduced form of nicotinamide adenine dinucleotide phosphate (NADPH) and riboses.

Normal

Uncooked corn starch

Many patients with type 1 diabetes require multiple insulin injections to manage their blood sugar levels. In such patients, nocturnal or early morning hypoglycemia is a recurring problem. On the other hand, carbohydrate-rich bedtime snacks tend to cause hyperglycemia in such individuals. One possible solution is to provide a bedtime snack containing 5 g of uncooked starch. Uncooked starch is very slowly digested and provides a low blood glucose peak in ~ 4 hours, which is sustained for ~ 7 hours. Uncooked starch is known to prevent nocturnal and early morning hypoglycemic incidents in both type 1 and type 2 diabetic patients, as well as in patients with glycogen storage diseases.

Foundations

Energy-independent and -dependent transport mechanisms

These transport mechanisms have been discussed in more detail in Chapter 6.

Energy-independent transport of solutes across biological membranes occurs down the concentration gradient either by simple (passive) or facilitated diffusion. In the latter case, a protein transporter facilitates either a unidirectional or a bidirectional transport. Many lipophilic molecules are transported by simple diffusion. Several nutrients, including glucose and amino acids, are transported by facilitated diffusion. Transport of solutes against a concentration gradient requires energy and is classified as either active or secondary active transport. In active transport, the chemical energy (usually that of ATP) is expended. An example of active transport is the Na^+-K^+ ATPase (see **Fig. 6.5**). In secondary active transport, one solute (an ion) is transported down its concentration gradient, and the resultant electrochemical gradient across the membrane is used to transport a second solute in either the same (symport) or opposite (antiport) direction against its concentration gradient. An example of symport is the cotransport of glucose (or galactose) and Na^+ by SGLT1 and that of antiport is the Na^+-Ca^{2+} exchanger.

Normal

Enterocytes

Enterocytes are simple columnar epithelial cells found in the small intestine and colon. Their apical surface is coated with a glycocalyx that contains digestive enzymes and microvilli, which dramatically increases their surface area. Enterocytes in the duodenum absorb iron, zinc, magnesium, calcium, most B vitamins, fats, and fat-soluble vitamins (A, D, E, and K); enterocytes in the jejunum absorb water-soluble vitamins, sugars, and amino acids; and enterocytes in the ileum absorb vitamin B_{12}, cholesterol, and bile salts. Enterocytes also secrete immunoglobulins into the lumen. Ions (and water by osmosis) are absorbed throughout the small intestine. Approximately 20% of water absorption occurs in the colon. Infection of enterocytes (often viral) leads to cell death and villous atrophy when cell loss exceeds cell production. As a result, digestion and absorption are impaired, and a net secretory state may occur. Infection also causes "leakiness" of the epithelium and dysfunction of certain enzymes. These changes may combine to cause a transient malabsorptive diarrhea until enterocyte replacement occurs.

Therapeutics

Familial renal glycosuria

In adults with normal blood glucose, of the approximately 180 g of glucose filtered each day through the kidneys, < 500 mg is actually excreted, and the rest is efficiently reabsorbed by the epithelial cells in kidney proximal tubules. The reabsorption is through secondary active transport mediated by the Na^+-glucose cotransporters, SGLT1 (10%) in the S3 segment and SGLT2 (90%) in the S1 segment. The SGLT transporters are encoded by SLC5 (solute carrier, family 5) genes. Normal glomerular filtration rate (GFR) of glucose is ~ 2.5 mg/mL/min/1.73 m^2. Therefore, when blood glucose levels are > 180 mg/dL, the reabsorption capacity of kidneys is exceeded, and glucose is detected in urine. Generalized dysfunction of proximal tubules (Fanconi-de Toni-Debré syndrome) can cause glycosuria along with excessive excretion of amino acids, phosphate, and bicarbonate. Glycosuria with normal blood glucose levels and in the absence of tubule disorders is characterized as familial renal glycosuria (FRG) and is associated with genetic defects in SLC5A2, which encodes SGLT2. FRG is considered a benign condition with urinary glucose excretion of < 10 g/1.73 m^2/d in heterozygotes. Homozygotes and compound heterozygotes have excretion rates > 10 g/ 1.73 m^2/d. It appears that expression of the SLC5A2 gene may be regulated by plasma glucose levels through the transcription factor, hepatic nuclear factor 1α (HNF1α). In type 2 diabetes, the expression of SLC5A2 is elevated. Administration of SGLT2 inhibitors (e.g., dapagliflozin) in such patients has been reported to raise the urinary glucose excretion to 70 g/d and normalize blood glucose with minimal salt wasting.

Therapeutics

Diabetes mellitus

Diabetes mellitus is a condition that causes hyperglycemia due to either decreased insulin secretion (type 1) or decreased insulin sensitivity of target tissues (type 2). Increased plasma glucose leads to increased glucose levels in tissue fluid and promotes the risk of infection. Elevated glucose levels also cause glycosuria, leading to polyuria and polydipsia. The main risk in uncontrolled diabetes is poor circulation to extremities which may necessitate amputations. Other complications include heart disease, stroke, blindness, kidney dysfunction, nervous system disorders, sexual dysfunction, and pregnancy complications. Individuals with type 1 diabetes are genetically predisposed and are sensitive to environmental damage of pancreatic β cells. Type 2 diabetes is a polygenic disorder and is strongly associated with obesity, hypertriglyceridemia, and insulin resistance.

The diagnosis of type 1 diabetes is made by conducting various blood tests:

1. Glycated hemoglobin (A_{1C}) test. Glycation refers to the nonenzymatic, covalent attachment of glucose to N-terminal amino acids of proteins. The A_{1C} test measures the percentage of hemoglobin with glucose covalently attached to N-terminal valine. This number is an indication of average blood sugar

levels over the previous 2 to 3 months. An $A_{1C} > 6.5\%$ is diagnostic of diabetes.

2. Random blood sugar level. A random blood test is taken and blood sugar measured. A value > 200 mg/dL (11.1 mmol/L) is suggestive of diabetes, especially if the patient has associated symptoms.

3. Fasting blood sugar test. The patient fasts overnight, and a blood sample is taken in the morning. A value > 126 mg/dL (> 7 mmol/L) on two separate occasions allows for a diagnosis of diabetes.

4. Estimated average glucose (eAG). The American Diabetes Association now recommends the use of aAG calculated from the A_{1C} values in the management of diabetes. eAG has the same units as the blood glucose level and corresponds to the A_{1C} levels as shown below.

HbA$_{1C}$ %	eAG (mg/dL)
6	126
7	154
8	183
9	212
10	240
11	269
12	298

5 Oral glucose tolerance test

Therapeutics
Glucose tolerance test
The glucose tolerance test is used to test for type 2 diabetes. It involves giving the patient a known oral dose of glucose, followed by an 8- to 12-hour fasting period. Measurements of plasma glucose levels are obtained before glucose administration and at intervals after, to determine how quickly plasma glucose levels fall and homeostasis is regained. Normal fasting plasma glucose levels are < 6.1 mmol/L. Glucose levels of 6.1 to 7.0 mmol/L are considered borderline and are indicative of impaired fasting glycemia. Measurements of plasma glucose taken after 2 hours should be < 7.8 mmol/L. Glucose levels of 7.8 to 11.0 mmol/L indicate impaired glucose tolerance; levels ≥ 11.1 mmol/L allow the diagnosis of diabetes.

Therapeutics
Metabolic syndrome
Metabolic syndrome is a combination of several disorders. Metabolic syndrome is diagnosed as the presence of any three of the following five parameters: (a) blood level of triglycerides > 150 mg/dL, (b) fasting glucose > 100 mg/dL, (c) plasma HDL cholesterol < 40 mg/dL (d) blood pressure > 130/85 mm Hg and (e) waist size > 40 in. in males and 35 in. in females. Patients with this syndrome are usually insulin resistant and at a higher risk for developing type 2 diabetes and coronary heart disease.

12.2 Gluconeogenesis: *De novo* Synthesis of Glucose

12.2.1 Overview

When blood glucose levels are low and glycogen stores have been depleted—usually due to fasting, starvation, intense exercise, or consumption of a low carbohydrate diet—the body relies heavily on gluconeogenesis to synthesize glucose *de novo* from pyruvate and other noncarbohydrate (and carbohydrate) carbon molecules. Key features of gluconeogenesis include the following:

- Gluconeogenesis takes place primarily in the liver (90%) and to a lesser degree in the kidneys and small intestine. Once new glucose has been synthesized in the liver, it is transported to the blood so that cells that are critically dependent on glycolysis for energy can continue to function. These include erythrocytes and cells of the brain, kidney, and exercising muscles.
- A comparison of gluconeogenesis and glycolysis (which breaks down glucose to pyruvate) shows that they have several enzymes and intermediates in common.
  - Gluconeogenesis involves the reversal of many of the reactions catalyzed by glycolytic enzymes, except for hexokinase/glucokinase, phosphofructokinase-1, and pyruvate kinase. These enzymes catalyze the three irreversible reactions of glycolysis and cannot be reversed due to the large energy barriers inhibiting their reversal (▶ Fig. 12.3a).
  - The key gluconeogenesis enzymes that allow cells to bypass these barriers are pyruvate carboxylase, phosphoenolpyruvate (PEP) carboxykinase, fructose 1,6-bisphosphatase, and glucose 6-phosphatase (▶ Fig. 12.3b).
  - Gluconeogenesis takes place in both the cytosol and the mitochondria, whereas glycolysis occurs in the cytosol only.
  - Importantly, gluconeogenesis and glycolysis are reciprocally regulated such that agents that activate one pathway inhibit the other (▶ Fig. 12.3c).
- In gluconeogenesis, six high-energy phosphate bonds (four ATP and two guanosine triphosphate [GTP]) are hydrolyzed to generate one molecule of glucose from two molecules of pyruvate.

12.2.2 Mechanism and Regulation of Gluconeogenesis (▶ Fig. 12.4)

Pyruvate Carboxylase

In the first step of gluconeogenesis, mitochondrial pyruvate is carboxylated to form oxaloacetate. This CO_2- and ATP-dependent reaction is catalyzed by pyruvate carboxylase—an enzyme that requires the cofactor biotin for its activity (▶ Fig. 12.5).

Modulators of pyruvate carboxylase's activity, as well as the disorders in which its activity is altered, are as follows:
- Pyruvate carboxylase is activated allosterically by acetyl coenzyme A (CoA)—the end product of fatty acid oxidation—whose levels increase during periods of fasting.
- Pyruvate carboxylase activity is increased by cortisol (a glucocorticoid hormone) via transcriptional induction.

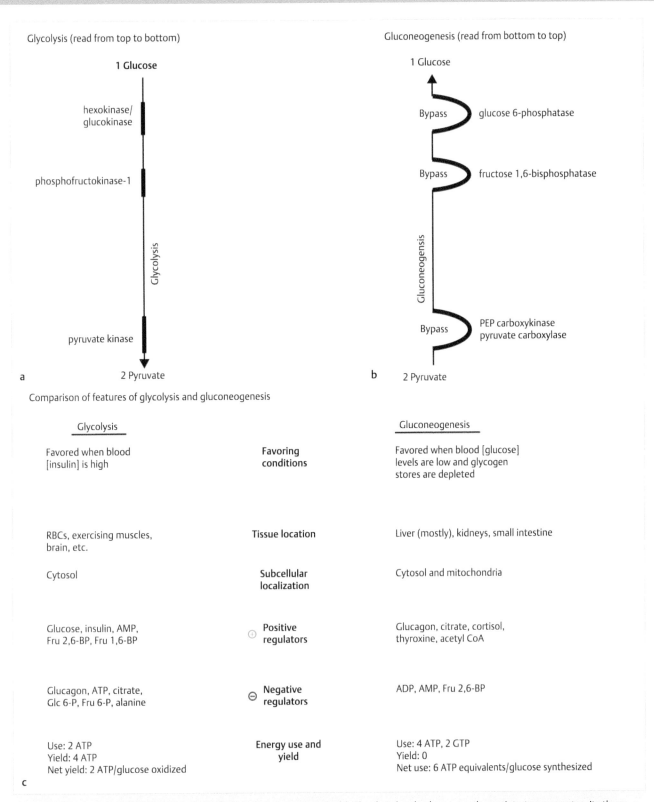

IV

Fig. 12.3 Comparison of key features of glycolysis and gluconeogenesis. (a) Glycolysis breaks down one glucose into two pyruvates. Its three irreversible reactions are catalyzed by hexokinase/glucokinase, phosphofructokinase-1, and pyruvate kinase. (b) Gluconeogenesis synthesizes one glucose from two pyruvates. The four enzymes— pyruvate carboxylase, phosphoenolpyruvate (PEP) carboxykinase, fructose 1,6-bisphosphatase (Fru 1,6-BP), and glucose 6-phospha-tase (Glc 6-P)—bypass the need for reversing the action of the three irreversible glycolytic enzymes. (C) Comparison of key features of glycolysis and gluconeogenesis. ADP, adenosine diphosphate; AMP, adenosine monophosphate; ATP, adenosine triphosphate; CoA, co-enzyme A; Fru 2,6-BP, fructose 2,6-bisphosphate; Fru 6-P, fructose 6-phosphate; GTP, guanosine triphosphate; RBCs, red blood cells.

187

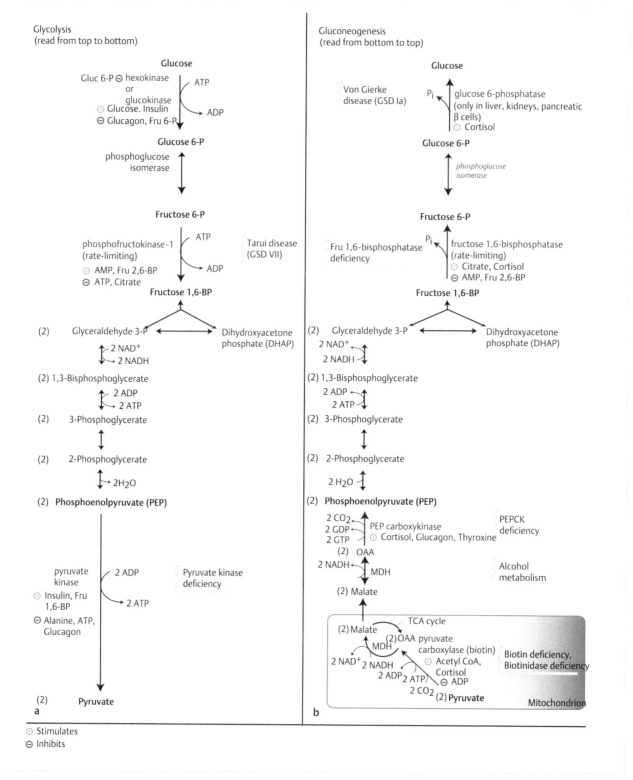

Fig. 12.4 Glycolysis versus gluconeogenesis. (**a**) Key reactions of glycolysis, points of regulation and associated disorders. (**b**) The reactions of gluconeogenesis, points of regulation, and associated disorders. Lines with a single arrowhead indicate irreversible reactions. Those with arrowheads on both ends indicate reversible reactions. ADP, adenosine diphosphate; AMP, adenosine monophosphate; ATP, adenosine triphosphate; BP, bisphosphate; CoA, coenzyme A; Fru, fructose; GDP, guanosine diphosphate; GSD, glycogen storage disease; MDH, malate dehydrogenase; NAD⁺, nicotinamide adenine dinucleotide; NADH, reduced form of nicotinamide adenine dinucleotide; OAA, oxaloacetate; P, phosphate; PEPCK, phosphoenolpyruvate carboxykinase; TCA, tricarboxylic acid.

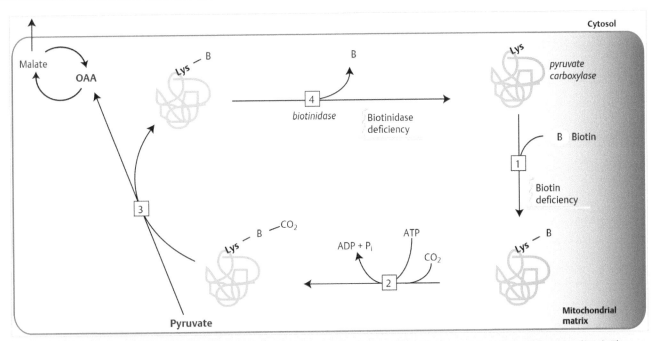

Fig. 12.5 Mechanism of action of pyruvate carboxylase. Pyruvate carboxylase (PC) transfers CO_2 to pyruvate to form oxaloacetate (OAA). The activity of PC requires the formation of a PC-biotin-CO_2 complex in the following manner: (1) Biotin is covalently linked to a lysine (Lys) residue on PC. (2) The hydrolysis of ATP drives the attachment of CO_2 to biotin in order to form the PC-biotin-CO_2 complex. (3) The latter then transfers CO_2 to pyruvate to generate OAA. (4) Biotinidase cleaves biotin from the lysine residue of PC, allowing it to be reused by another carboxylase. The activity of PC is reduced in individuals suffering from biotin deficiency or biotinidase deficiency.

Cortisol is a major stress-induced steroid hormone produced by the adrenal glands. Its levels are lower than normal in individuals with Addison disease (chronic adrenal insufficiency) and higher in those with Cushing syndrome.

○ Biotin deficiency is a disorder associated with a nutritional deficiency in biotin. It may be caused by large amounts of avidin (a protein found in raw egg whites), which binds to biotin and makes it unavailable for attachment to carboxylases.

○ Biotinidase deficiency is an autosomal recessive disorder marked by a deficiency in biotin. It is caused by a mutation in biotinidase. When biotinidase is defective, free biotin cannot be obtained from dietary biotin-bound proteins or recycled among the biotin-dependent carboxylases.

Mitochondrial and Cytosolic Malate Dehydrogenases

Because oxaloacetate cannot cross the inner mitochondrial membrane directly to enter the cytosol, an indirect method facilitated by the mitochondrial and cytosolic forms of malate dehydrogenase is used. The mitochondrial form is responsible for reducing oxaloacetate to malate which can be transported to the cytosol using the malate transporter. The cytosolic form of malate dehydrogenase then reoxidizes malate back into oxaloacetate. In doing so, NADH is oxidized to NAD^+ in the mitochondria, and NAD^+ is reduced to NADH in the cytosol. This NADH is utilized to generate glyceraldehyde 3-phosphate in the gluconeogenic pathway.

• If the levels of cytosolic NADH are greatly increased (as seen when alcohol metabolism is elevated), the equilibrium of the reaction catalyzed by the cytosolic malate dehydrogenase is switched to favor reduction of oxaloacetate to malate, which results in a decrease in gluconeogenesis.

Phosphoenolpyruvate Carboxykinase

The enzyme phosphoenolpyruvate carboxykinase (PEPCK) is present as cytosolic and mitochondrial isoforms that are equally expressed in humans.

1. The cytosolic form of the enzyme, PEPCK1, catalyzes the concurrent decarboxylation and phosphorylation of cytosolic oxaloacetate into PEP, utilizing both the energy and the phosphate group obtained from the hydrolysis of GTP to guanosine diphosphate.

• The transcription of PEP carboxykinase is induced by the hormones cortisol, glucagon, and thyroxine (see **Fig. 18.5**).

• The substrate of PEPCK1, oxaloacetate, is made exclusively in the mitochondrial matrix and cannot directly cross the inner mitochondrial membrane. Thus, it has to be converted into either aspartate (by an aminotransferase) or malate (by malate dehydrogenase) to be transported into cytoplasm, where it can be regenerated.

○ Transgenic mice overexpressing PEPCK1 in skeletal muscle are leaner and exhibit greater endurance and life span compared with control animals.

• The mitochondrial form of PEP carboxykinase (PEPCK2) converts oxaloacetate into PEP under conditions in which lactate is the predominant precursor for gluconeogenesis. Since the conversion of lactate to pyruvate yields NADH, cytosolic malate dehydrogenase reaction becomes unnecessary. So, oxaloacetate derived either from pyruvate or from TCA cycle is converted into PEP by the mitochondrial PEPCK2. PEP is then transported to the cytoplasm for the continuation of gluconeogenesis.

- PEPCK deficiency is a rare, early-onset autosomal recessive disorder caused by mutations in PEPCK1/2 that result in defective gluconeogenesis and hypoglycemia, failure to thrive, loss of muscle tone, and liver enlargement.

Fructose 1,6-Bisphophatase (Rate-Limiting)

Once fructose 1,6-bisphosphate has been synthesized from PEP (via a reversal of glycolytic reactions), fructose 1,6-bisphosphatase — the rate-limiting enzyme of gluconeogenesis—dephosphorylates fructose 1,6-bisphosphate into fructose 6-phosphate. Its activity is stimulated by cortisol and citrate but inhibited by adenosine monophosphate (AMP) and fructose 2,6-bisphosphate (see **Fig. 9.3**).

- The aforementioned molecules have the opposite effect on phosphofructokinase-1, the rate-limiting enzyme of glycolysis that catalyzes the reverse of fructose 1,6-bisphosphatase's reaction.
  - Fructose 1,6-bisphosphatase deficiency is a rare autosomal recessive disorder that develops in individuals with mutations that make this rate-limiting enzyme defective. In comparison, Tarui disease is an autosomal recessive disorder caused by mutations in the glycolytic enzyme phospho-fructokinase-1.

Glucose 6-Phosphatase

After fructose 6-phosphate is isomerized to glucose 6-phosphate, the latter is dephosphorylated by glucose 6-phosphatase to generate glucose. Glucose 6-phosphatase, whose activity is increased by cortisol, is not found in brain, adipose, or muscle tissue; therefore, gluconeogenesis cannot take place in these tissues. On the other hand, glucose 6-phosphatase *is* found in the liver, kidneys and small intestine The glucose 6-phosphatase complex is associated with the endoplasmic reticulum membrane with the active site of the enzyme facing the lumen. The enzyme complex involves a catalytic unit (G6PC) a glucose 6-phosphate transporter (G6PT/SLC37A4) and a glucose transporter which is not yet characterized. Studies with the recombinant protein reconstituted in liposomes have suggested that G6PT may function as an antiporter, exchanging glucose 6-phosphate for inorganic phosphate. Von Gierke disease (GSD type I) is an autosomal recessive disorder attributed to mutations that render glucose 6-phosphatase activity defective. Mutations in GRPC cause glycogen storage disease Ia (GSD Ia), whereas those in G6PT cause GSD Ib.

12.2.3 Cori Cycle and Precursor Molecules for Gluconeogenesis

Cori Cycle

The Cori cycle is a mechanism that links glycolysis in red blood cells and exercising muscles to gluconeogenesis in the liver (▶ Fig. 12.6). The lactate produced by anaerobic glycolysis in erythrocytes and exercising muscles is transported to the bloodstream and picked up by the liver to generate glucose via gluconeogenesis. The newly synthesized glucose is then sent back to the bloodstream and taken up by erythrocytes and exercising muscles. Although one turn of the Cori cycle is accompanied by a net loss of four ATP equivalents, it provides two key benefits:

1. It prevents the accumulation of lactate in erythrocytes and exercising muscles.
2. It regenerates glucose so that glycolysis can continue in the aforementioned cells/tissue.
3. It regenerates NADH (via lactate dehydrogenase) needed for gluconeogenesis.

Precursors

▶ Table 12.2 and ▶ Fig. 12.7 list the carbohydrate and noncarbohydrate sources of carbon molecules that can be used to synthesize glucose *de novo* via gluconeogenesis. The degradation of all three major energy nutrients (carbohydrates, lipids, proteins) provides precursor molecules for gluconeogenesis, but the following caveat must be considered:

- The fatty acid components of triacylglycerols are degraded into acetyl CoA, which cannot enter gluconeogenesis. However, the degradation of odd-numbered fatty acids generates propionate, which is converted to the TCA cycle

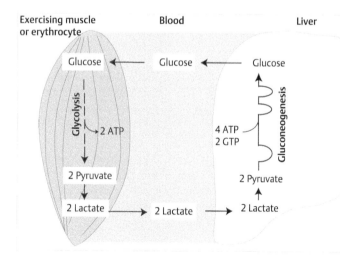

Fig. 12.6 **Cori cycle.** The Cori cycle links glycolysis in tissues that carry out anaerobic glycolysis, to gluconeogenesis in the liver. Its purpose is to prevent the accumulation of lactate in the cells that produce it and to regenerate the fuel (glucose) that these cells need in order to continue generating adenosine triphosphate (ATP) via glycolysis. The mechanism is as follows: lactate produced by exercising muscles (or red blood cells) is first expelled into the bloodstream and then taken up by the liver, where it is converted into glucose via gluconeogenesis. This newly formed glucose is then sent to the bloodstream, where it is retaken up by exercising muscles (or red blood cells) and used to generate more ATP via anaerobic glycolysis. GTP, guanosine triphosphate.

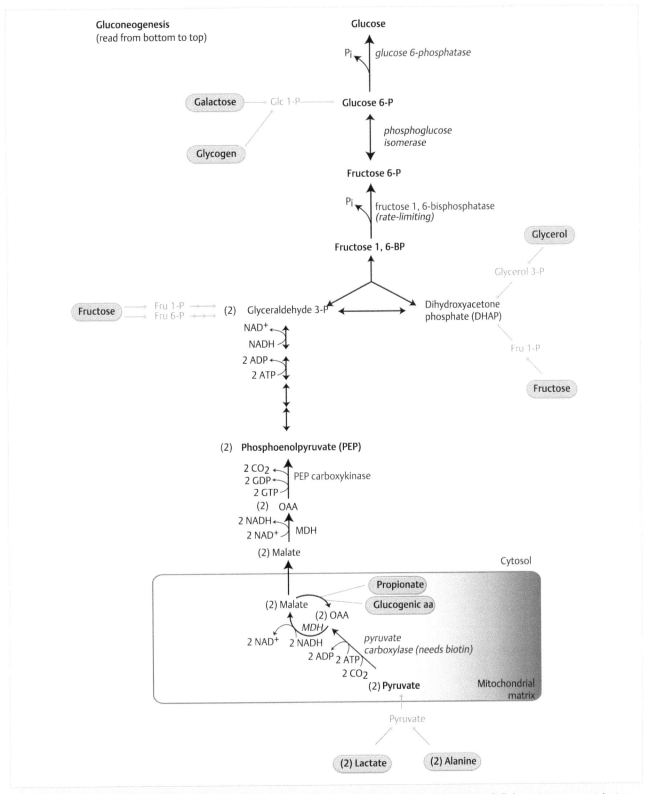

Fig. 12.7 Precursor molecules for gluconeogenesis. Gluconeogenesis can synthesize glucose from derivatives of all the major energy nutrients (carbohydrates, lipids, proteins). Hepatic gluconeogenesis uses lactate (reduced pyruvate), monosaccharides (fructose and galactose), glucogenic amino acids, and fat derivatives (glycerol, propionate). Of the 20 proteinogenic amino acids, all but two (leucine and lysine) are glucogenic (see **Fig. 15.6a**). aa, amino acids; ADP, adenosine diphosphate; ATP adenosine triphosphate; Fru, fructose; GDP, guanosine diphosphate; Glc, glucose; GTP, guanosine triphosphate; MDH, malate dehydrogenase; NAD⁺, nicotinamide adenine dinucleotide; NADH, reduced form of nicotinamide adenine dinucleotide; OAA, oxaloacetate; P, phosphate.

Table 12.2 Precursor molecules for gluconeogenesis

Precursor	Source	Point of entry of precursor
Fructose	Carbohydrate (sucrose) degradation	Glyceraldehyde 3-P (via a phosphorylated fructose intermediate)
Galactose	Carbohydrate (lactose) degradation	Glucose 6-P (via a phosphorylated glucose intermediate)
Glycogen	Carbohydrate degradation	Glucose 6-P (via glucose 1-P)
Glycerol	Lipid degradation	DHAP (via a phosphorylated glycerol intermediate)
Propionate	Degradation of odd-numbered fatty acids	TCA cycle intermediate (succinyl CoA), which is converted to malate
Lactate	Anaerobic glycolysis	Pyruvate (via oxidation of lactate)
Alanine	Protein degradation, pyruvate (via transamination)	Pyruvate (via deamination of alanine)
Amino acids (except leucine and lysine)	Protein degradation	TCA cycle intermediates, which are converted to malate

Abbreviations: DHAP, dihydroxyacetone phosphate; TCA, tricarboxylic acid cycle.

intermediate succinyl CoA and enters gluconeogenesis via its conversion to malate.

Normal
Fasting versus starving

Fasting is voluntarily not eating for varying lengths of time. The body adapts to this by depleting energy stores: glycogen stores in the liver in the first 16–18 hours, followed by lipolysis. In contrast, starvation occurs when body energy stores are essentially depleted, and the body resorts to utilizing essential tissues for energy. The result is a reduction in organ volume with gradual loss of function, loss of muscle mass, weakness, anemia, diarrhea, reduction in mental capacity, immune deficiency, and ultimately death.

Normal
Role of cortisol in fasting states

Cortisol is essential for survival during fasting states because of its proteolytic effects. During fasting, liver glycogen stores are used for glucose release to the blood but quickly become depleted. Gluconeogenesis is initiated using amino acids (from protein catabolism) in the presence of cortisol. However, if cortisol is deficient, death from hypoglycemia occurs. Plasma levels of cortisol during fasting are only slightly to moderately elevated (usually relative to the degree of initial hypoglycemia), but this elevation of cortisol is sufficient because cortisol has a permissive effect on key metabolic enzymes. Permissive effect may be seen as analogous to "priming." Corticosteroids prime metabolic pathways to respond to other hormones. For example, the effects of epinephrine on glycogen degradation and synthesis are greatly facilitated (potentiated) by cortisol. During fasting, the body also breaks down stored fat in adipose tissue into glycerol and fatty acids. Glycerol can then be converted to glucose in the liver. Cortisol enhances this lipolysis.

Therapeutics
Addison versus Cushing disease

Addison disease is the result of steroid hormone deficiency (i.e., a deficiency of cortisol, aldosterone, and androgens). It may be caused by hypothalamic or pituitary dysfunction, hormone receptor dysfunction, or more commonly, an autoimmune disease. Symptoms include fatigue, anorexia, weight loss, abdominal pain, infrequent menstruation, depression, and hyperpigmentation of the skin. Hypoglycemia may occur due to the lack of cortisol (↓ gluconeogenesis and ↑ peripheral glucose utilization). It is treated by the administration of synthetic steroids.

In contrast, Cushing syndrome is due to chronic glucocorticoid excess. Causes include tumors that produce excess adrenocorticotropic hormone (ACTH), adrenal tumors, and long-term corticosteroid use. Symptoms include the redistribution of body fat (fat affects trunk with relative sparing of the limbs ["buffalo hump"]), water retention (moon face, hypertension, edema), muscle wasting and weakness, thin skin, purple striae on the abdomen, osteoporosis, virilization, amenorrhea, and steroid-induced diabetes. Hyperglycemia occurs due to excess cortisol production. Primary treatment of Cushing syndrome is surgical removal of the causative tumors.

Normal
Diurnal variation in blood cortisol levels

Cortisol levels in the bloodstream display diurnal variation. Peak levels occur at around 8 am (5 to 23 mg/dL) and are at their lowest between midnight and 4 am. This phenomenon is utilized to minimize adrenocortical atrophy when giving glucocorticoid drugs: they are given when normal cortisol secretion is high and feedback inhibition is low (late morning), allowing the drug to be eliminated during the daytime and normal endogenous cortisol production to start early the following morning.

Normal

Hypoglycemia and hyperglycemia

Normal fasting blood glucose range is 70 to 100 mg/dL. Hypoglycemia develops at blood glucose levels of around 60 mg/dL, with symptoms such as tremors, hunger, sweating, and palpitations, progressing to confusion, drowsiness, seizures, coma, and death if blood glucose continues to fall. It is treated with the ingestion of a sugary drink if the patient is conscious, or by an injection of glucagon if the patient is unconscious. Hyperglycemia develops at sustained blood glucose levels above 180 mg/dL when the amount of glucose exceeds the capability of the kidneys to reabsorb it and glucose spills into the urine (glycosuria). There will also be increased thirst (polydipsia), headaches, difficulty concentrating, blurred vision, frequent urination (polyuria), fatigue, weight loss, nausea, and vomiting. Chronic hyperglycemia leads to poor wound healing; susceptibility to infection; accelerated atherosclerosis (deposition of fatty material on the arteries) causing strokes, coronary heart disease, and hypertension, as well as eye, kidney, and nerve disease (all seen in poorly controlled diabetes). Treatment may include insulin or other hypoglycemic drugs and regulation of carbohydrate intake.

Normal

Central nervous system and hypoglycemia

The brain and spinal cord require glucose for energy and are therefore sensitive to large decreases in plasma glucose levels. If there is a gradual decrease in blood glucose, the central nervous system (CNS) adapts by using ketones, but this adaptation requires several weeks. Hypoglycemia inhibits insulin synthesis and secretion, resulting in a decrease in the translocation of GLUT4 to the plasma membrane. This reduces glucose uptake in muscle and adipose tissue, thereby sparing glucose for the brain to use. GLUT3 in neural tissue is not affected by insulin; hence the brain can still use glucose in the absence of insulin.

Therapeutics

Biotin deficiency and biotinidase deficiency

Biotin is a coenzyme for carboxylase reactions. Therefore, it is essential for amino acid catabolism, gluconeogenesis, and fatty acid metabolism. When biotin levels are deficient, pyruvate accumulates because it is not converted to oxaloacetate due to reduced pyruvate carboxylase activity. Excess pyruvate is then converted to lactic acid, causing lactic acidosis, and to alanine. Deficiency of biotin manifests with rashes, brittle hair, hair loss, anemia, dermatitis, fungal infections, anorexia, lethargy, mild depression, muscle pains, and abnormal sensation (paresthesias). Biotin status can be determined by measuring the excretion of 3-hydroxyisovaleric acid and biotin in urine, or by measuring the activity of propionyl-CoA carboxylase in lymphocytes. Biocytin is the natural substrate of biotinidase and is used to measure biotinidase activity. Biotin and biotinidase deficiency are both treated by biotin replacement. For instance, biotin pills are readily available. Avoiding

uncooked egg white, which contains the biotin-binding protein avidin, is another way of preventing biotin malabsorption.

Therapeutics

Alcohol metabolism and hypoglycemia

Hypoglycemia may occur in alcoholics who rely on gluconeogenesis to maintain blood glucose levels. Alcohol (ethanol) is rapidly oxidized in the liver, producing an increase in NADH relative to NAD^+ in liver cells. Increased levels of NADH shift the lactate dehydrogenase reaction toward lactate and the cytosolic malate dehydrogenase reaction toward malate, thus preventing pyruvate and oxaloacetate from entering the gluconeogenesis pathway.

Therapeutics

Oral hypoglycemic drugs

Oral hypoglycemic drugs are useful in the treatment of type 2 (non-insulin-dependent) diabetes. Sulfonylurea drugs directly close ATP-sensitive K^+ channels on the surface of pancreatic β cells, causing membrane depolarization and increased insulin secretion. Biguanides decrease hepatic gluconeogenesis and the absorption of glucose from the gastrointestinal (GI) tract. Biguanides and thiazolidinediones also increase insulin sensitivity in skeletal muscle and adipose tissue. Because biguanides do not increase the release of pancreatic insulin, the risk of hypoglycemia is lower than with other sulphonylurea agents. α-Glucosidase inhibitors are competitive, reversible inhibitors of intestinal α-glucosidase, which causes delayed absorption of carbohydrates, thereby blunting postprandial hyperglycemia. Inhibitors of SGLT2 (e.g., canagliflozin, dapagliflozin) increase urinary excretion of glucose and thus help lower blood glucose levels.

Foundations

Acetyl CoA's effect on gluconeogenesis

Acetyl CoA, an allosteric activator of pyruvate carboxylase, links both glucose metabolism and fatty acid oxidation to the tricarboxylic acid (TCA) cycle. If the concentrations of both acetyl CoA and ATP are high, then oxaloacetate will be directed toward gluconeogenesis. However, if the acetyl CoA concentration is high but that of ATP is low, then oxaloacetate will be shunted to the TCA cycle to contribute to the production of ATP via oxidative phosphorylation.

Therapeutics

PEPCK deficiency

Phosphoenolpyruvate carboxykinase (PEPCK) deficiency is a rare autosomal recessive disorder of carbohydrate metabolism. PEPCK catalyzes the conversion of oxaloacetate into phosphoenolpyruvate. Symptoms include acidemia, hypoglycemia, loss of muscle tone, liver enlargement and impairment of its function, and failure to thrive.

IV

Therapeutics

Diabetic ketoacidosis

Diabetic ketoacidosis (DKA) is a life-threatening complication of diabetes (usually type 1 diabetes) that may occur following illness or inadequate/ inappropriate insulin therapy. In DKA, there is a severe shortage of insulin, so the body ceases to use carbohydrates as an energy source and starts using fatty acids, producing ketones (acetoacetate and β-hydroxybutyrate). Dehydration occurs (due to the osmotic diuresis caused by the excess glucose load in the renal tubules), followed by a metabolic acidosis and coma. Signs may include hyperventilation (to compensate for acidosis) and the breath smelling of ketones (sweet smell). Treatment involves giving insulin (replacement therapy), potassium (to correct losses due to dehydration), bicarbonate (to correct acidosis), and replacement fluids (to correct dehydration).

Therapeutics

Fructose 1,6-bisphosphatase deficiency

Fructose 1,6-bisphosphatase deficiency develops in individuals with rare mutations that make this rate-limiting enzyme defective. It presents in infancy or early childhood with hypoglycemia, lactic acidosis, ketosis, apnea (abnormal pauses in breathing), and hyperventilation triggered by fasting or ingestion of fructose, glycerol, or sorbitol.

Therapeutics

Von Gierke disease (glycogen storage disease I)

Von Gierke disease (a type I glycogen storage disease) is an autosomal recessive disorder. It has an incidence of 1 in 100,000 live births and is characterized by a deficiency of glucose 6-phosphatase activity. The activity of this enzyme is necessary for the release of free glucose into the bloodstream by the liver. Patients with Von Gierke disease exhibit marked fasting hypoglycemia due to their inability to replenish blood glucose after both glycogenolysis and gluconeogenesis. They also present with lactic acidosis (due to increased glycolysis) and an enlarged liver (hepatomegaly) due to the buildup of glycogen. Serum triglycerides are elevated (hyperlipidemia), as does uric acid due to both increased production (a depletion of phosphate leads to increased catabolism of purine nucleotides) and decreased excretion (lactate competes with urate for a common transporter). GSD Ia is the result of a loss of glucose 6-phosphatase catalytic unit (G6PC) while GSD Ib is caused by a defective glucose 6-phosphate transporter (G6PT).

Treatment of Von Gierke disease is by liver transplant or, if a suitable organ is not available, by surgical transposition of the portal vein. The latter operation redirects nutrient-rich blood from the intestine into the peripheral circulation; this at the same time improves the tissue supply with glucose and reduces glucose uptake in the liver. Uncooked cornstarch may be given to patients as a bedtime snack because it is broken down to glucose only slowly and thus keeps blood [glucose] up during the night.

12.3 Glycogen Metabolism

12.3.1 Glycogen

Glucose is stored in liver and skeletal muscle tissue as glycogen, a branched-chain homopolymer of glucose. Liver glycogen serves to regulate blood glucose levels, whereas muscle glycogen provides a fuel source for actively working muscles. The structure of glycogen consists of the following key features (▶ Fig. 12.8):

- Long chains in which glucose monomers are linked to each other via α-1,4 glycosidic bonds
- Branch points at every 8th to 10th glucose residue that are formed via α -1,6 glycosidic bonds between glucose monomers of separate chains
- Nonreducing ends identified by the presence of a terminal glucose monomer with a free hydroxyl group at carbon 4. Because glycogen chains are extended and degraded from their nonreducing ends, those that form a "tree" structure are rapidly extended or degraded, given that they contain a high number of nonreducing ends.
- The reducing end is identified as the glucose monomer that is covalently attached to glycogenin via its carbon 1 hydroxyl group. Glycogenin, a protein that catalyzes the formation of a short glycogen oligomer on itself, serves as a "primer" for glycogen synthesis and remains covalently attached to the glycogen molecule.
- Deficiencies in the synthesis or degradation of glycogen lead to a family of glycogen storage diseases, most of which are autosomal recessive (▶ Table 12.3). Those disorders that affect the breakdown of glycogen cause it to accumulate in organs such as the liver, which becomes enlarged (hepatomegaly). Consequently, the inability to maintain blood glucose levels manifests as hypoglycemia. Those disorders that affect the synthesis or degradation of glycogen cause patients to be highly dependent on dietary glucose rather than on their own stored form of glucose.

12.3.2 Glycogenesis versus Glycogenolysis

Glycogen is stored in cells as cytosolic granules, and the enzymes responsible for glycogen metabolism are also found in these granules. Several inherited deficiencies involving these metabolizing enzymes are responsible for some of the different glycogen storage diseases. Depending on which enzyme is deficient, these diseases can manifest as either storage of excessive levels of glycogen or the synthesis of glycogen of abnormal structure, or both.

Glycogenesis

This pathway for the synthesis of glycogen requires energy and three key events (▶ Fig. 12.9a):

1. **Trapping and activation of glucose:** Glucokinase/ hexokinase in the cytosol of hepatocytes and muscle cells catalyzes the phosphorylation of glucose into glucose 6-phosphate. This action traps this more polar form of glucose inside these cells.

Table 12.3 Disorders associated with deficiencies of enzymes in glycogen metabolism

Disorder No.	Disorder name	Defective enzyme	Pathway affected
GSD 0	–	Glycogen synthase	Glycogenesis: chain elongation
GSD I	von Gierke disease	Glucose 6-phosphatase	Glycogenolysis/gluconeogenesis: dephosphorylation of Glc 6-P to Glc
GSD II	Pompe disease	Acid maltase	Lysosomal glycogenolysis: release of Glc
GSD III	Cori disease	Debranching enzyme (a-1,6-glucosidase activity)	Glycogenolysis: Glc cleavage and release from branch point
GSD IV	Andersen disease	Branching enzyme (Glucosyl (4:6) transferase)	Glycogenesis: chain branching
GSD V	McArdle disease	Muscle glycogen phosphorylase	Glycogenolysis: Glc 1-P release
GSD VI	Hers disease	Liver glycogen phosphorylase	Glycogenolysis: Glc 1-P release

Abbreviation: GSD, glycogen storage disease.

IV

Glycogen structure

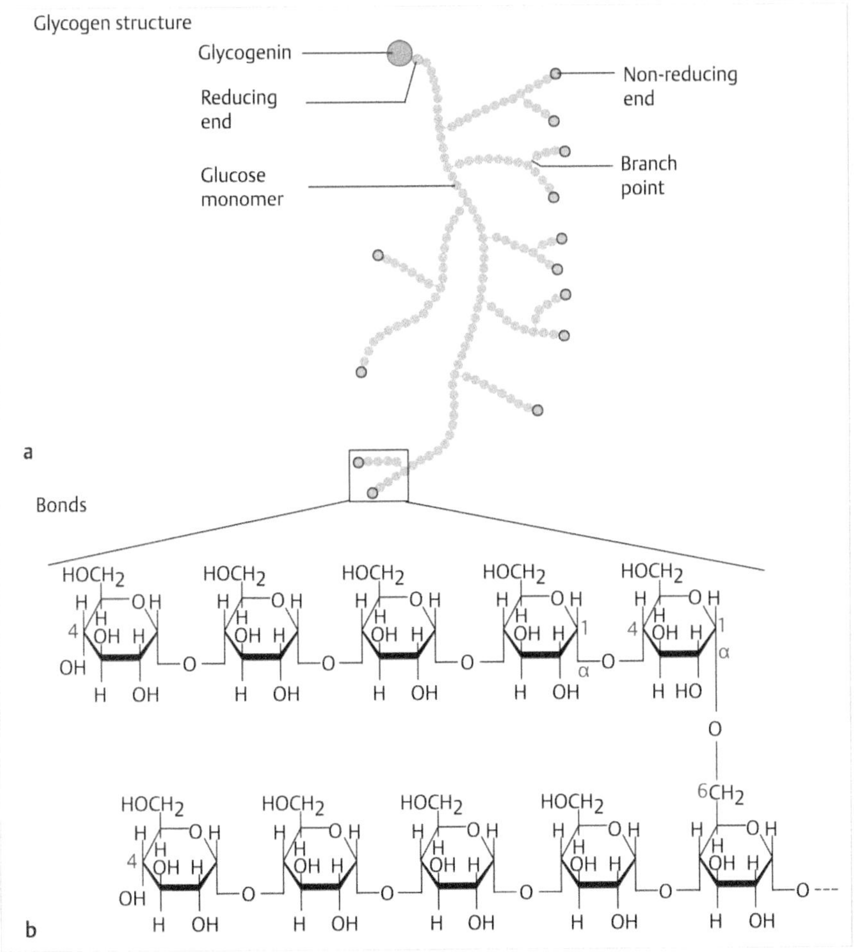

Fig. 12.8 Glycogen branch-chain homopolymer. (a, b) Glycogen is a branch-chain homopolymer of glucose molecules linked together via α-1,4 glycosidic bonds. However, at branch points, they are linked via α-1,6 glycosidic bonds. The reducing end of glycogen consists of a glucose monomer covalently attached to glycogenin. The nonreducing ends each contain a terminal glucose with a free hydroxyl group at carbon 4. Glycogen is degraded and extended from the nonreducing ends.

- Phosphoglucomutase then reversibly isomerizes glucose 6-phosphate into glucose 1-phosphate. Uridine diphosphate (UDP)-glucose pyrophosphorylase then transfers the glucose 1-phosphate to uridine triphosphate (UTP), which generates UDP-glucose (the active form of glucose) and releases pyrophosphate (PP_i). Hydrolysis of PP_i into two inorganic phosphates drives this reaction.

2. **Elongation of a glycogen "primer":** A preexisting glycogen oligomer serves as a primer to which individual glucose units are added. This primer can be a glycogen chain (with at least four glucose units) attached to glycogenin.

- Glycogen synthase—the rate-limiting enzyme of glycogenesis—catalyzes the transfer of glucose from UDP-glucose onto the nonreducing end of the glycogen chain. This results in the formation of α-1,4 glycosidic bonds between glucose molecules.
- Mutations in glycogen synthase result in a deficiency classified as glycogen storage disease type 0 (GSD 0). Patients with this disease do not store excess glucose in the liver. When mutations occur in the liver form of glycogen synthase, it manifests as fasting hypoglycemia, and hyperglycemia after feeding.

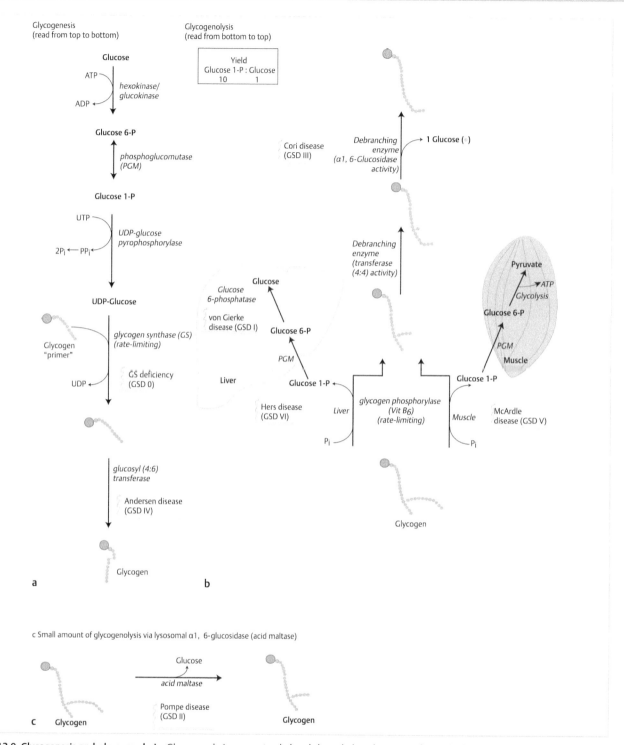

Fig. 12.9 Glycogenesis and glycogenolysis. Glycogen chains are extended and degraded at their nonreducing ends (C4-hydroxyl). **(a)** Glucose is phosphorylated to glucose 6-phosphate, which is then isomerized to glucose 1-phosphate. Glucose 1-phosphate is then transferred onto uridine triphosphate (UTP) to generate uridine diphosphate (UDP)-glucose and release pyrophosphate. UDP-glucose allows glucose to be transferred onto the nonreducing end of glycogen. **(b)** When glycogen is degraded, it generates glucose 1-phosphate and free glucose at a ratio of 10:1, respectively. Glycogen chains are degraded one glucose at a time by the vitamin B_6-dependent enzyme glycogen phosphorylase, which halts at four glucose residues from a branch point. This rate-limiting enzyme generates glucose 1-phosphate molecules, which are converted to glucose in hepatic tissue or to pyruvate (via glycolysis) in muscle tissue. Debranching enzyme, which has both transferase (4:4) activity and α-1, 6 glucosidase activity, transfers a block of three of the remaining four glucose residues to the nonreducing end of the main chain. It then cleaves the α-1,6 glycosidic bond of the remaining glucose, releasing it as free glucose. **(c)** A small amount of glycogen is degraded in lysosomes. ADP, adenosine diphosphate; ATP, adenosine triphosphate; GSD, glycogen storage disease; Pi, inorganic phosphate; PPi, pyrophosphate; PGM, phosphoglucomutase.

3. **Branching of glycogen chains:** When the glycogen chain reaches 11 residues, a fragment of the chain (about seven residues long) is broken off at an α-1,4 link and reattached elsewhere through an α -1,6 link by glucosyl (4:6) transferase (commonly known as the branching enzyme). The branching process increases the solubility of glycogen and also increases the number of terminal non-reducing ends.

- Andersen disease, also known as GSD type IV, is a rare disorder in which glucosyl (4:6) transferase is absent. This results in the formation of very long, unbranched chains in glycogen, which lowers its solubility.

Glycogenolysis

This pathway for the degradation of glycogen generates glucose in the form of glucose 1-phosphate and free glucose at a ratio of ~ 10:1. There are two key events that take place in glycogenolysis (▶ Fig. 12.9b):

1. **Chain shortening (release of glucose 1-phosphate):** The rate-limiting enzyme, glycogen phosphorylase, catalyzes the cleavage of glucose residues (one by one) as a molecule of glucose 1-phosphate from the nonreducing ends of glycogen. This occurs via phosphorolysis, a reaction in which the transfer of inorganic phosphate (P_i) onto the hydroxyl group of carbon 1 of the terminal glucose breaks the α -1,4 glycosidic bond.
   - Glycogen phosphorylase—which is active when phosphorylated and inactive when dephosphorylated— uses pyridoxal phosphate (vitamin B_6) as a cofactor.
   - Phosphorolysis of glucose residues continues down the chain until glycogen phosphorylase gets within four residues of the α -1,6 linkage of a branch point.
     - Hers disease, also known as GSD type VI, is a genetic disorder caused by a deficiency in the liver form of glycogen phosphorylase.
     - McArdle disease, also known as GSD type V, is a disorder caused by a deficiency in the muscle form of glycogen phosphorylase (myophosphorylase).
2. **Branch transfer and release of glucose:** Debranching enzyme uses its transferase (4:4) activity to transfer a block of three of the remaining four glucose residues to the nonreducing end of the main chain, forming an α -1,4 bond. Then this enzyme's α -1,6 glucosidase activity cleaves the α -1,6 bond of the single remaining glucose residue to release free glucose.

Fates of liver versus muscle glucose 1-phosphate. In the liver, glucose 1-phosphate molecules are converted to glucose 6-phosphate by the action of an epimerase and then to glucose by the action of glucose 6-phosphatase. Free glucose then enters the bloodstream. Myocytes in the muscle cannot hydrolyze glucose 6-phosphate and instead use it to generate energy via the glycolysis and TCA cycle. These different fates of glucose 1-phosphate are driven by the presence/absence of specific proteins in these tissues, as in the following examples:

- Hepatocytes express glucose 6-phosphatase: In the liver, glucose 1-phosphate is isomerized to glucose 6-phosphate, which is then dephosphorylated to form free glucose. The latter reaction is catalyzed by glucose 6-phosphatase.

- Muscle cells lack glucose 6-phosphatase activity: Although glucose 1-phosphate is also isomerized to glucose 6-phosphate in muscle cells the absence of hydrolysis in these cells causes glucose 6-phosphate to be metabolized to CO_2 by the glycolytic and TCA cycle pathways, which generate ATP.

Glycogenolysis in lysosomes. A small amount of glycogen (1 to 3% of total) is degraded in lysosomes by the enzyme acid maltase (acid α -glucosidase). This enzyme hydrolyzes both the α -1,4 and α -1,6 glycosidic linkages to release free glucose (see ▶ Fig. 12.9).

- Pompe disease (GSD II) is an autosomal recessive genetic disorder caused by a deficiency in acid maltase. This leads to glycogen accumulation in lysosomes of various tissues, especially the heart, liver, skeletal muscle, and the nervous system. Hypertrophic cardiomyopathy is a known feature of infantile onset form of Pompe disease. Enzyme replacement therapy (using alglucosidase alpha) is an effective treatment for this disease.

12.3.3 Regulation of Glycogen Metabolism

Careful control of liver glycogen metabolism is needed to maintain blood glucose at appropriate levels for glucose-dependent tissues like the brain and erythrocytes. Similarly muscle glycogen metabolism needs to be regulated to provide energy for exercising muscles. Control of glycogen metabolism involves the reciprocal regulation of the activities of glycogen synthase and glycogen phosphorylase—the rate-limiting enzymes of glycogenesis and glycogenolysis, respectively. A summary of the resulting effects are as follows (▶ Fig. 12.10):

- Glycogenesis is favored when blood glucose and insulin levels are high (as observed in the fed state) and cellular ATP levels are elevated (a signal of high energy). When glycogen synthesis is favored, the dephosphorylated forms of glycogen synthase (active) and glycogen phosphorylase (inactive; "b" form) predominate.
- Glycogenolysis is favored when blood glucose levels are low, but glucagon levels are high (as observed in the fasting state), and cellular Ca^{2+} and AMP levels are elevated (as seen in exercising muscles). When glycogen degradation is favored, the phosphorylated forms of glycogen synthase (inactive) and glycogen phosphorylase (active; "a" form) predominate.

Mechanism of Regulation by Insulin

When blood glucose levels are high, the β cells of the pancreas release insulin. Insulin then binds to its receptor tyrosine kinase on the surface of hepatocytes and muscle cells and triggers a signaling cascade that culminates in the activation of glycogen synthase and inactivation of glycogen phosphorylase. The four key proteins, and the mechanisms by which they promote glycogen synthesis in response to insulin, are as follows (▶ Fig. 12.11):

1. Protein kinase B (PKB)
2. GLUT4 (muscle and adipose cells only)
3. Glycogen synthase kinase 3 (GSK3)
4. Protein phosphatase1 (PP1)

IV

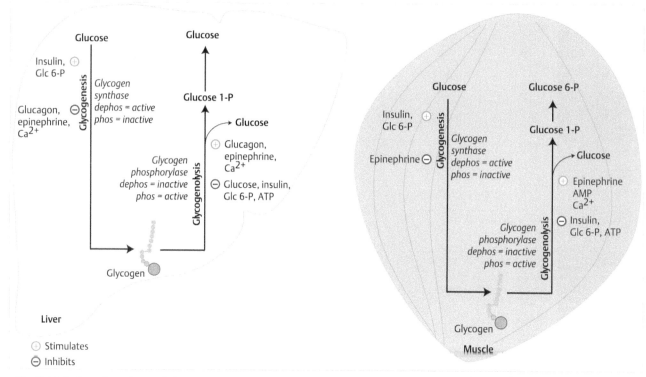

Fig. 12.10 Reciprocal regulation of glycogenesis and glycogenolysis. The regulators of glycogenesis and glycogenolysis in liver and muscle tissues are summarized. Note that glucagon exerts its effects on glycogen metabolism in liver cells only, whereas epinephrine affects both liver and muscle glycogen metabolism. ADP, adenosine diphosphate; AMP, adenosine monophosphate; ATP, adenosine triphosphate; Glc, glucose.

Signaling events downstream of the formation of the insulin-receptor complex activates PKB, which increases the uptake of glucose by muscle and adipose cells by increasing the number of GLUT4 glucose receptors that translocate to the plasma membrane. PKB also phosphorylates both PP1 (to activate it) and GSK3 (to inactivate it). Active PP1 then dephosphorylates glycogen synthase (to activate it) and dephosphorylates glycogen phosphorylase (to inactivate it). (In its inactive state, GSK3 is unable to phosphorylate and inhibit glycogen synthase.) Insulin also appears to promote the targeting of PP1 to glycogen particles which are the sites of action of glycogen synthase and glycogen phosphorylase.

- Diabetes mellitus type 2 is marked by reduced sensitivity to insulin (insulin resistance). This may be due to mutations in the insulin receptor and/or downstream signaling proteins, or downregulation of the insulin receptor triggered by chronically elevated insulin levels, which cause endocytosis and degradation of the insulin receptor that is not adequately replaced by the cell's translational machinery.
  - Rabson-Mendenhall syndrome: This is a very rare autosomal recessive disorder in which both alleles of the insulin receptor gene are defective, which manifests as insulin resistance.
  - Donohue syndrome (leprechaunism): This is a very rare autosomal recessive disorder characterized by mutations in the insulin receptor gene that produce a defective product. Patients with leprechaunism exhibit a more severe form of insulin resistance than those with Rabson-Mendenhall syndrome.

Mechanism of Regulation by Glucagon

When blood glucose levels are low, the α cells of the pancreas release glucagon. Glucagon then binds to its G protein–coupled receptor (GPCR) on the surface of hepatocytes (not muscle cells), which triggers a signaling cascade that leads to the inactivation of glycogen synthase and activation of glycogen phosphorylase. The enzymes and second messenger that mediate this effect are as follows (▶ Fig. 12.12):

1. G protein (trimeric)
2. Adenylate cyclase (AC) and the second messenger cyclic AMP (cAMP)
3. Protein kinase A (PKA)
4. Protein phosphatase 1 (PP1)
5. Phosphorylase kinase (PK)

Glucagon binding to its GPCR "turns on" its associated G protein, which then activates AC. AC then increases cellular cAMP levels, which activate PKA. Active PKA directly phosphorylates and inactivates glycogen synthase. In addition, active PKA phosphorylates PK to activate it. It also phosphorylates and activates the inhibitor 1 protein which inactivates PP1. Active PK (the "a" form) phosphorylates glycogen phosphorylase (to activate it). The result of glucagon signaling is an increase in blood glucose levels.

- Diabetes mellitus type 2 can also be associated with defects in the signaling events from the glucagon–GPCR complex.
- GSD IX is a disorder in which phosphorylase kinase is defective.

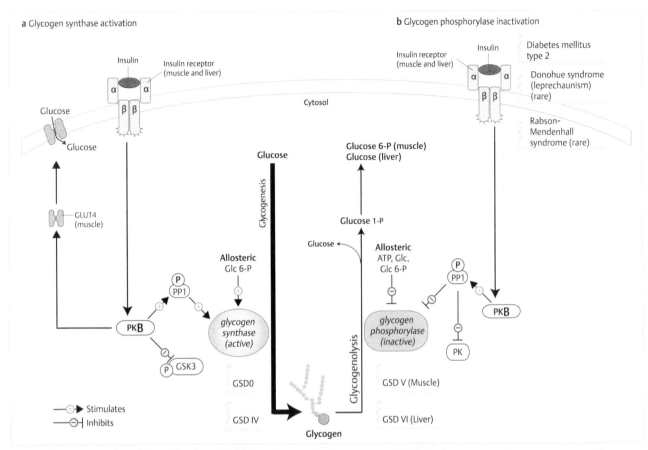

Fig. 12.11 Regulation of glycogen metabolism by insulin. In muscle and liver cells, the regulation of glycogenesis by insulin is mediated by phosphorylation and dephosphorylation events, respectively, catalyzed by protein kinase B (PKB) and protein phosphatase1 (PP1), which culminates in (a) the activation of glycogen synthase and (b) inhibition of glycogen phosphorylase. Glucose, glucose 6-phosphate, and ATP exert allosteric control over the activity of glycogen synthase and glycogen phosphorylase that favors glycogenesis. ATP, adenosine triphosphate; Glc, glucose; GSK3, glycogen synthase kinase 3; PK, phosphorylase kinase.

Other Regulators of Glycogen Metabolism

Epinephrine. This "fight or fight" hormone released by adrenal glands during periods of stress promotes the degradation of glycogen in both liver and muscle tissue via a signaling cascade that is identical to that of glucagon (i.e., GPCR → G protein → AC → cAMP → PKA; ▶ Fig. 12.12).

Allosteric regulators. Glucose 6-phosphate, glucose, ATP, Ca^{2+} and AMP.

- Glucose 6-phosphate allosterically activates glycogen synthase to stimulate glycogen synthesis (▶ Fig. 12.11). Conversely, glucose 6-phosphate and ATP allosterically inhibit glycogen phosphorylase. Due to the action of glucokinase, levels of glucose 6-phosphate are elevated in the liver after a meal. Free glucose is an allosteric inhibitor of glycogen phosphorylase in the liver but not in the muscle.
- In muscle cells, the breakdown of glycogen is stimulated by the allosteric activation of glycogen phosphorylase kinase by Ca^{2+} and glycogen phosphorylase by AMP—without the need for the activating phosphorylation of either enzyme. The levels of Ca^{2+} and AMP are especially elevated in exercising muscles because Ca^{2+} is released from the sarcoplasmic reticulum, and AMP is generated from ADP by the action of adenylate kinase when muscles contract.

Normal

Expression of hexokinase isoforms

Hexokinase exists in four major isoforms that differ in their tissue expression, affinity for glucose, product inhibition, and the sensitivity of gene expression to insulin. Hexokinases I through III are 100 kDa proteins that have a low Michaelis-Menten (K_m) for glucose, whereas HK-IV is a 50 kDa polypeptide with a several-fold higher K_m for glucose. HK-IV is also known as glucokinase and is the major enzyme for the phosphorylation of glucose as well as of fructose and mannose (see Chapter 9). Isozymes I through III are inhibited by the product glucose 6-phosphate, whereas glucokinase is not. Product inhibition of HK-I is antagonized by inorganic phosphate (P_i). On the other hand, P_i potentiates the product inhibition of HK-II and HK-III. HK-I and HK-II are associated with porin in the outer membrane of mitochondria, suggesting that the phosphorylation of glucose is coupled to the generation of ATP by oxidative phosphorylation. The expression of HK-II (muscle) and HK-IV (liver) is enhanced by insulin. Thus, in muscle, insulin seems to increase both the uptake and the utilization of glucose.

IV

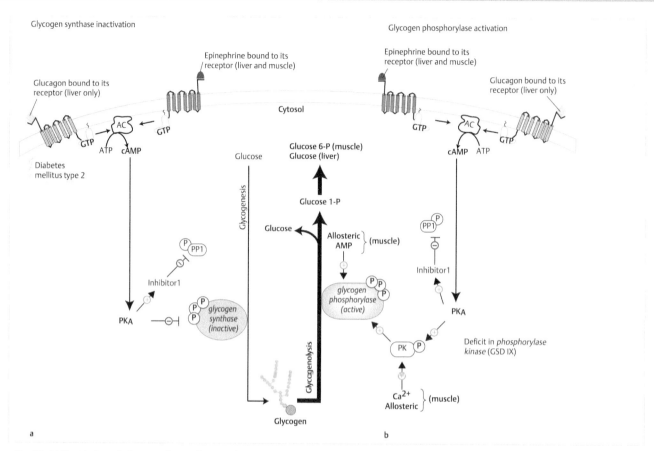

Fig. 12.12 Regulation of glycogenolysis. Glycogenolysis is regulated by glucagon (in liver cells only) and epinephrine (in liver and muscle cells) via signaling pathways that involve activation of their respective G protein-coupled receptor (GPCR), increase in cyclic adenosine monophosphate (cAMP) levels, activation of protein kinase A (PKA), and various phosphorylation/dephosphorylation events that result in (**a**) the inhibition of glycogen synthase and (**b**) activation of glycogen phosphorylase. Additional regulators of glycogenolysis include Ca^{2+} and AMP, which both activate glycogen phosphorylase. AC, adenylate cyclase; ATP, adenosine triphosphate; GSD, glycogen storage disease; GTP, guanosine triphosphate; PK, phosphorylase kinase; PP1, protein phosphatase1.

Therapeutics
GSD 0: deficiency in glycogen synthase

GSD 0 is a genetic disorder in which glycogen synthase is deficient. As a result, glucose cannot be stored as glycogen, making patients with this disorder highly dependent on glucose from the diet. These individuals are highly susceptible to hypoglycemia when fasting (e.g., during sleep). Therefore, they must eat frequently and are helped by the consumption of uncooked cornstarch at bedtime.. These patients may also experience periodic muscle cramping brought on by the lack of muscle glycogen.

Therapeutics
GSD IV/Andersen disease: deficiency in glucosyl (4:6) transferase (branching enzyme)

Andersen disease is an autosomal recessive disorder caused by a deficiency in glucosyl (4:6) transferase, the enzyme responsible for glycogen branching as it creates the α-1,6 bonds. As a result, individuals with this disorder possess longer chain glycogen with fewer branches than seen in normal individuals. A deficiency of glucosyl (4:6) transferase in the liver and spleen manifests as an enlargement of both organs (hepatosplenomegaly), scarring of the liver (cirrhosis), and death within 5 years after birth.

Foundations
Glycogen degradation via phosphorolysis versus hydrolysis

Degradation of glycogen for the most part involves sequential removal of glycosyl units from a linear polysaccharide chain. This is accomplished by phosphorolysis using the enzyme glycogen phosphorylase. In phosphorolysis, the α-1,4 glycosidic bond is cleaved using inorganic phosphate, yielding glucose 1-phosphate. However, phosphorylase cannot cleave the α-1,6 glycosidic bond at branch points. The debranching enzyme (α-1,6-glucosidase) uses hydrolysis to cleave this bond, yielding free glucose as the product. Phosphorolysis is energetically advantageous because the product is already phosphorylated and does not require further expenditure of ATP for activation.

Therapeutics

GSD VI/Hers disease: deficiency in liver glycogen phosphorylase

A reduction in glycogen phosphorylase activity prevents degradation of glycogen. As a result, glycogen accumulates in the liver and causes it to become extremely enlarged, and blood levels of glucose may be low. Patients with Hers disease, an autosomal recessive disorder, have a deficiency in liver glycogen phosphorylase. They present with enlarged livers and may or may not be hypoglycemic.

Therapeutics

GSD II/Pompe disease: deficiency in acid maltase

Pompe disease is an autosomal recessive disorder caused by a deficiency in lysosomal acid maltase (also known as acid α-glucosidase). The resulting accumulation of glycogen disrupts normal functioning of muscle and liver cells. There is progressive muscle weakness (myopathy) throughout the body, including the heart and skeletal muscle. Children with this disease often die of heart failure in infancy. Pompe disease is the only one of the glycogen storage disorders that results in lysosomal accumulation of glycogen.

Therapeutics

Enzyme replacement therapy

A recent development in the treatment of Pompe disease (GSD II) is enzyme replacement therapy using recombinant human acid α-glucosidase (e.g., Myozyme, Genzyme Corp., Cambridge, MA; Lumizyme, Genzyme). The recombinant enzyme is administered by intravenous infusion to infantile-onset patients with Pompe disease. The treatment improves the survival rate and reduces respiratory distress. Lumizyme (Genzyme) is approved by the US Food and Drug Administration (FDA) for treatment of children older than 8 years and when cardiac hypertrophy is absent. A drawback of this lifelong treatment is that it is quite expensive (average cost = $300,000 per year in 2013).

Therapeutics

GSD V/McArdle disease: deficiency in muscle glycogen phosphorylase

McArdle disease is an autosomal recessive disorder marked by a deficiency in muscle glycogen phosphorylase, the rate-limiting enzyme of glycogen degradation that cleaves glucose residues from glycogen for release as glucose 1-phosphate. Because they are unable to provide a sufficient supply of glucose to their muscles, individuals with this condition suffer from fatigue, severe muscle cramping, and muscle breakdown (rabdomyolysis) marked by myoglobin in the urine during intense exercise. Patients tolerate this disease fairly well by making appropriate reductions in strenuous physical activity. Intake of sucrose immediately prior to physical activity appears to improve exercise tolerance.

Therapeutics

GSD III/Cori disease: deficiency in debranching enzyme

An autosomal recessive disorder called Cori disease is caused by a deficiency in the α-1,6-glucosidase activity of the debranching enzyme in the muscle and liver. Individuals with this condition possess glycogen molecules that have a high number of short branches. They present with enlarged livers and mild hypoglycemia.

Therapeutics

GSD IX: deficiency in phosphorylase kinase

Phosphorylase kinase (PhK) is an enzyme that phosphorylates and activates glycogen phosphorylase to cause degradation of glycogen. PhK is made up of four subunits. Genetic defects in PhK lead to hypoglycemia and elevation of liver enzymes (ALT and AST) in plasma. The more common form of GSD-IX is due to mutations in the X-linked gene for PhK-α. Mutations in PhK-β and PhK-γ are also known. The clinical presentation of GSD-IX is similar to that of GSD-VI (Hers disease). The only treatment currently available is symptomatic and involves frequent carbohydrate-rich meals to counter hypoglycemia.

Foundations

Liver versus muscle glycogen phosphorylase

The liver and muscle isoforms of phosphorylase are products of separate genes located on chromosomes 14 and 11, respectively. Mutations in liver phosphorylase cause Hers disease (GSD VI), whereas those in the muscle enzyme cause McArdle syndrome (GSD V). Both of these disorders are inherited in an autosomal recessive fashion. These two enzymes also differ in their sensitivity toward some regulatory molecules. Both isoforms are activated by phosphorylation catalyzed by PhK and are subject to allosteric inhibition by ATP and glucose 6-phosphate. The muscle isoform is allosterically activated by AMP, which is a measure of low-energy status of the cell, by Ca^{2+}-calmodulin complex, and by G-actin, demonstrating a link between muscle contraction and energy production. The liver enzyme is inactivated by free glucose but is not affected by AMP. There is a third isozyme of phosphorylase in brain astrocytes that lacks the site for activating phosphorylation by PhK but is responsive to AMP. The brain does contain small amounts of glycogen.

Foundations

Ca^{2+}-calmodulin complexes

The muscle isozyme of phosphorylase is very sensitive to activation by Ca^{2+}. Calcium is released from the sarcoplasmic reticulum (SR) via the ryanodine receptors during muscle contraction in response to plasma membrane depolarization at the neuromuscular junctions. Calcium is also released into the sarcoplasm by the action of epinephrine acting through inositol triphosphate receptors on sarcoplasmic reticulum (see **Fig. 7.6**). Released Ca^{2+} binds to calmodulin, and the Ca^{2+}-calmodulin complex is capable of further activating phosphorylase *a*. The resultant degradation of glycogen provides the fuel for ATP generation and muscle contraction. Malignant hyperthermia is an inherited disorder characterized by functionally altered ryanodine receptors very sensitive to anesthetics and muscle relaxants. Reabsorption of mobilized Ca^{2+} requires a large expenditure of ATP and leads to hyperthermia in the muscle. Dantrolene is a muscle relaxant that binds to ryanodine receptors in the muscle to prevent the mobilization of Ca^{2+} and activation of phosphorylase *a*. Dantrolene is used to counteract malignant hyperthermia induced by general anesthesia in genetically susceptible patients.

Foundations

GPCRs: α- and β-adrenergic receptors

Adrenergic receptors are G protein–coupled receptors that mediate the action of epinephrine and related compounds (see Chapter 7). They are classified into α and β types. The former generally produce excitatory effects on smooth muscle, whereas the latter typically produce an inhibitory effect. (Note: In cardiac muscle, β-adrenergic receptors are excitatory.) They are further classified into subtypes based on their sensitivity to specific antagonists. The $α_1$ agonists (e.g., norepinephrine) act through the phosphoinositide pathway to cause smooth muscle contraction, whereas $α_2$ agonists (e.g., clonidine) act via the cAMP pathway to cause a similar effect. The β receptors generally act through the cAMP pathway. Different β receptor subtypes produce cardiac stimulation, bronchodilation, and lipolysis. Beta-blocker drugs (e.g., propranolol, metoprolol) act on $β_1$ receptors to slow heart rate and lower blood pressure. Glucagon acts via its own receptor in liver and adipose tissue through the cAMP pathway.

Foundations

Hormone-signaling cascades

The concentrations of hormones in the bloodstream as well as in tissues are often very low (in the nM range). The target cells also express relatively low numbers of receptors (a few thousand per cell). In spite of this limitation, the final response achieved in terms of metabolic pathways turned on or off can be rather large. Such amplification is achieved through signaling cascades. Taking GPCR signaling as an example, the cascade involves the binding of a hormone (e.g., glucagon, epinephrine) to its receptor, activation of G_s, stimulation of adenylate cyclase to produce cAMP, activation of PKA by cAMP, phosphorylation, and stimulation (or inhibition) of a target enzyme by PKA leading to up- or downregulation of a metabolic pathway. Each step in this cascade is capable of initiating multiple occurrences of the next step immediately downstream. It is thus easy to envision signal amplification at each stage of this cascade.

Normal

Neoplasia versus hyperplasia versus hypertrophy

Hypertrophy refers to an increase in the cell mass without any increase in cell number. Both hyperplasia and neoplasia involve an increase in cell proliferation. The difference between the two is that, whereas normal physiological control mechanisms still operate in hyperplasia, they are bypassed in neoplasia.

Therapeutics

Skin cell hyperplasia: acanthosis nigricans

An increase in circulating insulin manifests as acanthosis nigricans (skin hyperpigmentation) in skin folds in the neck, armpit, groin, and so forth, due to skin hyperplasia.

Foundations

G proteins

G proteins can bind to guanine nucleotides such as GTP and GDP. They are active when bound to GTP and inactive when bound to GDP. There are two major classes of G proteins: heterotrimeric G proteins (e.g., G_s, G_i, G_q) and monomeric G proteins (e.g., RAS, RAB). Trimeric G proteins participate in GPCR-mediated signaling pathways, whereas monomeric G proteins mediate receptor tyrosine kinase pathways.

12.4 Fructose and Galactose Metabolism

12.4.1 Overview

The monosaccharides fructose and galactose are metabolized primarily in the liver to generate intermediates that are used in glycolysis (in the fed state) or gluconeogenesis (in the fasting or starved state).

Fructose is primarily obtained from the cleavage of the dietary disaccharide sucrose (found in fruits, table sugar, and honey) into fructose and glucose (▶ Fig. 12.13a). Fructose is also obtained from the diet as a free monosaccharide from honey and a variety of fruits, but especially from foods sweetened with high-fructose corn syrup (e.g., sodas). The uptake of fructose from the diet is mediated by the actions of sucrase and GLUT5, which are found on the apical surface of epithelial cells that line the small intestine:

- Sucrase cleaves sucrose into fructose and glucose.
- GLUT5 facilitates the transport of fructose into epithelial cells that line the small intestine. The exit of fructose from these cells into the bloodstream, however, is facilitated by GLUT2 (▶ Fig. 12.13b). Fructose is then picked up by those tissues whose cells express either GLUT5 or GLUT2 (see ▶ Fig. 12.1 and ▶ Fig. 12.2).

In hepatocytes, ovaries, and seminal vesicles, fructose is generated from glucose via the polyol pathway, as follows (▶ Fig. 12.13c):

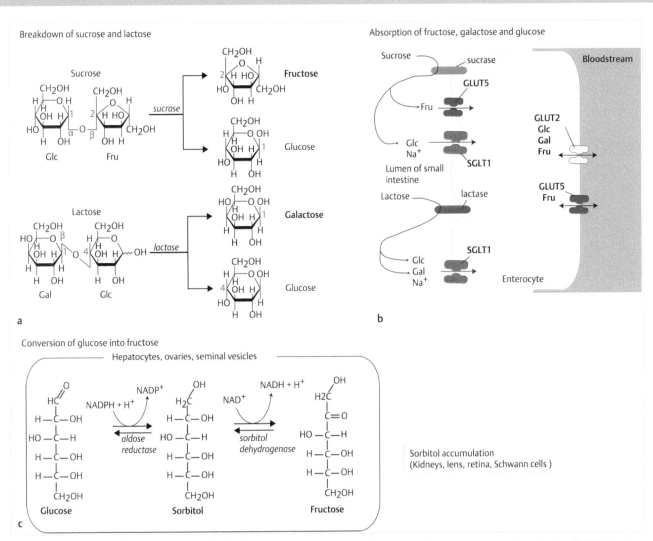

Fig. 12.13 Source and absorption of fructose and galactose. (a) The breakdown of sucrose by the enzyme sucrase generates fructose (Fru) and glucose (Glu); the breakdown of lactose by the enzyme lactase generates galactose (Gal) and glucose. **(b)** Sucrase and lactase—which are located on the apical surface of epithelial cells of the small intestine-cleave their substrates to release fructose, galactose, and glucose. The absorption of fructose is facilitated by glucose transporter 5 (GLUT5), whereas the absorption of galactose and glucose is facilitated by sodium-glucose transporter 1 (SGLT1). GLUT2 facilitates the export of these three monosaccharides into the bloodstream. GLUT5 is also present to facilitate the export of fructose. **(C)** The polyol pathway converts glucose into fructose in two steps in hepatocytes, ovaries, and seminal vesicles. The first step is catalyzed by aldose reductase and the second by sorbitol dehydrogenase. NADPH, reduced form of nicotinamide adenine dinucleotide phosphate; SI, small intestine.

- Aldose reductase catalyzes the NADPH-dependent reduction of glucose to sorbitol (a polyol/polyalcohol).
- Sorbitol dehydrogenase then catalyzes the NAD$^+$-dependent oxidation of sorbitol to fructose.
  - Sorbitol accumulates in cells that lack sorbitol dehydrogenase, such as those of the kidney, lens, and retina, and Schwann cells. As such, accumulation of sorbitol, an osmotically active compound, triggers the influx of water into affected cells, causing them to swell. This type of damage manifests as retinopathy, cataracts, and peripheral neuropathy, particularly under hyperglycemic conditions such as diabetes.

Galactose is obtained when the enzyme lactase breaks down the disaccharide lactose (found in milk products) into galactose and glucose (▶ Fig. 12.13a). Galactose and glucose are transported into epithelial cells of the small intestine via SGLT1 and transported out to the bloodstream via GLUT2 (▶ Fig. 12.13b).

- Another source of galactose is from the lysosomal breakdown of the complex carbohydrates found on glycolipids and glycoproteins. Transporters specific for neutral hexoses, N-acetylhexosamines and acidic monosaccharides have been identified on lysosomal membranes.

Mechanism of Fructose Metabolism

The metabolism of fructose (fructolysis) is similar in many respects to the metabolism of glucose (glycolysis) in that they both involve the following events (▶ Fig. 12.14):

Cellular entrapment via phosphorylation. Fructokinase catalyzes the ATP-dependent phosphorylation of fructose into fructose 1-phosphate, trapping it inside hepatocytes. (Similarly, glucose is phosphorylated by hexokinase/glucokinase, but at carbon 6, to form glucose 6-phosphate).

- Essential or benign fructosuria is an autosomal recessive disorder caused by a deficiency in fructokinase. Fructose is

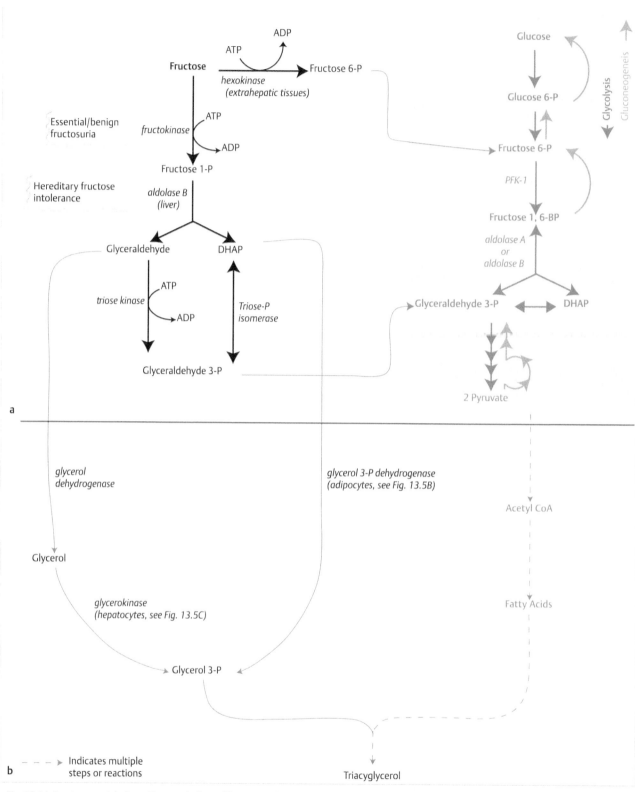

Fig. 12.14 Fructose metabolism. The metabolism of fructose is closely linked to the metabolism of glucose via glycolysis/gluconeogenesis. (**a**) In liver cells, fructose is metabolized to glyceraldehyde 3-phosphate, an intermediate that can be utilized for glycolysis or gluconeogenesis. Defects in fructokinase and aldolase B are respectively associated with essential/benign fructosuria and the more damaging hereditary fructose intolerance. In extrahepatic tissues, fructose is phosphorylated by hexokinase into fructose 6-phosphate, another intermediate that can be utilized for glycolysis or gluconeogenesis. (**b**) Fructose is more readily converted to fat than glucose because fructose's metabolism bypasses the rate-limiting step of phosphofructokinase-1 (PFK-1). Catabolism of fructose yields the two precursors necessary for t rig lyceride synthesis, namely, glycerol 3-phosphate and free fatty acids. ADP, adenosine diphosphate; ATP, adenosine triphosphate; CoA, coenzyme A; DHAP, dihydroxyacetone phosphate; P, phosphate.

excreted in the urine of these patients because it cannot be trapped in hepatocytes via phosphorylation.

- In extrahepatic tissues (e.g., muscle), fructose is phosphorylated by hexokinase at carbon 6 to generate fructose 6-phosphate. However, the K_m for fructose is significantly higher than that for glucose. Fructose 6-phosphate is an intermediate in glycolysis/gluconeogenesis and, depending on the energy needs of the cell, is used to generate energy or glucose.

Splitting of a six-carbon sugar into two three-carbon molecules. Aldolase B—found mainly in the liver—splits fructose 1-phosphate into glyceraldehyde and dihydroxyacetone phosphate (DHAP). Both products are then converted into glyceraldehyde 3-phosphate, another intermediate of glycolysis/gluconeogenesis, by triose kinase and triose phosphate isomerase, respectively. Aldolase B can also split fructose 1,6-bisphosphate into DHAP and glyceraldehyde 3-phosphate, just like aldolase A.

- Hereditary fructose intolerance is a severe autosomal recessive disorder caused by a deficiency in aldolase B. The resulting accumulation in fructose 1-phosphate sequesters much of the cell's phosphate, which inhibits glycogen phosphorylase (and thus glycogenolysis) and virtually stops ATP synthesis in the liver. The reduction in ATP levels prevents the maintenance of normal ionic gradients and leads to osmotic damage to hepatocytes. The low energy charge also inhibits gluconeogenesis and leads to hypoglycemia. Signs and symptoms of this disorder manifest when an infant is weaned of milk products and given fructose-containing foods.
- Fructose is metabolized more rapidly than glucose in the liver because fructose metabolism bypasses the rate-limiting phosphofructokinase-1 (PFK-1) step essential for glucose metabolism.
- Cleavage of fructose 1-phosphate generates glyceraldehyde, which is readily converted to glycerol 3-phosphate by the action of alcohol dehydrogenase and glycerol kinase (an enzyme present in the liver but not in adipose tissue). Glycerol 3-phosphate provides the backbone for triglyceride synthesis (▶ Fig. 12.14b).

Mechanism of Galactose Metabolism

The metabolism of galactose generates two key molecules: glucose 6-phosphate (an intermediate of glycolysis/gluconeogenesis) and UDP-galactose, which is critical for the synthesis of lactose, glycolipids, glycoproteins, and glycosaminoglycans. The mechanism of galactose metabolism involves the following events (▶ Fig. 12.15):

Cellular entrapment via phosphorylation. Galactokinase (GALK) catalyzes the ATP-dependent phosphorylation of galactose on carbon 1 to generate galactose 1-phosphate. As with the phosphorylation of glucose and fructose, the phosphorylation of galactose allows it to be trapped within the cell so that it can be metabolized further.

- Galactokinase deficiency is an autosomal recessive disorder in which GALK is defective. This results in the accumulation of galactose and galactitol (in the lens of the eyes and neural tissue). The symptoms of this disorder, which is also known as galactosemia type 2, manifest when infants ingest milk.
- Galactitol, the reduced form of galactose, accumulates when galactose levels are chronically high, and like sorbitol, it is osmotically active.

Uridine monophosphate (UMP) exchange. Galactose 1-phosphate uridyltransferase (GALT) catalyzes the transfer of UMP from UDP-glucose (leaving glucose 1-phosphate) onto galactose 1-phosphate (forming UDP-galactose). The glucose 1-phosphate is then converted to glucose 6-phosphate (by phosphoglucomutase) and utilized in glycolysis or gluconeogenesis.

- Classic galactosemia is an autosomal recessive disorder in which GALT is defective. It causes galactose 1-phosphate and galactitol to accumulate in the cells of the lenses, liver, nerves, and kidneys. This resulting damage to affected tissues manifests as cataracts, liver damage, and severe mental retardation. Signs and symptoms appear within a few days of starting breast or formula milk.
- Epimerization of the newly formed UDP-galactose by UDP-galactose 4-epimerase (GALE) regenerates UDP-glucose.
- Epimerase deficiency is a rare autosomal recessive disorder caused by a defect in GALE and leads to a milder form of galactosemia.

UDP-glucose and UDP-galactose. The "activated" or UDP-bound form of glucose can be obtained from glucose 1-phosphate and UTP via the action of UDP-glucose pyrophosphorylase (a glycogenesis enzyme). UDP-galactose is used to synthesize lactose (in mammary glands) or to attach galactose to glycolipids, glycoproteins, and glycosaminoglycans.

Therapeutics
High-fructose corn syrup and obesity

Consumption of high-fructose corn syrup (HFCS) has increased by 4000%, from 1.5 lb per capita yearly intake in 1970 to 63 lb in 2000. Although fructose raises blood sugar less than sucrose (glycemic index of 32 vs 92), it is more efficiently converted into fat because its metabolism bypasses the rate-limiting step of PFK-1. Therefore, it has been hypothesized that fructose consumption may contribute to obesity and to insulin resistance. However, it should be noted that the fructose content of HFCS is 55%, which is only slightly greater than that of sucrose (50%). Thus, the increased rate of obesity in the U.S. in the past 50 years may have more to do with increased calorie consumption than with fructose consumption alone.

Therapeutics
Semen and seminal vesicles

Spermatozoa of many species, including humans, appear to use fructose rather than glucose as the primary energy nutrient. Fructose is the major carbohydrate in the seminal plasma and contributes to seminal motility. It is produced by the seminal vesicles from glucose via sorbitol (polyol pathway). In addition to GLUT3, sperm cells display GLUT5 transporters that are specific for fructose. The rate of production of fructose by the seminal vesicles appears to be under the influence of serum testosterone. In patients with asthenozoospermia (infertility due to reduced sperm motility), sperm motility correlates with corrected seminal fructose level (seminal fructose multiplied with logarithm of sperm count).

IV

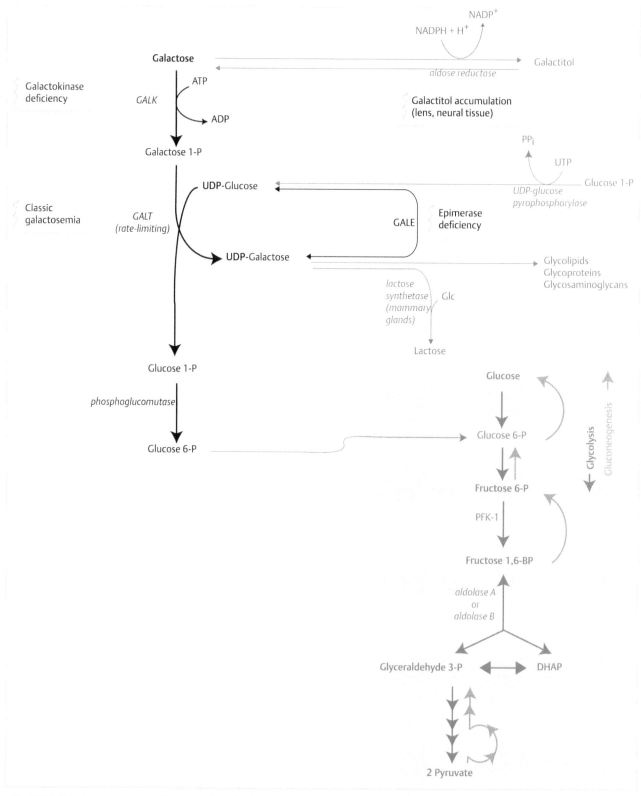

Fig. 12.15 Galactose metabolism. The metabolism of galactose generates glucose 6-phosphate, an intermediate that can be used in glycolysis, gluconeogenesis, and even the pentose phosphate pathway. Defects in galactokinase (GALK) and the rate-limiting galactose 1-phosphate uridyltransferase (GALT) are respectively associated with galactokinase deficiency and classic galactosemia. Galactose can also be converted to the osmotically active galactitol, which accumulates in lens and neural tissue when galactose levels are chronically high. Galactose metabolism requires uridine diphosphate (UDP)-glucose and releases UDP-galactose. The latter can be used to regenerate the former via UDP-galactose-4-epimerase (GALE) (which is hampered in epimerase deficiency) or utilized in pathways that generate lactose (in mammary glands) or generate glycosylated biomolecules (e.g., glycolipids, glycoproteins, and glycosaminoglycans). UDP-glucose is also generated in the glycogenesis pathway (see **Fig. 12.9**) via the action of UDP-glucose pyrophosphorylase. ADP, adenosine diphosphate; ATP, adenosine triphosphate; DHAP, dihydroxyacetone phosphate; Glc, glucose; NADPH, reduced form of nicotinamide adenine dinucleotide phosphate; P, phosphate; PPi, pyrophosphate; UTP, uridine triphosphate.

Therapeutics

Lactose intolerance

Lactose intolerance is an inability to digest lactose in dairy products caused by a deficiency (partial or total) of lactase. In a large majority of individuals, small intestinal lactase expression starts to decrease by the age of 2 or 3 years and reaches a minimum by age 10. Lactase persistence is due the dominant expression of the persistence allele in individuals who are lactose tolerant. Without lactase, lactose remains in the intestinal lumen, where it presents an osmotic load, resulting in diarrhea. Excess gas is also produced by microbial fermentation of the luminal lactose to methane and hydrogen gas. The symptoms of lactose intolerance can be minimized in lactose-intolerant individuals by either limiting their intake of dairy products, consuming lactase-containing foods, or oral ingestion of drugs (e.g., Lactaid) with a meal that is high in dairy.

Therapeutics

Galactosemia

Classic galactosemia (galactose in the blood) occurs when the conversion of galactose to glucose 1-phosphate is prevented due to galactose 1-P uridyltransferase (GALT) deficiency. Symptoms in neonates include failure to thrive, liver failure, sepsis, and bleeding. In the milder, Duarte variant form of the disease, there is 5–25% residual GALT activity in erythrocytes. Nonclassic galactosemia occurs when the conversion of galactose to galactose 1-phosphate is prevented due to a defect in galactokinase (GALK) or when UDP-galactose cannot be epimerized to UDP-glucose due to a defect in UDP-galactose epimerase (GALE). Galactose and galactitol (formed from galactose by aldose reductase in the polyol pathway only when there is galactosemia) accumulate in the blood and urine (galactosuria). Galactitol deposition in the eye leads to cataracts in early infancy. In addition, GALT deficiency leads to hepatomegaly. Cataracts are preventable if the disorder is detected early and galactose intake is restricted. Newborns in the USA are routinely screened for galactosemia.

Therapeutics

Sugar alcohols and cataracts in diabetic patients (diabetic retinopathy)

One mechanism by which cellular levels of the sugar alcohol (polyol) sorbitol are reduced is by the action of sorbitol dehydrogenase, an enzyme that converts sorbitol into fructose. Cells such as the lens and retina of the eye do not express sorbitol dehydrogenase and are therefore susceptible to the effects of sorbitol—an osmotically active compound that cannot freely cross membranes. When sorbitol accumulates in the cells, it triggers the influx of water into the affected cells, which swell (which applies pressure to surrounding cells/tissue) or burst (which destroys cells). Sorbitol accumulation is prevalent in individuals with chronic hyperglycemia (e.g., diabetics) and presents as cataracts, retinopathy, and peripheral neuropathy.

Therapeutics

Fructokinase deficiency—essential fructosuria

Fructosuria is the presence of high concentrations of fructose in urine. It is often caused by genetic mutations that create deficiencies in enzymes involved in fructose metabolism. For instance, an asymptomatic autosomal recessive disorder called essential fructosuria (a benign condition) is marked by a hepatic deficiency in fructokinase, an enzyme that phosphorylates fructose into fructose 1-phosphate. As a consequence, fructose accumulates and is excreted in urine.

Therapeutics

Aldolase B deficiency—hereditary fructose intolerance

Hereditary fructose intolerance is a destructive autosomal recessive disorder caused by a deficiency in hepatic aldolase B, an enzyme that cleaves fructose 1-phosphate into glyceraldehyde and dihydroxyacetone phosphate (DHAP). Without this enzyme, fructose and fructose 1-phosphate accumulate. The latter sequesters cellular phosphorus, which is necessary for critical phosphorylation reactions (e.g., generation of ATP). This condition damages the liver and may lead to kidney disease/failure. Individuals with this condition present with low blood levels of phosphorus (hypophosphatemia) and glucose (hypoglycemia) and have a low tolerance for foods high in fructose and sucrose.

Therapeutics

Detecting reducing sugars in urine

Sugars with a free oxygen on the anomeric carbon (e.g., most aldoses, including glucose) can reduce ferric or cupric ions and are therefore called reducing sugars. This property can be utilized to measure glucose in biological fluids using Benedict's reagent (copper sulfate). When the cupric (Cu^{2+}) ions in Benedict's reagent are reduced to cuprous (Cu^+) ions by reducing sugars such as glucose or galactose, the reagent changes color from blue to red or reddish brown. Disaccharides such as lactose and maltose (but not sucrose) can reduce Benedict's reagent. Fructose (a ketose) is not a reducing sugar per se but tautomerizes to an aldose under the alkaline conditions of Benedict's reagent. Early clinical methods for the diagnosis of diabetes mellitus utilized this test to detect the presence of glucose in urine. When plasma glucose levels are > 180 mg/dL, the capacity of renal proximal tubules to resorb glucose is exceeded, and glucose spills over into urine.

Normal

Lactose synthetase

Lactose synthetase is a complex of two proteins, β-D-galactosyltransferase and α-lactalbumin. The presence of α-lactalbumin (which is found only in lactating mammary glands and whose synthesis is increased in response to the hormone prolactin) alters the activity of β-D-galactosyltransferase by lowering its K_m for glucose such that it efficiently transfers galactose from UDP-galactose onto glucose to form lactose. In the absence of α-lactalbumin, β-D-galactosyltransferase instead transfers galactose onto *N*-acetyl-D-glucosamine to form *N*-acetyllactosamine. α-Lactalbumin can also bind metal ions such as Ca^{2+} and Zn^{2+} and act as a tumoricidal agent.

12.5 Pentose Phosphate Pathway

The pentose phosphate pathway (also known as the pentose shunt or hexose monophosphate shunt) is another means by which cells oxidize glucose. However, instead of generating ATP, NADH, and pyruvate like the oxidation of glucose via glycolysis, the pentose phosphate pathway oxidizes the phosphorylated form of glucose to produce the molecules boldfaced in the following reaction summary:

3 Glucose 6-P + 6 NADP⁺ → 3 Ribulose 5-P → 2 Fructose 6-P + Glyceraldehyde 3-P + 3 CO₂ + 6 NADPH + 6 H⁺

Two of its key products, ribulose 5-phosphate and NADPH, function as follows:
- **Ribulose 5-P:** This pentose can be isomerized into ribose 5-phosphate, which provides the sugar backbone for nucleotide biosynthesis.
- **NADPH:** This reduced coenzyme is critical for reductive biosyntheses (e.g., fatty acid and steroid syntheses) and for other reductive reactions that protect cells against damage by oxidizing agents and infection (▶ Fig. 12.16).

12.5.1 Mechanism

The pentose phosphate pathway occurs in the cytosol in two phases: the irreversible oxidative phase and the reversible non-oxidative (regenerative) phase (▶ Fig. 12.17).

Oxidative phase: 1 Glucose 6-P + 2 NADP⁺ + H₂O → 1 Ribulose 5-P + 1 CO₂ + 2 NADPH + 2 H⁺

Nonoxidative phase: 3 Ribulose 5-P ↔ 2 Fructose 6-P + Glyceraldehyde 3-P

Oxidative phase: The three irreversible reactions of this phase carry out the oxidation of glucose 6-phosphate into ribulose 5-phosphate while generating 2 NADPH and 1 CO₂. The latter two molecules are generated by the actions of the following enzymes:

- **Glucose 6-phosphate dehydrogenase (G6PD):** This enzyme catalyzes the committed, rate-limiting reaction that oxidizes glucose 6-phosphate into 6-phosphoglucono-δ-lactone. In doing so, it reduces NADP⁺ to NADPH. G6PD is highly specific for NADP⁺ and is inhibited by high levels of the product NADPH.
- **6-Phosphogluconolactone hydrolase:** Also known as gluconolactonase, this enzyme hydrolyzes 6-phosphogluconolactone to 6-phosphogluconate.
- **6-Phosphogluconate dehydrogenase:** This enzyme, which also uses NADP⁺, catalyzes the third reaction in which 6-phosphogluconate is decarboxylated to form ribulose 5-phosphate. In doing so, the carbon from the carbon 1 position is lost as CO₂, and NADP⁺ is reduced to NADPH.
  - NADPH can be used to regenerate the reduced form of glutathione (G-SH) through the action of glutathione reductase. G-SH is an antioxidant that serves as a coenzyme for glutathione peroxidase, an enzyme that detoxifies hydrogen peroxide (H₂O₂) by converting it into water (▶ Fig. 12.17). In red blood cells, this detoxification reaction is particularly important because it helps to protect membrane lipids from oxidative damage.
  - G6PD deficiency is an X-linked genetic defect that affects a significant number of people—particularly those of African descent. Individuals with this deficiency present with hemolytic anemia when the demand for the already low levels of NADPH is elevated. Demand for NADPH goes up when an individual contracts an infection, consumes fava beans, or takes oxidizing medications (e.g., antimalarials, sulfonamides, some antibiotics, and some antipyretics; see ▶ Table 12.4).

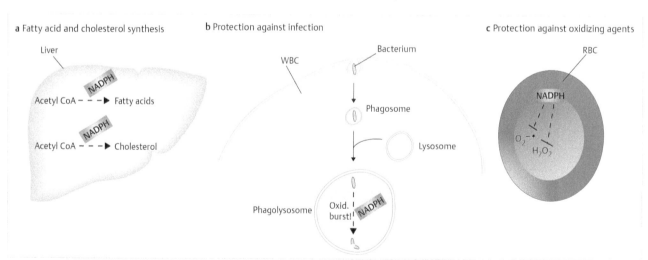

Fig. 12.16 Roles for NADPH in cellular processes. Nicotinamide adenine dinucleotide phosphate (NADPH) provides the reducing power in key processes such as **(a)** the synthesis of fatty acids and cholesterol, **(b)** protection against infection, **(c)** Regeneration of reduced glutathione required for detoxification of hydrogen peroxide. CoA, coenzyme A; Oxid. burst, oxidative burst; RBC, red blood cell; WBC, white blood cell.

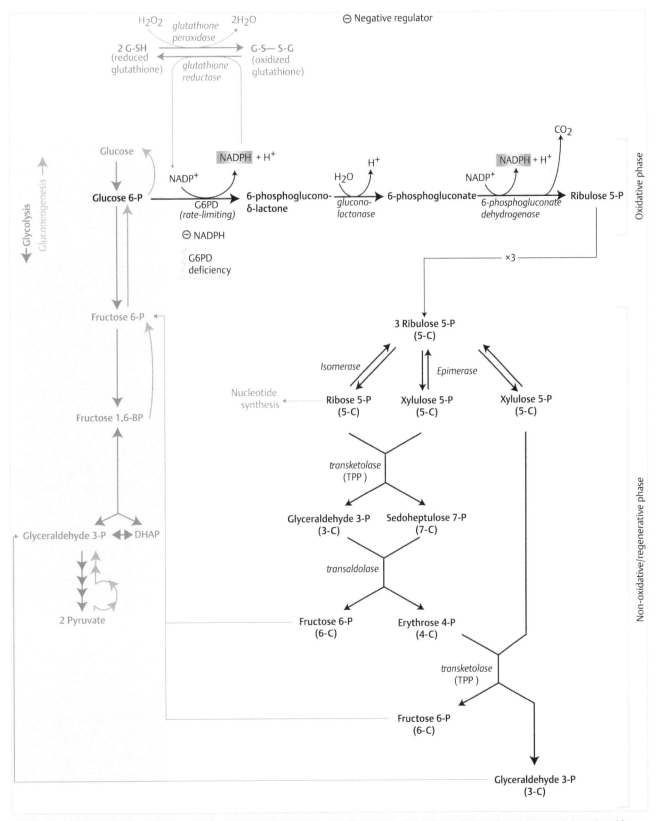

Fig. 12.17 Pentose phosphate pathway: oxidative and regenerative. Glucose 6-phosphate is oxidized to ribulose 5-phosphate and the reduced form of nicotinamide adenine dinucleotide phosphate (NADPH) during the oxidative portion of the pentose phosphate pathway, which is reduced in glucose 6-phosphate dehydrogenase (G6PD) deficiency. Isomerization of ribulose 5-phosphate generates ribose 5-phosphate, a substrate critical for the synthesis of nucleotides. NADPH is used by glutathione reductase to generate reduced glutathione, which is essential for glutathione peroxidase's neutralization of hydrogen peroxide (H_2O_2) to water. During the regenerative part of this pathway, three ribulose 5-phosphates are used to produce two fructose 6-phosphates and one glyceraldehyde 3-phosphate, which are used to regenerate glucose 6-phosphate, given that they are intermediates in the glycolysis/gluconeogenesis pathway. C, carbon; DHAP, dihydroxyacetone phosphate; P, phosphate; TPP, thiamine pyrophosphate; × 3, three times.

Table 12.4 Oxidizing medications

Medication class	Examples	Clinical use/Application
Antibiotics	Sulfamethoxazole Chloramphenicol	Urinary tract infections, cerebral abscesses due to staphylococci, bacterial meningitis (chloramphenicol can cause bone marrow toxicity and is not used much anymore)
Antipyretics	Acetanilide	Metabolized to paracetamol (acetaminophen), which has antipyretic activity (however, acetanilide causes cyanosis due to the formation of methemoglobin and is no longer used)
Antimalarials	Primaquine	Malaria, pneumocystis pneumonia, methemoglobinemia
Sulfonamides	Dapsone	Leprosy, dermatitis herpetiformis, pneumocystis pneumonia, acne, hemolysis, methemoglobinemia

Nonoxidative phase: Also known as the regenerative phase, it consists of a series of reversible reactions that start with the isomerization and epimerization of three molecules of ribulose 5-phosphate, followed by reactions in which two- and three-carbon segments are transferred between intermediates. The end result is the production of two fructose 6-phosphates and one glyceraldehyde 3-phosphate. The following are key features of the two enzymes that catalyze the transfer reactions:

1. **Transketolase:** This enzyme requires thiamine pyrophosphate as a coenzyme and catalyzes the transfer of two-carbon segments.
   - Mutations in the transketolase-like gene (*TKLT1*) have been implicated in neurodegenerative disease, diabetes, and cancer.
   - Transketolase activity in erythrocytes is used as a tool to determine the vitamin B_1 (thiamine) status of an individual

2. **Transaldolase:** This enzyme catalyzes the transfer of three-carbon segments.

Modulation of Oxidative and Nonoxidative Phases in Response to Cellular Demands

High demand for ribose 5-phosphate: In actively dividing cells, for which the demand for ribose 5-phosphate for nucleotide synthesis is high, the oxidative phase is favored. As a result, ribulose 5-phosphate is preferentially isomerized to ribose 5-phosphate (over epimerization to xylulose 5-phosphate).

- Because the reactions of the nonoxidative phase are reversible, it is possible to synthesize ribose 5-phosphate from fructose 6-phosphate and glyceraldehyde 3-phosphate without going through the oxidative phase of the pathway.

Demand for NADPH: When the demand for NADPH is greater than that for ribose 5-phosphate, the products of the nonoxidative phase (fructose 6-P and glyceraldehyde 3-P) are channeled into the gluconeogenic pathway for conversion into glucose 6-phosphate and reentry into the pentose phosphate pathway. However, defects in enzymes that facilitate their conversion to glucose 6-phosphate redirect fructose 6-P and glyceraldehyde 3-P into the glycolytic pathway (▶ Fig. 12.17).

- In lactating mammary gland and adipose tissue (which synthesize fatty acids), the activity of the pentose phosphate pathway is very high. Fatty acid synthesis requires a very active source of reducing power, given that 14 to 16 NADPHs are needed for every fatty acid (i.e., 16-carbon palmitate) made from acetyl CoA. Approximately half of these NADPHs come from the pentose phosphate pathway. Lung and liver also exhibit moderately high activity of the pentose phosphate pathway.

- In phagocytic cells (e.g., white blood cells engaged in killing bacteria), the activity of the pentose phosphate pathway is also very high. In white blood cells, NADPH is needed for the respiratory burst (or oxidative burst) response to invading microorganisms (▶ Fig. 12.18). In short, respiratory burst produces O_2-derived free radicals, which lead to the formation of the bacteria-killing agents H_2O_2 and hypochlorite (bleach). NADPH is also used in these cells to regenerate reduced glutathione (G-SH), which is needed for the neutralization of excess H O produced in response to invading bacteria.

Normal

NADPH in nitric oxide synthesis

Nitric oxide synthases (NOSs) are enzymes containing heme and flavin nucleotides that generate nitric oxide (NO) while oxidizing l-arginine to l-citrulline. The reaction requires two molecules of O_2 and 1.5 molecules of NADPH. The enzyme has three major isoforms: neuronal (NOSI), inducible (NOSII or iNOS), and endothelial (NOSIII or eNOS). NO is an important signaling molecule that uses cGMP as its second messenger. The NOSI product acts as a neurotransmitter, the NOSII product is antimicrobial, and NO produced by NOSIII acts as a vasodilator and an inhibitor of platelet aggregation.

Normal

Glutathione: a protective agent

Glutathione is γ-glutamylcysteinylglycine, in which the γ-carboxyl group of glutamate is in an amide linkage with the a-amino group of cysteine. In its reduced form (free SH), glutathione acts as a protective scavenging agent against hydrogen peroxide and other strong oxidizing agents. In red blood cells, if these agents are not neutralized, they will oxidize hemoglobin iron to the ferric state and also oxidize membrane lipids. Methemoglobin cannot carry oxygen, and the membranes will become very fragile leading to hemolysis. Thus, reduced glutathione helps to keep hemoglobin in the Fe^{2+} state (via the action of methemoglobin reductase) and helps to maintain red blood cell membrane integrity. It can be used up, however, and when fully converted to G-S-S-G (the oxidized form), it no longer functions as a protective agent.

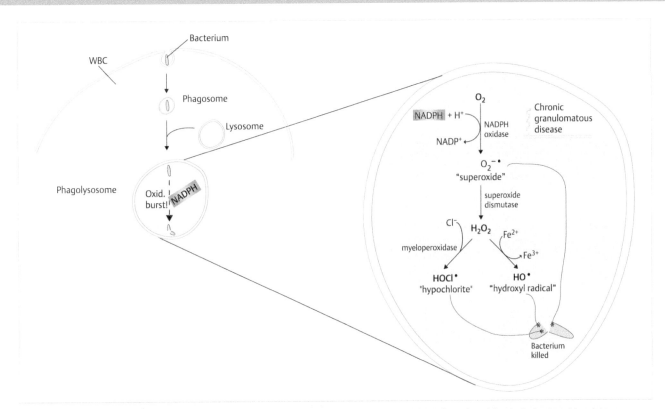

Fig. 12.18 Respiratory burst. The phagocytic white blood cells engaged in killing bacteria utilize the reduced form of nicotinamide adenine dinucleotide phosphate (NADPH) in the respiratory burst (or oxidative burst) response to invading microorganisms. This response produces O_2-derived free radicals, which lead to the formation of the bacteria-killing agents H_2O_2 and hyperchlorite (bleach). NADPH is also used in these cells to regenerate reduced glutathione (G-SH), which is needed for the neutralization of excess H_2O_2 that enters the cytosol (see ▶ Fig. 12.17). Oxid. burst; oxidative burst; WBC, white blood cell.

Therapeutics
Oxidizing drugs
The cytochrome P-450 drug metabolizing system consists of several cytochrome P-450 s (CYP) and NADPH-cytochrome P-450 reductase (CPR). In human liver, the ratio of CYP:CPR is 4:1, making the CPR rate-limiting. Thus, many CYP isozymes compete for the electrons provided by CPR. This competition for electrons from NADPH is a basis for adverse drug interactions among drugs metabolized by different CYP isozymes.

Normal
Fava beans and H_2O_2
In X-linked deficiency of glucose 6-phosphate dehydrogenase (G6PD), the erythrocytes are susceptible to rupture due to oxidative stress. Such stress can be induced by oxidant drugs and also by the ingestion of fava beans (particularly in people of Middle Eastern descent). Fava bean toxicity (favism) causes acute hemolysis, jaundice, headache, nausea, fever, and methemoglobinemia. Fava beans contain oxidizing agents such as divicine, isouramil, and convicine. Erythrocytes require an intact glutathione (GSH) system to detoxify H_2O_2 generated by divicine and other components of fava beans. Regeneration of GSH, which requires NADPH, is defective in G6PD deficiency.

12.6 Modified Carbohydrates in Glycosylated Biomolecules

In addition to their use as a source of energy, carbohydrates are important structural components of various biomolecules, such as glycoproteins, glycolipids, glycosaminoglycans, and proteoglycans. In addition to neutral monosaccharides, the carbohydrates found in these biomolecules include acidic monosaccharides and amino sugars (▶ Fig. 12.19):

- *Acidic monosaccharides* are sugars that have been modified to include a carboxylic acid group. They include D-glucuronic acid (GlcA) and L-iduronic acid (IdoA), which are derived from D-glucose, and D-galacturonic acid (GalA), which is derived from D-galactose.
  - Of noteworthy mention is *N*-acetylneuraminic acid (Neu5Ac), which is also known as sialic acid or NANA. It is a nine-carbon acidic sugar derived from mannose (six carbons) and pyruvate (three carbons).

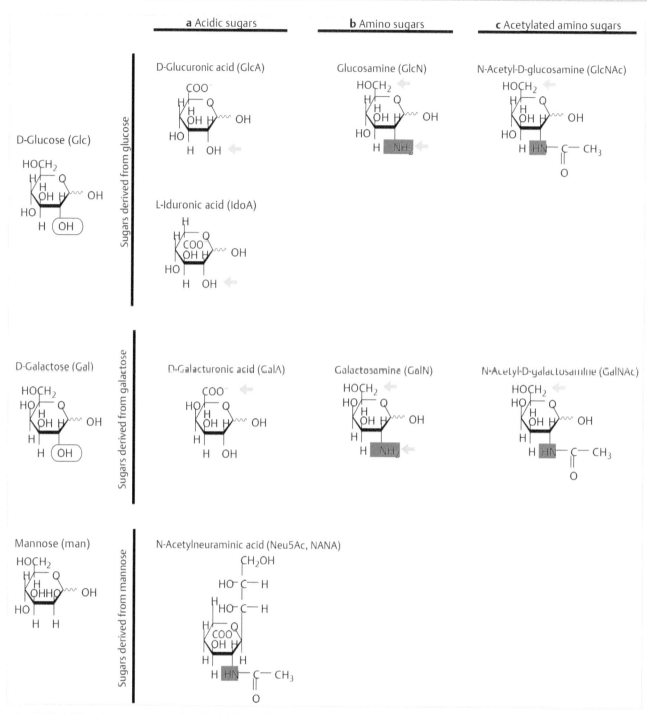

Fig. 12.19 Acidic and amino monosaccharides. (a) The acidic sugars are derived from glucose and galactose by changing the functional group of carbon 6 to a carboxylic acid group (highlighted yellow). (b) The amino sugars are derived from glucose and galactose by changing the hydroxyl group attached to carbon 2, to an amino group (highlighted pink). (c) Acetylation of the amino group on glucosamine or galactosamine generates their N-acetylated forms. Acetyl coenzyme A (CoA) is the donor of the acetyl group. The green arrow indicates sites of sulfation.

- *Amino sugars* are modified versions of sugars in which a hydroxyl group is replaced by an amino group. Examples include glucosamine (GlcN) and galactosamine (GalN), which are often acetylated to form N-acetyl-d-glucosamine (GlcNAc) and N-acetyl-d-galactosamine (GalNAc), respectively.

The following four key biomolecules contain unmodified, acidic, and amino sugars:

1. **Glycoproteins:** These are proteins that are attached to a short, branched, heteropolysaccharide chain via O- and N-glycosidic bonds (► Fig. 12.20, ► Fig. 12.21a).
   - In an O-glycosidic bond, the heteropolysaccharide is attached to the hydroxyl oxygen of a serine or threonine residue.
   - In an N-glycosidic bond, the heteropolysaccharide is attached to the amide nitrogen of an asparagine residue. The heteropolysaccharide residue that forms the N-glycosidic

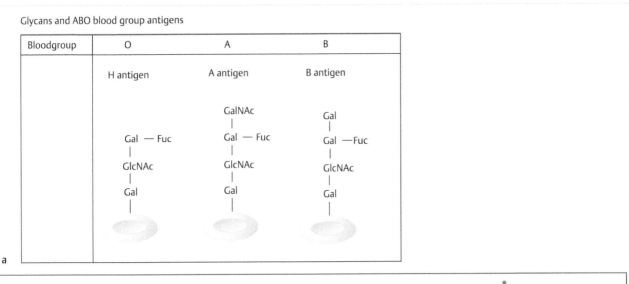

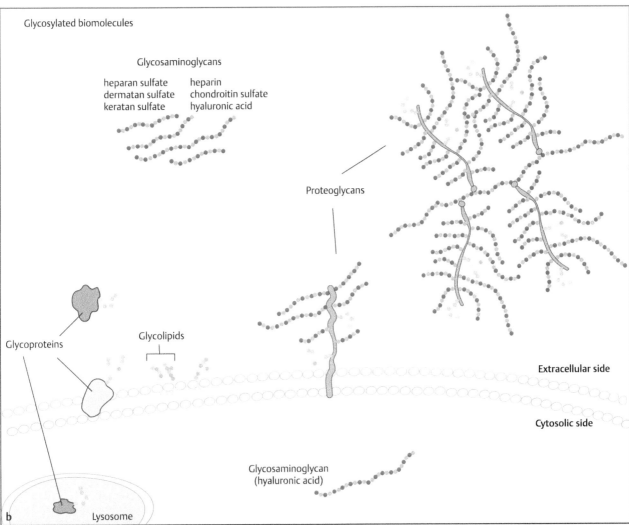

Fig. 12.20 Glycosylated biomolecules. (a) Glycans form the basis of the ABO blood group typing. They are antigenic determinants on membrane glycoproteins and glycolipids. Initially, the H antigen is formed. An additional sugar is then added by a glycosyltransferase specified by the allele in the ABO blood group locus. When the allele present is *N*-acetylgalactosamine transferase, an A group antigen is made. When it is a galactosyltransferase, a B group antigen is made. When both alleles are present, an AB blood group results, and the absence of both alleles yields an O blood group. **(b)** Glycoproteins, glycolipids, glycosaminoglycans, and proteoglycans are composed of unmodified and modified sugars. Fuc, fucose; Gal, galactose; GlcNAc, *N*-acetyl-D-glucosamine.

IV

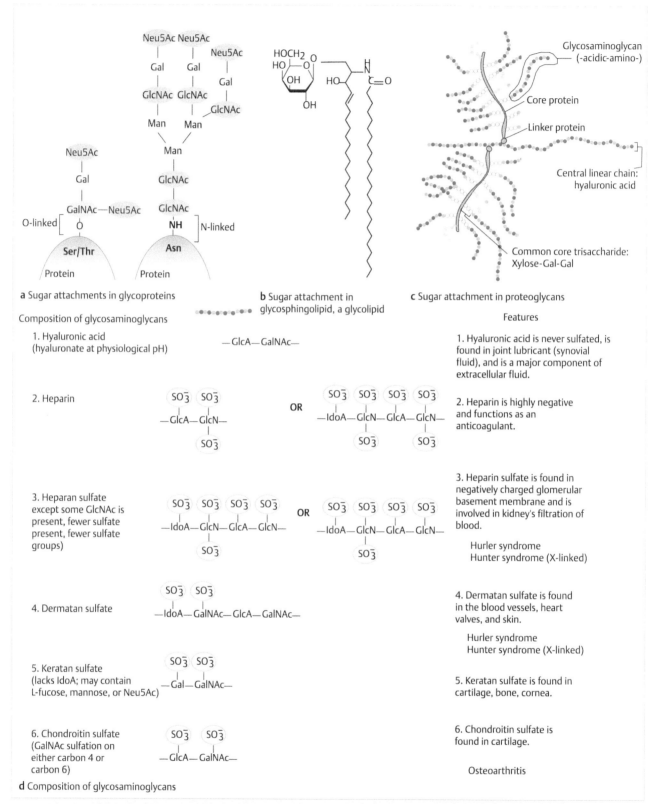

a Sugar attachments in glycoproteins

b Sugar attachment in glycosphingolipid, a glycolipid

c Sugar attachment in proteoglycans

Composition of glycosaminoglycans

Features

1. Hyaluronic acid (hyaluronate at physiological pH)	—GlcA—GalNAc—	1. Hyaluronic acid is never sulfated, is found in joint lubricant (synovial fluid), and is a major component of extracellular fluid.
2. Heparin	SO_3^- SO_3^- —GlcA—GlcN— SO_3^- **OR** SO_3^- SO_3^- SO_3^- SO_3^- —IdoA—GlcN—GlcA—GlcN— SO_3^- SO_3^-	2. Heparin is highly negative and functions as an anticoagulant.
3. Heparan sulfate except some GlcNAc is present, fewer sulfate present, fewer sulfate groups)	SO_3^- SO_3^- SO_3^- SO_3^- —IdoA—GlcN—GlcA—GlcN— SO_3^- **OR** SO_3^- SO_3^- SO_3^- SO_3^- —IdoA—GlcN—GlcA—GlcN— SO_3^-	3. Heparin sulfate is found in negatively charged glomerular basement membrane and is involved in kidney's filtration of blood. Hurler syndrome Hunter syndrome (X-linked)
4. Dermatan sulfate	SO_3^- SO_3^- —IdoA—GalNAc—GlcA—GalNAc—	4. Dermatan sulfate is found in the blood vessels, heart valves, and skin. Hurler syndrome Hunter syndrome (X-linked)
5. Keratan sulfate (lacks IdoA; may contain L-fucose, mannose, or Neu5Ac)	SO_3^- SO_3^- —Gal—GalNAc—	5. Keratan sulfate is found in cartilage, bone, cornea.
6. Chondroitin sulfate (GalNAc sulfation on either carbon 4 or carbon 6)	SO_3^- SO_3^- —GlcA—GalNAc—	6. Chondroitin sulfate is found in cartilage. Osteoarthritis

d Composition of glycosaminoglycans

Fig. 12.21 Sugar attachments in glycosylated molecules. (a) In glycoproteins, sugars are attached to serine/threonine residues via an *O*-glycosidic bond or asparagine residues via an *N*-glycosidic bond. The first five sugars in an *N*-linked heteropolysaccharide are two GlcNAc and three mannose residues. (b) This glycosphingolipid (a glycolipid) is attached to Gal via an *O*-glycosidic bond. (c) This proteoglycan is composed of a central chain of hyaluronic acid to which linker and core proteins are attached. Most of the glycosaminoglycans are attached to the core protein via a trisaccharide of xylose and two galactose molecules. (d) Summary of the sugar com position, degree of sulfation, functional features, and clinical correlates of six types of glycosaminoglycans. Asn, asparagine; Gal, galactose; GalNAc, *N*-acetyl-D-galactosamine; GlcA, D-glucuronic acid; GlcN, glucosamine; GlcNAc, *N*-acetyl-D-glucosamine; IdoA, L-iduronic acid; Man, mannose; Neu5Ac, *N*-acetylneuraminic acid; Ser, serine; SO_3^-, sulfate group; Thr, threonine.

bond is always GlcNAc, and this residue is attached to another GlcNAc and three mannose (Mann) residues, forming the core of all *N*-linked glycoproteins. Glycoproteins are glycosylated posttranslationally in the rough endoplasmic reticulum and the Golgi apparatus and distributed to different locations to carry out their various functions, as follows:

- Cell surface: Glycoproteins found on the surface of cells include integrins and antibodies (▶ Fig. 12.20a). They respectively function in cell adhesion and the immune response.
- Blood plasma: Except for albumin, the majority of proteins found in plasma (the fluid component of blood) are glycoproteins. They play a role in the immune response, blood clotting, transport, and modulating the activities of enzymes.
- Lysosome: The hydrolytic enzymes that digest old cells or food components in lysosomes are glycoproteins.

2. **Glycolipids**: These are lipids that are attached to carbohydrate residues. They are found on the outer leaflet of plasma membranes, where they serve to stabilize the membrane and participate in cell adhesion (▶ Fig. 12.20b, ▶ Fig. 12.21b).

- Glycosphingolipids, such as cerebroside, are built on a ceramide lipid moiety that consists of a long-chain amino alcohol (sphingosine) in an amide linkage to a fatty acid. In comparison, glycoglycerolipids, such as seminolipid, are built on a diacyl or acylalkylglycerol lipid moiety.
- Most animal glycolipids are glycosphingolipids. Gangliosides, found in the nervous system, are acid glycosphingolipids that contain sialic acid.

Normal

Glycocalyx

The outer leaflet of many biomembranes is covered with a carbohydrate shell (glycocalyx), created by the presence of glycolipids and glycosylated proteins (glycoproteins). The glycocalyx has three key functions: (1) Protection: The carbohydrate shell protects membrane components from mechanical injury or premature enzymatic degradation. (2) Cell adhesion: The glycocalyx enables cells to make stable contacts with other cells, an important function for tissue formation and fertilization. (3) Cell identification: The glycocalyx allows the body to differentiate its own healthy cells from foreign and diseased cells.

- Glycosphingolipids are degraded from the non-reducing end, one carbohydrate residue at a time, by exoglycosidases. Additional activator proteins, called saposins, aid in the presentation of sugars to lysosomal enzymes. Deficiencies in the exoglycosidases can cause glycolipid storage disorders (sphingolipidoses) with serious consequences (▶ Fig. 12.22).

1. **Glycosaminoglycans**: These long, unbranched heteropolysaccharides contain repeating disaccharide units composed primarily of an acidic monosaccharide and an amino sugar. The six physiologically relevant glycosaminoglycans include heparan sulfate, dermatan sulfate, heparin, keratan sulfate (which does not contain an acid sugar), chondroitin sulfate, and hyaluronic acid (which is not sulfated) (▶ Fig. 12.20b, ▶ Fig. 12.21d).

Therapeutics

Deficiencies in lysosomal hydrolytic enzymes

Lysosomes contain 50 to 60 soluble hydrolytic enzymes to degrade a variety of macromolecules. Many of the deficiencies in lysosomal degradative enzymes are due to genetic defects in their expression. Deficiency of hexosaminidase A, which digests sphingolipids (derivatives of fatty acids), is the underlying cause of the autosomal recessive disorder Tay-Sachs disease. Deficiencies in α-1,4-glucosidase, an enzyme that degrades glycogen, leads to the glycogen storage disorder Pompe disease. Deficiencies in enzymes that degrade glycosaminoglycans cause a host of disorders collectively called mucopolysaccharidoses (▶ Fig. 12.23), which include Hurler syndrome and Hunter syndrome. Both are marked by accumulations of heparin sulfate and dermatan sulfate. Hurler syndrome is an autosomal recessive disorder marked by a deficiency in α-L-iduronidase. Within 1 year after birth, patients present with coarse facial features, enlarged tongue, upper airway obstruction, mental retardation, corneal clouding, cardiomyopathy, hepatosplenomegaly, and developmental delay. Hunter syndrome is an X-linked disorder caused by a deficiency in iduronate sulfatase. These patients present with signs and symptoms similar to Hurler syndrome but of varying severity (mild to severe). Additionally, Hunter syndrome patients do not show signs of corneal clouding.

Key features of glycosaminoglycans include the following:
- They carry a large negative charge due to the acid sugar's carboxylic acid group (which is negatively charged at physiological pH) and varying amounts of sulfuric acid esterified to the sugars. The strong negative charge allows glycosaminoglycans to be heavily hydrated (i.e., bound to lots of water), which is key to the slippery or elastic nature of the fluids and connective tissue in which they are found.
- Mucopolysaccharidoses are a family of inherited disorders marked by defects in lysosomal hydrolases that degrade heparan sulfate or dermatan sulfate. These disorders include the autosomal recessive Hurler syndrome and the X-linked recessive Hunter syndrome (▶ Fig. 12.23).

2. **Proteoglycans**: These large protein–carbohydrate molecules (5% protein/95% carbohydrate) are composed of a central linear chain of hyaluronic acid to which core protein chains are attached (▶ Fig. 12.20, ▶ Fig. 12.21c). These core proteins serve as the site of attachment for multiple glycosaminoglycans, giving it its "bottlebrush" shape. A trisaccharide of xylose and two galactose molecules is commonly found at the site of attachment between the core protein and a glycosaminoglycan. (Xylose forms an *O*-glycosidic bond to a serine residue of the protein.) Proteoglycans are an essential constituent of the extracellular matrix (ECM), where they perform the following functions:
- Bind to cations and water
- Associate with other ECM components, such as fibronectin and elastin
- Control the movement of molecules through the ECM

IV

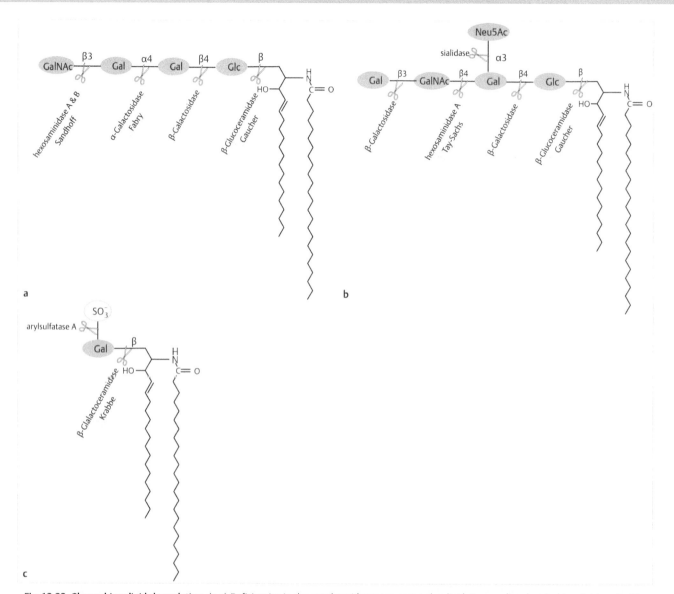

Fig. 12.22 Glycosphingolipid degradation. (a–c) Deficiencies in the exoglycosidases can cause glycolipid storage disorders (sphingolipidoses) with serious consequences. For instance, defects in hexosaminidase A cause Tay-Sachs disease with severe neurodegeneration and death within the first 5 years of life. In Sandhoff disease, both hex-osaminidase A and B are defective. Deficiency of a-galactosidase results in Fa bry disease, which causes severe pain, cornea l clouding, and renal and cerebrovascular disease. Lack of β -glucoceramidase can cause early-onset Gaucher disease with neurodegeneration and hepatosplenomegaly. Loss of β -galactoceramidase results in Krabbe disease with glycolipid accumulation in brain and loss of myelin. Gal, galactose; Glc, glucose; GlcNAc, N-acetyl-D-glucosamine; Neu5Ac, N-acetylneuraminic acid; SO⁻3, sulfate group; β3, α4, β4 are the specific types of bonds between the carbohydrate molecules.

Therapeutics
I-Cell disease

The hydrolytic enzymes of lysosomes are glycoproteins that contain mannose residues. After their synthesis in the rough endoplasmic reticulum (RER), the mannose residues on these proteins need to be phosphorylated for the proteins to be properly sorted through the *cis*- and *trans*-Golgi to the lysosomes. In I-cell disease, the enzyme N-acetylglucosamine-1-phosphotransferase (GlcNAc-PT) is deficient. As a result, all lysosomal hydrolases fail to be sorted properly and are instead secreted out into the bloodstream. Detection of lysosomal

hydrolases in the plasma distinguishes between defective synthesis and defective sorting.

Therapeutics
Osteoarthritis

Osteoarthritis is a noninflammatory degenerative joint disease caused by wear and tear on the joints. The articular cartilage becomes depleted, destroying chondroitin sulfate, and there are bony outgrowths at the margins. It commonly affects the

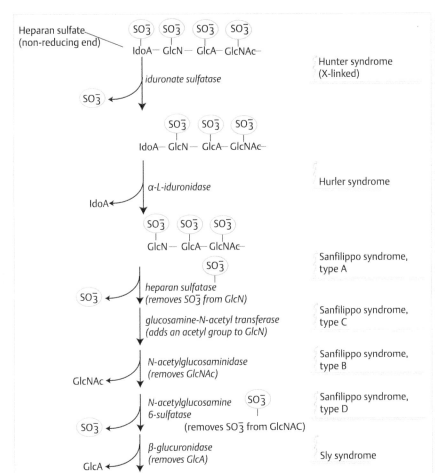

Fig. 12.23 Glycosaminoglycan degradation. Enzymes involved in the removal of sulfate groups and acidic or amino sugars during glycosaminoglycan degradation. The sugars are removed from the nonreducing ends. An endo-β-glucuronidase first cleaves large chains into smaller fragments, and each monosaccharide is then removed from the nonreducing end. N- and O-sulfate groups must first be removed before exoglycosidases can act. An unusual feature of heparin sulfate degradation is that this process also involves a synthetic step. After removal of the N-sulfate residue on GlcNSO⁻₃, the nonacetylated glucosamine must first be N-acetylated using acetyl CoA before α-N-acetylglucosaminidase can cleave this residue. Disorders (known as mucopolysaccharidoses) associated with defects in particular degradation enzymes are noted. GlcA, D-glucuronic acid; GlcN; glucosamine; GlcNAc, N-acetyl-D-glucosamine; IdoA, L-iduronic acid; SO⁻₃, sulfate group.

joints of the hand, hip, and knee and the zygapophyseal (facet) joints of the cervical and lumbar spine, causing pain, stiffness, and joint instability. Loss of hyaluronic acid (hyaluronan), an anionic non-sulfated glycosaminoglycan that is not covalently attached to any protein, from the synovial fluid of the joints

has also been implicated in osteoarthritis. Oral administration of chondroitin sulfate and glucosamine, alone or in combination, as well as injection of hyaluronic acid into the joints have provided limited benefit in the treatment of osteoarthritis.

13 Fatty Acid Metabolism

13.1 Lipids: Overview

Lipids are an extremely heterogeneous class of compounds that serve as the following:

1. **Fuel stores:** Lipids stored in adipose tissue as triacylglycerols (fats) are a major source of energy. They contain 9 kcal/g of energy, which is more than twice the amount contained in carbohydrates and proteins.
2. **Structural components:** Lipids are the primary components of cellular membranes and are critical for maintaining their structural integrity and function.
3. **Signaling molecules:** Lipids serve as signaling molecules that affect pathways that control cellular processes, such as cell growth, survival, and the immune response.
4. **Miscellaneous:** Brown adipose tissue functions in generating heat (thermogenesis), white adipose tissue provides insulation, and lipid components of bile play a role in the digestion of fat in the small intestine.

13.1.1 Lipid Classification

Lipids are divided broadly into two groups: the fatty acid derivatives and the isoprene derivatives (isoprenoids).

1. **Fatty acid derivatives:** These lipids contain fatty acids, that is, carboxylic acids with long, usually unbranched hydrocarbon chains that may be saturated (i.e., zero double bonds) (▶ Fig. 13.1a-1) or unsaturated (≥ 1 double bond). This group of lipids is further classified based on the core/backbone molecule to which the fatty acid chains are attached:
   - Glycerolipids contain one to three fatty acid chains attached to a glycerol backbone (▶ Fig. 13.1a-2) via ester bonds. Examples include mono- (▶ Fig. 13.1b-1), di-, and triacylglycerol.
   - Glycerophospholipids contain two fatty acid chains attached to a phosphorylated glycerol backbone; the phosphate group may also be esterified to another compound, such as an amino or sugar alcohol. Examples include phosphatidic acid (▶ Fig. 13.1b-2, ▶ Fig. 13.2), phosphatidylcholine, phosphatidylserine, phosphatidylethanolamine, and phosphatidylinositol.
   - Sphingophospholipids contain ceramide, a molecule made up of one fatty acid chain attached to sphingosine (▶ Fig. 13.1a-3, ▶ Fig. 13.2, ▶ Fig. 13.3) via an amide bond. In addition, they contain a phosphate group that is both attached to sphingosine and esterified to an amino or sugar alcohol. When the amino alcohol is choline, the resulting molecule is called sphingomyelin (▶ Fig. 13.1b-3, ▶ Fig. 13.2, ▶ Fig. 13.3).
   - Glycosphingolipids (also known as glycolipids) contain ceramide, to which one or more sugar residues are attached. Examples include cerebrosides (▶ Fig. 13.1b-4, ▶ Fig. 13.2, ▶ Fig. 13.3, ▶ Fig. 13.4) and gangliosides.
   - Eicosanoids are derived from the 20-carbon fatty acid arachidonic acid (see ▶ Fig. 13.13). Examples include prostaglandins, thromboxanes, leukotrienes, and hydroxy- and hydroperoxy fatty acids.

2. **Isoprene derivatives (isoprenoids):** These lipids are composed of multiple 5-carbon isoprene units that are linked
together to form linear chains or cyclic structures (▶ Fig. 13.1c-1). They include the lipid-soluble vitamins (A, D, E, K), ubiquinone (coenzyme Q), cholesterol, and the steroid hormones (▶ Fig. 13.1c-2). The metabolism of cholesterol and the steroid hormones is discussed in Chapter 14.

13.1.2 Acetyl Coenzyme A

Acetyl coenzyme A (acetyl CoA)—the "activated" form of acetic acid—is composed of an acetyl group attached to coenzyme A (CoA) via a high-energy thioester bond (▶ Fig. 13.2a, b). It is the most central molecule in lipid metabolism because it is generated in the mitochondrial matrix from the oxidative decarboxylation of pyruvate and from the degradation of fatty acids (via β-oxidation) and certain amino acids, and used as follows (▶ Fig. 13.2c):

- Acetyl CoA is the major precursor for the synthesis of fatty acid–derived lipids, isoprene-derived lipids (see Chapter 14), and ketone bodies (water-soluble compounds that serve as an energy source under conditions of starvation).
- Acetyl CoA is used to generate adenosine triphosphate (ATP) via entry into the tricarboxylic acid (TCA) cycle.

Normal
Fatty acid chain length

Fatty acids may be classified based on the number of carbon atoms into four types: short-chain fatty acids (SCFAs) contain fewer than 6 carbons, medium-chain fatty acids (MCFAs) have 6 to 12 carbons, long-chain fatty acids (LCFAs) have 13 to 20 carbons, and very long chain fatty acids (VLCFAs) contain 22 or more carbons.

13.2 Synthesis of Fatty Acids

Fatty acid synthesis takes place in liver, adipose tissue and lactating mammary gland. It involves the use of acetyl CoA to synthesize palmitate, a 16-carbon, saturated fatty acid. Fatty acid synthesis depends on the cooperative efforts of mitochondrial and cytosolic reactions, which can be divided into three phases (▶ Fig. 13.3):

- **Phase I—Cytosolic entry of acetyl CoA:** Because acetyl CoA is formed in the mitochondrial matrix, it must be transported to the cytosol to be used in the formation of fatty acid chains. The citrate shuttle is the transport mechanism that transfers acetyl units from the mitochondrial matrix to the cytosol.
- **Phase II—Generation of malonyl CoA:** An important substrate in fatty acid synthesis is malonyl CoA. The enzyme acetyl CoA carboxylase generates malonyl CoA by carboxylating acetyl CoA.
- **Phase III—Fatty acid chain formation:** Fatty acid synthase is the enzyme that catalyzes a series of seven reactions that incorporate acetyl CoA and malonyl CoA into a 16-carbon fatty acid chain.

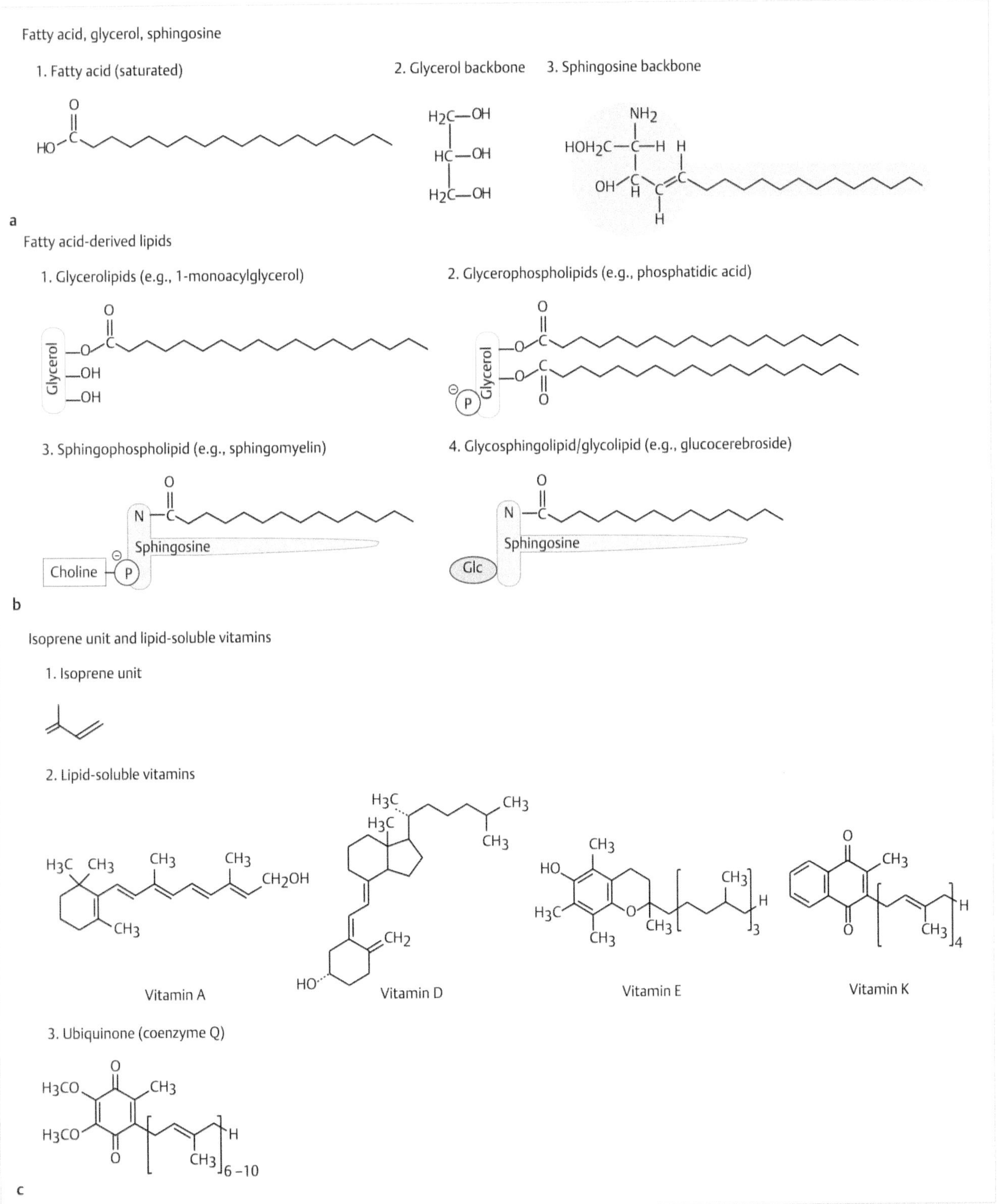

Fatty acid, glycerol, sphingosine

1. Fatty acid (saturated)   2. Glycerol backbone   3. Sphingosine backbone

a

Fatty acid-derived lipids

1. Glycerolipids (e.g., 1-monoacylglycerol)   2. Glycerophospholipids (e.g., phosphatidic acid)

3. Sphingophospholipid (e.g., sphingomyelin)   4. Glycosphingolipid/glycolipid (e.g., glucocerebroside)

b

Isoprene unit and lipid-soluble vitamins

1. Isoprene unit

2. Lipid-soluble vitamins

Vitamin A   Vitamin D   Vitamin E   Vitamin K

3. Ubiquinone (coenzyme Q)

c

Fig. 13.1 **Classification of lipids.** (a) Fatty acids are carboxylic acids with long, unbranched hydrocarbon chains that can be found attached to glycerol or sphingosine backbones. (b) Lipids that fall under the class of fatty acid derivatives include (1) glycerolipids (which contain one to three fatty acid chains attached to glycerol)(2) glycerophospholipids (which contain two fatty acid chains and a phosphate group attached to glycerol; some may also have an amino or sugar alcohol esterified to the phosphate group) (3) sphingophospholipids, and (4) glycosphingolipids (glycolipids); the latter two have a phosphate group or sugar residues attached to sphingosine, respectively. Some sphingophospholipids may have an amino or sugar alcohol esterified to their phosphate residue. (c) Isoprene-derived lipids such as vitamins A, D, E, and K and ubiquinone (coenzyme Q), are composed of multiple isoprene units linked together to form linear chains and cyclic structures.

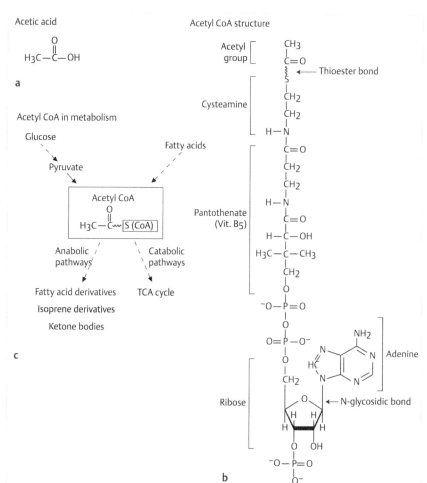

Fig. 13.2 Acetyl coenzyme. (a) Acetyl coenzyme A (acetyl CoA) is the "activated" form of the two-carbon building block acetic acid. **(b)** Acetyl CoA is composed of an acetyl group attached to coenzyme A via a high-energy thioester bond. **(c)** Acetyl CoA is formed from the oxidative decarboxylation of pyruvate and the degradation of fatty acids (via β-oxidation). It serves as the precursor for the synthesis of lipids (e.g., fatty acid-derived and isoprene-derived lipids) and ketone bodies. Acetyl CoA also enters the tricarboxylic acid (TCA) cycle to contribute to the production of adenosine triphosphate (ATP) via oxidative phosphorylation.

13.2.1 Mechanism

Phase I—Cytosolic Entry of Acetyl CoA via the Citrate Shuttle

Acetyl CoA is formed in the mitochondrial matrix, but it must be present in the cytosol in order for it to be used as a substrate in fatty acid biosynthetic reactions. Because it cannot directly cross the mitochondrial membrane, a special ATP-dependent transport mechanism called the citrate shuttle is employed to carry out the following two key functions (▶ Fig. 13.3):

1. **Transport acetyl CoA out of the mitochondria and into the cytosol.**
   - The citrate shuttle begins with the condensation of acetyl CoA with oxaloacetate to generate citrate. This step is catalyzed by the TCA cycle enzyme citrate synthase (step 1 in ▶ Fig. 13.3).
   - Citrate is then transported out of the mitochondrial matrix into the cytosol with the aid of a citrate transporter located in the inner mitochondrial membrane (step 2 in ▶ Fig. 13.3).
   - In the cytosol, citrate is converted back to acetyl CoA and oxaloacetate by ATP citrate lyase via a reaction that uses CoA and the energy from the hydrolysis of ATP into adenosine diphosphate (ADP) and inorganic phosphate (P_i) (step 3 in ▶ Fig. 13.3). Acetyl CoA can now be used to

synthesize fatty acids in the cytosol, and oxaloacetate is reduced to malate by malate dehydrogenase as the reduced form of nicotinamide adenine dinucleotide (NADH) is oxidized to nicotinamide adenine dinucleotide (NAD⁺) (step 4 in ▶ Fig. 13.3).
   - The activity of ATP citrate lyase is induced by glucose and insulin and negatively regulated by polyunsaturated fatty acids and leptin.

2. **Regenerate the TCA cycle intermediate oxaloacetate in the mitochondrial matrix.**
   - In order for the citrate shuttle to continue to operate, oxaloacetate must be regenerated in the mitochondrial matrix. This occurs via two possible mechanisms, one of which produces the reduced form of nicotinamide adenine dinucleotide phosphate (NADPH), an electron-carrying molecule that provides the reducing power for the synthesis of fatty acid chains.
   - In one mechanism, malate is transported into the mitochondrial matrix with the aid of the malate-α-ketoglutarate transporter (also located in the inner mitochondrial membrane) (step 5 in ▶ Fig. 13.3). The latter brings one malate into the matrix while simultaneously transporting one α-ketoglutarate out into the cytosol (not shown). In the matrix, malate is oxidized to oxaloacetate by malate dehydrogenase via a reaction that reduces NAD⁺ to NADH (step 6 in ▶ Fig. 13.3).

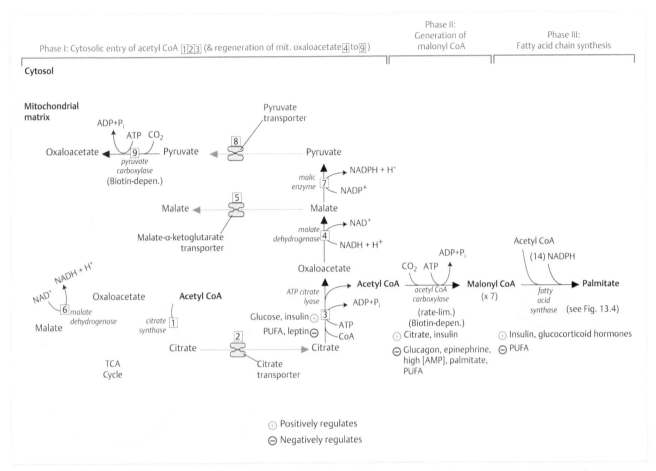

Fig. 13.3 Events required for the synthesis of fatty acids. Phase I. The citrate shuttle is a transport system designed to transport acetyl coenzyme A (acetyl CoA) from the mitochondrial matrix into the cytosol, where it can then be used to synthesize fatty acids. The citrate shuttle involves (1) the mitochondrial condensation of acetyl CoA with oxaloacetate to form citrate, (2) the transport of citrate out into the cytosol, and (3) the splitting of citrate into acetyl CoA and oxaloacetate. The latter is catalyzed by ATP citrate lyase. Steps 4 through 9 outline the two manners in which oxaloacetate is regenerated in the mitochondrial matrix. **Phase II.** Once in the cytosol, acetyl CoA is converted to malonyl CoA via the action of acetyl CoA carboxylase, a biotin-dependent enzyme. **Phase III.** Acetyl CoA, 7 malonyl CoA, and 14 NADPH are used by fatty acid synthase to generate the 16-carbon fatty acid, palmitate. ADP, adenosine diphosphate; AMP, adenosine monophosphate; ATP, adenosine triphosphate; NAD, nicotinamide adenine dinucleotide; NADH, reduced form of nicotinamide adenine dinucleotide; NADP, nicotinamide adenine dinucleotide phosphate; NADPH, reduced form of nicotinamide adenine dinucleotide phosphate; PUFA, polyunsaturated fatty acids; TCA, tricarboxylic acid.

• In an alternative mechanism, cytosolic malate is converted to pyruvate by malic enzyme via a reaction that reduces NADP⁺ to NADPH (step in 7 ▶ Fig. 13.3). Pyruvate is then transported into the mitochondrial matrix with the aid of the pyruvate transporter (located in the inner mitochondrial membrane) (step 8 in ▶ Fig. 13.3) and carboxylated into oxaloacetate (step 9 in ▶ Fig. 13.3). The hydrolysis of ATP to ADP and P_i provides the energy for this carboxylation reaction, which is catalyzed by pyruvate carboxylase.
  ○ Pyruvate carboxylase requires biotin for its activity.

Phase II—Generation of Malonyl CoA by Acetyl CoA Carboxylase

Once acetyl CoA is regenerated in the cytosol, it is carboxylated into malonyl CoA by acetyl CoA carboxylase (ACC) (▶ Fig. 13.3).

This rate-limiting, ATP-dependent reaction is summarized as follows:

$$Acetyl\ CoA + CO_2 + ATP \rightarrow Malonyl\ CoA + ADP + P_i$$

• When active, ACC is dephosphorylated and exists as a multimer. In its inactive form though, ACC is phosphorylated and exists as an inactive dimer.
• ACC requires biotin as a cofactor and is subject to regulation by metabolites, hormones, and end products, as follows:
  ○ ACC is allosterically activated by citrate and activated by insulin via a mechanism that promotes ACC's dephosphorylation.
  ○ ACC is inhibited by agents that promote its phosphorylation. These agents include glucagon and epinephrine (hormones that are elevated in the fasting state), high adenosine monophosphate (AMP) levels (which

IV

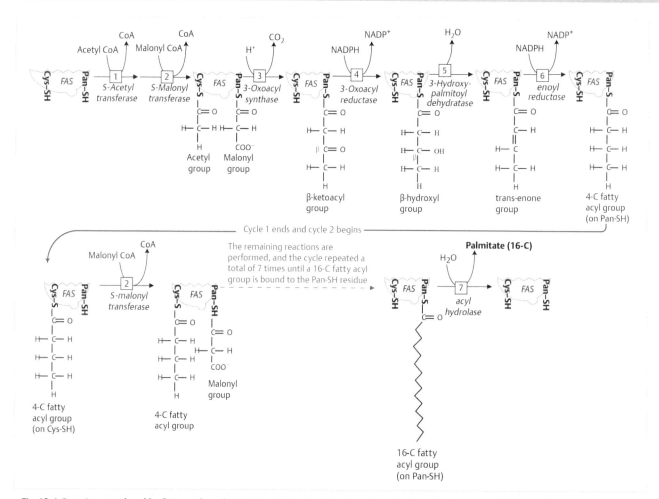

Fig. 13.4 Reactions catalyzed by fatty acid synthase. Fatty acid synthesis occurs in fatty acid synthase (FAS), a homodimeric enzyme complex that catalyzes seven reactions, six of which serve to condense an acetyl group and malonyl group into a β-ketone, then reduce the β-ketone into a fatty acyl group that has two carbons added after each cycle. These reactions are repeated until a 16-carbon palmitic group is formed. A total of seven cycles of the six reactions are performed and are followed by the seventh reaction, which releases palmitate. The substrates are moved between reaction centers by binding to a cysteine residue (Cys-SH) and phosphopantetheine (Pan-SH) residue of FAS. CoA, coenzyme A; NADP, nicotinamide adenine dinucleotide phosphate; NADPH, reduced form of nicotinamide adenine dinucleotide phosphate.

are reflective of a low-energy state), and an excess of the fatty acid biosynthesis end product palmitate. Additionally, the expression of ACC is suppressed by diets rich in polyunsaturated fatty acids (PUFA).

Malonyl CoA is essential for fatty acid synthesis because it serves not only as a substrate but as a regulator of this process. Specifically, malonyl CoA inhibits carnitine acyltransferase I (see ► Fig. 13.7a)—the rate-limiting enzyme of fatty acid degradation. In doing so, malonyl CoA prevents fatty acid synthesis and degradation from occurring simultaneously.

Phase III—Fatty Acid Chain Formation via Fatty Acid Synthase

The actual formation of fatty acid chains is carried out by fatty acid synthase (FAS), a large homodimeric enzyme complex that catalyzes six distinct enzymatic reactions in seven cycles,

followed by a seventh distinct reaction, to generate palmitate from acetyl CoA and malonyl CoA. A summary of this reaction follows.

1 Acetyl CoA + 7 Malonyl CoA + 14 NADPH + 14 H⁺ → Palmitate + 14 NADP⁺ + 7 CO₂ + 8 CoA + 6 H₂O

The seven distinct enzymatic reactions are designed to achieve three main goals (► Fig. 13.4):

1. **Condensation** (reactions 1 through 3):
   - In the first cycle, the two-carbon acetyl group of acetyl CoA is transferred (1) to a cysteine residue (Cys-SH) of FAS, forming a thioester bond. This transfer is catalyzed by the S-acetyl transferase activity of FAS.
   - In a similar fashion, the three-carbon malonyl group of malonyl CoA is transferred (2) to the phosphopantetheine residue (Pan-SH) of the acyl carrier protein of FAS, also forming a thioester bond. This

transfer is catalyzed by the *S*-malonyl transferase activity of FAS.

- The 3-oxoacyl synthase activity of FAS then transfers (3) the acetyl group from the cysteine residue to malonate and decarboxylates malonate (releasing CO_2) to generate a four-carbon β-ketoacyl group.

2. **Reduction** (reactions 4 through 6):
- The β-ketoacyl group is reduced (4) to a β-hydroxyl group by the 3-oxoacyl reductase activity of FAS. In this reaction, NADPH is oxidized to NADP+.

  NADPH. The synthesis of palmitate uses a large amount (14) of NADPH, which it gets from the following sources:
  - *Malic enzyme* (net 1 NADPH): When malic enzyme catalyzes the oxidation of malate to pyruvate, 1 NADPH is produced.
  - *Pentose phosphate pathway* (net 2 to 12 NADPH): When the phosphorylated form of glucose (glucose 6-phosphate) is converted to ribulose 5-phosphate, 2 NADPH molecules are produced. If the demand for NADPH is greater than the demand for ribulose 5-phosphate (a precursor for nucleotide synthesis), the latter is used to regenerate glucose 6-phosphate, which reenters the pentose phosphate pathway to ultimately produce 12 NADPH (see **Fig.12.17**).
  - *Folate-dependent pathway* (net 1 to 2 NADPH): In proliferating cells, the oxidation of N^5-N^{10}-methylene-tetrahydrofolate to N^{10}-formyl-tetrahydrofolate by methylenetetrahydrofolate dehydrogenase also contributes a significant portion of cytosolic NADPH pool.
- The elimination (5) of H_2O from the β-hydroxyl group to generate a trans-enone (marked by the double bond between carbons 2 and 3), followed by its reduction (6) to a hydrocarbon (via a reaction that oxidizes another NADPH to NADP+), generates a four-carbon fatty acyl group attached to the Pan-SH residue of FAS.

  Repeat reactions six more times. This four-carbon fatty acyl group is transferred from the Pan-SH residue to the cysteine residue of FAS. As such, the fatty acyl residue (rather than a new acetyl group) is used as the substrate for condensation with additional malonate groups bound to the Pan-SH residue.
- The remaining reactions are repeated for a total of seven cycles. Consequently, the four-carbon fatty acyl group elongates by two carbons in each cycle until the 16-carbon palmitate group is generated (▶ Table 13.1).

3. **Product release** (reaction 7): Once the fatty acyl residue contains 16 carbons, the acyl hydrolase (thioesterase) activity of FAS uses H_2O to cleave the thioester bond between the palmitate residue and the Pan-SH residue to release palmitate.

13.2.2 Elongation of Palmitate and Desaturation of Fatty Acids

Elongation. Palmitate is converted into longer-chain fatty acids in the smooth endoplasmic reticulum (SER) or mitochondria. The fatty acid chains are lengthened two-carbon units at a time via reactions similar to those catalyzed by fatty acid synthase. As such, NADPH is used for the reduction steps, but the two-

Table 13.1 Summary of reactants and fatty acyl group carbons generated and used in each of the seven cycles catalyzed by fatty acid synthase

Cycle #	Substrates and reducing equivalents	Fatty acyl size
1	1 Acetyl CoA + 1 Malonyl CoA + 2 NADPH	4-carbon fatty acyl group
2	4-carbon fatty acyl group + 1 Malonyl CoA + 2 NADPH	6-carbon fatty acyl group
3	6-carbon fatty acyl group + 1 Malonyl CoA + 2 NADPH	8-carbon fatty acyl group
4	8-carbon fatty acyl group + 1 Malonyl CoA + 2 NADPH	10-carbon fatty acyl group
5	10-carbon fatty acyl group + 1 Malonyl CoA + 2 NADPH	12-carbon fatty acyl group
6	12-carbon fatty acyl group + 1 Malonyl CoA + 2 NADPH	14-carbon fatty acyl group
7	14-carbon fatty acyl group + 1 Malonyl CoA + 2 NADPH	16-carbon fatty acyl group (palmitate group)

Abbreviations: CoA, coenzyme A; NADPH, reduced form of nicotinamide adenine dinucleotide phosphate.

carbon units are donated by malonyl CoA in the SER and by acetyl CoA in mitochondria.

Desaturation. The desaturation of fatty acids introduces double bonds into their hydrocarbon tails. These reactions, which require NADPH and cytochrome b_5 reductase, are catalyzed in the SER by acyl CoA desaturases. Humans possess four distinct acyl CoA desaturases (Δ^4, Δ^5, Δ^6, and Δ^9) in the SER membranes that can introduce double bonds between carbons 4–5, 5–6, 6–7, or 9–10 of fatty acid chains.

- The Δ^9-desaturase is primarily responsible for the synthesis of monounsaturated fatty acids, whereas the other desaturases are involved in the synthesis of polyunsaturated ω-6 and ω-3 fatty acids from the essential fatty acids, linoleic acid (18:2ω6) and α-linolenic acid (18:3ω3).
- Fatty acids containing double bonds beyond carbons 9 and 10 cannot be endogenously generated and must be obtained in the diet (e.g., ω-3 fatty acids).

13.2.3 Regulation of Fatty Acid Synthesis

Regulation of mammalian fatty acid synthesis occurs at multiple levels—ATP citrate lyase, acetyl CoA carboxylase (ACC), fatty acid synthase, and the desaturases. The activities of these lipogenic enzymes are induced by a low-fat, high-carbohydrate diet and are 25- to 100-fold higher in the fed state when compared to the fasting state.

- **Regulation of ATP citrate lyase.** This enzyme appears to be stabilized and stimulated by phosphorylation at multiple sites. Its gene expression is induced by glucose/insulin. This induction, however, is counteracted by polyunsaturated fatty acids and by the adipocyte-derived hormone, leptin.
- **Regulation of ACC.** This committed and rate-limiting step of fatty acid synthesis is regulated by modulating the

interconversion of ACC between the inactive dimer form and the active multimer form, and also at the level of its gene expression. Cytosolic citrate, the supplier of acetyl CoA, promotes the formation of the active multimeric form, whereas long-chain fatty acyl CoAs inactivate the enzyme by promoting the dissociation of the multimer. Glucagon and epinephrine cause protein kinase A (PK-A)–mediated phosphorylation of ACC, which inhibits the formation of the active multimer. On the other hand, insulin stimulates protein phosphatase 1-mediated dephosphorylation of ACC, which favors multimer formation. Palmitate stimulates an AMP-activated protein kinase (AMPK), which, then phosphorylates and inactivates ACC.

- **Regulation of fatty acid synthase.** The expression of FAS is induced by insulin and glucocorticoid hormones and is suppressed by dietary polyunsaturated fatty acids.
- **Regulation of desaturases.** The expression of all desaturases is also induced by insulin and suppressed by dietary poly unsaturated fatty acids. Dietary cholesterol induces the expression of Δ^9-desaturase, whereas it suppresses that of the other desaturases.

Normal
Essential fatty acids

Because humans cannot perform *de novo* synthesis of ω-6 and ω-3 fatty acids, they need to obtain such fatty acids or their precursors from the diet. Two such precursors, linoleic acid (18:2ω6) and α-linolenic acid (18:3ω3) (see ▶ Fig. 3.2) are termed essential fatty acids. The ω-6, polyunsaturated fatty acid, arachidonic acid (20:4ω6) can be synthesized by elongation and desaturation of linoleic acid (18:2ω6) and serves as the precursor of several eicosanoid compounds (e.g., prostaglandins, thromboxanes, leukotrienes) (see ▶ Fig. 3.7) The ω-3 polyunsaturated fatty acids eicosapentanoic acid (EPA, 20:5ω3) and docosahexanoic acid (DHA, 22:6ω3) can similarly be synthesized from α-linolenic acid (18:3ω3). Both EPA and DHA (which may also be directly obtained from oily fish) appear to play a role in ocular health and may protect against age-related macular degeneration and diabetic retinopathy. Other beneficial effects of EPA and DHA have been noted in the maintenance of cognitive functions, neuronal survival, leptin secretion, insulin sensitivity, and regulating inflammation.

Normal
Sites of *de novo* fatty acid biosynthesis

In humans, the major sites of fatty acid synthesis are liver, adipose tissue, mammary glands, and fat deposits in muscle. However, it should be noted that *de novo* lipogenesis is suppressed by dietary fat. When dietary fat constitutes > 30% of calorie intake, < 10% of fatty acids secreted by the liver are of endogenous origin. In most other mammals, except rodents, adipose tissue is the primary site of *de novo* lipogenesis. In rodents, the liver is a major contributor to lipogenesis. All mammals exhibit significant levels of fatty acid biosynthesis in lactating mammary glands.

Therapeutics
Fatty liver and alcoholics

Alcoholic fatty liver develops in individuals consuming large amounts (> 60 g) of alcohol per day on a prolonged basis. Multiple mechanisms have been proposed for the development of fatty liver. Alcohol metabolism increases hepatic [NADH]:[NAD⁺] ratio, thus increasing the formation of glycerol 3-phosphate and thereby triacylglycerol synthesis. It also inhibits fatty acid oxidation and the secretion of very low-density lipoproteins (VLDL) by the liver and promotes free radical formation and oxidative stress. In initial stages, alcoholic fatty liver disease is reversible through abstinence and moderation. If unchecked, it progresses to alcoholic hepatitis and eventually to cirrhosis.

Foundations
Medium-chain fatty acid synthesis in lactating mammary gland

Approximately 20% of the fatty acids in milk fat are derived by endogenous synthesis in the epithelial cells of the lactating mammary gland. A different isoform of acyl hydrolase (thioesterase II) in this tissue causes early termination of the fatty acid synthase (FAS) cycle, resulting in the release of medium-chain fatty acids (8 to 12 carbons long) for incorporation into milk fat. Lipids containing such shorter fatty acids are easier to digest and oxidize by infants.

13.3 Fatty Acid Storage and Release

13.3.1 Biosynthesis of Triacylglycerols

Fatty acids are stored in adipocytes as triacylglycerols, which are composed of three fatty acid chains attached to a glycerol backbone. Their synthesis occurs in the cytosol of cells of the small intestine and those of liver and adipose tissues. A common aspect of triacylglycerol synthesis in all three of the aforementioned tissues is that they all use the "activated" form of fatty acids, fatty acyl CoA, to build triacylglycerols.

The free form of fatty acids and the glycerol backbone are obtained from various sources, as follows:

- **Free fatty acids:** Cells of the small intestine take up fatty acids released from the digestion of dietary triacylglycerols (▶ Fig. 13.5a) Hepatocytes, on the other hand, synthesize fatty acids *de novo* from acetyl CoA (▶ Fig. 13.5b). Adipocytes, however, absorb fatty acids released when triacylglycerols from diet-derived chylomicrons and liver-derived very low density lipoproteins (VLDL) are hydrolyzed by capillary lipoprotein lipase (▶ Fig. 13.5c).
  - Fatty acyl CoA is then generated in each of these tissues by the attachment of CoA to free fatty acids via a reaction catalyzed by fatty acyl CoA synthetase. This reaction involves the hydrolysis of ATP into AMP and PPᵢ. The energy

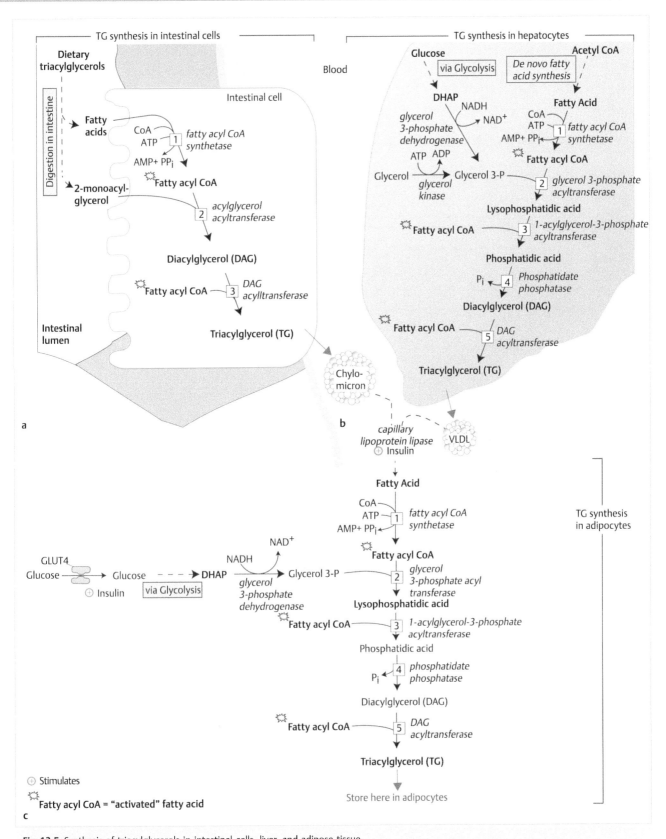

Fig. 13.5 Synthesis of triacylglycerols in intestinal cells, liver, and adipose tissue.
(a) Intestinal cells utilize diet-derived fatty acids and 2-monoacylglycerol to generate triacylglycerols (TGs). The latter are then packaged into chylomicrons for transport through blood. AMP, adenosine monophosphate; ATP, adenosine triphosphate; CoA, coenzyme A. (b) Hepatocytes utilize newly synthesized fatty acids and glycerol 3-phosphate to generate TGs, which are then packaged into very low-density lipoproteins (VLDLs) for transport through blood. ADP, adenosine diphosphate; DHAP, dihydroxyacetone 3-phosphate; NAD$^+$, nicotinamide adenine dinucleotide; NADH, reduced form of nicotinamide adenine dinucleotide. (c) Adipocytes obtain fatty acids from circulating chylomicrons and VLDLs (via the action of capillary lipoprotein lipase, which is stimulated by insulin) and use them to build TGs on a glycerol 3-phosphate backbone. GLUT4, glucose transporter 4; P$_i$, inorganic phosphate; PP$_i$, pyrophosphate.

requirement for fatty acid activation is considered to be two ATP equivalents because it takes two phosphorylation steps to convert AMP back to ATP.

- **Glycerol backbone:** Cells of the small intestine use 2-mono-acylglycerol obtained from the digestion of dietary triacylglycerols as the source of the glycerol backbone to which two fatty acid chains are added (▶ Fig. 13.5a). In contrast, liver and adipose tissue use glycerol 3-phosphate as the source of the glycerol backbone to which three fatty acid chains are attached. However, glycerol 3-phosphate is obtained from different precursors in liver and adipose tissues.
  - Liver: The phosphorylation of glycerol by glycerol kinase generates glycerol 3-phosphate, and the reduction of the glycolytic intermediate dihydroxyacetone 3-phosphate (DHAP) by glycerol 3-phosphate dehydrogenase also produces glycerol 3-phosphate.
  - Adipose: Because adipose tissue lacks glycerol kinase, its supply of glycerol 3-phosphate comes solely from the reduction of DHAP by glycerol 3-phosphate dehydrogenase.

Mechanism of Triacylglycerol Synthesis in Intestinal Cells

In the intestinal lumen (▶ Fig. 13.5a) digestive enzymes break down dietary triacylglycerols into free fatty acids and 2-mono-acylglycerol. The latter two are then taken up by intestinal epithelial cells, where the following reactions occur:

1. Fatty acyl CoA synthetase "activates" fatty acids by attaching them to CoA, forming fatty acyl CoAs.
2. Acylglycerol acyltransferase then transfers the acyl residue from a fatty acyl CoA to the carbon-1 hydroxyl group of 2-monoacylglycerol. This reaction generates diacylglycerol (DAG).
3. DAG acyltransferase then transfers the acyl residue from a second fatty acyl CoA onto the carbon-3 hydroxyl group of DAG. This generates triacylglycerol.
   - These triacylglycerols are then packaged with apolipoproteins and other lipids into chylomicrons for release into the bloodstream via lymph.

Mechanism of Triacylglycerol Synthesis in Liver

In hepatocytes (▶ Fig. 13.5b) enzymes involved in fatty acid synthesis generate their free fatty acids via *de novo* synthesis from acetyl CoA. They then generate triacylglycerols via the following reactions:

1. Fatty acyl CoA synthetase "activates" the free fatty acids by attaching them to CoA, forming fatty acyl CoAs.
   Glycerol 3-phosphate in hepatocytes is obtained when glycerol kinase phosphorylates glycerol or when DHAP is reduced.
2. Glycerol 3-phosphate acyltransferase then transfers the acyl residue from a fatty acyl CoA onto the carbon 1 hydroxyl of glycerol 3-phosphate, generating lysophosphatidic acid (1-acylglycerol-3-phosphate).
3. Next, 1-acylglycerol-3-phosphate acyltransferase transfers the acyl residue from a second fatty acyl CoA to the carbon 2 hydroxyl of lysophosphatidic acid, generating phosphatidic acid (1,2-acylglycerol-3-phosphate).

4. Cleavage of phosphatidic acid's phosphodiester bond, which releases P_i and generates DAG, is catalyzed by phosphatidate phosphatase, which uses water to cleave the phosphodiester bond.
5. DAG acyltransferase then transfers the acyl residue from a third fatty acyl CoA onto the carbon 3 hydroxyl of DAG, generating triacylglycerol.
   - These triacylglycerols are packaged into VLDLs for release into the bloodstream.
   - DAG acyltransferase is a potential therapeutic target in the treatment of obesity and type 2 diabetes.

Mechanism of Triacylglycerol Synthesis in Adipose Tissue

In the capillaries that supply adipose tissue and muscle, triacylglycerols packaged within chylomicrons and VLDLs are cleaved by capillary lipoprotein lipase into two free fatty acids and monacylglycerol. Capillary lipoprotein lipase is secreted by adipocytes, but it lines the walls of capillaries, where it carries out its function.

- Insulin stimulates adipocytes to secrete capillary lipoprotein lipase.
- Capillary lipoprotein lipase is activated by apolipoprotein C-II, a protein found on the outer shell of mature chylomicrons (see **Fig. 14.7a**).
1. In adipocytes (▶ Fig. 13.5c), fatty acyl CoA synthetase "activates" fatty acids by attaching them to CoA, forming fatty acyl CoAs.

Because adipocytes lack glycerol kinase, they obtain glycerol 3-phosphate through the reduction of DHAP.

- Insulin promotes an increase in the absorption of glucose via glucose transporter 4 (GLUT4) and thus increases the amount of glycerol 3-phosphate produced for use in triacylglycerol synthesis in adipocytes.

The remaining four steps to generate triacylglycerol in adipocytes are identical to steps 2, 3, 4, and 5 in hepatocytes.

- These triacylglycerols are then stored within the adipose tissue.

13.3.2 Hydrolysis of Triacylglycerols for Fatty Acid Release

When energy is needed, triacylglycerols are degraded into glycerol and fatty acid residues, the latter of which are transported to cells/tissues for β-oxidation—a catabolic process that cleaves fatty acid residues two carbons at a time to yield acetyl CoA, the reduced form of flavin adenine dinucleotide ($FADH_2$), and NADH. Tri-, di-, and monoacylated glycerolipids are degraded by three main lipases contained within adipocytes (▶ Fig. 13.6a, **bottom**):

1. **Hormone-sensitive lipase** hydrolyzes triacylglycerol into a free fatty acid and diacylglycerol. The activity of this enzyme is controlled by various hormones, as follows:
   - Glucagon, epinephrine, and norepinephrine activate hormone-sensitive lipase.
   - Insulin inhibits the activity of hormone-sensitive lipase.
2. **Lipoprotein lipase** hydrolyzes diacylglycerol into a free fatty acid and monoacylglycerol. (In contrast, the capillary form of

IV

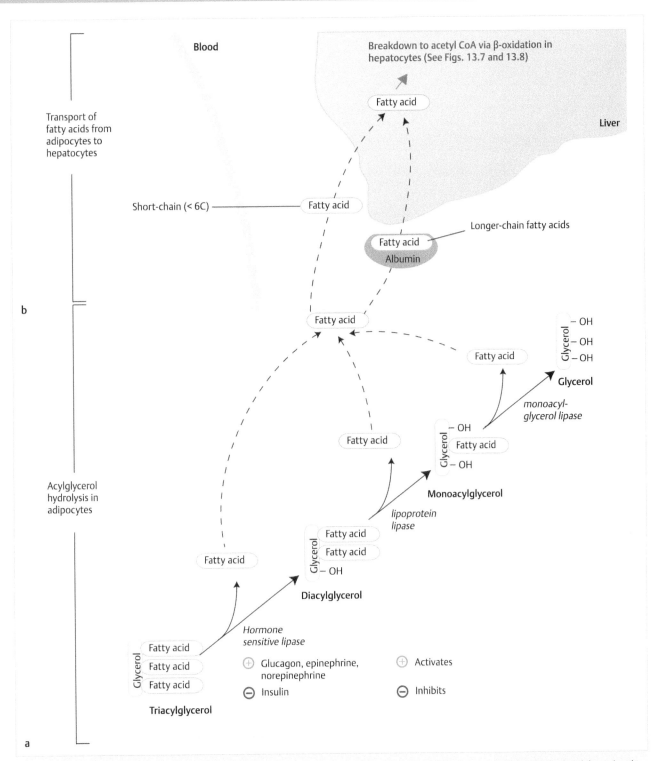

Fig. 13.6 Lipases that catalyze the hydrolysis of acylglycerols. (a, *bottom***)** In adipose tissue, triacylglycerols are hydrolyzed into diacylglycerol and a free fatty acid by hormone-sensitive lipase. This enzyme is activated by glucagon, epinephrine, and norepinephrine but is inhibited by insulin. Diacylglycerol is hydrolyzed to monoacylglycerol and a free fatty acid by lipoprotein lipase. Monoacylglycerol is hydrolyzed to glycerol and a free fatty acid by monoacylglycerol lipase. **(b,** *top***)** Free fatty acids are then sent to the liver for degradation. Short-chain fatty acids are soluble in blood, but longer-chain fatty acids must bind albumin for transport through blood. CoA, coenzyme A.

lipoprotein lipase hydrolyzes triacylglycerol into two fatty acids and monoacylglycerol.)

3. **Monoacylglycerol lipase** hydrolyzes monoacylglycerol into a free fatty acid and glycerol.

Transport and release. Short-chain (fewer than six carbons) fatty acids are soluble in blood. However, longer-chain free fatty acids are not. They are therefore bound to albumin for transport through blood (▸ Fig. 13.6b, **top**).

Foundations

Mechanism of hormone-sensitive lipase regulation

Hormone-sensitive lipase is the initial degradative enzyme of triacylglycerol catabolism in the adipose tissue. The activity of this enzyme is upregulated by phosphorylation carried out by protein kinase A. As seen in Chapter 9, protein kinase A (see **Fig. 9.6**) is activated by hormones such as glucagon and epinephrine that raise cellular levels of cyclic adenosine monophosphate (cAMP). Conversely, hormone-sensitive lipase is down-regulated by dephosphorylation carried out by protein phosphatase 1. This phosphatase is activated by insulin. Thus, glucagon and epinephrine promote lipolysis in adipocytes, whereas insulin inhibits it. It is noteworthy that these hormones have the opposite effect on acetyl CoA carboxylase, the rate-limiting step of fatty acid biosynthesis (see Section 13.2.3).

Normal

Perilipin

Perilipins are a family of homologous proteins that coat the surface of lipid storage droplets in adipocytes and in muscle and regulate lipolysis by restricting access to hormone-sensitive lipase (HSL). Five members of this family, perilipins 1 through 5, have been identified in humans. Perilipin 1 (also known as perilipin A) is expressed in mature adipocytes, and its overexpression inhibits lipolysis, whereas a knockout of its expression promotes lipolysis. Like HSL, perilipin A is a substrate for protein kinase A (PK-A), and phosphorylation changes its conformation to allow the association of activated HSL with the lipid droplets. Adipocyte-specific overexpression of perilipins could be a therapeutic strategy in the treatment of obesity.

Normal

Synthetic fats—olestra

Triacylglycerols are composed of a glycerol backbone attached to three fatty acid chains. In comparison, the synthetic fat olestra (Olean) is composed of a sucrose backbone attached to six to eight fatty acids. The resulting bulkiness of olestra prevents it from being absorbed by the small intestines and it is excreted in stool without providing any caloric value to the consumer. However, ingestion of olestra disrupts the absorption of lipid-soluble vitamins (e.g., A, D, E, K) because they are easily dissolved in olestra and are also therefore excreted without being absorbed. Individuals who consume high amounts of olestra-containing products (especially seen in snacks that have "low/zero" fat, such as potato chips) may be subject to vitamin deficiencies, abdominal cramps, bloating, and diarrhea.

13.4 Catabolism of Fatty Acids

β-Oxidation is a catabolic pathway that takes place in the mitochondrial matrix of liver cells. It cleaves fatty acid chains two carbons at a time to yield two-carbon acetyl CoA molecules, $FADH_2$, and NADH. The events that must occur in order for cells

to degrade fatty acids and harness the energy they contain is divided into two phases:

- **Phase I: Transport of free fatty acids into the mitochondrial matrix:** Although short-chain fatty acids (SCFAs) and medium-chain fatty acids (MCFAs) can diffuse directly into mitochondria, long-chain fatty acids (LCFAs) and very long-chain fatty acids (VLCFAs) cannot. LCFAs can only be transported from the cytoplasm into the mitochondria with the aid of the carnitine shuttle. VLCFAs are oxidized in peroxisomes until they are the length of LCFAs.
- **Phase II: β-Oxidation of fatty acids:** In general, typical fatty acids (i.e., those with an even number of carbons and zero double bonds) and atypical fatty acids (those with an uneven number of carbons and/or double bonds) are catabolized either completely or partially by β-oxidation.

13.4.1 Phase I: Transport of Long-Chain Fatty Acids into Mitochondrial Matrix via the Carnitine Shuttle

1. Cytosolic LCFAs are first "activated" by attachment to CoA (via a thioester bond) to form fatty acyl CoA (▶ Fig. 13.7a) This ATP-dependent reaction is catalyzed by fatty acyl CoA synthetase. The fatty acyl CoAs can now move into the intermembrane space.
   - Fatty acyl CoA synthetase is located in the outer mitochondrial membrane but catalyzes its reaction on the cytoplasmic side of the membrane.
2. Carnitine palmitoyltransferase I (CPT I) transfers the fatty acyl residue from fatty acyl CoA to carnitine. This reaction generates fatty acylcarnitine in the intermembrane space. This enzyme is also known as carnitine acyltransferase.
   - CPT I is the rate-limiting enzyme of fatty acid degradation and is inhibited by malonyl CoA (a substrate of fatty acid synthesis). It is located in the outer mitochondrial membrane but catalyzes its reaction on the side facing the intermembrane space.
   - Primary carnitine deficiency is marked by reduced levels of intracellular carnitine due to either nutritional deficiency (e.g., in vegans or during total parenteral nutrition) or a deficiency of plasma membrane Na-dependent carnitine transporter.
3. Carnitine-acylcarnitine translocase (CACT) is an antiporter that transports one fatty acylcarnitine into the mitochondrial matrix while simultaneously exporting one carnitine molecule out (from the CPT II reaction yet to be discussed) and into the intermembrane space.
4. Carnitine palmitoyltransferase II (CPT II) then transfers the fatty acyl residue from fatty acylcarnitine to CoA. This reaction generates fatty acyl CoA and carnitine in the matrix. Fatty acyl CoA is then acted upon by enzymes involved in the β-oxidation of fatty acids.
   - CPT II is located in the inner mitochondrial membrane and catalyzes its reaction on the matrix side of the membrane.
   - Defects in muscle CPT II are more common and are associated with another type of secondary carnitine deficiency known as CPT II deficiency.
   - Secondary carnitine deficiency due to an accumulation of acylcarnitines can occur because of a variety of metabolic

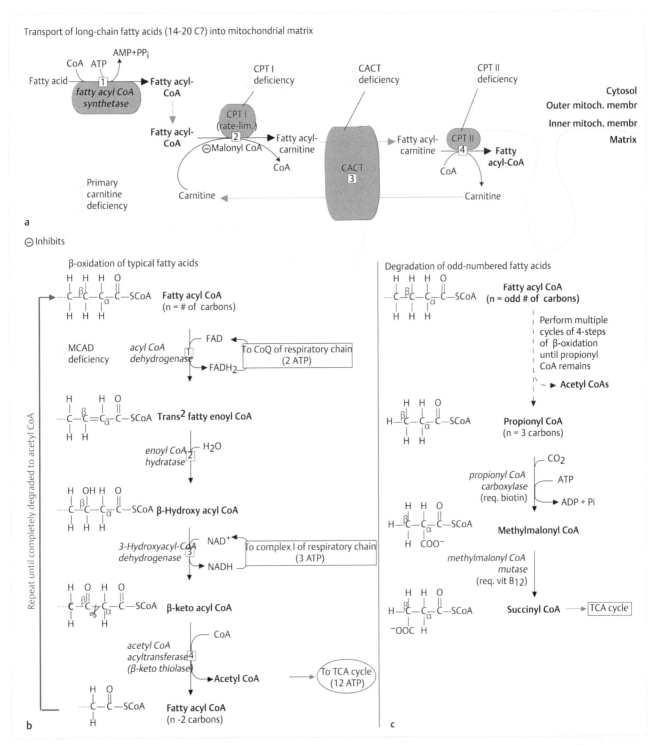

Fig. 13.7 Carnitine shuttle and degradation of typical and odd-numbered fatty acids. (a) Free fatty acids residing in the cytosol are "activated" via attachment of coenzyme A (CoA) by fatty acyl CoA synthetase. The resulting fatty acyl CoA moves through the outer mitochondrial membrane and into the intermembrane space. Here the rate-limiting enzyme carnitine palmitoyltransferase I (CPT I) transfers the fatty acyl groups from CoA onto carnitine, forming fatty acylcarnitine. CPT I is inhibited by malonyl CoA. Fatty acylcarnitine enters the mitochondrial matrix through the carnitine-acylcarnitine translocase in exchange for carnitine. Once inside the mitochondrial matrix, the fatty acyl residue of fatty acyl carnitine is transferred back onto CoA, reforming fatty acyl CoA and carnitine. This reaction is catalyzed by carnitine palmitoyltransferase II (CPT II), which is bound to the inner mitochondrial membrane. The fatty acyl CoA can now be acted on by the enzymes that carry out the β-oxidation of fatty acids. AMP, adenosine monophosphate; ATP, adenosine triphosphate; CACT, carnitine-acylcarnitine translocase; PPi, pyrophosphate. (b) Typical fatty acids are degraded by the four steps of b-oxidation, which yields FADH2, NADH, and acetyl CoA, molecules that contribute to ATP production. FADH2, reduced form of flavin adenine dinucleotide; MCAD, medium-chain acyl CoA dehydrogenase; NADH, reduced form of nicotinamide adenine dinucleotide. (C) Odd-numbered fatty acids undergo rounds of β-oxidation until their last three carbons form propionyl CoA. The propionyl residue is carboxylated to methylmalonyl CoA, which is then isomerized to succinyl CoA, an intermediate of the tricarboxylic acid (TCA) cycle, via enzymes that require biotin or cobalamin (vitamin B_{12}) for their activity.

disorders, including a deficiency of CACT or CPT II, fatty acid oxidation disorders such as medium-chain acyl CoA dehydrogenase (MCAD) deficiency, and organic acidemias. Acylcarnitines also inhibit the reabsorption of free carnitine in the kidneys.

13.4.2 Phase II: β-Oxidation of Fatty Acids

Typical fatty acids

Typical long-chain fatty acids, such as those with saturated and even-numbered carbon chains, are completely broken down by the four steps of β-oxidation (▶ Fig. 13.7b) Each round, which is centered on a fatty acid's β-carbon, produces acetyl CoA (which enters the TCA cycle) and the reduced coenzymes $FADH_2$ and NADH. $FADH_2$ delivers electrons to the electron transport chain at coenzyme Q/ubiquinone, and NADH does so at complex I. The four steps involved in each round of β-oxidation of typical fatty acids are as follows:

1. Acyl CoA dehydrogenase oxidizes the β-carbon (two positions from the carbonyl) of fatty acyl CoA. This reaction produces $FADH_2$ and an enone (conjugated alkene and ketone) called *trans*-enoyl-CoA.
   - $FADH_2$ can generate two ATPs via oxidative phosphorylation (Chapter 11).
   - There are four types of acyl CoA dehydrogenases that act on fatty acids of different chain lengths. They include short-chain acyl CoA dehydrogenase (SCAD), medium-chain acyl CoA dehydrogenase (MCAD), long-chain acyl CoA dehydrogenase (LCAD), and very long chain acyl CoA dehydrogenase (VLCAD).
   - MCAD deficiency develops in patients with inherited defects in MCAD and is the most commonly observed disorder associated with the step.
2. Enoyl CoA hydratase then saturates the alkene via the addition of H_2O at the β-carbon to generate β-hydroxyacyl CoA.
3. 3-Hydroxyacyl CoA dehydrogenase then oxidizes the β-carbon, forming β-ketoacyl CoA and producing NADH.
   - NADH can generate three ATPs via oxidative phosphorylation (see Chapter 11).
4. Acetyl CoA acyltransferase (also known as β-ketothiolase) attaches the sulfur atom of CoA to the ketone formed from the cleavage of acetyl CoA from the fatty acyl chain. The remaining fatty acyl CoA chain is thus shortened by two carbons.
   - Acetyl CoA can generate 12 ATP via entry into the TCA cycle.

These four reactions are repeated until the typical fatty acid is completely broken down to acetyl CoA. The catabolism of 16-carbon palmitic acid can generate 129 molecules of ATP.

Atypical fatty acids

Odd-numbered fatty acids. Atypical fatty acids, such as those with an odd number of carbons, undergo multiple rounds of β-oxidation until three carbons remain in the form of propionyl CoA (▶ Fig. 13.7c) The mechanism from then on involves the actions of a carboxylase and mutase, as follows:
- Propionyl CoA carboxylase, which requires biotin for its activity, carboxylates propionyl CoA in an ATP-dependent reaction that generates methylmalonyl CoA.
- Methylmalonyl CoA mutase, which requires adenosylcobalamin (a derivative of vitamin B_{12}) for its activity, isomerizes methylmalonyl CoA into succinyl CoA (an intermediate of the TCA cycle).

Unsaturated fatty acids. Atypical fatty acids containing unsaturated carbon chains (i.e., ≥ 1 double bond) undergo β-oxidation until a disruptive alkene is reached. Further oxidation of these types of fatty acids require intervening reactions that convert the disruptive alkene to an oxidizable enone. These steps are catalyzed by two types of enzymes (▶ Fig. 13.8a):
1. Reductase (e.g., enoyl CoA reductase), which reduces double bonds that cannot be isomerized
2. Isomerase (e.g., enoyl CoA isomerase), which moves the disruptive double bond to form the enone

Very long chain fatty acids (VLCFAs). Atypical fatty acids, such as those with chain lengths greater than 20 carbons, are degraded by β-oxidation in peroxisomes rather than in the mitochondrial matrix. Key differences in the β-oxidation reactions of these two organelles are as follows (▶ Fig. 13.8b):
- In peroxisomes, the first step is catalyzed by a flavin adenine dinucleotide (FAD)–containing acyl CoA oxidase rather than an acyl CoA dehydrogenase as seen in mitochondria. When $FADH_2$ is formed in peroxisomes, it is oxidized to FAD during the conversion of water to hydrogen peroxide (H_2O_2) which can be detoxified by catalase. This is in contrast to mitochondrial $FADH_2$, whose electrons are transferred to electron-transferring flavoprotein (ETF), and then via ETF:ubiqinone reductase to ubiquinone.
  - Likewise, NADH and acetyl CoA generated in peroxisomes by fatty acid β-oxidation are not directly coupled to ATP production. NADH is reoxidized using the peroxisomal and cytosolic forms of a lactate dehydrogenase shuttle. The acetyl units are exported into the cytoplasm either as acetylcarnitine or as free acetate. When the VLCFAs are shortened to fewer than 20 carbons, they are sent to mitochondria for further degradation via β-oxidation.
- Zellweger syndrome and infantile Refsum disease are associated with defects in the biogenesis and assembly of peroxisomes, respectively.
- X-linked adrenoleukodystrophy (ALD) is associated with defects in the ALD protein (*ABCD1* gene product) that transports VLCFA CoAs into peroxisomes.
- Adult Refsum disease is associated with a defective α-hydroxylase, an enzyme involved in the peroxisomal degradation (via α-oxidation, which removes a single carbon) of the branched-chain fatty acid phytanic acid (▶ Fig. 13.8c).

▶ Table 13.1 contains a list of some of the disorders associated with defects in the catabolism of fatty acids in mitochondria and peroxisomes.

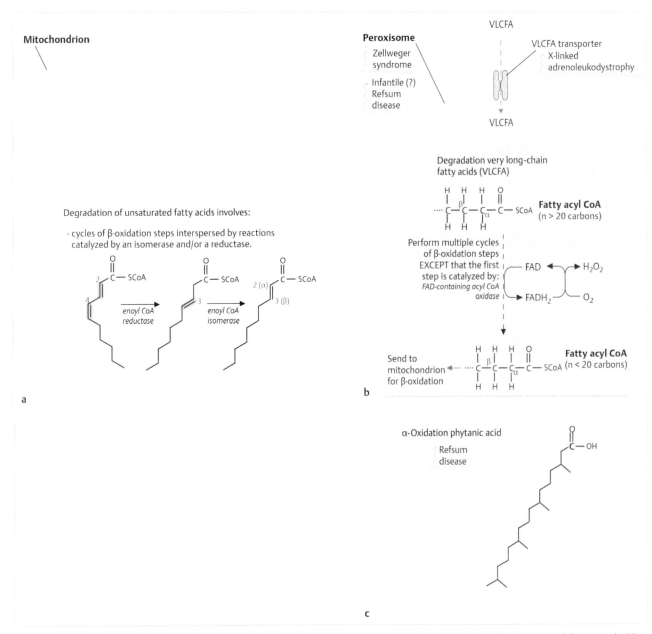

Mitochondrion

Degradation of unsaturated fatty acids involves:

- cycles of β-oxidation steps interspersed by reactions catalyzed by an isomerase and/or a reductase.

enoyl CoA reductase

enoyl CoA isomerase

a

Peroxisome

Zellweger syndrome

Infantile (?) Refsum disease

VLCFA

VLCFA transporter
X-linked adrenoleukodystrophy

VLCFA

Degradation very long-chain fatty acids (VLCFA)

Fatty acyl CoA (n > 20 carbons)

Perform multiple cycles of β-oxidation steps EXCEPT that the first step is catalyzed by: *FAD-containing acyl CoA oxidase*

FAD ← → H_2O_2

FADH₂ ← → O_2

Send to mitochondrion for β-oxidation ←

Fatty acyl CoA (n < 20 carbons)

b

α-Oxidation phytanic acid

Refsum disease

C — OH

c

Fig. 13.8 Degradation of the unsaturated and very long chain fatty acids. (a) Unsaturated fatty acids undergo β-oxidation until disruptive double bonds are formed. When needed, enoyl coenzyme A (CoA) reductase and enoyl CoA isomerase, respectively, reduce and isomerize these disruptive double bonds to create the correct conjugated alkene that can be degraded further by b-oxidation. **(b)** β-oxidation of very long chain fatty acids (VLCFAs) takes place in peroxisomes. The first reaction is catalyzed by an FAD-containing acyl CoA oxidase. Once the fatty acid chain is reduced to fewer than 20 carbons, it is sent to mitochondria for further b-oxidation. FAD, flavin adenine dinucleotide; FADH₂, reduced form of flavin adenine dinucleotide. **(c)** Phytanic acid, a branched-chain fatty acid, is degraded in peroxisomes via the mechanism of α-oxidation. Several of the disorders associated with defects in peroxisomal degradation of fatty acids are noted.

Therapeutics

Carnitine deficiencies

Carnitine is a derivative of the amino acid lysine. Although small amounts of carnitine can be synthesized by the liver and the kidney, the diet is a major source of carnitine found in skeletal muscle. Primary carnitine deficiency may be caused by strict vegan diets, defects in hepatic synthesis of carnitine, defects in carnitine uptake from the bloodstream, or defects in renal reabsorption. This results in symptoms that range from mild muscle cramping to severe muscle weakness and

death. Genetic deficiencies in carnitine palmitoyltransferase II (CPT II) expression, particularly in the cardiac and skeletal muscle, can lead to cardiomyopathy and myoglobinuria following prolonged exercise. On the other hand, deficiencies of carnitine palmitoyltransferase I (CPT I) or carnitine-acylcarnitine translocase (CACT) in the liver are rare and frequently lethal at a young age. Dietary supplementation with carnitine appears to be helpful in milder cases of fatty acid translocation defects.

Table 13.1 A partial list of disorders associated with defects in the catabolism of fatty acids in mitochondria and peroxisomes

Disorder	Causes	Associated organelle
Primary carnitine deficiency	Conditions that lead to low intracellular carnitine levels; conditions include defects in plasma membrane carnitine transporter, insufficient dietary supply of carnitine, and defects in hepatic synthesis of carnitine	—
CPT I deficiency	Defect in carnitine palmitoyltransferase I (CPT I)	Mitochondria
CACT deficiency	Defect in carnitine-acylcarnitine translocase (CACT)	Mitochondria
CPT II deficiency	Defect in carnitine palmitoyltransferase II (CPT II)	Mitochondria
MCAD deficiency	Defect in medium-chain acyl coenzyme A dehydrogenase (MCAD)	Mitochondria
Zellweger syndrome	Defect in biogenesis of peroxisomes	Peroxisome
Infantile Refsum disease	Defect in assembly of peroxisomes	Peroxisome
X-linked adrenoleukodystrophy	Defect in transport of very long chain fatty acids into peroxisomes	Peroxisome
Adult Refsum disease	Defect in degradation of phytanic acid	Peroxisome

Note: Carnitine palmitoyltransferase is also known as carnitine acyltransferase.

Foundations

Energy cost of unsaturation in fatty acids

The double bonds in unsaturated fatty acids provide obstacles to the normal process of β-oxidation. Such obstacles are overcome by the action of enoyl CoA reductase (which converts a 2, 4-dienoyl CoA into 3-enoyl CoA), and enoyl CoA isomerase (which converts 3-enoyl CoA into 2-enoyl CoA) (see ▶ **Fig. 13.8a**). There is however, an energy cost associated with this special management. The reaction catalyzed by enoyl CoA reductase uses NADPH as a cofactor. As mitochondrial NADPH is equivalent to NADH, this decreases the energy yield of β-oxidation by three ATP molecules. Similarly, the formation of 2-enoyl CoA by enoyl CoA isomerase bypasses the first step of β-oxidation catalyzed by acyl CoA dehydrogenase, resulting in the loss of production of an FADH$_2$. As a result, the ATP yield decreases by two molecules.

Therapeutics

Jamaican vomiting sickness

Hypoglycin A (L-α-amino-methylenecyclopropylpropionic acid) is a toxin in the unripe fruit of the akee tree (*Blighia sapida* Köenig) that is native to West Africa and was introduced to Jamaica in 1776. Ingestion of akee fruit causes Jamaican vomiting sickness with vomiting, generalized weakness, altered consciousness, and death. Clinical features include hypoglycemia, intractable vomiting, abdominal pain, and lethargy. Metabolism of hypoglycin A generates products that conjugate and sequester carnitine and coenzyme A. As a result, the transport and β-oxidation of long-chain fatty acids becomes inhibited. As in the case of inherited disorders of fatty acid oxidation, increased utilization of glucose and decreased gluconeogenesis (due to nonactivation of pyruvate carboxylase) result in hypoglycemia. Increases in small chain fatty acids and dicarboxylic acids cause metabolic acidosis. Increased levels of octanoic acid, a known mitochondrial poison, may contribute to the lethargy and central nervous system effects.

Therapeutics

X-Linked adrenoleukodystrophy

X-Linked adrenoleukodystrophy (ALD) is an inherited demyelination disorder due to defects in the transport of VLCFA CoAs into peroxisomes. It causes abnormal accumulation of lignoceric acid (24:0) and cerotic acid (26:0) in brain and adrenals of affected children. The defect is the result of a deficiency of ALD protein, the product of the *ABCD1* gene and a peroxisomal VLCFA CoA transporter. The symptoms include weakness and stiffness in the legs, impaired vision, and behavioral problems. Females who inherit a defective copy of the *ABCD1* gene on one of their X chromosomes may exhibit symptoms of adrenomyeloneuropathy (AMN) rather than ALD in their middle age. Symptoms of AMN include progressive neuropathy, paraparesis (loss of motor function) and adrenal insufficiency. ALD was popularized by a book and a movie titled *Lorenzo's Oil*, the story of a young patient with ALD named Lorenzo Odone. The title refers to the nutritional protocol, containing rapeseed and olive oils, developed by the patient's father, Augusto, a layperson, to slow the progression of the disease. Rapeseed oil contains erucic acid (20:1), which decreases the accumulation of VLCFA by apparently inhibiting their synthesis. Current treatment protocols also include cortisol administration. A lentiviral vector-based hematopoietic stem cell gene therapy with recombinant *ABCD1* gene shows some promise.

Foundations
Breakdown of biomolecules to succinyl CoA

One of the end products of the β-oxidation of odd-numbered fatty acids is propionyl CoA, which is converted via methylmalonyl CoA to succinyl CoA, an intermediate of the TCA cycle. Although acetyl CoA is not a precursor for gluconeogenesis, succinyl CoA can be converted to glucose via oxaloacetate. It may be recalled in this context that succinyl CoA is also generated during the degradation of the amino acids methionine, threonine, valine, and isoleucine (see **Fig. 15.9**).

Therapeutics
α-Oxidation, phytanic acid, and adult Refsum disease

Phytanic acid (3,7,11,15-tetramethylhexadecanoic acid) (▶ Fig. 13.8c) derived from chlorophyll, is a branched-chain fatty acid that humans obtain from dairy products, ruminant animal (e.g., cows, goats, sheep) fats, and certain types of fish. It cannot be broken down by β-oxidation due to the presence of the 3-methyl group. It is the only known substrate for catabolism by α-oxidation in peroxisomes in which a single carbon is removed from the carboxyl end to generate 2-methyl-branched pristanic acid (2,6,10,14-tetramethylpentadecanoic acid), which can be further broken down by peroxisomal and mitochondrial β-oxidation. A deficiency of phytanoyl CoA hydroxylase causes adult Refsum disease (ARD), leading to an accumulation of phytanoic acid. ARD is an autosomal recessive neurologic disease, and patients present with peripheral polyneuropathy, cerebellar ataxis, retinitis pigmentosa, anosmia, and hearing loss.

Therapeutics
Infantile Refsum disease

Infantile Refsum disease is an autosomal recessive disorder within the Zellweger spectrum and is caused by mutations in the genes for peroxins– proteins required for normal peroxisome assembly. Affected infants have decreased cerebral myelination and a loss of hearing and vision.

Normal
Omega oxidation of fatty acids

This alternative to the β-oxidation of fatty acids takes place in the endoplasmic reticulum (ER) and is catalyzed by the cytochrome P-450 system. ω-Oxidation involves the omega (ω)-carbon (which is positioned at the end opposite to that of the carboxyl group of a fatty acid) and generates dicarboxylic fatty acids. The ω-carbon is oxidized to an alcohol and then to a carboxylic acid via an aldehyde intermediate. This is normally a minor pathway. However, in patients with medium-chain acyl CoA dehydrogenase (MCAD) deficiency, the accumulated medium-chain fatty acids undergo ω-oxidation to medium-chain dicarboxylic acids (C6 through C10). The latter and their conjugates with carnitine and glycine can be detected in the plasma and urine.

Therapeutics
Fatty acid oxidation disorders

Inherited disorders of fatty acid oxidation encompass deficiencies of a wide range of enzymes and proteins involved in the transport and β-oxidation of fatty acids. These include members of the carnitine shuttle, various acyl CoA dehydrogenases (VLCAD, LCAD, MCAD, and SCAD), as well as the trifunctional protein (TFP), which comprises the activities of enoyl CoA hydratase, 3-hydroxyacyl CoA dehydrogenase, and β-ketothiolase. All known disorders of fatty acid oxidation are inherited as autosomal recessive traits, and several are part of newborn screening programs by measurement of acylcarnitine profiles in blood spots. Of these, the most common is a deficiency of MCAD, with an incidence of 1 in 12,000. This can lead to secondary carnitine deficiency due to increased excretion of medium-chain acylcarnitines and acylglycines in the urine. In addition, the C8 fatty acid octanoic acid accumulates in the liver, acts as a mitochondrial poison, and can cause hyperammonemia by interfering with the urea cycle. Some of the MCFAs undergo ω-oxidation, leading to the formation of medium-chain dicarboxylic acids and their conjugates with carnitine and glycine. Metabolic acidosis is the result of an overload of mono- and dicarboxylic acids in plasma. The inability of liver to use fatty acids for fuel makes it dependent on glucose as an energy source and limits gluconeogenesis (due to the low activity of pyruvate carboxylase as a result of reduced levels of its activator, acetyl CoA, as well as due to reduced ATP production) and can cause severe hypoglycemia. It appears likely that MCAD deficiency is in fact responsible for several instances of previously reported cases of Reye syndrome and sudden infant death syndrome (SIDS).

13.5 Ketone Bodies

Excessive β-oxidation of fatty acids occurs in states of fasting and starvation and causes an elevation in acetyl CoA levels. These acetyl CoA molecules are condensed with each other in hepatic mitochondria to produce ketone bodies.

- Ketone bodies are the water-soluble and acidic compounds known as acetoacetate, β-hydroxybutyrate, and acetone. Their accumulation lowers the pH of blood.
- Ketone bodies are produced only in the liver and serve as an important energy source for peripheral tissues during periods of prolonged (> 24 h) fasting.

13.5.1 Ketone Body Synthesis in Hepatocytes

The series of reactions in ketone body synthesis—which are similar to those of cholesterol synthesis—condense three acetyl CoA molecules together to form 3-hydroxy-3-methylglutaryl CoA (HMG CoA). HMG CoA is then converted to acetoacetate,

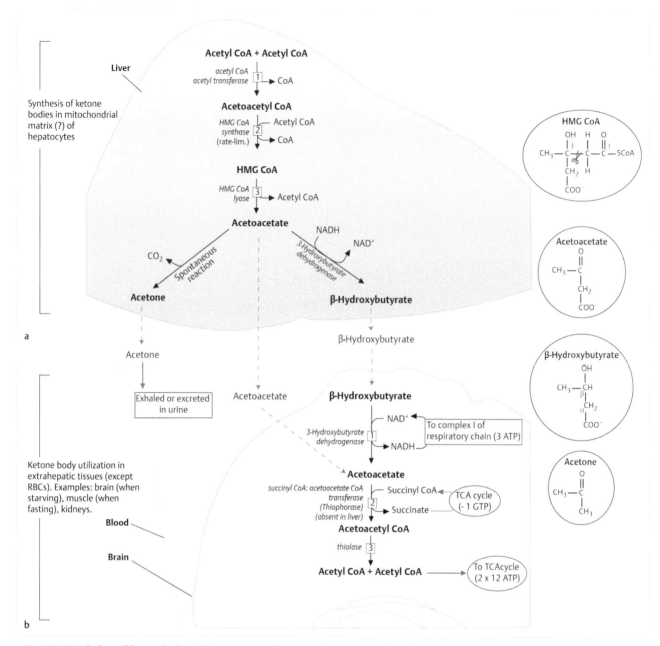

Fig. 13.9 Metabolism of ketone bodies. (a) Condensation of two acetyl coenzyme A (acetyl CoA) to generate acetoacetyl CoA, followed by the latter's condensation with a third acetyl CoA (by the rate-limiting HMG CoA synthase), creates 3-hydroxy-3-methyl-glutaryl CoA (HMG CoA). HMG CoA is cleaved by HMG CoA lyase to form acetoacetate and acetyl CoA with the release of a proton. Acetoacetate is either spontaneously decarboxylated to acetone or reduced to β-hydroxybutyrate. These three ketone bodies are released into the bloodstream, where acetone is exhaled or excreted in urine, but acetoacetate and β-hydroxybutyrate are taken up by peripheral tissues. **(b)** In peripheral tissues, β-hydroxybutyrate is converted to acetoacetate in a reaction that generates the reduced form of nicotinamide adenine dinucleotide (NADH). Acetoacetate is converted to acetoacetyl CoA via the action of thiophorase, an enzyme that is absent in liver cells. Acetoacetyl CoA is cleaved into two acetyl CoA molecules, which enter the tricarboxylic acid (TCA) cycle. RBCs, red blood cells.

which is either reduced to β-hydroxybutyrate or spontaneously decarboxylated into acetone. The steps of ketone body synthesis in liver mitochondria are as follows (▶ Fig. 13.9a):

1. Acetyl CoA acyltransferase transfers an acetyl residue from one acetyl CoA onto the α-carbon of a second acetyl CoA molecule, generating acetoacetyl CoA.

2. HMG CoA synthase transfers another acetyl residue from a third acetyl CoA onto the β-ketone of acetoacetyl CoA, generating HMG CoA.

- HMG CoA synthase is the rate-limiting enzyme of ketone body synthesis.

3. HMG CoA lyase converts the carbon 3 hydroxyl group of HMG CoA into a β-ketone via a reaction that generates a proton, acetyl CoA, and acetoacetate.

- Acetoacetate can be spontaneously decarboxylated to generate acetone. Because the latter cannot be oxidized further, it enters the bloodstream and is exhaled (detected as a fruity odor) or excreted in urine.

- Alternatively, acetoacetate can be reduced to β-hydroxybutyrate by 3-hydroxybutyrate dehydrogenase in a reaction that oxidizes NADH to NAD⁺.

13.5.2 Ketone Body Breakdown and Utilization in Peripheral Tissues

Acetoacetate and β-hydroxybutyrate are released into the blood by the liver and are taken up by peripheral tissues such as muscle, kidney, and brain. Ketone bodies are then broken down via the following mechanism (▶ Fig. 13.9b):

1. 3-Hydroxybutyrate dehydrogenase oxidizes β-hydroxybutyrate back into acetoacetate via a reaction that reduces NAD⁺ to NADH.
   - NADH can then donate its electrons to complex I of the respiratory chain to generate three molecules of ATP.
2. Succinyl CoA: acetoacetate CoA transferase (also known as thiophorase) "activates" acetoacetate by transferring CoA from succinyl CoA onto acetoacetate. This reaction generates succinate and acetoacetyl CoA.
   - The conversion of succinyl CoA to succinate by the TCA cycle would normally generate one GTP (equivalent to one ATP). Therefore, the use of succinyl CoA to activate acetoacetate instead equates to a loss of one ATP.
   - Liver cells cannot break down ketone bodies because they lack succinyl CoA: acetoacetate CoA transferase (thiophorase).
3. Thiolase then converts acetoacetyl CoA into two molecules of acetyl CoA, which enter the TCA cycle to ultimately generate 12 ATP per acetyl CoA.

13.5.3 Energy Yield

- One acetoacetate yields 23 ATP (24 from 2 acetyl CoA, minus 1 lost due to activation of acetoacetate).
- One β-hydroxybutyrate yields 26 ATP (3 from NADH, 24 from 2 acetyl CoA, minus 1 lost due to activation of acetoacetate).

Foundations

Ketogenic amino acids

Leucine and lysine are purely ketogenic amino acids because they can be catabolized only to acetyl CoA and/or acetoacetate, whereas threonine, tryptophan, isoleucine, phenylalanine, and tyrosine are both keto- and glucogenic (see **Fig. 15.6**).

Normal

Fuel supplies during fasting and starvation

During the first several hours of fasting, the fuel sources are blood glucose followed by glycogen stores in muscle and in liver. As insulin levels fall and glucagon levels rise, hepatic gluconeogenesis leads to a large increase in the release of glucose by the liver. At the end of the first day of fasting, mobilization of fatty acids from triacylglycerols stored in adipose tissue begins. Muscle shifts to fatty acids for fuel due to a lack of uptake of glucose. After 3 days, hepatic ketone

body production starts to increase. Glycerol from lipolysis and glucogenic amino acids from proteolysis of rapidly turning over proteins supply precursors for continued gluconeogenesis. At this stage, ketone bodies provide a third of the fuel sources for brain and heart muscle. After 1 to 2 weeks of starvation, ketone bodies become the major fuel source for the brain, and the degradation of muscle slows down. After the depletion of triacylglycerol stores by the end of 2 to 3 months, proteins become the only remaining fuel source until death.

Normal

NADH:NAD⁺ ratio and ketone bodies

The two main ketone bodies are acetoacetate and β-hydroxybutyrate. Their interconversion is catalyzed by mitochondrial β-hydroxybutyrate dehydrogenase. The ratio of β-hydroxybutyrate to acetoacetate in blood depends on the redox state of hepatic mitochondria as defined by the NADH:NAD⁺ ratio. Although the plasma β-hydroxybutyrate:acetoacetate ratio is usually 1:1 after a meal, it can rise to 6:1 after prolonged (> 72 h) fasting, and it can go as high as 10:1 during acute diabetic ketoacidosis (DKA). In DKA, the enhanced catabolism of fatty acids leads to an increase in the redox state, which favors β-hydroxybutyrate production. A high NADH:NAD⁺ ratio also inhibits the TCA cycle and diverts acetyl CoA toward ketone body synthesis.

Therapeutics

Testing for ketones

Commercial tests for ketones in urine and blood employ Legal reaction, in which acetoacetate in a sample of urine or blood is reacted with nitroprusside (nitroferricyanide) reagent under alkaline conditions to produce a purple-colored complex on a test strip. The presence of glycine in the reagent allows the detection of acetone as well. Legal test is semiquantitative and does not measure β-hydroxybutyrate. Sulfhydryl drugs (e.g., the antihypertensive drug captopril) can cause false-positives in the nitroprusside test. The blood levels of β-hydroxybutyrate can be measured fairly accurately in the range of 0.1 to 6.0 mM using immobilized β-hydroxybutyrate dehydrogenase test strips (Abbott Precision Xtra, Abbott Laboratories, Abbott Park, IL). Blood levels of β-hydroxybutyrate in normal fasting subjects are < 0.5 mM, whereas they can be 1 mM or greater in patients with DKA.

Therapeutics

Ketoacidosis during starvation and diabetes

Physiological ketosis, with mild to moderately elevated ketone bodies in circulation, can occur in response to fasting during pregnancy and in infants. Prolonged exercise and ketogenic diets (high in fat) can also cause physiological ketosis. In both starvation and uncontrolled diabetes, there can be a pathological overproduction of ketone bodies because there is enhanced mobilization and catabolism of fatty acids induced by an increase in the glucagon:insulin ratio. Glucagon stimulates fatty acid mobilization from adipose through the stimulation of hormone sensitive lipase and promotes fatty acid import into hepatic mitochondria through lower levels of malonyl CoA production. Thus, glucagon promotes increased concentrations of acetyl CoA in hepatic mitochondria. Enhanced gluconeogenesis (again due to glucagon) leads to a depletion of oxaloacetate, which would normally condense with acetyl CoA to form citrate. As a consequence, ketone body production is favored. Both acetoacetate and β-hydroxybutyrate are relatively strong organic acids ($pK_a \sim 3.5$) and tend to lower the blood pH, causing acidosis. Excess ketone bodies are excreted in the urine (ketosis), and acetoacetate can also be spontaneously converted to acetone, which is exhaled, giving a characteristic "fruity odor" to the breath of individuals with uncontrolled diabetes that mimics the breath of someone who is intoxicated. Other causes of pathological ketoacidosis include toxic ingestion of ethanol, methanol, ethylene glycol or salicylates, and cortisol or growth hormone deficiency.

13.6 Membrane Lipids

On the cytosolic face of the smooth endoplasmic reticulum, fatty acids are used to synthesize glycerophospholipids and sphingophospholipids (collectively referred to as phospholipids), which are the structural components of cellular membranes. Sphingolipids are particularly abundant in the white matter of the central nervous system.

13.6.1 Metabolism of Glycerophospholipids

Synthesis of glycerophospholipids. Glycerophospholipids are made up of two fatty acyl residues and a phosphate group esterified to a glycerol backbone. The phosphate residue, in turn, can be esterified to amino or sugar alcohols (e.g., choline and inositol, respectively) to generate specific glycerophospholipids. The mechanisms for the synthesis of the various glycerophospholipids share two common features:

1. Diacylglycerol (DAG) is a common substrate.
2. Cytidine diphosphate (CDP) is attached to different alcohols to help them serve as substrates (e.g., CDP-ethanolamine, CDP-choline, and CDP-DAG) (▶ Fig. 13.10a).

The synthesis of glycerophospholipids occurs primarily through transfer reactions catalyzed by transferases, as follows (▶ Fig. 13.10b):

- Phosphatidylethanolamine is produced when ethanolamine phosphotransferase transfers phosphoethanolamine from CDP-ethanolamine onto the carbon 3 hydroxyl group of DAG.
- Phosphatidylserine is generated when ethanolamine is removed from phosphatidylethanolamine and replaced with serine. Phosphatidylserine can be converted back to phosphatidylethanolamine by the removal of CO_2.
- Phosphatidylcholine is generated when choline phosphotransferase transfers phosphocholine from CDP-choline onto the carbon 3 hydroxyl of DAG.

○ Alternatively, when choline levels are low, phosphatidylcholine is produced via a reaction in which methyl groups (CH_3) are added to phosphatidylethanolamine. These methyl groups are provided by *S*-adenosyl methionine (SAM).
- Phosphatidylinositol is generated when inositol is transferred to the carbon 3 hydroxyl of CDP-DAG. This reaction, which releases CMP, is catalyzed by CDP-DAG-inositol-3-phosphatidyl transferase.
- Phosphatidic acid (1, 2-diacylglycerolphosphate) is produced when the carbon 3 hydroxyl of DAG is phosphorylated (▶ Fig. 13.10a).

Degradation of glycerophospholipids. Phospholipases are enzymes that hydrolyze specific ester bonds within membrane-bound glycerophospholipids to trigger the release of their various components, as follows (▶ Fig. 13.10c):

- Phospholipase A_1 (PLA_1) hydrolyzes the ester bond between the carbon 1 hydroxyl and its fatty acyl group.
- Phospholipase A_2 (PLA_2) hydrolyzes the ester bond between the carbon 2 hydroxyl and its fatty acyl group.
- Phospholipase C (PLC) hydrolyzes the ester bond between the carbon 3 hydroxyl and the phosphate group.
- Phospholipase D (PLD) hydrolyzes the phosphatidyl ester bond between the sugar or amino alcohol and the phosphate group.

Once released, the fatty acid chains are degraded via β-oxidation.

Foundations

PLD and Alzheimer disease

Gene knockout of the Phospholipase D isoforms, PLD1 and PLD2, in mouse models of Alzheimer disease appears to be prevent the progression of the disease. Isoform-specific inhibitors of PLD, derived from the psychotropic agent, halopemide, have been developed and may help define the role of PLD in in the pathogenesis of Alzheimer disease.

Foundations

Plasmalogens

Plasmalogens are a type of glycerophospholipids that contain a fatty alcohol via a vinyl ether bond at the sn-1 position and an unsaturated fatty acid via an ester linkage at the sn-2 position. The head group is usually either a choline or an ethanolamine (see ▶ Fig. 3.6a). Plasmalogens may represent up to 18% of total phospholipid mass in humans and are highly expressed in the nervous system, but their function is not very clear. It has been proposed that they serve as antioxidants and free radical scavengers. Their biosynthesis involves both peroxisomes and endoplasmic reticulum. Peroxisomal disorders such as Zellweger syndrome and cerebral adrenoleukodystrophy cause impaired biosynthesis of plasmalogens. Prefrontal cortex regions of the brain of patients with Alzheimer disease contain significantly lower levels of choline plasmalogens.

Plasmalogens may also play a role in prostaglandin formation by providing arachidonic acid.

IV

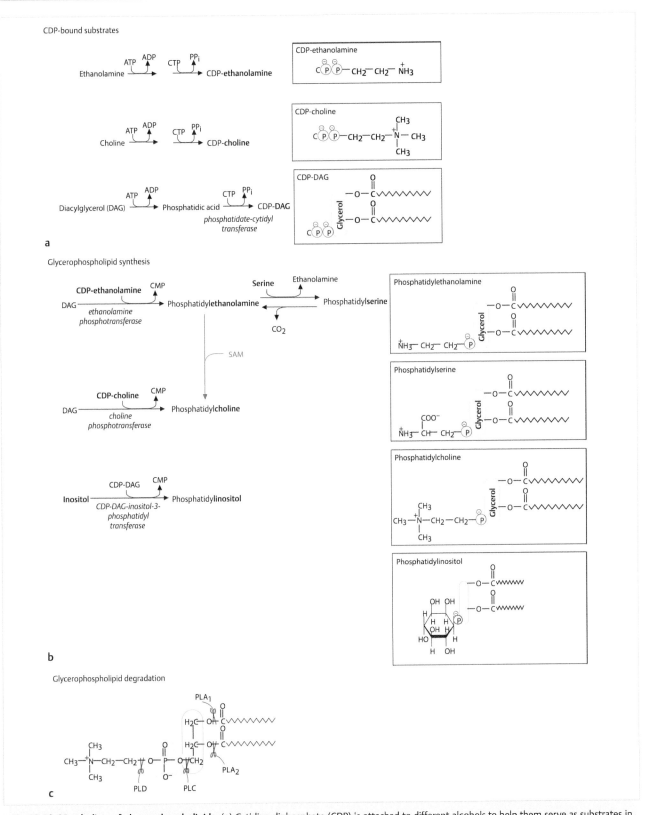

Fig. 13.10 Metabolism of glycerophospholipids. (a) Cytidine diphosphate (CDP) is attached to different alcohols to help them serve as substrates in the synthesis of glycerophospholipids. The mechanism for forming common CDP-bound alcohols, such as CDP-ethanolamine, CDP-choline, and CDP-diacylglycerol (DAG), is outlined here. (b) The synthesis of phosphatidylethanolamine, phosphatidylserine, phosphatidylcholine, and phosphatidylinositol is outlined here. (c) Glycerophospholipids are degraded by phospholipases (e.g., PLA$_1$, PLA$_2$, PLC, PLD) that cleave ester bonds at specific sites.

Table 13.2 Sphingolipidoses and their associated defective enzyme(s)

Sphingolipidosis	Defective enzyme	Effect
Niemann-Pick disease	Sphingomyelinase	Accumulation of sphingomyelin in brain and red blood cells; leads to seizures, ataxia; fatal before 3 years
Tay-Sachs disease	Hexosaminidase A	Accumulation of gangliosides (GM₂) in neurons; leads to muscle atrophy, blindness (Sandhof disease is more rapid)
Sandhof disease	Hexosaminidase A and B	Similar to Tay-Sachs, but Sandhof disease progresses more rapidly than the former Tay-Sachs
Krabbe disease	β-Galactosidase	Accumulation of glycolipids in oligodendrocytes; leads to complete demyelination
Gaucher disease	β-Glucosidase	Accumulation of glucocerebrosides in liver, spleen, and red blood cells; leads to skeletal erosion
Fabry disease	α-Galactosidase	Accumulation of glycolipids in brain, heart, kidney; leads to rashes, kidney failure, peripheral neuropathy
Metachromatic leukodystrophy	Arylsulfatase A	Accumulation of sulfatides in neural tissue; leads to demyelination; nervous tissue stains brownish yellow with cresyl violet dye

Note: The most common symptoms of sphingolipidoses are mental retardation and enlargement of the liver and/or spleen. All listed disorders are autosomal recessive with the exception of Fabry disease (X-linked).

13.6.2 Metabolism of Sphingolipids

Sphingolipids are built on the long-chain amino alcohol sphingosine, whose components are derived from serine and palmitic acid. Addition of a fatty acyl chain to sphingosine generates ceramide (▶ Fig. 13.11a) the precursor molecule for the synthesis of sphingolipids such as sphingophospholipids and glycosphingolipids/ glycolipids.

- Sphingophospholipids are each composed of ceramide + phosphate + amino (or sugar) alcohol.
- Glycosphingolipids (glycolipids) are each composed of ceramide + sugar residues.

Synthesis and degradation of sphingolipids

Sphingolipids are degraded to ceramide in the lysosomes of the reticuloendothelial system (liver, spleen, and bone marrow). Sphingolipidoses are diseases that arise from genetic deficiencies in enzymes that degrade sphingolipids (▶ Table 13.3, ▶ Fig. 13.11, ▶ Fig. 13.12) The mechanisms by which various sphingolipids are formed and degraded are summarized as follows:

- Sphingomyelin is generated when phosphocholine or sometimes phosphoethanolamine is attached to ceramide.
  - Sphingomyelinase cleaves sphingomyelin into phosphocholine and ceramide in the lysosomes. Niemann-Pick disease is a lysosomal storage disorder associated with a defect in sphingomyelinase. It is marked by the accumulation of sphingomyelin in spleen, liver, lungs, bone marrow and brain. It leads to seizures and ataxia and can be fatal before 3 years of age.
- Gangliosides are produced when two or more sugars and *N*-acetylneuraminic acid (Neu5Ac or sialic acid) are added to ceramide.
  - Hexosaminidases A and B cleave the glycosidic bond linking the amino sugar *N*-acetyl-D-galactosamine (GalNAc) and galactose (▶ Fig. 13.12).
  - Tay-Sachs disease is caused by defective hexosaminidase A and manifests as accumulation of ganglioside GM₂ in neurons. It leads to muscle atrophy and blindness.

- Sandhoff disease, which is caused by defects in both hexosaminidase A and B, progresses more rapidly.
- Cerebrosides such as galactocerebroside and glucocerebroside are produced when a sugar (e.g., galactose or glucose, respectively) is attached to ceramide.
  - β-Galactosidase (β-galactoceramidase) cleaves the glycosidic bond between galactose and ceramide. A defect in β-galactosidase leads to Krabbe disease. This disorder is marked by accumulation of glycolipids in oligodendrocytes, which leads to complete demyelination.
  - β-Glucosidase cleaves the glycosidic bond between glucose and ceramide. Gaucher disease is caused by a defective β-glucosidase (β-glucoceramidase). Accumulation of glucocerebrosides in liver, spleen, and red blood cells, and skeletal erosion, are observed in patients with this disorder.
- Globosides are formed when three or more sugars along with the amino sugar GalNAc are attached to ceramide.
  - α-Galactosidase cleaves the glycosidic bond between two galactose residues. Fabry disease develops when α-galactosidase is defective. It is marked by the accumulation of glycolipids in brain, heart, and kidney and leads to rashes, kidney failure, and peripheral neuropathy.
- Sulfatides are generated when sulfate residues are transferred to cerebrosides. Phospho-adenosine-5′-phosphosulfate (PAPS) serves as the donor of these sulfate residues.
  - Arylsulfatase A cleaves sulfate groups from sulfatides. Metachromatic leukodystrophy is caused by a defect in arylsulfatase A. It is marked by the accumulation of sulfatides in neural tissue and leads to demyelination. Nervous tissue stains brownish yellow with cresyl violet dye.

13.7 Eicosanoids

13.7.1 Overview

Eicosanoids are a group of signaling molecules that mediate many of the body's defense mechanisms, such as pain, inflammation, allergic response, and blood clotting. They are synthe-

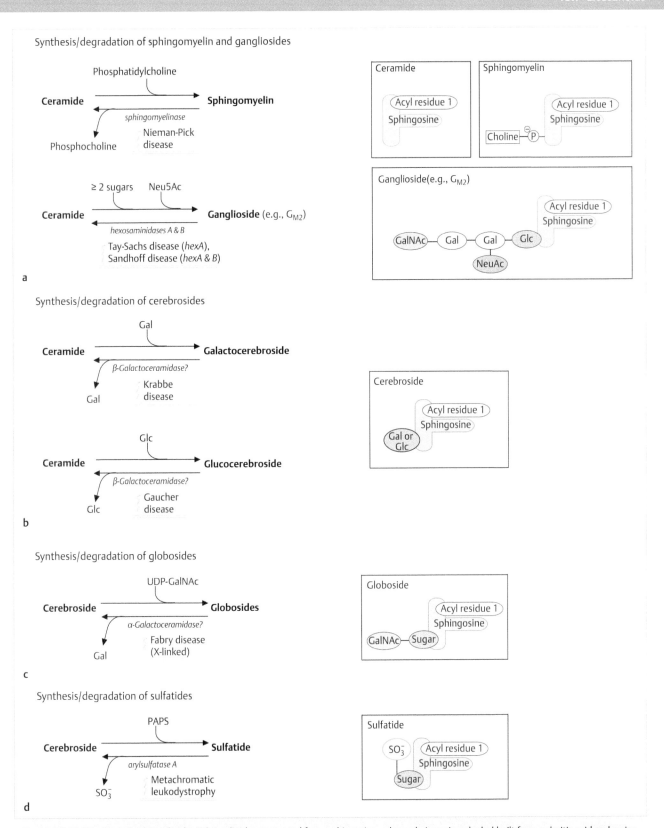

Fig. 13.11 Metabolism of sphingolipids. Sphingolipids are created from sphingosine, a long-chain amino alcohol built from palmitic acid and serine. Attachment of a fatty acid to the carbon 2 amino group of sphingosines in an amide linkage produces ceramide. (**a**) Adding phosphocholine to ceramide generates sphingomyelin. Adding sugars, either unmodified or modified, to ceramide gives rise to glycosphingolipids (glycolipids) such as gangliosides (**a**), cerebrosides (**b**), globosides (**c**), and sulfatides (**d**). Sulfate groups are donated by phospho-adenosine-5′-phospho-sulfate (PAPS). The sphingolipidoses associated with defects in particular enzymes are noted. UDP, uridine diphosphate.

IV

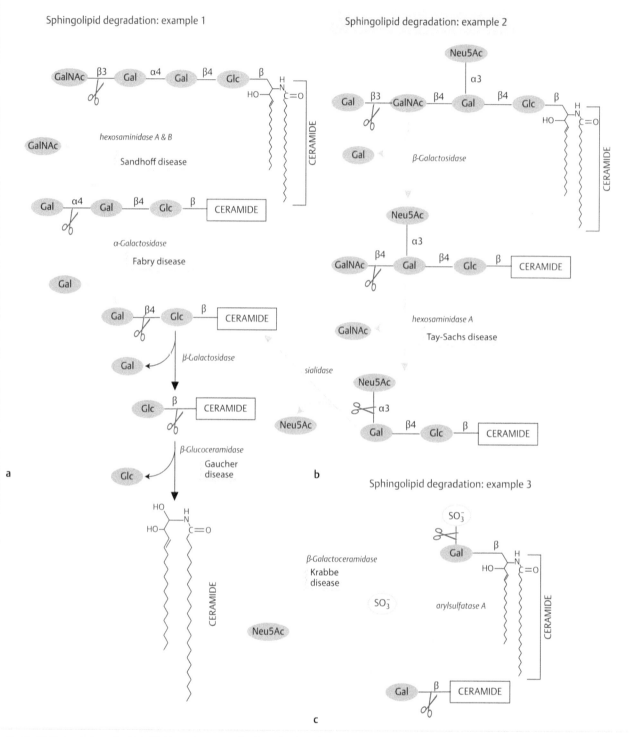

Fig. 13.12 Degradation of sphingolipids and associated sphingolipidoses. (a-c) Schematic of the enzymes and disorders associated with the degradation of three examples of sphingolipids.

sized from 20-carbon unsaturated fatty acids containing three, four, or five double bonds (Greek *eicosa* = 20). Eicosanoid production is not limited to a single organ or tissue.

- The most common precursor of eicosanoids is arachidonic acid (20:4ω6). This fatty acid is formed by the elongation and desaturation of the essential fatty acids linoleic (18:2ω6) and γ-linolenic (18:3ω6) acid (▶ Fig. 13.13).
- Other precursors of eicosanoids include dihomo-γ-linolenic acid (20:3ω6) and the ω-3 fatty acid, eicosapentanoic acid (EPA, 20:5ω3).
- Because arachidonic acid is stored in cells in the form of membrane glycerophospholipids, it can be released by the action of an inducible cytosolic phospholipase A_2 (PLA_2) (▶ Fig. 13.13).
  - Corticosteroids act as antiinflammatory agents by inhibiting the activity of PLA_2, which prevents its induction by external stimuli. Additionally, corticosteroids such as dexamethasone and corticosterone repress tumor necrosis factor (TNF)–induced expression of *PLA_2* gene and inhibit the production of all eicosanoids.

13.7.2 Classes

There are four main classes of eicosanoids (▶ Fig. 13.13):
1. **Prostaglandins (PGs):** These contain a five-membered ring structure with variable substitutions, and with one to three double bonds outside the ring. The naming convention of individual prostaglandins includes a capital letter designation after PG to indicate the specific ring structure, followed by a subscript that specifies the number of double bonds outside the ring, and the letter α or β to indicate the stereospecificity of the hydroxyl group, if present, at position 9 at the top of the ring (e.g., $PGF_{2\alpha}$, PGI_2).
2. **Thromboxanes (TXs):** These contain a six-membered oxane ring structure. The naming of individual thromboxanes includes a capital letter designation after TX to indicate the ring substitutions, followed by a numerical subscript to indicate the number of nonring double bonds (e.g., TXB_2).
3. **Hydroxyeicosatetraenoic acids (HETEs):** These are formed from arachidonate by the action of 5-, 12-, or 15-lipoxygenases via the corresponding hydroperoxy intermediates. Examples include 5-HETE, 12-HETE, and 15-HETE.
4. **Leukotrienes (LTs):** These derive their name from the fact that they contain three conjugated double bonds and were originally discovered in leukocytes. The naming of various types of leukotrienes includes a capital letter designation after LT, followed by the total number of double bonds (e.g., LTD_4).

13.7.3 Eicosanoid Metabolism

The release of arachidonate from phospholipids by phospholipase A_2 is the rate-limiting step for the following two pathways through which eicosanoids are produced from arachidonic acid.
1. **Cyclooxygenase (COX) pathway** leads to the formation of prostaglandins and thromboxanes via unstable intermediates, PGG_2 and PGH_2. This occurs via reactions catalyzed by prostaglandin H (PGH) synthase—a heme-containing dioxygenase that exhibits both cyclooxygenase

and peroxidase activities. There are two isozymes of PGH synthase called COX1 and COX2. COX1 is constitutively expressed in many tissues, whereas COX2 is inducible by growth factors and cytokines.
   Key features of COX reactions include the following (▶ Fig. 13.13):
   - The cyclooxygenase activity of PGH synthase forms PGG_2 from arachidonate.
   - PGG_2 is then converted to PGH_2 by the peroxidase activity of PGH synthase.
   - PGH_2 is then rapidly converted into other prostaglandins, prostacyclin, and thromboxanes by additional enzymes present in specific tissues.
     - Many nonsteroidal antiinflammatory drugs (NSAIDs) inhibit both isozymes of COX, thus reducing inflammation, fever, and pain by decreasing prostaglandin production. They also inhibit blood clotting by inhibiting thromboxane production.
     - Aspirin (acetylsalicylic acid) is an irreversible inhibitor of COX enzymes. Aspirin covalently modifies the enzyme's protein structure by acetylating a serine residue in the active site.
2. **Lipoxygenase pathway** leads to HETEs and leukotrienes via unstable intermediates called HPETEs (hydroperoxyeicosatetraenoic acids).

13.7.4 Effects of Eicosanoids

Most eicosanoids are fairly short-lived, so they tend to act in a paracrine fashion. They signal through G protein–coupled receptor pathways and alter the levels of secondary messengers, as follows:
- PGE_2 signaling increases cellular cAMP levels.
- $PGF_{2\alpha}$ signaling causes an increase in cGMP levels.
- Thromboxane signaling, however, tends to decrease the levels of cAMP (▶ Fig. 13.14a) and cGMP.

The specific roles of eicosanoids in mediating the body's defense mechanisms are summarized as follows:

Prostaglandins are the mediators of inflammation and pain. They generally cause:
- vasodilation through vascular smooth muscle relaxation and
- an increase in vascular permeability, leading to edema.
  - PGE_2 can cause uterine smooth muscle contractions and has been used clinically to induce labor.

Thromboxanes act to facilitate blood clotting by enhancing vasoconstriction and promoting platelet aggregation (▶ Fig. 13.14a).
- PGI_2 (prostacyclin) interferes with blood clotting by interfering with thromboxane's action. Prostacyclin, which is produced by the endothelial cells of the blood vessel wall, is relatively long-lived compared with other prostaglandins and is known as the circulating prostaglandin.

HETEs, especially 5-HETE, affect neutrophils and eosinophils (▶ Fig. 13.14b). It mediates chemotaxis, stimulates adenylate cyclase, and induces polymorphonuclear leukocytes to degranulate and release hydrolytic enzymes such as elastase, myeloperoxidase, cathepsins, and defensins.

Leukotrienes are more stable than prostaglandins. They are the mediators of the allergic response and are involved in the development of asthma. Leukotrienes are usually produced

IV

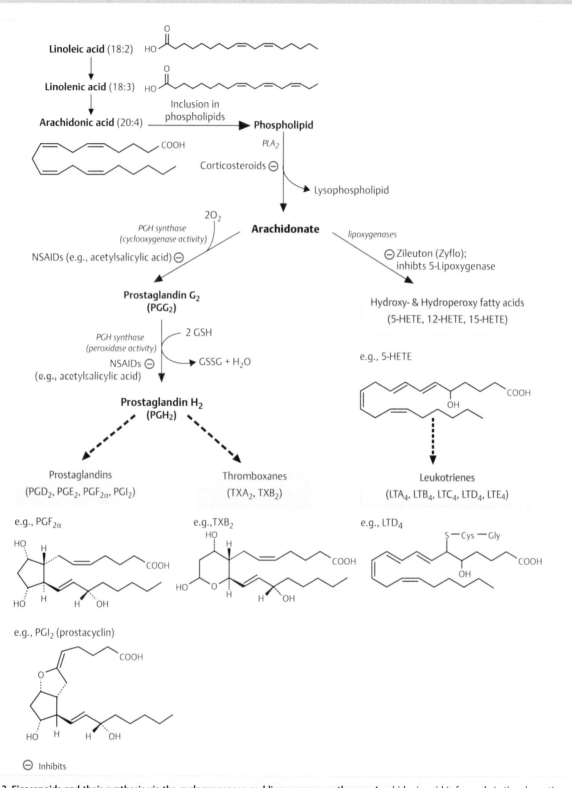

Fig. 13.13 Eicosanoids and their synthesis via the cyclooxygenase and lipoxygenase pathways. Arachidonic acid is formed via the elongation and saturation of the essential fatty acids linoleic acid and γ-linolenic acid. The 20-carbon arachidonate is incorporated into membrane glycerophospholipids and released by the action of phospholipase A_2 (PLA_2). PLA_2 is inhibited by corticosteroids. Metabolism of freed arachidonate by the cyclooxygenase (COX) pathway generates prostaglandin H_2 (PGH_2) via the action of PGH synthase. This enzyme is inhibited by nonsteroidal antiinflammatory drugs (NSAIDs) such as aspirin (acetylsalicyclic acid). PGH_2 is then converted to prostaglandins and thromboxanes. On the other hand, metabolism of arachidonate by the lipoxygenase pathway generates hydroxyeicosatetraenoic acids (HETEs) and leukotrienes. GSH, reduced glutathione; GSSG, oxidized glutathione.

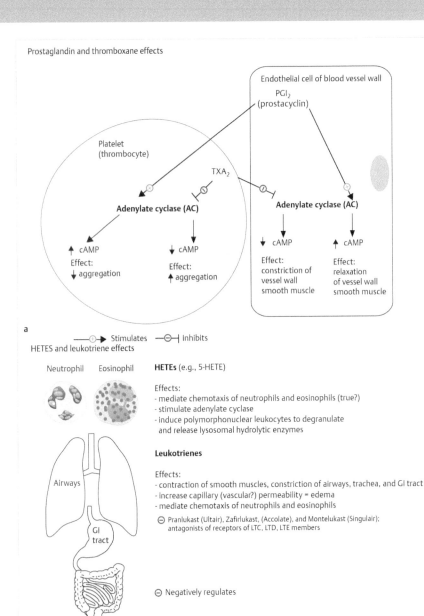

Prostaglandin and thromboxane effects

Fig. 13.14 Effects of eicosanoids. (a) Thromboxanes (e.g., TXA_2) inhibit the production of cyclic adenosine monophosphate (cAMP) by adenylate cyclase. In doing so in platelets and endothelial cells of blood vessel walls, thromboxanes facilitate blood clotting by promoting platelet aggregation and enhancing vasoconstriction. **(b)** Summarized are the effects of hydroxyeicosatetraenoic acids (HETES) and leukotrienes on neutrophils, eosinophils, the airways, and the gastrointestinal (GI) tract.

IV

within minutes after an allergic stimulus (e.g., binding of IgE to receptors on the surface of mast cells) and are called mediators of immediate hypersensitivity.

- Leukotrienes are produced only in cells of myeloid lineage, such as neutrophils, eosinophils, mast cells, macrophages, basophils, and monocytes.
- Production of leukotrienes is regulated at multiple levels, such as cytosolic phospholipase A_2 ($cPLA_2$), 5-lipoxygenase (5-LO), and leukotriene C_4 synthase (LTC_4S). $cPLA_2$ is activated by divalent cations such as Ca^{2+} and by phosphorylation on serine residues (usually mediated by mitogen-activated protein kinases). Activated enzyme relocalizes from the cytoplasm to the nuclear envelope, which is the source of its substrate phospholipids.
  - LTs promote smooth muscle contraction, constriction of pulmonary airways, trachea, and intestine, and increased capillary permeability, resulting in edema.
  - LTC, LTD, and LTE members, such as LTC_4, LTD_4, and LTE_4, are described as slow-reacting substances of anaphylaxis

(SRS-A) or cysteinyl LTs. They cause a slowly evolving but protracted contraction of smooth muscles in the airways and gastrointestinal tract.
  - Plasma enzymes rapidly convert LTC_4 to LTD_4 and then slowly to LTE_4. As such, LTD_4, for example, increases in the allergic response.
  - LTB_4 helps mediate chemotaxis of neutrophils and eosinophils.
  - LTs are much more potent than histamine in contracting non-vascular smooth muscles of the bronchi and intestine.

Pharmaceuticals that target eicosanoid metabolism

Several drugs for asthma and allergies target eicosanoid synthesis:
- Zileuton is a 5-lipoxygenase inhibitor that blocks the production of LTC, LTD, and LTE members, as well as LTB_4 and 5-HETE.

- Pranlukast, zafirlukast, and montelukast are antagonists of LTC, LTD, and LTE member receptors.
- Steroidal antiinflammatory drugs such as hydrocortisone, prednisone, and betamethasone appear to act by blocking LT and HETE production by inhibiting phospholipase A_2 levels so as to interfere with the mobilization of arachidonic acid.

Therapeutics
Nonsteroidal antiinflammatory drugs

NSAIDs such as aspirin, ibuprofen, and naproxen are multibillion-dollar over-the-counter (OTC) pharmaceuticals.

Therapeutics
Selective COX2 inhibitors

Prostaglandins produced by the action of COX1 help gastric mucosa to secrete mucus, which protects the mucosal layer from damage due to acid. NSAIDs, by inhibiting prostaglandin production, increase the risk of development of gastric ulcers. Selective COX2 inhibitors such as celecoxib and rofecoxib have been developed that do not inhibit COX1 and are therefore less prone to gastric injury while still being effective regulators of pain and inflammation. However, some COX2 inhibitors (e.g., rofecoxib) have been found to cause a higher rate of incidence of thrombotic cardiovascular events due to continued production of thromboxane in the presence of a decreased prostacyclin (PGI_2) synthesis.

Therapeutics
Anticoagulative potency of aspirin

Most NSAIDs inhibit COX1 and COX2 in the platelets, and as a result, platelets lose the ability to aggregate and cannot initiate hemostasis. When the NSAID treatment is withdrawn, thromboxane production resumes and so does clotting ability. Aspirin, however, covalently modifies COX1 and COX2 and permanently suppresses the production of thromboxanes. The only way to overcome the inhibitory effect of aspirin is to synthesize new prostaglandin H (PGH) synthase. Because platelets lack nuclei, new enzyme synthesis requires the formation of new platelets (the normal turnover rate for platelets is 7 days). When aspirin is withdrawn, platelet thromboxane levels continue to be reduced, and the antithrombotic effect is now exacerbated by the resumed production of circulating prostacyclin in the endothelium.

Therapeutics
Aspirin-induced asthma

Aspirin-induced asthma is the result of enhanced conversion of arachidonate into leukotrienes when COX enzymes are disabled.

Therapeutics
Patent (open) ductus arteriosus

The ductus arteriosus is a small blood vessel that connects the pulmonary artery to the aortic arch during fetal development. It allows blood from the right ventricle to bypass the nonfunctioning lungs and mix with oxygenated blood leaving the left ventricle. Prostaglandins, specifically PGE_1 (Alprostadil), are responsible for the patency of the ductus arteriosus. It should close spontaneously shortly after birth. In some preterm infants, however, the ductus arteriosus remains open. Medications that block the synthesis of prostaglandins can be used to help achieve a faster closure. These include indomethacin, a nonselective inhibitor of both COX1 and COX2.

Therapeutics
Prostaglandin E_1

Prostaglandin E_1 goes by the pharmaceutical name alprostadil.

Normal
Lipoxins, resolvins, and protectins

Lipoxins, resolvins, and protectins (also called neuroprotectins) are essential fatty acid–derived mediators of active resolution of inflammation. Lipoxins (e.g., LXA4) are made from arachidonic acid ($20:4\ \omega6$). Eicosapenatanoic acid ($20:5\omega3$) serves as the precursor of the E series of resolvins (e.g., RvE1, RvE2), whereas docosahexanoic acid ($22:6\omega3$) is the precursor of the D series of resolvins (e.g., RvD1, RvD2) and protectins (e.g., protectin D1). Their biosynthesis is aspirin triggered and is catalyzed by acetylated COX2. These compounds oppose the proinflammatory action of prostanoids and have been shown to reduce dermal inflammation and peritonitis; stimulate resolution of neutrophil trafficking; block LTB_4-induced chemotaxis and degranulation of polymorphonuclear leukocytes and LTD_4-induced vasoconstriction; and have beneficial effects in animal models of stroke, Alzheimer disease, and asthma. Lipoxins, resolvins, and protectins may help explain the potent antiinflammatory effects of aspirin and also some of the documented benefits of ω-3 fatty acids. Stable analogues of these compounds that resist metabolic inactivation are currently being developed as a new genus of pharmacological agents in the treatment of pathological inflammation.

14 Cholesterol and Steroid Metabolism

14.1 Isoprenoids

Isoprenoids are a class of lipids that, like the fatty acid–derived lipids, are synthesized from the two-carbon molecule acetyl coenzyme A (CoA). Lipids that are classified as isoprenoids include the following (▶ Fig. 14.1):

- Steroids (e.g., cholesterol, bile acids, steroid hormones)
- All or portions of structures of lipid-soluble vitamins (e.g., vitamins A, D, E, K)
- Others such as ubiquinone/coenzyme Q (which plays a role in the mitochondrial electron transport chain), dolochol (which acts as a carrier of sugars during the assembly of *N*-glycosylated proteins), the isoprenoid tail of heme A, and the prenyl groups found attached to various proteins that facilitate their anchorage to cellular membranes and are essential for their maturation and function.

The building block for the synthesis of all isoprenoids is an acetyl CoA–derived molecule called isopentenyl pyrophosphate (IPP), also known as "active" isoprene (▶ Fig. 14.1) The five carbons of IPP are obtained from three acetyl CoA molecules, and when multiple IPP units are linked together, they form linear and/or cyclic molecules. For instance:

- Six IPP units can be condensed into a tetracyclic (four-ring) structure called a sterane (▶ Fig. 14.2a) and the side chain of sterols. The sterane structure is a hallmark component of all steroids (▶ Fig. 14.2b).

Foundations

Sources of acetyl CoA

Acetyl CoA, the precursor for isoprenoid biosynthesis, is generated in the mitochondria from multiple sources, such as oxidative decarboxylation of pyruvate, β-oxidation of fatty acids, and catabolism of several amino acids, as detailed in **Fig. 15.6a**. It is transported into the cytoplasm by the citrate shuttle, as described in **Fig. 13.3**.

Foundations

Prenylated proteins

Prenylation is a type of covalent lipid modification of certain proteins. It involves the addition of a farnesyl (three isoprene units) or a geranylgeranyl (four isoprene units) group to cysteine residues at or near the C-terminus of proteins. Examples of prenylated proteins include nuclear lamins, some

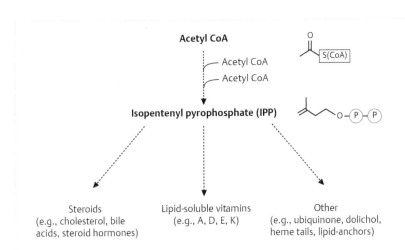

Fig. 14.1 Isoprenoids. Three acetyl coenzyme A (CoA) molecules are used to generate an "active" isoprene called isopentenyl pyrophosphate (IPP). This five-carbon IPP serves as the building block for the synthesis of all isoprenoids, including steroids and lipid-soluble vitamins.

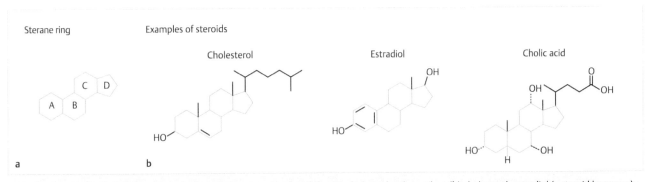

Fig. 14.2 Steroids. All steroids contain the four-ring sterane structure (**a**) and include molecules such as (**b**) cholesterol, estradiol (a steroid hormone), and cholic acid (a bile acid). *Note:* Sterols are steroid molecules with hydroxyl groups.

protein kinases, and monomeric G proteins such as RAS and related proteins. Because of the hydrophobic nature of the prenyl group, the modification promotes membrane association of prenylated proteins. Such lipid anchoring to the plasma membrane is necessary for the signal-transducing role of proteins such as RAS. Prenylation is a prerequisite for proper maturation of nuclear lamin A. It appears to play an important role in protein–protein interactions as well.

14.2 Cholesterol

14.2.1 Structure

Cholesterol—the most important steroid—is a critical component of plasma membranes and serves as a precursor for the synthesis of a variety of essential biomolecules, such as bile acids, steroid hormones, and vitamin D. Cholesterol is composed of 27 carbons, one hydroxyl (OH) group, and one double bond distributed within its structure, as follows (▶ Fig. 14.3):

- The sterane ring is composed of 17 carbons.
- The methyl-branched side chain at carbon 17 (C-17) is made up of eight carbons.
- The two methyl groups at C-10 and C-13 account for two carbons.
- There is an OH group at C-3.
- There is a double bond between C-5 and C-6.

14.2.2 Cholesterol Synthesis

The human body synthesizes ~ 750 mg of cholesterol per day. The synthesis of cholesterol takes place in the cytosol and endoplasmic reticulum (ER) of nucleated cells in all tissues. The largest amounts, however, are synthesized by the liver, small intestine, adrenal cortex, ovaries, testes, and skin in many animals. In humans, the liver accounts for only 10–15% of total cholesterol synthesis. The rest comes from the extrahepatic tissues. The overall pathway of cholesterol synthesis is summarized by the following equation:

$$18 \text{ Acetyl CoA} + 18\text{ATP} + 16\text{NADPH} + 16\text{H}^+ + 4\text{O}_2$$
$$\rightarrow \text{Cholesterol} + 16\text{NADP}^+ + 18\text{ADP} + 18\text{P}_i$$

The synthesis of cholesterol involves numerous steps, which can be divided into two phases:

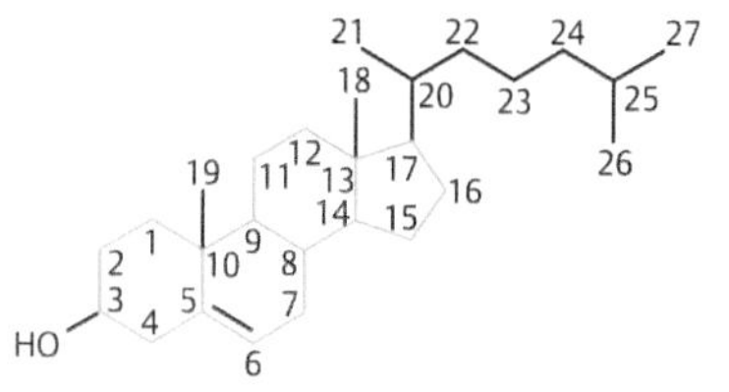

Cholesterol

Fig. 14.3 **Structural features of cholesterol.** Cholesterol is a 27-carbon molecule; 17 carbons make up the sterane ring (green), 8 carbons are found in the methyl-branched side chain at carbon 17 (C-17), and 2 carbons are found in the methyl (CH$_3$) groups at C-10 and C-13. An OH group is located at C-3, and a double bond exists between C-5 and C-6.

Phase I: Conversion of Acetyl CoA into Isopentenyl Pyrophosphate (▶ Fig. 14.4a, b)

- The first two reactions condense three acetyl CoAs into 3-hydroxy-3-methylglutaryl CoA (HMG CoA) in the cytoplasm. These reactions are similar to those that generate mitochondrial HMG CoA for the synthesis of ketone bodies (see **Fig. 13.9**).
- HMG CoA reductase, the rate-limiting enzyme of cholesterol synthesis, utilizes two molecules of the reduced form of nicotinamide adenine dinucleotide phosphate (NADPH) for its conversion of HMG CoA to mevalonate (step 3). Although HMG CoA reductase is embedded in the membrane of the ER, its catalytic domain extends into the cytoplasm, where it carries out its enzymatic activity.
- The activity of HMG CoA reductase is stimulated by the hormones insulin and thyroxine and inhibited by glucagon, sterols, high adenosine monophosphate (AMP) concentration, vitamin E, and statins.
- Mevalonate is then converted to IPP in three steps, the first two being adenosine triphosphate (ATP)-dependent.

Phase II: Conversion of Isopentenyl Pyrophosphate into Cholesterol (▶ Fig. 14.4a, b, c)

- Sequential head-to-tail condensation of three IPP units form farnesyl pyrophosphate (FPP).
- Head-to-head condensation of two FPP molecules, which is dependent on NADPH to form squalene, a 30-carbon linear molecule is catalyzed by an enzyme localized to the ER. Subsequent steps in the pathway also take place in the ER.
- Oxygen is used in the cyclization of squalene into lanosterol, a 30-carbon, OH-containing cyclic sterol. NADPH also provides the reducing power for these reactions.
- Lanosterol is then converted in multiple steps involving oxidative demethylation, isomerization, and reduction into cholesterol, a 27-carbon cyclic molecule. NADPH again provides the reducing power for these reactions.
- Enzymes that catalyze the reactions that convert lanosterol to cholesterol are the targets of antifungal agents such as miconazole and ketoconazole.

14.2.3 Regulation of Cholesterol Synthesis

Cholesterol synthesis is regulated mainly through HMG CoA reductase, the enzyme that converts HMG CoA to mevalonate (▶ Fig. 14.4a). The activity, phosphorylation/dephosphorylation state, expression, and rate of degradation of HMG CoA reductase are modulated by insulin and thyroxine, glucagon, cholesterol and its derivatives, a family of drugs called statins, and elevated AMP levels, as follows:

1. **Direct inhibition**
   - Direct inhibitors of HMG CoA reductase activity (in vitro) include free fatty acids, bile acids, and oxysterols (which are created by the addition of oxygen or hydroxyl groups to cholesterol).

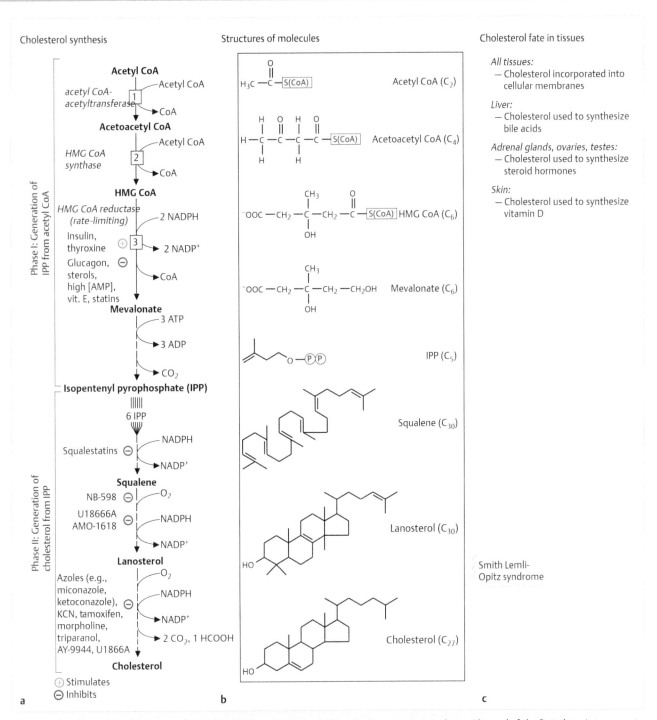

Cholesterol synthesis

Structures of molecules

Cholesterol fate in tissues

All tissues:
— Cholesterol incorporated into cellular membranes

Liver:
— Cholesterol used to synthesize bile acids

Adrenal glands, ovaries, testes:
— Cholesterol used to synthesize steroid hormones

Skin:
— Cholesterol used to synthesize vitamin D

IV

Fig. 14.4 Cholesterol synthesis. (a) Pathway. **(b)** Structures. Cholesterol biosynthesis occurs in two phases. The goal of the first phase is to convert acetyl coenzyme A (CoA) into isopentenyl pyrophosphate (IPP). The steps involved are as follows: (1) Two acetyl CoA molecules are condensed to form acetoacetyl CoA in a reaction catalyzed by acetyl CoA acetyltransferase. (2) 3-Hydroxy-3-methylglutaryl (HMG) CoA synthase transfers the acetyl residue of a third acetyl CoA onto acetoacetyl CoA, generating HMG CoA. (3) HMG CoA reductase, the rate-limiting enzyme, utilizes two molecules of the reduced form of nicotinamide adenine dinucleotide phosphate (NADPH) to convert HMG CoA into mevalonate. The activity of HMG CoA reductase is stimulated by the hormones insulin and thyroxine and inhibited by glucagon, sterols, high adenosine monophosphate (AMP) concentrations, vitamin E, and statins. Through multiple steps that utilize three adenosine triphosphates (ATPs), mevalonate is converted to the IPP. The goal of the second phase is to convert the 5-carbon IPP into the 27-carbon cholesterol. Multiple reactions, in which NADPH is used, convert 6 IPPs into the 30-carbon linear molecule squalene. Two reactions then utilize O_2 and NADPH to convert squalene into the cyclic 30-carbon sterol lanosterol. Multiple steps then convert lanosterol into the 27-carbon cholesterol via reactions that use O_2 and NADPH. Three carbons from lanosterol are removed in the form of two CO_2 and one HCOOH (formic acid). Several pharmaceuticals target various enzymes involved in the conversion of lanosterol to cholesterol. Mutations in 7-dehydrocholesterol reductase, the terminal step in cholesterol synthesis, cause Smith-Lemli-Opitz syndrome. **(C)** The uses of cholesterol in various tissues are summarized here. ADP, adenosine diphosphate; KCN, potassium cyanide.

- HMG CoA reductase activity is pharmacologically inhibited by statins, a family of compounds that compete with its substrate, HMG CoA, for binding to the enzyme's active site (▶ Fig. 14.5a). Common statin drugs include lovastatin, simvastatin, pravastatin, atorvastatin, and fluvastatin.

2. **Covalent modification:** HMG CoA reductase is inactive when phosphorylated and active when dephosphorylated (▶ Fig. 14.5b).

   - Conditions of low energy, marked by high AMP levels, stimulate the phosphorylation and inhibition of HMG CoA reductase by AMP-activated protein kinase (AMPK).
   - Glucagon inhibits HMG CoA reductase by preventing its dephosphorylation.
   - Insulin activates HMG CoA reductase by promoting its dephosphorylation.

3. **Modulation of transcription:** The HMG CoA reductase gene contains a consensus sequence known as the sterol regulatory element (SRE) in its promoter region. This allows its transcription to be regulated by a family of transcription factors called sterol regulatory element–binding proteins (SREBP) (▶ Fig. 14.5c).

   - The inactive precursor form of SREBP (~ 125 kDa) is an integral ER membrane protein that exists in complex with another protein called SREBP cleavage-activating protein (SCAP). In the presence of cholesterol or oxysterols, the SREBP–SCAP complex is retained in the ER due to interaction with another ER protein known as INSIG. As a result, the rate of transcription of HMG CoA reductase is low.
   - Low sterol levels promote the release of the SREBP–SCAP complex from the ER to the Golgi apparatus, where SREBP undergoes sequential proteolysis to release the active mature form of SREBP (~ 68 kDa). Mature SREBP dimerizes and translocates to the nucleus to stimulate the transcription of the HMG CoA reductase gene and other SREBP-dependent genes of the pathway.
   - Insulin and thyroxine (a thyroid hormone) have been shown to increase the rate of synthesis of HMG CoA reductase.

4. **Modulation of translation**

   - The rate of translation of HMG CoA reductase mRNA to protein is reduced by γ-tocotrienol (a member of the vitamin E family) and oxylanosterols (e.g., 24(S), 25-oxidolanosterol).

5. **Modulation of protein turnover:** In the presence of cholesterol and/or oxysterols, HMG CoA reductase associates with INSIG, which causes polyubiquitination of HMG CoA reductase protein. This leads to its extraction from the ER and rapid degradation in the 26S proteasome complex.

   - Degradation of HMG CoA reductase is enhanced by sterols (including methylated sterols), oxysterols, tocotrienols, unidentified nonsterol isoprenoid derivative(s) of mevalonate, and the bisphosphonate SR-12813.

Normal

Role of liver in cholesterol homeostasis

The liver plays a vital role in whole-body cholesterol homeostasis. It accounts for a significant portion of endogenous cholesterol synthesis and is the primary organ responsible for elimination of cholesterol from the body. Most of the dietary cholesterol is delivered to the liver via chylomicron remnants, and the liver assembles very low-density lipoproteins (VLDL), which are metabolized in the bloodstream to low-density lipoproteins (LDL). The liver is also a major source of nascent high-density lipoproteins (HDL). Lastly, the liver accounts for the bulk of clearance of lipoproteins from the blood and secretes both cholesterol and bile acids (the end products of cholesterol catabolism) into bile.

Therapeutics

Atherosclerosis

Atherosclerosis is a hardening of the arteries caused by the formation of fatty plaques containing cholesterol and other lipids along blood vessel walls. As a result, the flow of oxygenated blood through the vessels is restricted and may be completely obstructed when plaque rupture leads to thrombosis. Thus, an individual with atherosclerosis is at risk for myocardial infarction and stroke.

Therapeutics

Inhibitors of HMG CoA reductase: statins

Statins are drugs that lower plasma total cholesterol levels by 20 to 60%. They are potent competitive inhibitors of HMG CoA reductase, the rate-limiting enzyme of cholesterol synthesis. However, their hypocholesterolemic effect is predominantly due to an increase in the SREBP maturation pathway, leading to enhanced LDL receptor–mediated clearance of plasma cholesterol. Examples of statin drugs include lovastatin, simvastatin, pravastatin, atorvastatin, and fluvastatin. In concert with a low-lipid diet, statins are taken by individuals with hypercholesterolemia to lower their risk of developing heart disease, heart attacks, and strokes. It should be noted that statin treatment leads to a large compensatory overproduction of HMG CoA reductase protein, which remains inactive in the presence of statins. It is speculated that isolated myotoxic side effects of high-dose statin treatment may be due to decreased formation of ubiquinone or prenylated proteins in the muscle.

Therapeutics

Late-stage inhibitors of cholesterol synthesis

Azole-based antimycotics are routinely used to combat fungal infections. N-substituted imazoles (e.g., miconazole, ketoconazole, fluconazole, itraconazole) act by interfering with the synthesis of ergosterol, which is necessary for the integrity of the plasma membrane of fungal cells, by inhibiting cytochrome P-450–dependent 14α-demethylation of lanosterol. At higher doses, these drugs also affect mammalian 14α-demethylase (CYP-51A1) activity as well. Other cytochrome P-450–dependent enzymes are targets of azole-based drugs. Ketoconazole has been shown to inhibit cholesterol 7α-hydroxylase (CYP-7A1), the first and rate-limiting step of bile acid biosynthesis. Triparanol, progesterone, and tamoxifen inhibit FAD-dependent sterol Δ^{24}-reductase, which converts desmosterol into cholesterol. The antiestrogen

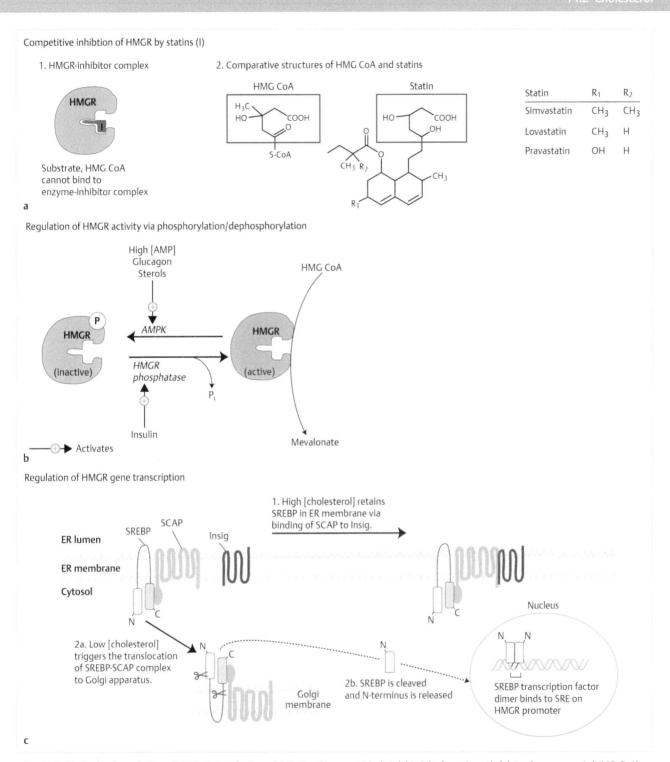

Fig. 14.5 **Methods of regulation of HMG CoA reductase.** (a) Statins (I) competitively inhibit 3-hydroxy-3-methylglutaryl coenzyme A (HMG CoA) reductase (HMGR). (b) HMGR is phosphorylated and inactivated by adenosine monophosphate (AMP)–activated protein kinase (AMPK). HMGR is dephosphorylated and activated by HMGR phosphatase. (c) High levels of cholesterol retain sterol regulatory element–binding protein (SREBP) in the membrane of the endoplasmic reticulum (ER). Low concentrations of cholesterol, however, trigger the release of SREBP from the ER membrane to the nucleus via Golgi apparatus, where it stimulates the transcription of the *HMGR* gene via binding to a sterol regulatory element (SRE) in HMGR's promoter region. SCAP, SREBP cleavage-activating protein.

drugs (e.g., tamoxifen, anastrozole) are inhibitors of aromatase as well. The epileptogenic steroid U18666A is an inhibitor of oxidosqualene cyclase, sterol Δ^{8-7} isomerase, and Δ^{24}-reductase. It also inhibits intracellular cholesterol trafficking similar to that seen in Niemann-Pick type C disease. Another epileptogenic agent, AY9944, is a potent inhibitor of Δ^{7}-reductase. Antipsychotic drugs (e.g., haloperidol, clozapine, risperidone) appear to induce dyslipidemia, in part, through an inhibition of Δ^{7}-reductase, Δ^{8-7} isomerase, and Δ^{14}-reductase activities. The fungal-derived squalestatins are the most potent and selective inhibitors of squalene synthase. The allylamine, NB-598, is a selective inhibitor of squalene epoxidase.

Normal
Cytochrome P-450 and drug interactions
Cytochrome P-450 (CYP-51) enzymes are responsible for more than 20 reactions needed to convert the linear isoprenoid squalene into cholesterol. CYP enzymes are also involved in the metabolism of many xenobiotics, including statin drugs that inhibit HMG CoA reductase. Lovastatin, atorvastatin, simvastatin, and fluvastatin, for example, are metabolized by CYP-3A4, CYP-2C8, and CYP-2C9. Agents that inhibit CYP enzymes cause abnormal increases in plasma concentrations of certain statins and increase the possibility of toxic side effects, such as myopathy and rhabdomyolysis. Such inhibitors include not only drugs such as itraconazole, clarithromycin, and cyclosporine but also citrus juices such as grapefruit juice. On the other hand, agents that induce CYP enzymes (e.g., rifampicin, carbamazepine, and the dietary supplement St. John's wort) decrease the plasma levels of statins.

Foundations
Kinetics of statin-mediated inhibition
All statins share an HMG-like moiety in their structures, which allows them to compete for the active site of HMG CoA reductase (▶ Fig. 14.5a-2). While the enzyme's K_m for HMG CoA is ~ 4 μM, the K_i values for statins are in the range of 5 to 45 nM, making them very potent competitive inhibitors of HMG CoA reductase activity. It may be recalled that a competitive inhibitor increases the apparent K_m of an enzyme for its substrate without affecting the V_{max}. Three of the statins on the market, lovastatin, simvastatin, and pravastatin, are fermentation-derived fungal or bacterial products, whereas several fluorophenyl-substituted statins (e.g., fluvastatin, atorvastatin, rosuvastatin) are completely synthetic products.

Normal
Isopentenyl pyrophosphate and farnesyl/geranyl lipids
The conversion of isopentenyl pyrophosphate (IPP) into squalene involves intermediate products such as geranyl pyrophosphate (GPP, C-10) and farnesyl pyrophosphate (FPP, C-15). IPP is first isomerized to another 5-C compound, dimethylallyl pyrophosphate (DMAPP). Condensation of an IPP with a DMAPP yields GPP. Addition of another DMAPP to GPP produces FPP. Condensation of two FPP molecules results in the formation of squalene. A by-product, geranylgeranyl pyrophosphate (GGPP, 20-C), is generated by the addition of a DMAPP to an FPP. Both FPP and GGPP are substrates for protein prenyltransferases, which covalently modify certain proteins. FPP also serves as a substrate for *cis*-prenyltransferase, leading to the formation of dolichol, and for *trans*-prenyltransferase, leading to the synthesis of the side chain of coenzyme Q (ubiquinone).

14.3 Cholesterol Storage and Transport

14.3.1 Storage: As Cholesterol Esters
Cholesterol has a very low solubility in water of only 0.01 mg/100 mL (0.01 mg/dL). This allows it to reside within the hydrophobic environment of the plasma membrane and some internal membranes such as the ER. When in excess, cholesterol is esterified to a fatty acid to generate an even more hydrophobic molecule called a cholesterol ester (▶ Fig. 14.6), which is stored in lipid droplets in the cytoplasm.
- The esterification of cholesterol is catalyzed by acyl CoA: cholesterol acyltransferase (ACAT).

14.3.2 Transport: In Lipoproteins
Despite the hydrophobic characteristics of free (unesterified) cholesterol, as well as its ester, normal blood cholesterol concentrations range from 150 to 200 mg/dL—which is 15,000 to 20,000 times greater than cholesterol's solubility in water. This

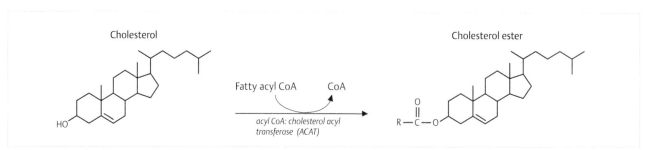

Fig. 14.6 Esterification of cholesterol. Acyl CoA:cholesterol acyltransferase (ACAT) catalyzes the esterification of a fatty acid to cholesterol. This generates a cholesterol ester, which is more hydrophobic than the free cholesterol. Cholesterol esters are stored in lipid droplets in the cytoplasm.

high concentration of cholesterol in blood is made possible by plasma lipoproteins, which are three-dimensional circular structures that solubilize large amounts of cholesterol (free and esterified), as well as triacylglycerols and fat-soluble vitamins (▶ Fig. 14.7).

Lipoproteins therefore contribute to the metabolism of lipids by serving as their transport vehicle. The structure of lipoproteins is generally composed of the following:

- **Outer shell:** Made up of a monolayer of phospholipids, free cholesterol, and one or more proteins called apolipoproteins. Apolipoproteins serve as structural components, as enzyme activators and as ligands that bind to specific cell surface receptors.
- **Inner core:** Made up of a collection of hydrophobic neutral lipids such as triacylglycerols and cholesterol esters.

Types of Lipoproteins

There are five major lipoproteins, and they differ in size, density, and the relative amounts and types of lipid and protein they contain. For instance:

- The largest lipoproteins are the least dense due to a relatively high concentration of triacylglycerols.
- The smallest lipoproteins are the densest due to relatively high concentrations of proteins and phospholipids.

Listed in order from largest and least dense to smallest and most dense, the different types of lipoproteins are (▶ Fig. 14.7a-c): chylomicrons, very low-density lipoproteins (VLDL), intermediate-density lipoproteins (IDL), low-density lipoproteins (LDL), and high-density lipoproteins (HDL).

- Various disorders—either hyperlipoproteinemias or hypolipoproteinemias (▶ Table 14.1)—arise due to abnormalities in the synthesis and processing of lipoproteins.

Chylomicrons

These are the largest of the lipoprotein particles and are considered "exogenous" because they are assembled in the intestinal cells from diet-derived lipids. As such, chylomicrons are especially abundant in blood after a lipid-rich meal. They transport dietary triacylglycerols, cholesterol, and other lipids from the small intestine for uptake by muscle, adipose, and liver cells.

Chylomicrons contain apolipoproteins that include apoB-48, apoC-II, and apoE, and are processed in the body through the following mechanism (▶ Fig. 14.8a):

1. Nascent chylomicrons are first assembled in the intestines and secreted into the lymphatic circulation and then into the blood. The transport of chylomicrons from the intestines to the lymphatic system and blood is facilitated by the presence of apoB-48 on their outer layer. ApoC-II and apoE are acquired from HDL in the bloodstream.
2. The triacylglycerols in chylomicrons in the bloodstream are hydrolyzed rapidly by capillary lipoprotein lipase, an enzyme secreted by parenchymal cells such as adipocytes and distributed to the surface of endothelial cells lining the capillary beds. The activation of capillary lipoprotein lipase is triggered by the presence of apoC-II.
- Defects in apoC-II are associated with type I hyperlipoproteinemia in which chylomicrons accumulate. A deficiency in lipoprotein lipase also leads to type I hyperlipoproteinemia. Patients with these abnormalities

Table 14.1 Summary of hyper- and hypolipoproteinemia

Disorder type	Cause	Effects
Hyperlipoproteinemia		
Type I (familial hyperchylomicronemia)	Deficiency in apoC-II or defective lipoprotein lipase	Chylomicrons: ↑ Triacylglycerol: ↑
Type IIa and IIb (familial hypercholesterolemia)	LDL receptor is completely (IIa) or partially defective (IIb)	Cholesterol: ↑ Triacylglycerol: normal (IIa), ↑ (IIb) LDL: ↑ VLDL: ↑ (IIb)
Type III (familial dysbetalipoproteinemia)	Defect in apoE	Cholesterol: ↑ Chylomicron remnants: ↑ Triacylglycerol: ↑ IDL: ↑
Type IV (familial hypertriglyceridemia)	Reduction in the catabolism of VLDLs or increase in their synthesis	Cholesterol: ↑ (slightly) Triacylglycerol: ↑ VLDL: ↑
Type V	Combination of types I and IV	Chylomicrons: ↑ VLDL: ↑ Triacylglycerol: ↑ LDL: normal
Hypolipoproteinemia		
Tangier disease	Defect in transporter that supports cholesterol pickup by nascent HDLs	HDL: ↓
Abetalipoproteinemia	Lack of apoB-48 and apoB-100	Chylomicrons: ↓ VLDL, IDL, LDL: ↓
Hypoalphalipoproteinemia	Accelerated catabolism of apoA-I and apoA-II	HDL: ↓

Abbreviations: HDL, high-density lipoprotein; IDL, intermediate-density lipoprotein; LDL, low-density lipoprotein; VLDL, very low-density lipoprotein; t, elevated; ↓, decreased.

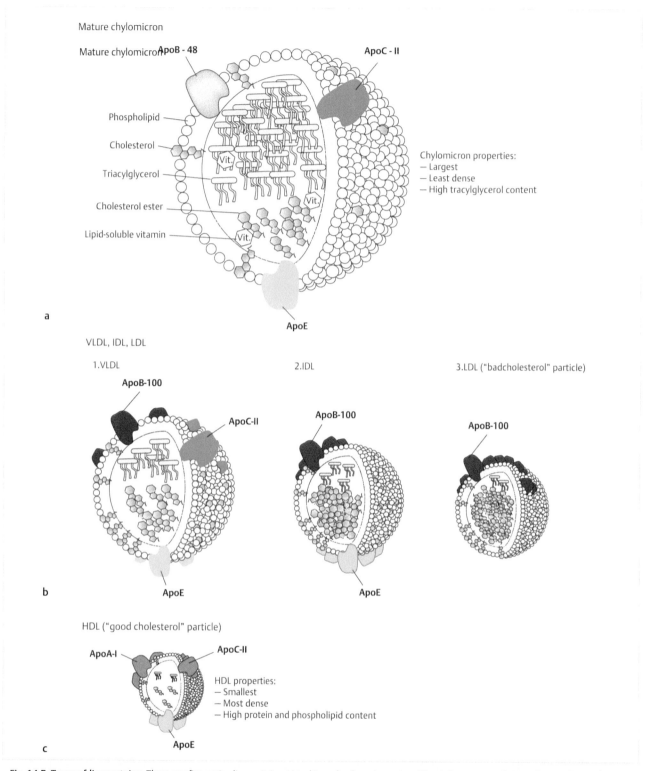

Mature chylomicron

Mature chylomicron ApoB - 48

ApoC - II

Phospholipid

Cholesterol

Triacylglycerol

Cholesterol ester

Lipid-soluble vitamin

Vit.

Vit.

Vit.

Chylomicron properties:
— Largest
— Least dense
— High tracylglycerol content

ApoE

a

VLDL, IDL, LDL

1.VLDL

ApoB-100

ApoC-II

ApoE

2.IDL

ApoB-100

ApoE

3.LDL ("badcholesterol" particle)

ApoB-100

b

HDL ("good cholesterol" particle)

ApoA-I

ApoC-II

HDL properties:
— Smallest
— Most dense
— High protein and phospholipid content

ApoE

c

Fig. 14.7 Types of lipoproteins. There are five major lipoproteins. Listed in order from largest and least dense to smallest and most dense, they are (**a**) chylomicrons, (**b**) very low-density lipoproteins (VLDLs), intermediate-density lipoproteins (IDLs), low-density lipoproteins (LDLs), and (**c**) high-density lipoproteins (HDLs). Only the major apolipoproteins associated with each particle are indicated.

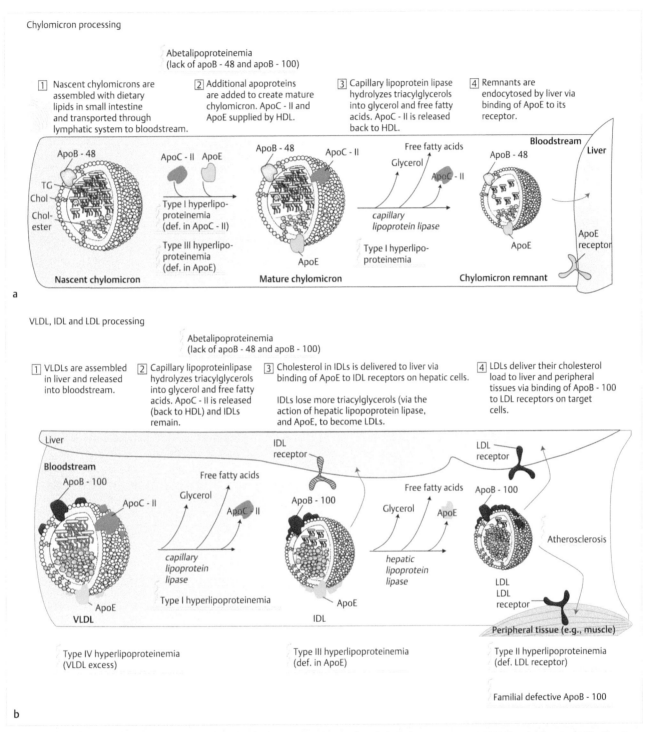

Fig. 14.8 Processing of chylomicrons, VLDL, IDL, and LDL. (a) The mechanism by which chylomicrons are processed and taken up by the liver is outlined here. Various disorders associated with apolipoprotein deficiencies and enzyme deficiencies are also noted. **(b)** The mechanisms by which very low-density lipoproteins (VLDL) are processed into intermediate-density lipoproteins (IDL) and low-density lipoproteins (LDL), and the uptake of the latter two are outlined here. Various disorders associated with abnormalities in lipoproteins, apolipoproteins, and receptors are also noted. Chol, cholesterol; TG, triacylglycerol.

IV

have plasma triacylglycerol concentrations that are excessively high (> 1000 mg/dL; normal is 50 to 150 mg/dL).

- The free fatty acids and glycerol released by the action of lipoprotein lipase are used by tissues, as follows:
  - Fatty acids are used to generate energy in muscle and used to synthesize triacylglycerol for storage in adipose tissue.
  - Glycerol is used by the liver to synthesize triacylglycerols or as a gluconeogenic substrate.
3. The cholesterol-rich chylomicron residual particles, known as remnants, retain apoE but not apoC-II and are endocytosed by the liver via binding of apoE to its receptor.
   - Defects in apoE are linked to type III hyperlipoproteinemia, which disrupts hepatic uptake of chylomicron remnants (and IDL).

VLDL, IDL, and LDL

VLDL, often referred to as the "endogenous" counterparts of chylomicrons, are synthesized in the liver. They transport triacylglycerols, cholesterol, and other lipids for uptake by muscle and adipose tissue. The apoproteins apoB-100, apoC-II, and apoE are found on the outer shell of VLDL (▶ Fig. 14.7b-1).

- Like chylomicrons, the triacylglycerols contained within VLDL are hydrolyzed by capillary lipoprotein lipase, which lines the walls of capillaries (▶ Fig. 14.8b).
- The activation of capillary lipoprotein lipase is triggered by apoC-II, and the free fatty acids released by its hydrolytic action are used by muscle and adipose cells for energy and storage, respectively. Glycerol, also released upon triacylglycerol hydrolysis, is taken up by the liver to synthesize triacylglycerols.
- Elevated levels of VLDL are associated with type IV hyperlipoproteinemia or may be observed in patients who are obese, diabetic, or abusing alcohol.

VLDL are processed and converted to IDL and LDL via the following mechanisms (▶ Fig. 14.8b):

- **IDL** are the remnant particles left after VLDL have unloaded most of their triacylglycerol content and released apoC-II (▶ Fig. 14.7b-2). Therefore, IDL contain only apoB-100 and apoE on their outer shells, and they have a higher concentration of cholesterol (free and in ester form) than VLDL.
  - Cholesterol from IDL is delivered to the liver via a mechanism facilitated by binding of apoE to IDL receptors on the surface of hepatic cells (▶ Fig. 14.8b).
  - Some of the IDL also exchange part of their lipids with nascent HDL (▶ Fig. 14.9).
  - IDL lose more triacylglycerol and all apoproteins except for apoB-100 through the action of hepatic lipase to become LDL.
- **LDL**, often referred to as "bad cholesterol" particles, are enriched in cholesterol (particularly cholesterol esters) and serve as the main carriers of cholesterol in human blood (▶ Fig. 14.7b-3).
  - LDL deliver their cholesterol load to liver and peripheral tissues via a mechanism in which apoB-100 (the only apolipoprotein present on LDL) binds to a cell surface receptor called the LDL receptor (▶ Fig. 14.8b). This triggers endocytosis of LDL, which are then degraded in

endosomes/lysosomes, releasing cholesterol, fatty acids (due to triacylglycerol degradation), and amino acids (due to protein degradation).
- High levels of blood LDL predispose an individual to atherosclerosis and the development of heart disease.

HDL

HDL (▶ Fig. 14.7c) are referred to as the "good cholesterol" particles because they mediate the transfer of cholesterol from peripheral tissues to the liver via a process called reverse cholesterol transport. Protein- and phospholipid-rich HDL are processed as follows (▶ Fig. 14.9):

1. Nascent, lipid-poor HDL particle containing apoA-I and phospholipid is synthesized by both the liver (70%) and the small intestine (30%). It acquires free cholesterol from liver and peripheral tissues through the action of ATP-binding cassette proteins, ABCA1 and ABCG1, and exists as a disc-shaped particle.
2. Lecithin:cholesterol acyltransferase (LCAT), whose activation is triggered by apoA-I, catalyzes the esterification of the acquired cholesterol by transferring the fatty acid from phosphatidylcholine (lecithin) onto cholesterol. As a result, HDL becomes spherical due to the increase in cholesterol esters within its core.
3. HDL transfers its cholesterol esters to VLDL, IDL, and LDL in exchange for triacylglycerols and phospholipids. These exchanges are facilitated by cholesterol ester transfer protein (CETP) and phospholipid transfer protein (PLTP). It also acquires several apoproteins from other lipoproteins in circulation (e.g., apoA-II, apoC-II, apoE).
4. HDL delivers its cholesterol load to the liver and to endocrine glands by a nonendocytic, selective uptake mechanism involving the scavenger receptor, SR-BI. In addition, SR-BI may also mediate endocytosis of cholesterol-rich HDL particles as a redundant mechanism.

In addition to its function of clearing cholesterol from peripheral tissues, HDL serves as a reservoir for apolipoproteins. For instance, HDL donates apoC-II and apoE to chylomicrons and accepts them when they are released during the processing of chylomicrons.

- A rare autosomal recessive disorder called Tangier disease is a type of hypolipoproteinemia. It is marked by excessively low levels of HDL due to defects in the ABCA1 transporter that aids in the uptake of cholesterol (and phospholipids) by nascent HDLs.

▶ Fig. 14.10 provides an overview of lipoprotein metabolism, and ▶ Table 14.1 provides a summary of disorders associated with lipoprotein metabolism.

14.3.3 Hypocholesterolemic Drugs

Several hypocholesterolemic drugs have been developed to effectively lower plasma LDL cholesterol, the major risk factor for atherosclerosis and coronary heart disease. The effects on lipoprotein/lipid levels, side effects, and contraindications/warnings of some of these pharmaceuticals are summarized in ▶ Table 14.2.

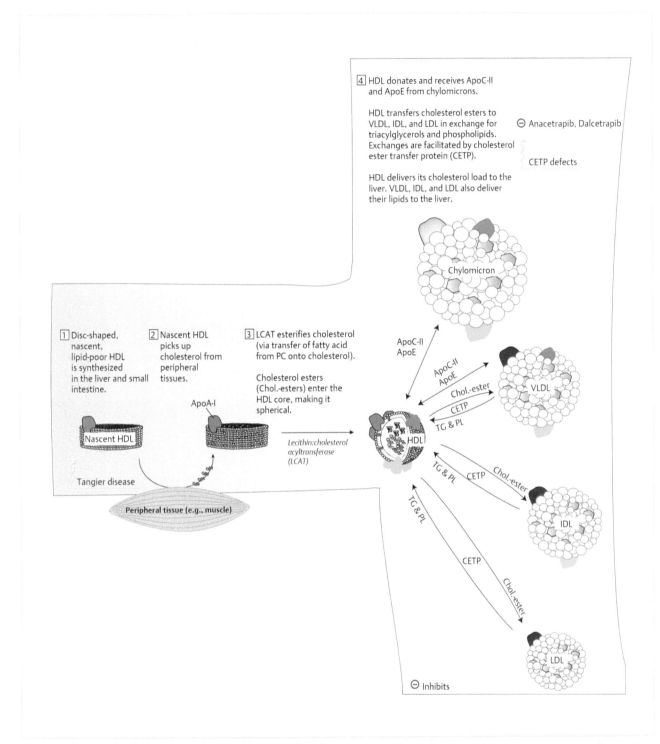

Fig. 14.9 High-density lipoprotein processing. The mechanism by which mature high-density lipoproteins (HDLs) are created and the methods by which HDLs exchange lipid and protein components with other lipoproteins are outlined here. IDL, intermediate-density lipoprotein; LDL, low-density lipoprotein; PC, phosphatidylcholine; PL, phospholipid; TG, triacylglycerol; VLDL, very low-density lipoprotein.

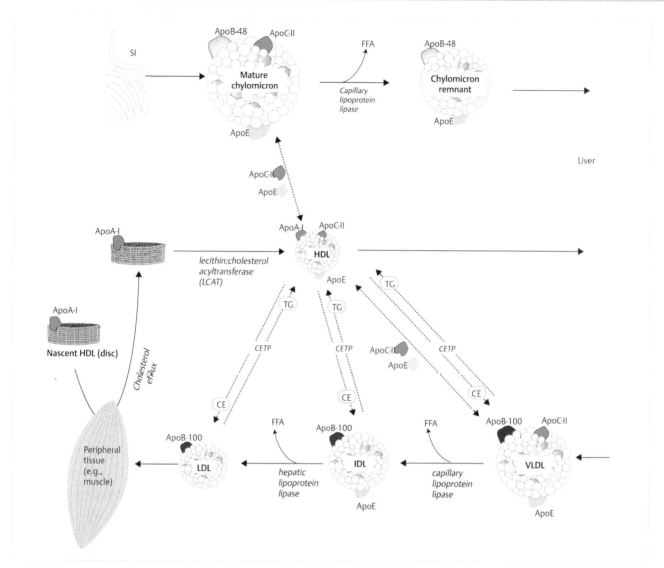

Fig. 14.10 Integration of lipoprotein processing. Overview of the integration of lipoprotein processing. CE, cholesterol ester; CETP, cholesterol ester transfer protein; CM, chylomicron; CMR, chylomicron remnant; FFA, free fatty acids; HLL, hepatic lipoprotein lipase; IDL, intermediate-density lipoprotein; LDL, low-density lipoprotein; LPL, lipoprotein lipase; TG, triacylglycerol.

Table 14.2 Hypocholesterolemic drugs: Effects and contraindications/warnings

Hypocholesterolemic agents	Lipid effects	Selected side effects	Selected contraindications/Warnings
HMG CoA reductase inhibitors (statins)	LDL ↓ HDL ↑ TAG ↓	Myopathy, ↑ liver enzymes	Active or chronic liver disease Concomitant use of certain drugs
Bile acid sequestrants	LDL ↓ HDL ↑ TAG nc or ↓	GI distress, constipation, impaired absorption of other drugs	Dysbetalipoproteinemia
Nicotinic acid (niacin)	LDL ↓ HDL ↑ TAG ↓	Flushing, hyperglycemia, hyperuricemia, hepatotoxicity	Chronic liver disease, severe gout, diabetes, peptic ulcer disease
Fibrates	LDL ↓ HDL ↑ TAG ↓	Dyspepsia, gallstones, myopathy	Severe renal or hepatic disease
Plant stanols	LDL ↓	Unknown	Unknown
Plant sterols	LDL ↓	Unknown	Unknown
CETP inhibitor (e.g., Anacetrapib) (clinical development abandoned)	LDL ↓ HDL ↑↑	Unknown	Chronic kidney disease, hypertension

Abbreviations: CETP, cholesterol ester transfer protein; GI, gastrointestinal; HDL, high-density lipoprotein; IDL, intermediate-density lipoprotein; LDL, low-density lipoprotein; nc, no change; TAG, triacylglycerol; VLDL, very low-density lipoprotein; ↑, elevated; ↓, decreased.

Normal
Lymphatic system

Lymph is a clear fluid that is essentially recycled plasma. The lymphatic system is part of the circulatory system, which carries the lymph in a single direction, toward the heart. The lymphatic system, consisting of lymph vessels and lymphoid tissue, plays an active role in the digestive and immune functions of the body. Lymph circulation helps remove the interstitial fluid from tissues, transport reconstituted lipids (e.g., chylomicrons) from the small intestine, and transport lymphocytes and antigen-presenting cells. The lymphoid tissue is an organized mass of white blood cells and connective tissue (e.g., thymus, bone marrow, lymph nodes). The lymph nodes act to trap and destroy circulating cancer cells. However, when overwhelmed, the lymphatic system may help spread the cancer through metastasis. Swelling of lymph nodes is observed in infections and cancer (e.g., non-Hodgkin lymphoma).

Foundations
Apolipoprotein functions

Apolipoproteins serve three important functions: they perform a structural role in stabilizing the structure of lipoproteins (e.g., apoB in LDL, apoA-I in HDL, and apoE in VLDL and some HDL), they are involved in the transport and redistribution of lipids among various tissues, and they serve as cofactors for enzymes that act on lipids (e.g., activation of lipoprotein lipase by apoC-II, LCAT by apoA-I and other apolipoproteins).

Therapeutics
Type I hyperlipoproteinemia (familial hyperchylomicronemia)

Type I hyperlipoproteinemia (also known as hyperchylomicronemia) is caused by an inability to hydrolyze the triacylglycerols in chylomicrons and VLDL. The underlying disorder could be either a primary deficiency of lipoprotein lipase or a deficiency of apoC-II, which is an essential member of the enzyme complex and is needed to activate lipoprotein lipase. Type I hyperlipoproteinemia is often recognized fortuitously by the creamy appearance of a routine blood sample. If the plasma is allowed to stand overnight at 4 °C, it separates into a creamy top layer with a clear infranatant layer. Whereas primary lipoprotein lipase deficiency manifests in hyperchylomicronemia very early in infancy, a deficiency of apoC-II presents clinically in postadolescence. In fact, the first patient with apoC-II deficiency was diagnosed when his plasma triglyceride levels fell sharply following a blood transfusion. Both types of deficiencies are recessively inherited and are characterized by fasting plasma triglyceride levels > 1000 mg/dL, abdominal pain, acute pancreatitis, and cutaneous eruptive xanthomas (yellow-colored fat deposits in skin). Interestingly, these patients do not appear to be at a higher risk for premature atherosclerosis. Treatment involves restriction of dietary fat intake to < 15% of total calories. Medium-chain triglycerides are permitted because they do not contribute to chylomicrons.

Therapeutics
Type II hyperlipoproteinemia (familial hypercholesterolemia)

Type II hyperlipoproteinemia, also known as familial hypercholesterolemia (FH), is an inherited metabolic disorder due to defects in the cellular uptake of LDL through the LDL receptor pathway. Receptor-mediated uptake is the major (75%) mechanism for the clearance of plasma LDL, and defects in this process lead to an accumulation of cholesterol in the blood and the subsequent development of atherosclerosis. Over 1000 mutations in the LDL receptor have been reported that impair its ability to recognize apoB-100 on LDL. FH is inherited in an autosomal dominant fashion, with homozygous or compound heterozygous patients having fasting plasma cholesterol levels > 800 mg/dL (normal plasma cholesterol = 130 to 200 mg/dL). In heterozygotes, values of 300 to 500 mg/dL are common. Untreated homozygous patients usually die of coronary artery disease (CAD) before teenage years, whereas heterozygous patients develop CAD by age 40. Xanthomas (deposits of cholesterol in skin and tendons), arcus senilis (corneal deposits of cholesterol around the iris), and angina pectoris (chest pain) are some of the physical symptoms of FH. Whereas heterozygous patients respond to diet and a combination of statins and bile acid–binding resins, the only effective treatments for homozygous patients are LDL apheresis (filtering LDL from plasma) and liver transplantation.

Therapeutics
Plasma cholesterol and atherosclerosis

Plasma cholesterol levels, particularly the levels of LDL cholesterol, are positively correlated with mortality due to cardiovascular disease. High LDL levels coupled with endothelial dysfunction lead to an influx of LDL into the arterial wall and its subsequent modification by reactive oxygen species (ROS). Unregulated uptake of modified LDL via the scavenger receptors by the macrophages results in the phenotype of foam cells. Death of foam cells contributes to the deposition of fat that initiates the development of arterial plaque leading to atherosclerosis.

Therapeutics
Combined hyperlipidemia

Combined hyperlipidemia (CHL), either inherited or acquired, is the most common form of dyslipidemia and affects one in five individuals. It is characterized by increases in plasma LDL and VLDL and a decrease in HDL. The acquired form may arise from metabolic syndrome (increases in plasma triglycerides, low HDL, insulin resistance, hypertension, and central obesity). The inherited or familial combined hyperlipidemia is probably a polygenic disorder involving polymorphisms in several proteins (e.g., apoA-I, apoC-III, apoA-IV, apoA-V). Individuals with CHL are susceptible to premature CAD. Diabetes, hyperthyroidism, and alcoholism exacerbate the CAD risk.

IV

IV

Therapeutics
Beneficial effects of HDL

HDL cholesterol (HDL-C) levels correlate positively with reduced risk of CAD in both men and women. Conversely, levels of HDL-C < 35 mg/dL are associated with an increased risk of CAD. The risk of heart disease decreases by 2 to 3% for each increase in HDL-C of 1 mg/dL. The beneficial effects of HDL are attributed chiefly to its ability to mediate reverse cholesterol transport from peripheral tissues to the liver. HDL may also play antioxidant and antiinflammatory roles. In general, women have higher levels of HDL-C than men. Weight loss, exercise, smoking cessation, and moderate consumption of alcohol (2 to 6 ounces/day) promote HDL-C levels. Among antihypercholesterolemic drugs, CETP inhibitors, fibrates, and niacin are known to raise HDL-C levels. Others, such as the antidiabetic thiazolidine compounds, estrogens, and ω-3 fatty acids, can also raise HDL-C. Certain mutations in apoA-I (e.g., apoA-I$_{Milano}$) and CETP also increase HDL-C levels. Familial hypoalphalipoproteinemia is the most common inherited disorder resulting in low HDL-C (< 35 mg/dL). Although the genetic causes remain to be uncovered, this disorder is characterized by a rapid catabolism of HDL and apoA-I. Tangier disease (a defect in the ABCA1 transporter that mediates efflux of cholesterol from peripheral cells to nascent HDL) and deficiencies of apoA-I or LCAT also cause a decrease in HDL-C. Other factors that contribute to a lowering of HDL-C are smoking, obesity, progestins, androgens, β-blockers, and high intake of polyunsaturated ω-6 fatty acids.

Therapeutics
Cholesterol-lowering drugs—statins

Statins mimic the structures of HMG CoA and mevalonate, the substrate and product of HMG CoA reductase. Because their affinity for the active site of reductase is several orders of magnitude greater than that of HMG CoA, statins are very potent competitive inhibitors of the rate-limiting enzyme of cholesterol biosynthesis. As a result of statin action, cellular levels of cholesterol fall, allowing the export of the SCAP–SREBP complex to the Golgi apparatus for processing and the release of the mature transcription factor. Mature SREBP enhances the rate of transcription of the SRE-containing LDL receptor gene. Increased levels of LDL receptor on hepatic membranes cause enhanced uptake of LDL cholesterol, leading to a lowering of plasma cholesterol levels.

Therapeutics
Cholesterol lowering drugs — PCSK9 inhibitors

PCSK9 (proprotein convertase subtlisin/kexin 9) is a serine protease in the bloodstream that regulates the levels of LDL receptors on a cell. It binds to the extracellular domain of the LDL receptor and traffics with it to the lysosome and tags the receptor for degradation rather than recycling back to the cell surface. PCSK9 inhibitors such as evolocumab (Repatha, Amgen, Thousand Oaks, CA) and alirocumab (Praulent, Sanofi-Aventis, Bridgewater, NJ and Regeneron, Tarrytown, NY) are monoclonal antibodies that bind to circulating PCSK9 and

prevent its interaction with the LDL receptor. As a result, LDL receptors are more likely to participate in multiple cycles of LDL delivery to the lysosomes contributing to the lowering of serum cholesterol.

14.4 Cholesterol Elimination via Bile Acid Metabolism

The liver contains a pool of cholesterol due to the deposition of cholesterol by lipoproteins. The sterane ring of cholesterol cannot be degraded; therefore, cholesterol can only be eliminated from the body in two ways:

1. Cholesterol is converted to bile acids in the liver and stored in bile.
2. Some free cholesterol and bile acids are excreted in feces.

14.4.1 Bile Acids and Salts

Bile is a lipid-emulsifying mixture produced by the liver and stored in the gallbladder. After a meal, bile enters the duodenum (upper intestine) to solubilize diet-derived lipids, making them easier to digest. Bile is composed of bile acids, cholesterol, phospholipids, fatty acids, proteins, bile pigments, and inorganic salts. Bile acids are synthesized from cholesterol and are characterized as follows (▶ Fig. 14.11a):

- A bile acid is a 24-carbon derivative of cholesterol that has a carboxylic acid group and two or more hydroxyl groups. It is often conjugated to an amino acid such as glycine or taurine via an amide bond.
- A bile salt is the ionized (deprotonated) form of a bile acid. A bile salt could be unconjugated or conjugated.
- Bile acids and bile salts are amphipathic molecules with hydrophilic and hydrophobic regions. This feature enables them to act as detergents that emulsify fat by forming mixed micelles in the intestinal lumen. In such micelles (▶ Fig. 14.11b), the hydrophobic region of the bile salts interacts with the hydrophobic region of the lipids, whereas the hydrophilic region faces the outer aqueous environment.
- Triacylglycerols in mixed micelles are accessible to breakdown by pancreatic lipase. Fatty acids, monoglycerides, cholesterol, and fat-soluble vitamins (A, D, E, K) form a dynamic equilibrium between the micellar form and the monomeric molecule form in the aqueous phase. Absorption into the intestinal epithelial cells occurs entirely from the monomeric form in the aqueous phase.
- Bile acids also act as signaling molecules that bind to and activate both cell surface receptors and nuclear receptors, the latter of which control the expression of multiple genes.

14.4.2 Bile Acid Metabolism

The metabolism of bile acids takes place in the liver, gallbladder, and small intestine, as follows (▶ Fig. 14.12a):

1. **Cholesterol is converted to primary bile acids (liver).** The synthesis of bile acids begins with the addition of an OH group to carbon 7 of cholesterol to generate

Cholesterol, bile acids and salts

Cholesterol

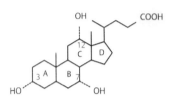

Bile acid (e.g., cholic acid)   Corresponding bile salt

Conjugated bile acid
(e.g. glycocholic acid)   Corresponding bile salt

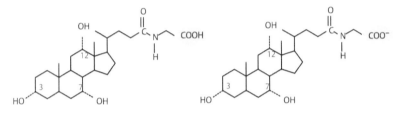

a

Mixed micelle

Phospholipid head group
Phospholipid fatty acid tails
Cholesterol
Triacylglycerol fatty
acid tails
Bile acid
Cholesterol ester

b

Fig. 14.11 Bile acids and salts. (a) Structures of cholesterol compared with examples of bile acids and bile salts. **(b)** Illustration of bile salt-containing mixed micelle, which is essential for the absorption of lipids and lipid-soluble vitamins by intestinal cells.

IV

7α-hydroxycholesterol. This rate-limiting step is catalyzed by 7α-hydroxylase, which has the following characteristics:
- It belongs to the microsomal cytochrome P-450 family of monooxygenases (*CYP7A1* gene product).
- It uses vitamin C as a cofactor.
- Its transcription is activated by cholesterol and inhibited by both primary and secondary bile acids.
  Subsequent addition of an OH group on carbon 12, removal of three carbons from the methyl-branched side chain, and the inclusion of a carboxylic group generate

primary bile acids known as chenodeoxycholic acid (dihydroxy acid) and cholic acid (trihydroxy acid) (▶ Fig. 14.12a). Both chenodeoxycholic acid and cholic acid act as inhibitors of 7α-hydroxylase.
- Bile acids, which have pK_a values of ~ 6, are not efficient emulsifiers of lipids because only 50% of them will be ionized (i.e., deprotonated and negatively charged) to bile salts at pH 6, the pH of the intestinal lumen.
2. **Bile acids are conjugated to amino acids.** To become a better emulsifier, the carboxyl group of a bile acid is

Bile metabolism in the liver, gallbladder, and small intestine

Structures of some molecules generated during bile metabolism

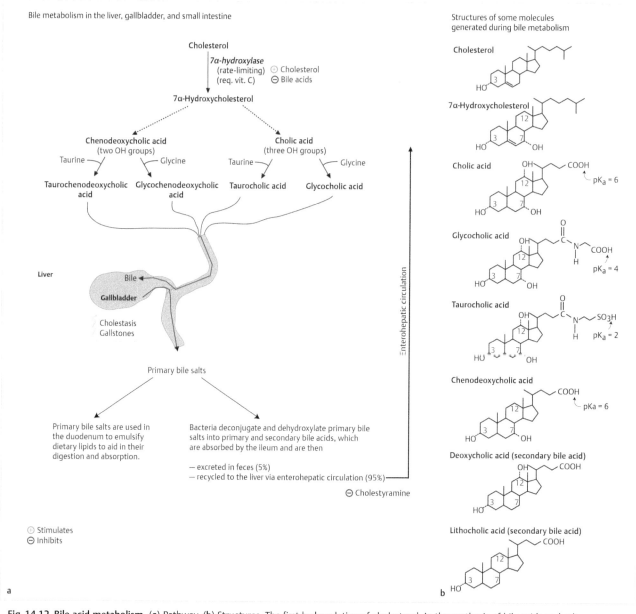

Fig. 14.12 Bile acid metabolism. (a) Pathway. (b) Structures. The first hydroxylation of cholesterol, in the synthesis of bile acids and salts, occurs on carbon 7 and is catalyzed by 7α-hydroxylase. This enzyme's activity is stimulated by cholesterol but inhibited by bile acids. Subsequent reactions convert 7α-hydroxycholesterol into primary bile acids. Bile acids are usually conjugated with glycine or taurine. These conjugated and unconjugated bile acids/salts are then sent to the gallbladder for storage in bile. Bile is secreted from the gallbladder into the intestine, where bile salts emulsify lipids (to aid in their digestion). Bile salts are also deconjugated and dehydroxylated by bacterial enzymes (The primary bile acids are dehydroxylated at the C-7 position to produce secondary bile acids.). The bile acids are reabsorbed in the ileum, where some (5%) are excreted in feces, and the rest (95%) are returned to the liver by the enterohepatic circulation. Nonabsorbable resins like cholestyramine bind to bile acids to promote their excretion rather than their return to the liver.

covalently attached via an amide bond to either glycine or taurine to generate a conjugated bile acid. Taurine, which is derived from cysteine, is a nonproteinogenic amino acid with a sulfate group.

- Bile acids conjugated to glycine have pK_a values of ~ 4 (▶ Fig. 14.12b). As such, they are good emulsifiers because essentially 100% of these molecules will be ionized in the intestinal lumen to bile salts.
- Bile acids conjugated to taurine have even lower pK_a values of ~ 2, due to the presence of the sulfate

group (▶ Fig. 14.12b). Therefore, they are the best emulsifiers as they are easily ionized in the intestinal lumen.

Once synthesized, primary bile acids are secreted from the liver into the gallbladder for storage in bile.

3. **Bile is released into the duodenum, where bile salts (1) aid in the digestion of lipids and (2) are metabolized to secondary bile acids by intestinal bacteria.**
   - In response to cholecystokinin released by the duodenal enteroendocrine cells (e.g., after a meal), bile is secreted

into the duodenum, where its bile salts emulsify lipids so that they can be digested and absorbed.

- Additionally, bacteria present in the intestines break down bile salts by deconjugating them (i.e., removing amino acid groups) and dehydroxylating them (i.e., removing OH at carbon 7). The dehydroxylation of these primary bile acids generates secondary bile acids, which are identified by the absence of an OH group on their carbon 7. Secondary bile acids also can inhibit 7α-hydroxylase.

4. **The bile acids are reabsorbed in the distal ileum and recycled**.
- Primary and secondary bile acids are then absorbed by the distal ileum (last section of the small intestine). A Na⁺-dependent active transport mechanism mediates the uptake of primary bile acids, whereas secondary bile acids are reabsorbed passively.
- Five percent of ileal bile acids, along with some cholesterol, are excreted in feces.
- Ninety-five percent of ileal bile acids, however, are returned to the liver via the enterohepatic circulation for reuse. Once in the liver, the primary and secondary bile acids undergo reconjugation.
- Ion-exchange resins such as cholestyramine and colestipol are bile-acid sequestrants that prevent the absorption and increase the percentage of bile acids that are excreted.

Therapeutics
Gallstones

Supersaturation of gallbladder bile with cholesterol results in the formation of gallstones that are crystals made up of cholesterol. Insufficient bile salt or phospholipid secretion or excess cholesterol secretion can lead to gallstone disease (cholelithiasis): cholesterol that normally occurs in bile needs bile salts to stay in solution. Continued disturbance of bile salt metabolism can lead to malabsorption syndromes, including steatorrhea and, in extreme cases, deficiency of fat-soluble vitamins. More than 500,000 cholecystectomies are done annually for treatment of symptomatic gallstones and associated complications. Oral ursodeoxycholic acid (an isomer of chenodeoxycholic acid) is a secondary bile acid that reduces cholesterol secretion into bile and improves biliary cholesterol solubility. It can be used to dissolve small to medium cholesterol gallstones. Studies show that ursodeoxycholic acid can reduce the incidence of gallstone formation in persons participating in a very-low-calorie diet program and after bariatric surgery. Prophylactic use of ursodeoxycholic acid can also be effective in the prevention of gallstone formation in patients having rapid weight reduction.

Therapeutics
Cholesterol-lowering drugs: bile acid–binding resins

Approximately 2,5 to 5 g of bile acids are present in enterohepatic circulation and undergo 6 to 8 complete cycles each day. The efficiency of their resorption is quite high (~ 95%). About 300 to 600 mg/d (~ 5%) are excreted in the feces. Interference with the enterohepatic circulation of bile acids leads to altered patterns of bile acid synthesis. Nonabsorbable bile acid–binding resins such as cholestyramine (Questran, Bristol-Myers Squibb, New York, NY) and colestipol (Colestid, Pfizer, New York, NY) cause a large increase in the excretion of bile acids. As a result, the rate of bile acid synthesis from cholesterol is stimulated by the induction of cholesterol 7α-hydroxylase (due to a release of feedback inhibition of this enzyme). The depletion of the liver cholesterol pool leads to an increase in hepatic uptake of LDL cholesterol by both receptor-dependent and receptor-independent mechanisms and lowers plasma cholesterol levels.

Therapeutics
Cholestasis and malabsorption of nutrients

Cholestasis (impaired bile flow), usually due to biliary obstruction, leads to maldigestion of lipid constituents of diet (steatorrhea) due to a decrease in bile salts in the intestinal lumen. Undigested fat traps lipid-soluble vitamins such as A, D, E, and K and causes their malabsorption.

14.5 Cholesterol Conversion to Steroid Hormones and Vitamin D

Steroid hormones are important signaling molecules that are synthesized from cholesterol. Unlike peptide hormones (which bind to their receptors on a cell's outer surface), steroid hormones enter target cells and bind to receptors located in the cytoplasm or nucleus. These receptors function as transcription factors when bound by steroid hormones to induce or repress the transcription of particular genes (▶ Fig. 14.13). Signaling pathways activated by steroid hormones regulate the following processes:
- Cell growth and differentiation into specific cell types
- The body's response to stress
- Metabolism of nutrients
- Allergic, inflammatory and immune responses

▶ Table 14.3 provides a list of common steroid hormones and the specific biological processes they affect.

Normal
Progesterone and pregnancy

Progesterone supports gestation (pregnancy) and embryogenesis and is also involved in the maintenance of the menstrual cycle. It regulates the voltage-gated Ca²⁺ channels on the spermatozoa, prepares the uterus for implantation, causes smooth muscle relaxation, and decreases maternal immune response. A decrease in progesterone levels precedes menstruation, labor, and lactation.

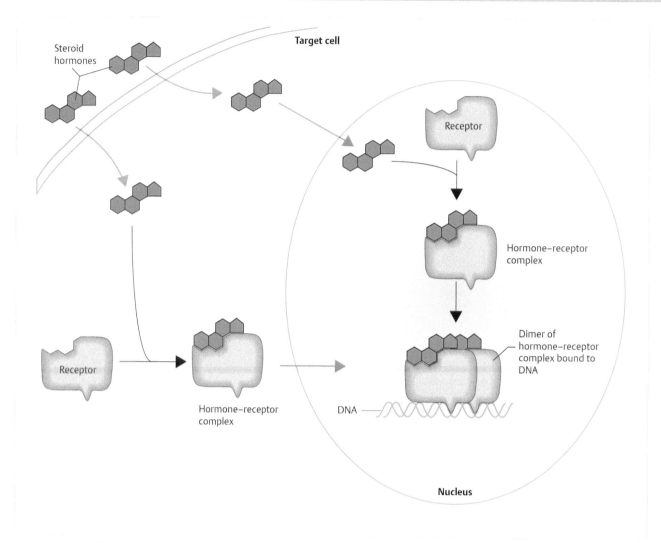

Fig. 14.13 Steroid hormone control of transcription. Steroid hormones enter target cells and bind to receptors in the cytoplasm or nucleus. Once formed, the hormone-receptor complex (as a dimer) binds to specific hormone response elements on DNA to regulate the transcription of specific genes.

Therapeutics

Glucocorticoids and infant respiratory distress syndrome

In normal-term infants, a burst of glucocorticoids preceding delivery alters the lung structure by stimulating the production of surfactant (mainly dimyristoyl phosphatidylcholine, DMPC), which allows the air spaces to expand. In preterm neonates, this process is defective, leading to infant respiratory distress syndrome (IRDS). IRDS can be prevented by giving glucocorticoids to expectant mothers.

Foundations

Metabolic modulation of steroid hormone effects

The response of target tissues to a steroid hormone is sometimes determined by further metabolism of the hormone. For example, mineralocorticoid target tissues such as the kidneys, colon, and parotid gland contain a receptor that has equal affinity for both mineralo- and glucocorticoids. These tissues avoid Na^+/H_2O retention induced by the much higher circulating levels of glucocorticoids by metabolizing cortisol to cortisone through the action of 11β-hydroxysteroid dehydrogenase. Cortisone has a much lower affinity for the mineralocorticoid receptor. Natural licorice root contains isoflavones, which are inhibitors of 11 β-dehydrogenase. Therefore, consumption of real licorice can lead to hypertension due to salt retention.

The androgenic potency of testosterone is amplified by its conversion to dihydrotestosterone (DHT) mediated by the enzyme 5α-reductase. DHT has a much higher affinity than testosterone for the androgen receptor. Finasteride, an inhibitor of 5α-reductase, prevents this potentiation. Finasteride has been used to treat benign prostatic hyperplasia. The drug has also been used to treat male pattern baldness, which is caused by the action of DHT in the scalp.

Table 14.3 Steroid hormones and their biological effects

Hormone class and examples	Sites of synthesis, distribution, and effects
Progestins	
Progesterone	• Synthesized in adrenal glands, ovaries, and testes • Distributed to uterus • Mediates implantation (nidation) and maintenance of pregnancy
Glucocorticoids	•
Cortisol Cortisone Corticosterone	• Synthesized in adrenal glands • Distributed to a large number of tissues and organs (e.g., muscle, liver) • Increases blood pressure and Na$^+$ uptake in kidneys • Mediates response to stress by increasing protein catabolism and gluconeogenesis and reducing inflammation
Mineralocorticoids	•
Aldosterone 11-Deoxycorticosterone	• Synthesized in adrenal glands • Distributed to kidney tubules, colon, and parotid gland • Increases Na$^+$/H$_2$O retention, K$^+$ excretion, and blood pressure
Estrogens	•
Estradiol Estrone	• Synthesized in ovaries (major), placenta, and adipose tissue • Distributed to primary and secondary reproductive organs • Mediates feminization, estrous cycle, and inhibits testosterone synthesis
Androgens	•
Testosterone 5α-Dihydrotestosterone Dehydroepiandrosterone (DHEA)	• Synthesized in adrenal glands, ovaries, and testes (major) • Distributed to primary and secondary reproductive organs and muscle • Mediates spermatogenesis, secondary male characteristics, bone maturation, and virilization

14.5.1 Steroid Hormone Synthesis

Steroid hormones are synthesized from cholesterol in the smooth endoplasmic reticulum of the adrenal cortex, ovaries, and testes. These tissues obtain cholesterol from circulating LDL and HDL, from *de novo* synthesis from acetyl CoA, or from cholesterol esters stored in cytoplasmic lipid droplets.

Mechanism of Steroid Hormone Synthesis

The synthesis of steroid hormones begins with the rate-limiting step catalyzed by desmolase, an enzyme that incorporates a carbonyl group (C=O) on the D ring of cholesterol and cleaves off a six-carbon piece of its side chain (between carbons 20 and 22), to form pregnenolone (▶ Fig. 14.14). Key characteristics about desmolase include the following:
- It is a member of the cytochrome P-450 family of monooxygenases and is therefore also known as P-450scc (scc: side chain cleavage), a product of the *CYP11A1* gene.
- It is only found in tissues that produce steroid hormones (e.g., gonads and adrenal cortex).
- Its expression is stimulated by adrenocorticotropic hormone (ACTH)—an anterior pituitary hormone that is secreted under stressful conditions.

Pregnenolone (an alcohol) is then generally converted to progesterone (an enone). Depending on the tissue in which it is synthesized, progesterone is converted to aldosterone (a mineralocorticoid), cortisol (a glucocorticoid), estradiol (an estrogen), and testosterone (an androgen), as described here:
1. **Adrenal cortex:** Progesterone is converted to aldosterone (in the zona glomerulosa), cortisol (in the zona fasciculata), and the adrenal androgens, dehydroepiandrosterone and

androstenedione (in the zona reticularis) (▶ Fig. 14.14a). Minor amounts of estradiol and testosterone may also be generated in the zona reticularis.
- Aldosterone is a mineralocorticoid that promotes the retention of Na$^+$ and H$_2$O in the kidneys, as well as excretion of H$^+$ and K$^+$. Excessive levels of aldosterone (as seen in patients with Conn syndrome) trigger an increase in blood volume, which leads to hypertension. Deficient levels of aldosterone, however, trigger the loss of an excessive amount of salt.
- Cortisol, also known as hydrocortisone, is a glucocorticoid that stimulates the breakdown of muscle, gluconeogenesis, and glycogen synthesis. Cortisol also has antiinflammatory and antiimmune properties.
- Elevated levels of cortisol are associated with Cushing syndrome, a condition marked by the accumulation of fat on the face and trunk. Increased cortisol production due to pituitary or adrenal tumors causes endogenous Cushing syndrome, whereas the chronic administration of corticosteroids may lead to exogenous Cushing syndrome.
- Reduced cortisol biosynthesis due to deficiencies in specific cytochrome P-450 enzymes in the steroid hormone biosynthetic pathway leads to congenital adrenal hyperplasia (CAH). CAH results from increased pituitary secretion of ACTH due to a lack of feedback inhibition on the hypothalamus by cortisol.
- Addison disease is a rare case of severe adrenal insufficiency due to either a malformation of or damage to the adrenal glands, resulting in a loss of both gluco- and mineralocorticoids.
2. **Ovaries:** Progesterone is either secreted (if synthesized in the ovary's corpus luteum) or converted into testosterone and then to estradiol (if synthesized outside the corpus

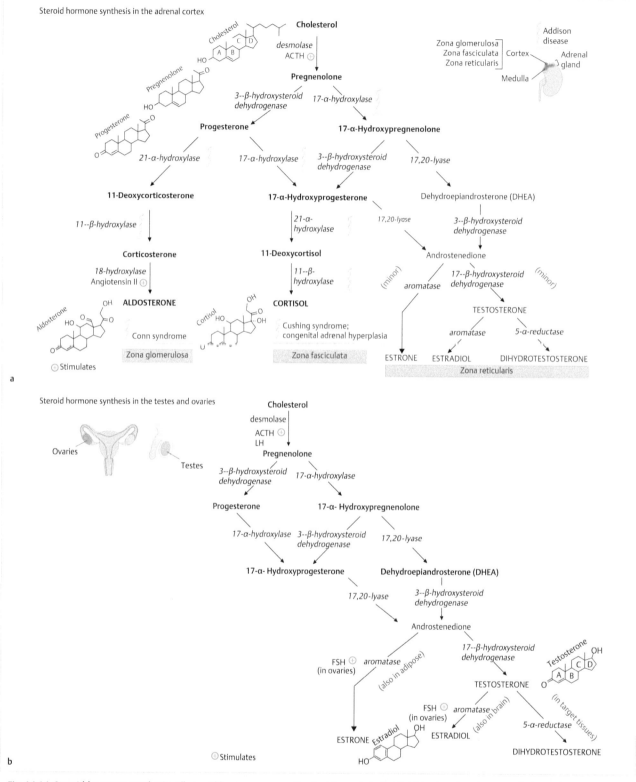

Fig. 14.14 Steroid hormone synthesis. All steroid hormones are synthesized from cholesterol. (**a**) In the adrenal cortex, cholesterol is converted to pregnenolone by desmolase and further metabolized into aldosterone and cortisol, as well as some estrogens (e.g., estradiol) and androgens (e.g., testosterone) in specific layers of the adrenal cortex (see top right image). The activity of desmolase is stimulated by adrenocorticotropic hormone (ACTH), and that of 18-hydroxylase is stimulated by angiotensin II. Various disorders associated with defective enzymes and abnormal production of aldosterone and cortisol are noted. (**b**) In the gonads (ovaries and testes), estrogens and androgens are synthesized via the same pathway observed in the adrenal cortex. The activity of desmolase is stimulated by both ACTH and luteinizing hormone (LH), and the activity of aromatase in ovaries is stimulated by follicle-stimulating hormone (FSH).

luteum) (▶ Fig. 14.14b). The adrenal androgens are also utilized as a precursor for estradiol.
- Estradiol contributes to the development of secondary female characteristics (feminine features), to the proliferative phase of the endometrium, and to ovulation.
- Progesterone is essential for the maintenance of a pregnancy.

3. **Testes:** Pregnenolone and the adrenal androgens are converted to testosterone and then to its more potent form, dihydrotestosterone (▶ Fig. 14.14b).
- Testosterone/dihydrotestosterone stimulates spermatogenesis and the development of secondary male characteristics (masculine features).

Several of the reactions that convert cholesterol into steroid hormones are catalyzed by hydrolases, dehydrogenases, and aromatase, which, when disrupted, lead to a host of disorders. General characteristics of these enzymes are as follows:

- **Hydroxylases:** They add OH groups to substrates. Like desmolase, they are members of the cytochrome P-450 family of hydroxylases.
  - The most common inherited defect (1 in 12,000 live births) is in 21-hydroxylase (▶ Fig. 14.14a). In the severe form, it leads to salt wasting (hyponatremia) and hypotension due to decreased production of aldosterone and hypoglycemia due to decreased production of cortisol. In females, this deficiency causes virilism (development of male secondary characteristics) due to an increased flow of intermediates into adrenal androgens.
  - A rare deficiency of 17α-hydroxylase causes a loss of cortisol as well as sex steroids. However, the decrease in cortisol is compensated for by increased production of corticosterone.
  - Defects in 11β-hydroxylase cause hypertension due to the accumulation of 11-decoxycorticosterone, which has mineralocorticoid activity. It also causes virilism in females.
- **Dehydrogenases:** They oxidize carbonyl groups (C=O) to hydroxyl groups (C-OH).
  - Deficiencies in 3β-hydroxysteroid dehydrogenase disrupt the production of progesterone and its downstream steroid hormones.
- **Aromatase:** Oxidizes the carbonyl group of testosterone into an OH and eliminates methyl groups to transform the A ring (first ring) of testosterone into a conjugated (aromatic) ring as seen in estradiol (▶ Fig. 14.14b).

Regulation by Hypothalamus and Pituitary Glands

Steroid hormone synthesis in the adrenal cortex and gonads is modulated by signals they receive from the hypothalamus, via the pituitary gland, as follows:

- **CRH and ACTH:** In response to various stressful stimuli (e.g., hypoglycemia, cold, exercise), the hypothalamus increases its synthesis and secretion of corticotropin-releasing hormone (CRH). The latter then triggers the release of adrenocorticotropic hormone (ACTH) by cells of the anterior pituitary gland (▶ Fig. 14.15a, b).

- ACTH positively affects the conversion of cholesterol to pregnenolone and stimulates the release of cortisol from the adrenal cortex (▶ Fig. 14.14).
- Elevated levels of cortisol suppress the release of CRH from the hypothalamus and ACTH by the anterior pituitary gland via a negative feedback mechanism.

- **GnRH, LH, and FSH:** Another molecule synthesized and secreted by the hypothalamus is gonadotropin-releasing hormone (GnRH). The latter stimulates the synthesis and secretion of follicle-stimulating hormone (FSH) and luteinizing hormone (LH) by the pituitary gland.
  - In females, LH stimulates the activity of desmolase, which converts cholesterol into pregnenolone, and FSH stimulates the activity of aromatase, which converts testosterone into estradiol (or androstenedione into estrone).
  - GnRH release by the female hypothalamus, as well as that of LH and FSH from the pituitary gland, is pulsatile in accordance with both the menstrual stage (follicular vs luteal) and ovarian estrogen and progesterone production (▶ Fig. 14.15b).
  - In males, LH stimulates the activity of desmolase, which leads to elevated production of testosterone. FSH promotes spermatogenesis.
- The release of GnRH, as well as LH and FSH in men, is also pulsatile (once every 90 minutes) and inhibited by elevated levels of testosterone and inhibin (a nonsteroidal hormone secreted by Sertoli cells of the testis).

14.5.2 Vitamin D

The effects of vitamin D are attributed to its active form, calcitriol (1,25-dihydroxycholecalciferol). Because the B ring of cholesterol's sterane structure is broken during the synthesis of vitamin D, the latter is not classified as a steroid. However, like all steroid hormones, vitamin D acts through binding to a nuclear receptor and altering the expression of target genes containing vitamin D response element (VDRE) sequences.

Mechanism

Cholecalciferol (vitamin D_3) is the inactive form of vitamin D that can be produced in skin from the photochemical cleavage of the B ring of 7-dehydrocholesterol (via UV irradiation of skin) or in intestinal cells from dietary ergocalciferol. Subsequent steps that take place in both the liver and the kidneys include the following (see **Fig. 1.7a, b**):

1. Cholecalciferol is first hydroxylated in the liver by 25-hydroxylase to generate 25-hydroxycholecalciferol.
2. 25-Hydroxycholecalciferol is then hydroxylated in the proximal tubules of the kidneys by 1α-hydroxylase to generate 1, 25-dihydroxycholecalciferol (calcitriol).
- The action of 1α-hydroxylase is stimulated by parathyroid hormone (PTH) and low blood concentrations of phosphate (PO_4^{3-}) but inhibited by calcitriol.
  Calcitriol binds to intracellular receptors (transcription factors) to influence the transcription of specific genes that (1) stimulate the absorption of Ca^{2+} and PO_4^{3-} from the intestines, (2) increase the reabsorption of

Hypothalamus and pituitary gland

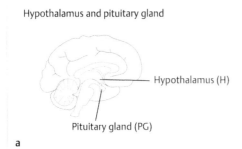

Hypothalamus (H)

Pituitary gland (PG)

a

Regulation of hormones synthesized and secreted by hypothalamus, pituitary gland, testes and ovaries

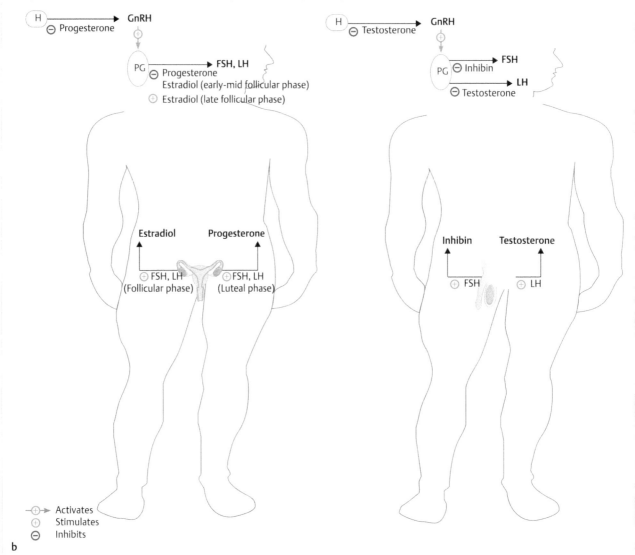

⊕→ Activates
⊕ Stimulates
⊖ Inhibits

b

Fig. 14.15 Regulation of steroid hormone synthesis. (a) Location of the hypothalamus and pituitary glands. **(b)** Relationship between hormones synthesized and secreted by the hypothalamus (H) and pituitary gland (PG) and hormones produced by the ovaries and testes. FSH, follicle-stimulating hormone; GnRh, gonadotropin-releasing hormone; LH, luteinizing hormone.

Ca^{2+} by the kidneys, and (3) promote resorption of Ca^{2+} from bone. The resulting effect of calcitriol is an elevation in blood Ca^{2+} and PO_4^{3-} levels for the maintenance of proper bone mineralization or bone density
(see **Fig. 1.7c**).

- Deficiencies in vitamin D can occur due to inadequate dietary intake, conditions that disrupt the absorption of lipids, poor functioning of the liver and kidneys, hypoparathyroidism, or lack of exposure to sunlight.
- Vitamin D deficiency manifests as brittle bones observed as rickets in children (marked by growth deficiency and skeletal deformities), osteomalacia in adults (marked by "pathological fractures"), and hypocalcemic tetany (involuntary muscle contractions due to low blood Ca^{2+}).

Normal

Steroid hormones and globulins

Steroid hormones are transported in the blood complexed to specific carrier proteins. The human corticosteroid-binding globulin (CBG) is a glycosylated globulin that belongs to the serine protease inhibitor (SERPIN) family of proteins. CBG is involved in the transport and release of the majority (80 to 90%) of plasma glucocorticoid hormones and also progesterone. Sex steroids such as testosterone, dihydrotestosterone, and estradiol are transported by the homodimeric glycoprotein, sex steroid hormone binding globulin (SHBG), and to a lesser extent by albumin. Whereas SHBG is only partially saturated in women, its binding sites are mostly occupied by testosterone in men. Both CBG and SHBG are made mostly in the liver.

Normal

Rennin-angiotensin-aldosterone system (RAAS)

The renin–angiotensin–aldosterone system (RAAS) controls blood pressure and fluid balance. Kidneys release the enzyme renin into circulation when a low blood volume is sensed. Renin cleaves the zymogen angiotensinogen (made by the liver) into angiotensin I, which is subsequently proteolytically processed into the vasoconstrictor angiotensin II in lung capillaries by angiotensin-converting enzyme (ACE). Angiotensin II stimulates the release of vasopressin from the pituitary gland and the mineralocorticosteroid hormone aldosterone from the adrenal cortex. Aldosterone acts on the kidneys to increase Na^+ and water resorption, thus raising the blood pressure and volume. ACE inhibitors are widely used in the treatment of hypertension. Vasopressin acts as a vasoconstrictor, stimulates thirst, and increases water retention in the kidneys.

Normal

Cortisol suppression of the immune system

Glucocorticoids such as cortisol cause immunosuppression by inhibiting both cellular and humoral immune response. They induce the production of i-κBα inhibitory protein, which helps sequester the transcription factor nuclear factor kappa B (**NF-κB**) in inactive cytoplasmic complexes. **NF-κB** is necessary for the synthesis of many cytokines, such as interleukin (IL)-2, which are needed for T cell proliferation. Cortisol also promotes T cell apoptosis. Decreased IL-2 and its receptor lead to an inhibition of clonal expansion of B lympocytes as well.

IV

15 Protein and Amino Acid Metabolism

15.1 Proteins

Proteins are biomolecules that carry out cellular work; they are the gears, motors, and machines of life. The functions of proteins include the following:

- Serving as enzymes, which are biological catalysts that catalyze chemical reactions with extreme specificity. Thus, proteins have a hand in the synthesis of almost every molecule in a living organism (including the synthesis of other proteins).
- Imparting structure to tissues, such as muscle, connective tissue, bone, and hair
- Mediating communication between cells as well as between cells and the extracellular environment by serving as messengers (cell signals). These include hormones, such as insulin and glucagon.
- Protective function as antibodies which bind to foreign molecules
- Acting as transport or storage molecules (e.g., hemoglobin and ferritin)

15.2 Amino Acids

Amino acids, the most basic unit of peptides and proteins, are nitrogen-containing carboxylic acids. When they attach to each other via peptide bonds, they form oligopeptides (2–50 amino acids) or polypeptides (> 50 amino acids) which are also known as proteins. There are 20 natural amino acids that are commonly used in the synthesis of new proteins in the body (▶ Table 15.1).

- In addition to playing a role in protein synthesis, the 20 natural amino acids also serve as precursors for several important biological molecules, including hormones, neurotransmitters, nucleotides and porphyrins (see Chapter 16).

- 10 of the natural amino acids are considered "essential" because they can only be obtained from the diet or by recycling of endogenous proteins. The remaining 10 are referred to as nonessential because, in addition to being supplied by the diet and endogenous protein degradation, these amino acids can be synthesized when needed by *de novo* biosynthetic pathways in mammals (▶ Table 15.2).
  - It should be noted that there are > 400 species of bacteria in the adult human intestinal tract, and they do contribute to the amino acid pool by supplying some of both nonessential and essential amino acids (e.g., Gly, Glu, Ala, Pro, Val, His, Lys, Thr).

Foundations

Proteinogenic amino acids

The 20 amino acids listed in ▶ Table 15.1 all participate in protein synthesis in mammals. An additional amino acid that is observed in selenoproteins (e.g., glutathione peroxidase) is selenocysteine (Sec), in which selenium replaces the sulfur normally found in Cys. Sec is considered the 21st amino acid. Sec synthesis occurs after a special tRNA Ser(Sec) is already charged with Ser. Selenocysteine synthase then converts the Ser on the tRNA to Sec. Pyrrolysine (Pyl) is the 22nd proteinogenic amino acid found only in some methane-producing bacteria. Other nonstandard amino acids found in animal proteins, such as hydroxyproline and hydroxylysine, are generated by posttranslational modifications.

Normal

Conditionally essential amino acids

Arg, which is synthesized via reactions of the urea cycle, is considered "conditionally essential" for premature infants. The poorly functioning urea cycle in premature infants cannot keep

Table 15.1 Essential and nonessential amino acids

Essential (10) (use mnemonic: PVT TIM HALL)	Nonessential (10)
Phenylalanine (Phe, F), Valine (Val, V), Threonine (Thr, T), Tryptophan (Trp, W), Isoleucine (Ile, I), Methionine (Met, M), Histidine (His, H), Arginine (Arg, R)*Leucine (Leu, L), Lysine (Lys, K),	Alanine (Ala, A) Aspartate (Asp, D) Asparagine (Asn, N)* Cysteine (Cys, C)* Glutamate (Glu, E) Glutamine (Gln, Q)* Glycine (Gly, G)* Proline (Pro, P)* Serine (Ser, S)* Tyrosine (Tyr, Y)*

Note: The amino acids marked by asterisks are termed conditionally essential because they become essential only under certain conditions.

Table 15.2 Proteolytic enzymes: Classification

Enzyme class	Class functions and examples
Exopeptidase	Attacks the protein's termini • Aminopeptidases attack the N-terminus (e.g., aminopeptidase N) ○ A subclass of aminopeptidases called dipeptidylpeptidases (DPP) remove dipeptides from the amino terminus (e.g., prolyl dipeptidase or DPP-4) • Carboxypeptidases attack the C-terminus (e.g., carboxypeptidase A) • Dipeptidases attack a dipeptide (amino acid pair) (e.g., renal dipeptidase)
Endopeptidase (proteinase or protease)	Attacks within the protein • Serine proteases contain a catalytic Ser residue (e.g., trypsin, chymotrypsin, and elastase) • Cysteine proteases contain a catalytic Cys residue (e.g., caspases and lysosomal cathepsins) • Aspartate proteases contain a catalytic Asp residue (e.g., pepsin, renin, and some lysosomal proteases) • Metalloproteases contain a catalytic metal ion such as Zn^{2+} (e.g., carboxypeptidase A, collagenase, and angiotensin-converting enzyme)

up with their body's demand for arginine, so this amino acid must be obtained from the diet. Arg also becomes a conditionally essential amino acid in persons with inherited defects in any of the urea cycle enzymes, excepting arginase. Similarly, Cys, which is synthesized from Met via homocysteine, can become conditionally essential if either of the enzymes needed for converting homocysteine to Cys is defective. Tyr can become an essential amino acid in patients with phenylketonuria, which is the result of defects in the conversion of Phe to Tyr.

The term *amino acid pool* refers to the population of free amino acids that are distributed throughout the body. This pool is maintained by the metabolism of proteins and amino acids, as follows (▶ Fig. 15.1):

1. It is constantly depleted by the synthesis of 300–400 g of proteins/day, and it is constantly replenished by the degradation of a similar amount of proteins/day.
2. It obtains amino acids from the digestion of food and proteins secreted into the gastrointestinal tract. These amino acids undergo absorption from the digestive tract into the bloodstream.

IV

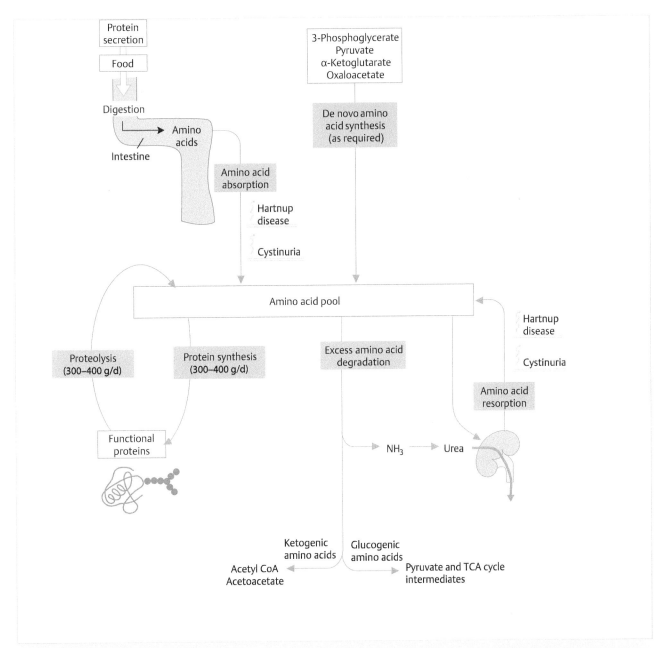

Fig. 15.1 Protein and amino acid metabolism. The amino acid pool is the population of free amino acids that are distributed throughout the body. It is constantly depleted and replenished by the respective synthesis and degradation of proteins. It is primarily supplied with amino acids from absorption of digested proteins from the intestine and from resorption of amino acids by the kidneys. When required, it acquires nonessential amino acids from *de novo* synthesis. When the amino acid pool is in excess, amino acids are degraded into pyruvate and tricarboxylic acid (TCA) cycle intermediates or degraded to acetyl coenzyme A (acetyl CoA) and acetoacetate. The nitrogen released during amino acid degradation is converted to urea and excreted in urine.

3. When required, nonessential amino acids are supplied to the pool via *de novo* synthesis.
4. When the amino acid pool is in excess, amino acids are degraded either into reactants or intermediates of the tricarboxylic acid (TCA) cycle for the purpose of generating energy or molecules that serve as precursors for the *de novo* synthesis of glucose and lipids.
   - The nitrogen component of degraded amino acids cannot be used for the aforementioned processes; therefore, it is converted to urea and excreted from the body in urine.

15.3 Protein Metabolism

15.3.1 Protein Synthesis (Translation)

Proteins are synthesized as linear polypeptides on ribosomes in the cytosol. The basis for the specificity of many antibiotics is due to the differences between the components of prokaryotic and eukaryotic protein synthesis systems. This section focuses primarily on protein degradation. A detailed description of protein synthesis mechanisms in prokaryotes and eukaryotes is found in Chapter 19.

15.3.2 Protein Degradation (Proteolysis)

Proteins are generally too large to be directly absorbed and are therefore degraded to amino acid building blocks by proteolytic enzymes (▶ Table 15.2). These enzymes are primarily described according to their site of attack, as follows:
- **Exopeptidases:** attack outside the protein at the C- or N-terminus
- **Endopeptidases (called proteinases or proteases):** attack within the protein at specific sites. Proteases are further described in terms of their reaction mechanism, which is dependent on the catalytic amino acid residue within their active site (▶ Table 15.2, ▶ Fig. 15.2).

Therapeutics

Hartnup disease and cystinuria

The transport of amino acids into and out of cells is mediated by protein transporters. Autosomal recessive diseases such as Hartnup disease and cystinuria are associated with defects in the transporters for particular amino acids, causing them to be concentrated in urine. For instance, Hartnup disease is caused by a defect in a transporter for nonpolar or neutral amino acids (e.g., tryptophan), which is primarily found in the kidneys and intestine. It manifests in infancy as failure to thrive, nystagmus (abnormally rapid and repetitive eye movement), intermittent ataxia (lack of muscle coordination), tremor, and photosensitivity. Cystinuria, on the other hand, is caused by a defect in the transport system responsible for the uptake of the dimeric amino acid cystine and the dibasic amino acids Arg, Lys, and ornithine. (Cystine is formed when two Cys are oxidized and linked by a disulfide bond.) This defect results in the formation of cystine crystals or stones in the kidneys (renal calculi), which can be identified via a positive nitroprusside test. Patients with this condition present with renal colic (abdominal pain that comes in waves and is linked to kidney stones).

15.3.3 Control of Proteolysis

Protein degradation, which takes place intracellularly or extracellularly, is controlled as follows:
- **Intracellular proteolytic control:** Proteolytic enzymes are controlled through "marking" mechanisms that tag their protein substrate for degradation. This keeps intracellular enzymes from indiscriminately degrading functional proteins. There are two modes of intracellular degradation:
  - *Lysosomal degradation.* Many intracellular proteases are sequestered in lysosomes. The > 50 types of hydrolyases within the lysosome are capable of degrading all intracellular macromolecules, such as proteins, lipids, and oligo/polysaccharides. These enzymes are active at the

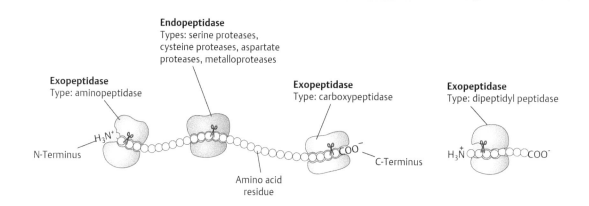

Fig. 15.2 Proteolytic enzymes. Proteolytic enzymes catalyze the cleavage of peptide bonds only at very specific sites. Exopeptidases recognize one of the protein termini such that aminopeptidases attack at the N-terminus, whereas carboxypeptidases attack at the C-terminus. Dipeptidases break peptide bonds between dipeptides exclusively (the enzyme binds to both N- and C-termini). Endopeptidases (proteases) catalyze the cleavage of peptide bonds within the protein.

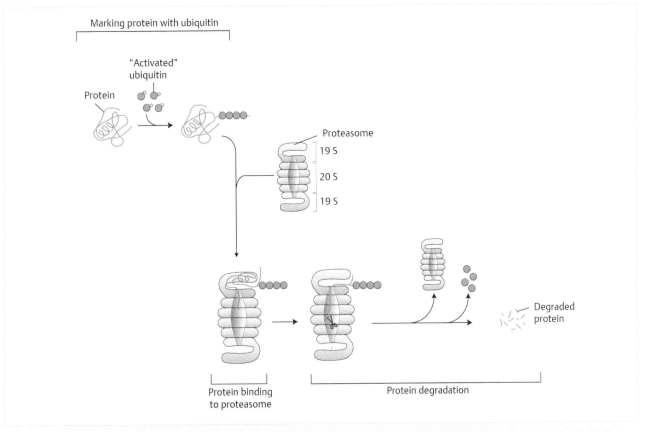

Fig. 15.3 Proteasomal degradation. Proteasomes are cytoplasmic protein complexes that degrade ubiquitinated proteins. Once target proteins are ubiquitinated, the 19S particle of the proteasome binds the ubiquitinated protein and unfolds it in an ATP-dependent manner. The protein then enters the large 20S catalytic nucleus of the proteasome, where it is degraded.

acidic pH of the lysosome (pH = 5) but not at the cytoplasmic pH (pH = 7). This characteristic protects functional proteins from degradation in case of lysosomal rupture.

○ *Proteasomal degradation.* The 26S proteasomes are large cytoplasmic protein complexes that degrade proteins tagged with polyubiquitin (▶ Fig. 15.3). Proteasomes are composed of a catalytic, barrel-shaped core (20S core), which is flanked on both ends by 19S particles that seal the openings. Proteins cannot enter the core unless they are tagged by a chain of small, 76-amino acid polypeptides called ubiquitin. The 19S particle of the proteasome binds the polyubiquitinated protein and unfolds it in an ATP-dependent manner. The linear protein is moved into the catalytic 20S core of the proteasome, where it is degraded.

• **Extracellular proteolytic control:** Proteins are degraded extracellularly (e.g., in the gastrointestinal tract) by proteolytic enzymes that are secreted as needed. These enzymes are often secreted as inactive precursors called zymogens, which must be activated by other enzymes via proteolytic cleavage. For instance, the serine protease trypsin is secreted from the pancreas into the small intestine as trypsinogen. Trypsinogen can be activated either by enteropeptidase or by already active trypsin (▶ Fig. 15.4).

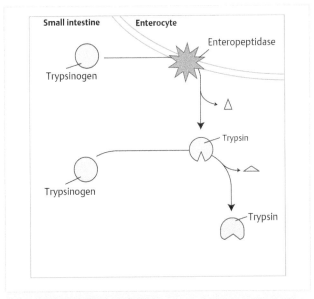

Fig. 15.4 Trypsinogen activation to trypsin. The inactive proenzyme trypsinogen is secreted by the pancreas into the small intestine for activation to trypsin. This occurs when enteropeptidase, an enzyme on the surface of enterocytes, cleaves a six-peptide sequence (hexapeptide) from the N-terminus of trypsinogen. The resulting β-trypsin then activates other trypsinogen molecules through autocatalytic cleavage at two sites.

Therapeutics
Protease inhibitors as drugs

Protease inhibitors are an important class of drugs that are effective against external (e.g., viral infections) as well as internal (e.g., hypertension, cancer) causes of disease. Inhibitors of human immunodeficiency virus (HIV) protease (e.g., Crixivan, Merck, Whitehouse Station, NJ; Truvada, Gilead, Foster City, CA), either by themselves or in combination with reverse transcriptase inhibitors, are effective in the treatment of acquired immunodeficiency syndrome (AIDS). Other protease inhibitors are useful in the treatment of hepatitis C infection. Angiotensin-converting enzyme (ACE) inhibitors, such as enalapril and lisinopril, are used to lower blood pressure. Other protease inhibitors are under development for conditions such as thrombosis (factor Xa inhibitors), Alzheimer disease (γ-secretase inhibitors), and diabetes (dipeptidylpeptidase-4 inhibitors).

Therapeutics
Sorting of lysosomal hydrolases

Lysosomes acquire proteins and organelles to be degraded by autophagy, phagocytosis, and endocytosis. Many of the hydrolytic enzymes of the lysosomes are glycoproteins tagged with mannose 6-phosphate, which helps to sort specific proteins to lysosomes through the Golgi apparatus via late endosomes. The details of this process are as follows: Lysosomal hydrolases are synthesized in the rough endoplasmic reticulum and are transported through the Golgi apparatus to be packaged into late endosomes. The endosomes mature into or fuse with lysosomes. The proteins destined for lysosomes are marked with mannose 6-phosphate (M6P) residues on their N-linked oligosaccharides. M6P receptor proteins in the trans–Golgi network recognize these tagged proteins and assemble them into clathrin-coated vesicles that bud from the trans–Golgi network for delivery to the endosomes. The phosphorylation of mannose residues is performed by N-acetylglucosamine-1-phosphotransferase (GlcNAc-PT). In inclusion-cell (I-cell) disease, the gene that encodes GlcNac-PT is defective; as a result, instead of being targeted to the lysosomes, the hydrolases are secreted and can be detected in circulation.

Therapeutics
Regulation of digestive enzyme secretion

The release of several gastrointestinal hormones is triggered by the components of food, the distension of the stomach upon food intake, and neural stimulation. These hormones, in turn, regulate the secretion of digestive enzymes. The hormone gastrin, produced by G cells of the antral mucosa, stimulates the secretion of acid by parietal cells and of pepsinogen by chief cells of the stomach. In the acidic environment of the stomach, pepsinogen cleaves itself into active pepsin, which then cleaves more pepsinogen into pepsin. In the stomach, pepsin digests dietary proteins into peptides. Another hormone, somatostatin, produced by D cells of the antral

mucosa, acts to inhibit gastrin and acid release. Secretin, produced by S cells of the duodenum, also inhibits gastrin release while stimulating pancreatic secretion of fluid and bicarbonate. Cholecystokinin, produced by I-cells of the duodenum, stimulates the release of pancreatic enzymes, including trypsinogen, chymotrypsinogen, carboxypeptidase, and aminopeptidase. Trypsinogen is proteolytically activated by duodenal enteropeptidase to trypsin, which then helps in further activation of trypsinogen.

Foundations
Catalytic triad in serine proteases

The catalytic mechanism of serine proteases such as chymotrypsin and trypsin involves a catalytic triad of three amino acids: Ser, His, and Asp. The hydroxyl group of Ser and the nitrogen of His participate in the cleavage of peptide bonds, whereas Asp hydrogen bonds with His to facilitate catalysis. Hydrogen bonding of Asp-COOH and His-H allows His-N to deprotonate Ser-OH, which then initiates a nucleophilic attack on the carbonyl C of the peptide bond, generating a tetrahedral intermediate. The active site is restored by the participation of water.

15.4 Amino Acid Metabolism
15.4.1 Amino Acid Synthesis

The 10 nonessential proteinogenic amino acids are synthesized *de novo* from molecules derived from glucose 6-phosphate. All of these amino acids (with the exception of Glu), are synthesized via reactions that involve the transfer of an amino group (transamination) to a keto acid. Amino acids that share common biosynthetic precursors are grouped together in the following families (▶ Fig. 15.5, ▶ Table 15.3):

- **Aromatic family:** The aromatic His is synthesized in plants and bacteria via the transamination of the pentose phosphate pathway metabolite, ribose 5-phosphate. While the rate of synthesis of His in humans is quite low, gut bacteria could be a source of this amino acid. Another member of this family, Tyr, is synthesized via the hydroxylation of the essential amino acid Phe. (In microorganisms and plants, Phe is synthesized via the Shikimate pathway, which requires the use of erythrose 4-phosphate—a derivative of ribose 5-phosphate.)
- **Serine family:** Amino acids in this family are synthesized from the glycolytic metabolite, 3-phosphoglycerate. Transamination of 3-phosphoglycerate generates Ser, which can then be converted to Cys (whose sulfur atom comes from Met) or Gly.
- **Pyruvate family:** Ala, the only amino acid in this family, is generated from the transamination of pyruvate.
- **Aspartate family:** Amino acids in this family are synthesized from the TCA cycle metabolite, oxaloacetate. Transamination of oxaloacetate generates Asp, which undergoes reductive amination for conversion to Asn.
- **Glutamate family:** Synthesis of amino acids in this family starts from the TCA cycle metabolite α-ketoglutarate.

IV

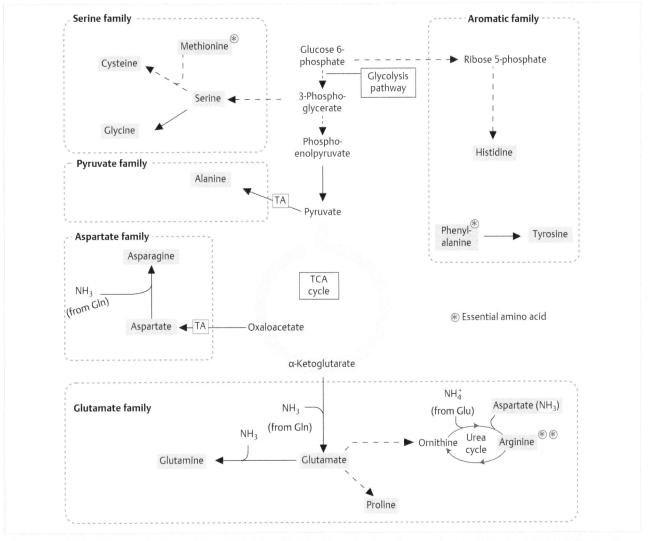

Fig. 15.5 Amino acid synthesis: overview. Amino acids are synthesized from derivatives of glucose 6-phosphate via the transfer of amino groups onto carboxylic acids. With the exception of glutamate, all amino acids are synthesized via transamination (TA) of the keto acid. The serine family is synthesized from intermediates of the glycolysis. (The essential amino acid methionine donates its sulfur to serine to form cysteine.) Histidine is synthesized from ribose 5-phosphate. Tyrosine is not considered essential, but it is formed from the hydroxylation of phenylalanine, an essential amino acid. The glutamate and aspartate families are synthesized from intermediates in the tricarboxylic acid (TCA) cycle. Aspartate (formed from pyruvate) is used to generate asparagine. Glutamate is formed via reductive amination of α-ketoglutarate. Glutamate is then used to produce glutamine, proline, and arginine. Essential amino acids are indicated with a star. Double stars indicate that arginine is a conditionally essential amino acid.

Table 15.3 Summary of synthesis of nonessential amino acids (AAs)

Members of family	Summary of synthesis
Aromatic family: includes AAs synthesized from ribose 5-phosphate and Phe	
His, Tyr	Ribose 5-P → His
	Phe → Tyr
Serine family: includes AAs synthesized from 3-phosphoglycerate	
Ser, Cys, Gly	3-Phosphoglycerate → Ser → Cys or Gly
Pyruvate family: includes AAs synthesized from pyruvate	
Ala	Pyruvate → Ala
Aspartate family: includes AAs synthesized from oxaloacetate	
Asp, Asn	Oxaloacetate → Asp → Asn
Glutamate family: includes AAs synthesized from α-ketoglutarate	
Glu, Gln, Pro, Arg*	α-Ketoglutarate → Glu → Gln, Pro, or Arg

*Arg: the synthesis of Arg from Glu involves the urea cycle.

Reductive amination of α-ketoglutarate generates Glu, which can be converted to Gln via an ATP-dependent amination. Alternatively, Glu can be converted to Pro or Arg. The synthesis of Arg, however, involves reactions of the urea cycle.

15.4.2 Amino Acid Degradation (▶ Table 1504)

Seven of the proteinogenic amino acids are described as ketogenic because their degradation produces acetyl coenzyme A (acetyl CoA) or acetoacetate (▶ Fig. 15.6). These two molecules serve as precursors for the generation of ketone bodies and lipids. On the other hand, 18 of the 20 proteinogenic amino acids are described as glucogenic because they can be degraded to pyruvate or to intermediates of the TCA cycle (▶ Fig. 15.7, ▶ Fig. 15.8, ▶ Fig. 15.9, ▶ Fig. 15.10). These molecules serve as precursors for the synthesis of glucose via gluconeogenesis. It is important to note the following:
1. Lys and Leu are purely ketogenic.
2. Thr, Trp, Ile, Phe, and Tyr are both keto- and glucogenic.

All amino acids contain nitrogen in the amino group bound to the α-carbon. Six of the 20 proteinogenic amino acids also contain nitrogen in their side chains (Trp, Asn, Gln, His, Lys, Arg) (see ▶ Fig. 15.6; orange-colored amino acids). The amino groups of amino acids are removed as ammonia/ammonium ion (NH_3/NH_4^+) via two types of reactions: transaminations and deaminations.
- Transaminations are catalyzed by a group of enzymes known as aminotransferases (transaminases), which all require the cofactor pyridoxal phosphate (a derivative of vitamin B_6) for

their activity. Pyridoxal phosphate (PLP) is covalently linked to the side chain of a specific Lys residue on the aminotransferase and helps to shuttle the amino group from an amino acid to a keto acid.
- Deaminations are catalyzed by variety of enzymes that carry out three types of deaminations:
  1. Eliminating (nonoxidative) deamination in which ammonia is released
  2. Oxidative deamination in which ammonia is released and NAD^+ is reduced to NADH
  3. Hydrolytic deamination in which ammonia is released via a hydrolytic reaction with water

Normal
Nitrogen balance

Nitrogen balance is the difference between intake and excretion of nitrogenous compounds. Most of the nitrogen in the body is incorporated into macromolecules, such as proteins and nucleic acids. A positive nitrogen balance (+ NB) signifies an anabolic state, and growth and is commonly seen during childhood, pregnancy, and convalescence. A negative nitrogen balance (–NB) signifies a catabolic state and occurs as a result of malnutrition, amino acid imbalance, and terminal diseases such as cancer.

An individual's nitrogen balance can be assessed by determining the person's blood urea nitrogen (BUN) levels, which are normal at 7 to 20 mg/dL (2.5 to 7.1 mmol/L).

NB = Nitrogen intake – Nitrogen loss

Healthy adult NB: Nitrogen intake = Nitrogen loss

+ NB = Nitrogen intake > Nitrogen loss

–NB = Nitrogen loss > Nitrogen intake

Table 15.4 Summary of degradation of amino acids (AAs)

Amino acids and degradation products	Degradation mechanisms
AAs degraded to pyruvate: Ala, Trp, Ser, Gly, Thr, Cys (▶ Fig. 15.7)	• Ala is transaminated directly to pyruvate because pyruvate is the keto acid of Ala ○ Trp is converted to Ala • Ser undergoes an eliminating deamination directly to pyruvate ○ Gly is converted to Ser ○ Thr is converted to Gly (and acetyl CoA) • Cys undergoes metabolism to pyruvate via complex reaction mechanisms
AAs degraded to α-ketoglutarate: Glu, Gln, Pro, His, Arg (▶ Fig. 15.8)	• Glu undergoes oxidative deamination or transamination to α-ketoglutarate because the latter is the keto acid of Glu ○ Arg is converted to Glu via the urea cycle ○ Gln is converted to Glu via hydrolytic deamination of its side chain ○ His undergoes a nonoxidative deamination, and its imidazole ring is oxidized to formiminoglutamate; transfer of the formimino group to tetrahydrofolate (THF) produces Glu ○ Pyrrole ring of Pro is oxidized to contain a double bond (N=C), which is then saturated; oxidation opens up the ring, forming glutamate semialdehyde, which is oxidized to Glu
AAs degraded to succinyl CoA: Ile,* Val,* Met, Thr (▶ Fig. 15.9)	• Ile, Val, Met, and Thr are degraded via separate pathways that generate a common intermediate, propionyl CoA, which is then converted to succinyl CoA
AAs degraded to fumarate: Tyr, Phe, Asp (▶ Fig. 15.10)	• Tyr is oxidized to break its ring and form maleylacetoacetate, which is then rearranged to fumarylacetoacetate; the latter is then hydrolyzed to produce fumarate (and acetoacetate) – Phe is converted to Tyr
AAs degraded to oxaloacetate: Asp, Asn (▶ Fig. 15.10)	• Asp is transaminated directly to oxaloacetate because oxaloacetate is the keto acid of Asp • Asn is converted to Asp via hydrolytic deamination of its side chain
Degradation to acetyl CoA and acetoacetate Lys, Leu,* Thr, Tyr, Ile* (▶ Fig. 15.7, ▶ Fig. 15.9, ▶ Fig. 15.10)	• Lys and Leu are each degraded via separate pathways to acetyl CoA and acetoacetate • Lys never donates an amino group in transamination reactions • When Thr is converted to Gly, acetoacetate is released • Degradation of Tyr generates fumarate and acetoacetate • The degradation of Ile generates succinyl CoA and acetyl CoA

Abbreviations: HMG CoA, 3-hydroxy-3-methylglutaryl coenzyme A. *Branched-chain amino acids.

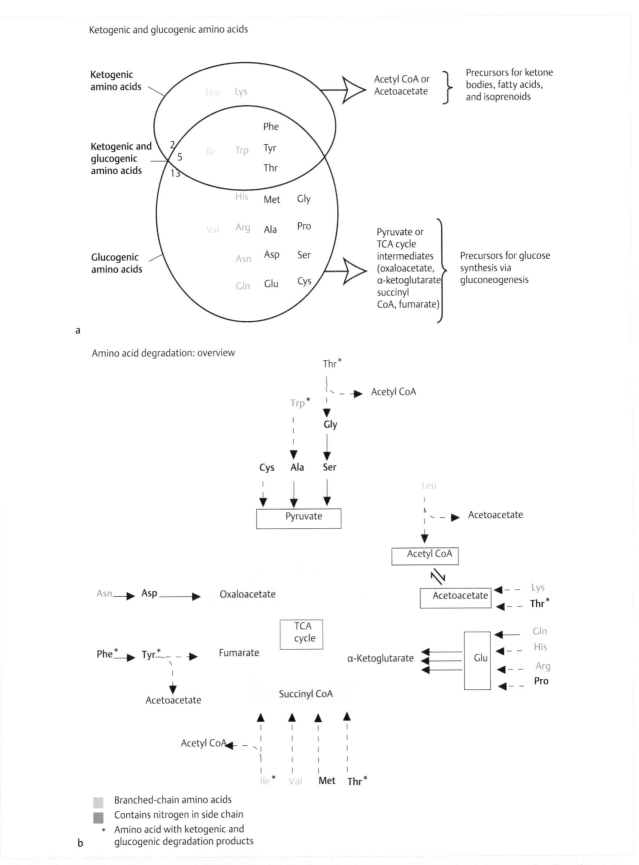

Fig. 15.6 Proteinogenic amino acids: ketogenic and glucogenic. (a, b) All 20 amino acids contain an α-carbon bound to a carboxylic acid, an amino group, and a side chain. The ketogenic amino acids are degraded to acetyl coenzyme A (acetyl CoA) or acetoacetate. The glucogenic amino acids are degraded to pyruvate or four intermediates of the tricarboxylic acid (TCA) cycle (oxaloacetate, α-ketoglutarate, succinyl CoA, and fumarate). Dashed arrows indicate more than one reaction step. Asterisks (*) denote those amino acids that are both ketogenic and glucogenic.

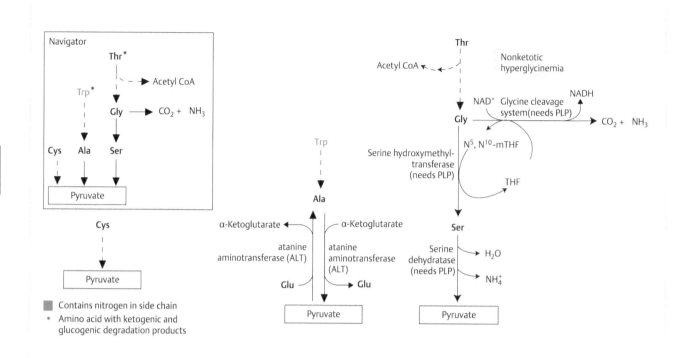

Fig. 15.7 Degradation of amino acids to pyruvate. Cys is degraded to pyruvate via several reactions (dashed arrow). Trp is converted to Ala via several reactions. Via a transamination reaction, Ala is converted to pyruvate, while α-ketoglutarate is converted to Glu. Thr is converted to Gly via a series of reactions that release acetyl coenzyme A (acetyl CoA). Gly is converted to Ser via a reaction that involves tetrahydrofolate (THF) derivatives. Ser is converted to pyruvate via a reaction that releases ammonium ion and water and is catalyzed by a pyridoxal phosphate (PLP)-dependent enzyme. Alternatively, Gly can be degraded to CO_2 and ammonia via a reaction that involves THF derivatives and is catalyzed by an enzyme (called the glycine cleavage complex) that requires PLP for its activity. Nonketotic hyperglycinemia is associated with defects in the glycine cleavage system. (Dashed arrows indicate more than one reaction step.) Orange color denotes amino acids that contain nitrogen in their side chains. Asterisks (*) denote those amino acids that are both ketogenic and glucogenic.

Foundations

Glycine encephalopathy

Glycine encephalopathy (GCE), formerly known as nonketotic hyperglycinemia, is caused by inherited defects in the multiprotein glycine cleavage complex (GCC) located in mitochondria. GCC cleaves Gly into ammonia and CO_2 during the pyridoxal phosphate-dependent conversion of tetrahydrofolate to N^5, N^{10}-methylene tetrahydrofolate. Defects in the genes encoding any of the four proteins of GCC can cause neonatal, infantile, mild-episodic, or late-onset forms of GCE. The classical neonatal form is characterized by hypotonia and apnea, leading to death. Patients with the infantile form of the disease exhibit seizures and severe mental retardation. Mild mental retardation in childhood and episodes of delirium and chorea are features of the mild-episodic form. Patients with the late-onset form of GCE present with progressive spastic diplegia and optic atrophy in childhood but do not exhibit seizures or mental retardation. A finding of Gly concentration in cerebrospinal fluid that is > 10% of the value in plasma is usually diagnostic of the typical GCE. Plasma levels of organic acids such as propionic acid and methylmalonic acid are usually normal. The diagnosis may be confirmed by an assay of GCC activity in liver biopsy samples. Prenatal diagnosis involves the GCC assay in chorionic villus samples.

15.4.3 Notable Derivatives of Amino Acids (▶ Fig. 15.11)

S-Adenosylmethionine (SAM) and homocysteine (▶ Fig. 15.12a).

Met is the precursor for the synthesis of Cys. The pathway of conversion of Met to Cys proceeds via two important intermediates, S-adenosylmethionine (SAM) and homocysteine.

- Homocysteine is an independent risk factor in atherosclerotic vascular disease.
- S-Adenosylmethionine is the "activated" methyl donor for many biological methylation reactions, as summarized in ▶ Fig. 15.12a.

Catecholamine neurotransmitters (▶ Fig. 15.12b). Tyr is a precursor for the synthesis of catecholamine neurotransmitters, such as dopamine, norepinephrine, and epinephrine, as well as the melanin pigments. The synthesis of catecholamines requires the use of tetrahydrobiopterin (THB), vitamin C, and SAM.

Serotonin (▶ Fig. 15.12c). Trp is the precursor for niacin and the hormone serotonin (5-hydroxytryptamine), which regulates pain perception, appetite, and mood. Many antidepressant drugs are inhibitors of serotonin reuptake in the synapses. Serotonin can be converted to melatonin in the pineal gland. Melatonin is thought to regulate sleep as well as the estrus cycle in mammals.

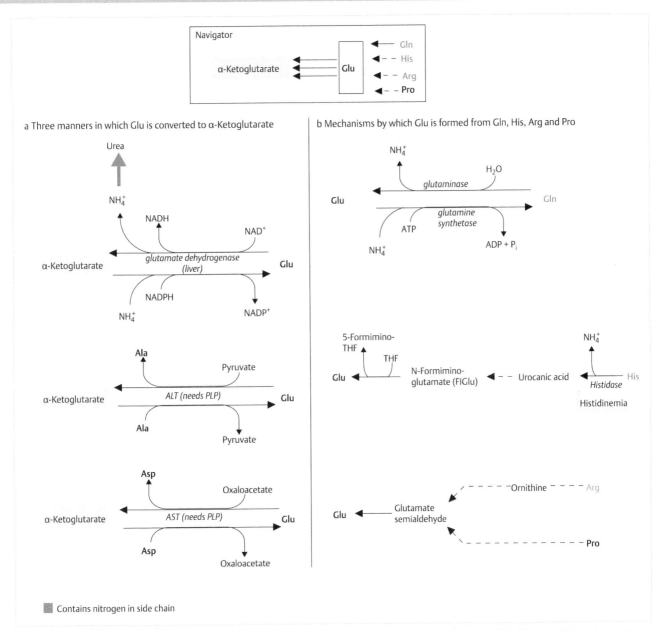

IV

a Three manners in which Glu is converted to α-Ketoglutarate

b Mechanisms by which Glu is formed from Gln, His, Arg and Pro

Contains nitrogen in side chain

Fig. 15.8 Degradation of amino acids to α-ketoglutarate. (a) Removal of the amino group of Glu generates α-ketoglutarate. This occurs via three possible mechanisms: (1) oxidative deamination by glutamate dehydrogenase, which releases ammonium ion (NH^+_4); (2) transfer of the amino group to pyruvate by alanine aminotransferase (ALT), which generates Ala; (3) transfer of the amino group to oxaloacetate by aspartate aminotransferase (AST), which generates Asp. (b) Gln undergoes hydrolytic deamination to Glu, releasing ammonium ion. His is broken down to Glu via a series of reactions that include a nonoxidative deamination by histidase, which releases ammonium (NH^+_4), and one that requires tetrahydrofolate (THF). Defects in histidase are associated with histidinemia. The breakdowns of Arg and Pro to Glu intersect at a common intermediate, glutamate semialdehyde. Arg conversion to ornithine involves the urea cycle. Dashed arrows indicate more than one reaction step. Orange color denotes amino acids that contain nitrogen in their side chains. ADP, adenosine diphosphate; ATP, adenosine triphosphate; PLP, pyridoxal phosphate.

Therapeutics

Aminotransferases in the clinical setting

Aminotransferases are normally located in the mitochondria and the cytoplasm of many cells, particularly in liver, kidney, intestine, and muscle. An increase in the levels of these enzymes in the bloodstream is diagnostic of damage to tissues. The two clinically important aminotransferases are alanine aminotransferase (ALT), also known as serum glutamate-pyruvate transaminase (SGPT), and aspartate aminotransferase (AST), also known as serum glutamate-oxaloacetate transaminase (SGOT). Serum ALT is increased in viral hepatitis, liver cell necrosis, and prolonged circulatory collapse. Serum AST is increased 6 to 8 hours after a myocardial infarction. It is also increased in biliary cirrhosis, liver cancer, pancreatitis, mononucleosis, alcoholic cirrhosis, and strenuous exercise. Serum ALT is a more specific diagnostic of liver disease than AST.

IV

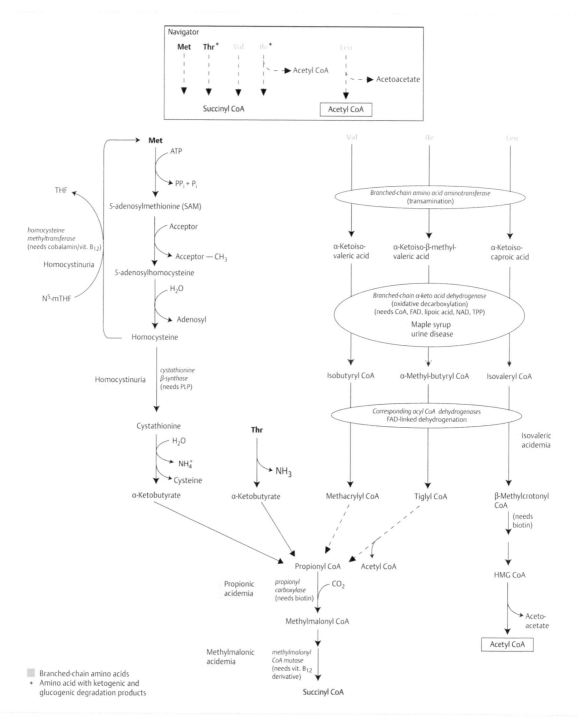

Fig. 15.9 Degradation of amino acids to succinyl coenzyme A (succinyl CoA), acetoacetate, and acetyl CoA. The degradation of Met to homocysteine includes the adenosine triphosphate (ATP)–dependent activation of Met into S-adenosylmethionine (SAM). Homocysteine can then be converted back to Met or used in the synthesis of Cys. The branched-chain amino acids Val, Ile, and Leu are degraded via reactions that begin with a transamination, followed by an oxidative carboxylation (by branched-chain α-keto acid dehydrogenase), and then a flavin adenine dinucleotide (FAD)–linked dehydrogenation. Branched–chain amino acids are not degraded in the liver due an absence of the required aminotransferase. Instead, they are degraded mainly in the muscle, kidney and brain. The degradation of Met, Thr, Val, and Ile generates succinyl CoA (and acetyl CoA in Ile degradation). Leu degradation generates both acetyl CoA and acetoacetate. The disorders associated with defects in certain enzymes are indicated. They include homocystinuria, propionic acidemia, methylmalonic acidemia, maple syrup urine disease, and isovaleric acidemia. Dashed arrows indicate more than one reaction step. Asterisks (*) denote those amino acids that are both ketogenic and glucogenic. HMG, 3-hydroxy-3-methylglutaryl; NAD+, nicotinamide adenine dinucleotide; PLP, pryridoxal phosphate; TPP, thiamine pyrophosphate.

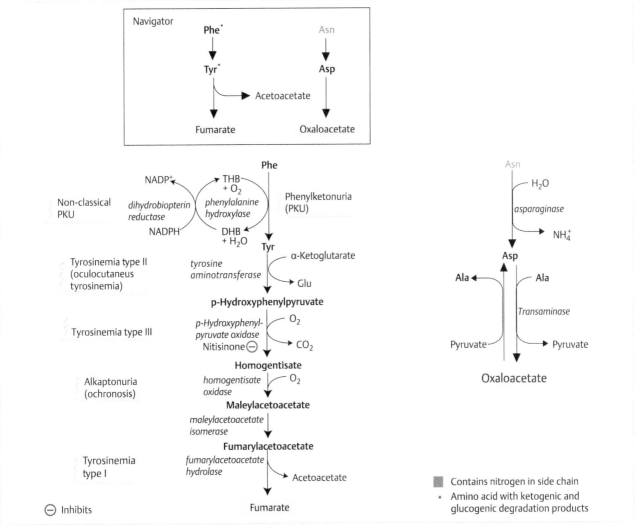

Fig. 15.10 Amino acid degradation to fumarate and oxaloacetate. Hydroxylation of Phe generates Tyr via a reaction that requires oxygen and tetrahydrobiopterin (THB). Phenylketonuria (PKU) is associated with a defect in phenylalanine hydroxylase, and nonclassical PKU is associated with defects in the production of THB by dihydrobiopterin (DHB) reductase. Tyrosine's ring structure is then broken down into fumarate and acetoacetate via a series of reactions. The disorders associated with defects in enzymes that catalyze these reactions include tyrosinemias types I through III and alkaptonuria. The drug nitisinone is used in the treatment of alkaptonuria and tyrosinemia type I because of its inhibitory effects on *p*-hydroxphenylpyruvate oxidase. Orange color denotes amino acids that contain nitrogen in their side chains. Asterisks (*) denote those amino acids that are both ketogenic and glucogenic. NADP+, nicotinamide adenine dinucleotide phosphate; NADPH, reduced form of nicotinamide adenine dinucleotide phosphate.

Therapeutics

Histidinemia

Histidinemia is characterized by increased levels of His in plasma. Increased blood levels of histamine and imidazole may also be found. It is caused by autosomal recessive mutations in the gene (*HAL*) that encodes histidase, which metabolizes His to urocanic acid. Histidase is mainly expressed in liver and skin. Although histidinemia is a benign condition in most patients, it may exacerbate the effects of fetal or neonatal hypoxia, leading to behavioral problems and learning disorders.

Foundations

Mitochondrial respiration

Mitochondrial respiration requires the intermediates in the tricarboxylic acid cycle—that is, the carboxylic acids that are present in mitochondria only in small amounts. They are regenerated by the oxidation of acetyl coenzyme A (acetyl CoA) to CO_2. These intermediates are also consumed by anabolic pathways (see **Fig. 10.5**) and therefore must be regenerated by anaplerotic reactions. The most important anaplerotic reactions are the degradation of the glucogenic amino acids.

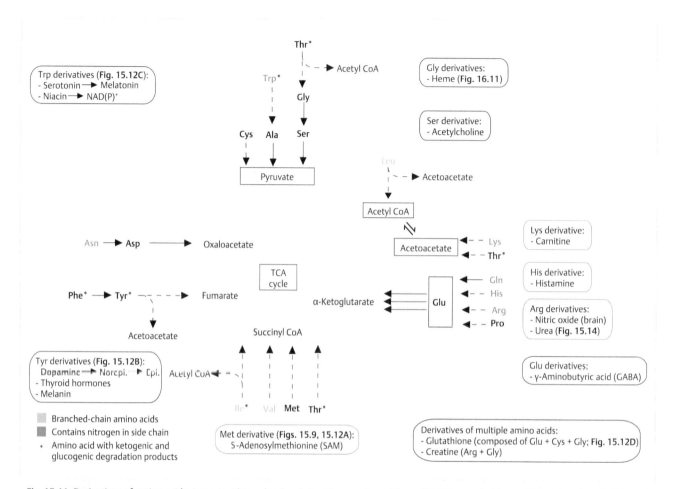

Fig. 15.11 Derivatives of amino acids. Important biomolecules derived from amino acids are listed in rounded boxes. The pathways and additional details for some are provided by the referenced figures. Dashed arrows indicate more than one reaction step. Orange color denotes amino acids that contain nitrogen in their side chains. Asterisks (*) denote those amino acids that are both ketogenic and glucogenic. CoA, coenzyme A; TCA, tricarboxylic acid cycle.

Foundations

Keto acid dehydrogenase enzyme complexes

Branched-chain α-keto acid dehydrogenase (BCKD), which is involved in the metabolism of branched-chain amino acids such as Val, Leu, and Ile, belongs to the same family of large multisubunit enzyme complexes as pyruvate dehydrogenase and α-ketoglutarate dehydrogenase. Each complex in eukaryotes contains ~100 subunits arranged into three functional entities: E1 [thiamine pyrophosphate (TPP)–dependent dehydrogenase], E2 (dihydrolipoyl transacetylase), and E3 (dihydrolipoyl dehydrogenase). The complex requires five cofactors derived from vitamins: TPP (thiamine, vitamin B_1), lipoic acid, coenzyme A (pantothenate, vitamin B_5), flavin adenine dinucleotide (FAD; riboflavin, vitamin B_2), and nicotinamide adenine dinucleotide (NAD+; niacin, vitamin B_3).

Therapeutics

Maple syrup urine disease

Maple syrup urine disease (MSUD) is a rare autosomal disease resulting from a deficiency of branched-chain α-keto acid dehydrogenase (BCKD) activity. The hallmark of the disease is the presence of branched-chain amino acids and their α-keto derivatives in the urine of patients, giving it the characteristic odor of burnt maple sugar. These compounds also accumulate in the blood, causing toxic effects on brain function and mental retardation. Treatment involves feeding a synthetic diet limiting branched-chain amino acids (Val, Leu, Ile). In some forms of mild MSUD, the activity of BCKD may be restored to normal by thiamine supplementation of the diet.

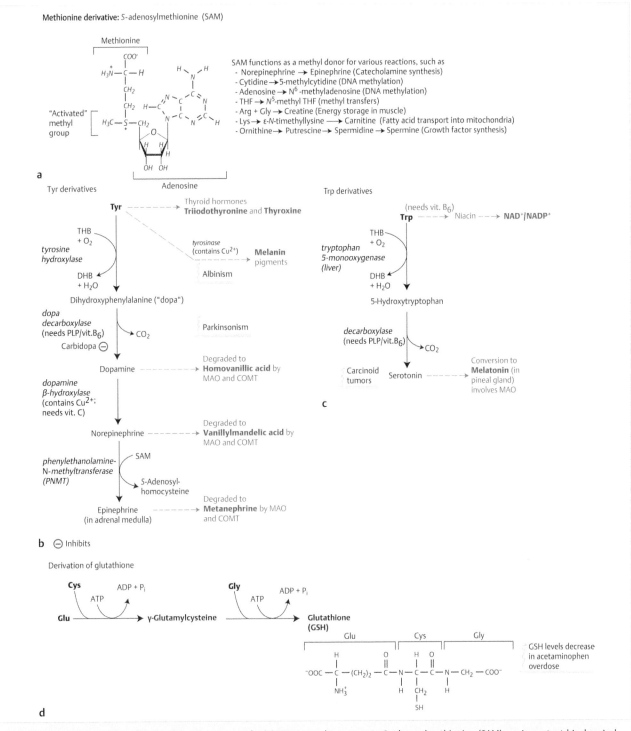

Fig. 15.12 Specific examples of derivatives of amino acids. (a) Met is used to generate *S*-adenosylmethionine (SAM), an important biochemical agent in methyl transfer reactions. SAM is used as the methyl donor in such diverse processes as catecholamine synthesis, DNA methylation, energy storage in muscle, cell proliferation, and mitochondrial transport of fatty acids. SAM is also a precursor for Cys via the intermediate homocysteine (see ▶ Fig. 15.9). **(b)** Tyr is a precursor for the synthesis of catecholamine neurotransmitters, such as dopamine, norepinephrine, and epinephrine, in adrenal and neuronal cells. This pathway uses the cofactors tetrahydrobiopterin (THB), vitamin C, pyridoxal phosphate (PLP), and the methyl donor SAM. Tyr also serves as a precursor for the synthesis of thyroid hormones and melanin pigments. **(c)** Trp is converted to 5-hydroxytryptophan by an enzyme that uses THB as a cofactor. 5-Hydroxytryptophan is, in turn, decarboxylated to serotonin. Serotonin can then be converted to melatonin. Trp also serves as a precursor for niacin. **(d)** The reduced form of glutathione (GSH) is derived from Glu, Cys, and Gly. Disorders associated with each amino acid's derivative pathway are noted. They include albinism, carcinoid tumors, and acetaminophen overdose. ADP, adenosine diphosphate; ATP, adenosine triphosphate; COMT, catechol-*O*-methyltransferase; DHB, dihydrobiopterin; MAO, monoamine oxidase; NAD⁺, nicotinamide adenine dinucleotide; NADP⁺, nicotinamide adenine dinucleotide phosphate; THF, tetrahydrofolate.

IV

Therapeutics
Isovaleric acidemia

Isovaleric acidemia is the result of a deficiency of isovaleryl CoA dehydrogenase, an enzyme involved in Leu catabolism. Increased levels of isovaleric acid are toxic to the brain, and symptoms in affected infants include lethargy, vomiting, and seizures. The buildup of isovaleric acid also causes a distinctive odor of sweaty feet. Treatment of this autosomal recessive disorder involves restriction of Leu intake and administration of Gly or carnitine to conjugate and excrete excess isovaleric acid.

Therapeutics
Propionic acidemia

Propionic acidemia is a rare autosomal recessive disorder resulting from a deficiency of biotin-dependent propionyl CoA carboxylase, which converts propionyl CoA into methylmalonyl CoA. Propionic acid is a product of catabolism of Met, Thr, Val, and Ile. It is also produced by β-oxidation of fatty acids with an odd number of carbons and by catabolism of the side chain of cholesterol. In the normal course of metabolism, propionyl CoA is eventually converted to succinyl CoA and enters the TCA cycle. Propionic acid or its nonnatural metabolites appear to be toxic to basal ganglia; affected infants are lethargic, fail to thrive, and exhibit vomiting and seizures. Propionic acidemia manifests as ketosis, which is often accompanied by increased blood levels of glycine (ketotic hyperglycinemia) and ammonia, which may contribute to the encephalopathy. 2-Methylcitrate, which is formed by the citrate synthase catalyzed condensation of propionyl CoA with oxaloacetate, is excreted in the urine. 2-Methylcitrate is toxic to energy production in mitochondria and inhibits isocitrate dehydrogenase and glutamate dehydrogenase. By these actions, 2-methylcitrate may contribute to the encephalopathy seen in both propionic acidemia and methylmalonic acidemia. Treatment includes restriction of intake of relevant amino acids (Met, Thr, Val, and Ile) and administration of carnitine and biotin. Oral antibiotics are given to reduce microbial production of propionic acid in the intestinal tract.

Therapeutics
Methylmalonic acidemia

Methylmalonic acidemia is caused by a deficiency of methylmalonyl CoA mutase and results in an accumulation of methylmalonic and propionic acids and their metabolites in plasma. The symptoms of this disorder as well as the accumulation of metabolites, including 2-methylcitrate, in blood and urine mirror those of propionic acidemia. Methylmalonyl CoA mutase is a cobalamin (vitamin B_{12})-dependent enzyme. Treatment includes restriction of Met, Val, Ile, and Thr and supplementation with carnitine and vitamin B_{12}.

Therapeutics
Consequences of hyperhomocysteinemia and homocystinuria

Hyperhomocysteinemia and homocystinuria result from defective metabolism of homocysteine due to vitamin deficiencies (B_6, B_{12}, and folic acid) or due to inherited defects in enzymes such as cystathionine β-synthase. Hyperhomocysteinemia is considered an independent risk factor in atherosclerotic heart disease and stroke, as well as in other disorders, such as eye lens dislocation, osteoporosis, and mental retardation. Vitamin supplementation of diet has, in some cases, normalized plasma homocysteine levels.

Foundations
Tetrahydrofolate pool

A very important member of the one-carbon donor pool is tetrahydrofolate (THF), which is formed from dietary folate via dihydrofolate. The conversion of dihydrofolate to THF is catalyzed by dihydrofolate reductase, which is a target for the antifolate class of antitumor drugs, such as methotrexate. THF exists in several active forms, such as N^5-methyl THF; N^5-formimino THF; N^{10}-formyl THF; N^5, N^{10}-methylene THF; and N^5, N^{10}-methynyl THF. They play important roles in the biosynthesis of Gly, Ser, Met, purines, and deoxythymidine monophosphate (dTMP) (see Chapter 16). Trimethoprim, an antibiotic used to treat urinary tract infections, shows 30,000-fold greater specificity toward bacterial dihydrofolate reductase compared to the mammalian enzyme.

Therapeutics
Phenylketonuria

Defects in the activity of phenylalanine hydroxylase activity cause phenylketonuria (PKU), the most common inborn error of amino acid metabolism. Phe in these patients is instead converted to phenylpyruvate and then to phenyllactate and to phenylacetate. The latter two compounds disrupt neurotransmission and block amino acid transport in the brain as well as myelin formation, resulting in severe impairment of brain function. The patient's urine may have a musty odor due to phenylacetate. Synthesis of the pigment melanin, which is a product of Tyr, is also impaired. This defect was the first one to be included in newborn screening for inherited metabolic disorders. Treatment involves limiting Phe intake in infants. Pregnant women with PKU also need to limit their Phe intake. More than 80% of dietary protein for PKU patients is supplied by a synthetic formula that is supplemented with Tyr. Secondary PKU is the result of a deficiency in tetrahydrobiopterin (THB), which is an essential cofactor of phenylalanine hydroxylase. Defects in either the synthesis or the regeneration of THB lead to secondary PKU.

Foundations

Tetrahydrobiopterin/dihydrobiopterin

Tetrahydrobiopterin (THB) is an essential cofactor in the hydroxylations of the aromatic amino acids, Phe, Tyr, and Trp, as well as in the production of nitric oxide (NO) from Arg. It is biosynthesized from GTP via a pathway involving three enzymes and is regenerated by the reduced form of nicotinamide adenine dinucleotide phosphate (NADPH)–dependent reduction of dihydrobiopterin catalyzed by dihydropteridine reductase. Defects in the biosynthesis or regeneration of THB can lead to secondary phenylketonuria (PKU). The pathways for the production of monoamine neurotransmitters (dopamine, norepinephrine, and serotonin) from Tyr and Trp are also disrupted when THB is deficient, leading to neurologic dysfunction. Synthetic THB, sapropterin (Kuvan, BioMarin, Novato, CA) is used in the treatment of secondary PKU.

Therapeutics

Tyrosinemias

Tyrosinemia is characterized by elevated blood levels of Tyr. Transient tyrosinemia in newborns is the result of delayed expression of enzymes involved in the catabolism of Tyr. Hereditary infantile tyrosinemia (tyrosinemia type I) is the result of a defect in the gene encoding fumarylacetoacetate hydrolase, an enzyme in the pathway of Tyr catabolism to fumarate (see ▶ Fig. 15.10). Infants with this disorder have a distinctive cabbage-like odor and develop severe liver failure unless promptly treated. They excrete succinylacetone, a compound derived from fumarylacetoacetate, in their urine. Succinylacetone is toxic to the liver and kidneys. It interferes with the TCA cycle, causes renal tubule dysfunction, and inhibits the biosynthesis of heme at the level of δ-aminolevulinic acid (δ-ALA) dehydratase (porphobilinogen synthase). Tyrosinemia type II is caused by a deficiency of tyrosine aminotransferase, which generates p-hydroxyphenylpyruvate from Tyr. Patients with this disorder exhibit photophobia and skin lesions on their palms and soles. Tyrosinemia type III is the result of a defect in p-hydroxyphenylpyruvate oxidase and is characterized by intermittent ataxia. Of the three types of tyrosinemia, type I is the most common and used to require liver transplantation. In recent times, nitisinone, a reversible inhibitor of p-hydroxyphenylpyruvate oxidase, has emerged as the front-line treatment for type I tyrosinemia. Nitisinone prevents the formation of fumarylacetoacetate, which is the precursor for toxic succinylacetone.

Therapeutics

Alkaptonuria

Alkaptonuria is due to a defect in homogentisate oxidase, an enzyme in the Tyr degradative pathway (see ▶ Fig. 15.10). It causes homogentisic acid to accumulate. Autooxidation of homogentisic acid (with light) and polymerization of products produce dark-colored pigments in urine. Black pigmentation in the intervertebral disks of patients with degenerative arthritis and ochronosis (darkened sclera) are also observed.

Therapeutics

Albinism and tyrosinase

Albinism is a disease due to a severe lack of melanin. Conversion of tyrosine to melanin is blocked due to defects in the enzyme tyrosinase (or in the transport of tyrosine), resulting in partial or complete absence of normal pigment in skin, hair, and eyes (oculocutaneous albinism).

Therapeutics

Parkinsonism

Parkinson disease is the result of a loss of conversion of dihydroxyphenylalanine ("dopa") to the neurotransmitter dopamine in the brain due to destruction of neural tissue. The disease causes tremors and difficulties in movement. The most common treatment is the administration of levodopa (L-dopa) because dopamine itself cannot cross the blood–brain barrier. To limit inadvertent uptake of L-dopa by nonbrain tissues, carbidopa is coadministered. Carbidopa inhibits dopa decarboxylase to prevent the uptake of "dopa" by peripheral tissues. The infantile form of Parkinson disease is due to defects in tyrosine hydroxylase.

Normal

Catecholamine degradation by MAO and COMT

Catecholamines are short-lived signaling molecules. Monoamine oxidase (MAO) and catechol O-methyltransfersase (COMT) are the enzymes involved in the degradation of dopamine into homovanillic acid (HVA) and both norepinephrine and epinephrine into vanillylmandelic acid (VMA). The levels of VMA in urine are measured in patients suspected of having pheochromocytomas. In these patients, the adrenal glands overproduce catecholamines. MAO also converts serotonin into 5-hydroxyindoleacetic acid, which is excreted in urine. MAO inhibitors such as hydrazines, phenethylamines, and benzamides act as antidepressants due to their ability to inhibit rapid degradation of monoamine neurotransmitters in the synaptic cleft. Some show higher specificity toward dopamine catabolism and are used to treat Parkinson disease.

Normal

Histamine

Histamine is a hydrophilic, vasoactive amine that is synthesized from His and stored in cytoplasmic granules until specific signals cause its release. It is produced by the action of histidine decarboxylase in mast cells as well as in enterochromaffin-like (ECL) cells, and enteric nerve fibers in the stomach. Histamine is released from mast cells in response to allergen/ immunoglobulin E (IgE) complexes. Binding of histamine to H_1 receptors in different tissues leads to vasodilation and hypotension, bronchoconstriction, separation of endothelial cells, and edema. Histamine is responsible for hives, pain, and itching due to insect stings, allergic rhinitis, and motion sickness. Antihistamines bind to H_1 receptors and act as inverse agonists (they bind to the same site as histamine but exert the opposite

IV

pharmacological effect). Histamine, released from ECL cells after stimulation by gastrin and acetylcholine, binds to H_2 receptors on parietal cells of gastric mucosa to stimulate acid secretion. H_2 receptor antagonists (e.g., cimetidine, ranitidine) block histamine stimulation of parietal cells and inhibit acid secretion.

IV

Therapeutics
Serotonin

Serotonin (5-hydroxytryptamine), synthesized from Trp, is a neurotransmitter that controls appetite, mood, and sleep. Although it is present in the central nervous system (CNS), the majority of serotonin in the body may be found in the enterochromaffin cells in the gastrointestinal tract, where it regulates bowel motility. This neurohormone also plays a role in bladder control, ejaculatory latency, platelet aggregation, and cardiovascular function. These varied effects are mediated through multiple subtypes of G protein–coupled serotonin receptors. In the CNS, serotonin action is terminated by its reuptake via one or more monoamine transporters in the presynaptic neuron. Drugs that interfere with the reuptake process, such as tricyclic antidepressants, amphetamine, cocaine, and selective serotonin reuptake inhibitors (SSRIs), prolong serotonin action and are effective in the treatment of anxiety and depression.

Therapeutics
Carcinoid tumors

Carcinoid tumors occur mostly in the midgut (ileum) and the respiratory tract. A small fraction (~10%) of these tumors overproduce serotonin, which causes diarrhea, flushing, wheezing, and abdominal cramping. Urinary excretion of 5-hydroxy indole acetic acid, a product of serotonin catabolism, is elevated in these cases.

Normal
Thyroglobulin and thyroid hormones

Thyroglobulin is a 660 kDa protein made by follicular cells of the thyroid gland and utilized to produce the hormones thyroxine (T_4) and triiodothyronine (T_3). Thyroglobulin contains ~120 Tyr residues, some of which can be iodinated to generate monoiodo- and diiodotyrosines. T_4 is made by coupling two diiodotyrosines, whereas T_3 is made by coupling a diiodotyrosine to a monoiodotyrosine. T_3 is more potent than T_4 but has a shorter half-life in circulation. T_3 can also be generated from T_4 by the action of a deiodinase in target tissues. Patients diagnosed with hyperthyroidism disorders (e.g., Graves disease) are treated with agents such as carbimazole and propylthiouracil, which block iodination of thyroglobulin by thyroperoxidase in the follicular lumen to decrease the production of T_4 and T_3.

Foundations
Creatinine

A small fraction (1 to 2%) of phosphocreatine in the muscle is nonenzymatically converted, by cyclization, to creatinine, which is excreted in urine. Under conditions of kidney dysfunction or muscle degeneration, the levels of creatinine in serum are elevated (normal range = 0.6 to 1.3 mg/dL). Creatinine clearance rate (C_{cr}) refers to the volume of plasma clearance of creatinine per unit time, and a decrease in its value is an accurate indicator of renal disease. C_{cr} is calculated by measuring creatinine concentration in serum and a 24-hour pooled sample of urine [(urine creatinine × urine volume)/ serum creatinine]. The normal range for C_{cr} is 90 to 130 mL/min.

Therapeutics
Glutathione and acetaminophen detox

Glutathione (γ-glutamylcysteinylglycine, GSH) is a tripeptide containing Gly, Cys, and Glu. Whereas Gly is linked to Cys through a regular peptide bond, the amide linkage between Cys and Glu involves the γ-carboxylic group of Glu. Glutathione serves as a major antioxidant and can detoxify hydrogen peroxide to water by serving as a cofactor for glutathione peroxidase. In the process, an oxidized form of glutathione, GSSG, is generated that contains two molecules of GSH in a disulfide linkage. Regeneration of GSH from GSSG requires the action of glutathione reductase. GSH is also used to conjugate hydrophobic drugs or their metabolites (e.g., acetaminophen) to render them more polar. An overdose of acetaminophen can deplete GSH levels. In such cases, N-acetylcysteine, which can be converted to Cys by cells, is administered to restore GSH levels. Glutathione also participates in the transport of amino acids into cells by a mechanism known as the γ-glutamyl cycle. In this process, the Glu residue of GSH is transferred to the extracellular amino acid (X) by γ-glutamyl transpeptidase (GGT). The dipeptide product (Glu-X) is transported inside the cell by an amino acid transporter, where it is hydrolyzed to release X. GGT is also involved in the formation of leukotriene D_4 from leukotriene C_4. Elevated serum levels of GGT are a marker for hepatobiliary dysfunction.

15.5 Urea Cycle

15.5.1 Overview

There is no mechanism to store amino acids in the body. They must be either synthesized or obtained from the diet. Excess amino acids are rapidly degraded or excreted.

- The removal of nitrogen in the form of ammonia from an amino acid leaves the carbon skeleton, which can be utilized either as an energy source or as a precursor for gluconeogenesis or other products.
- Ammonia must be disposed of because even small amounts can be toxic to the CNS. Detoxification of ammonia is accomplished through its conversion to urea by the liver.

Urea

Urea is a compound that contains two amino groups (NH_2) linked by a carbonyl group (C=O) and is produced by the urea cycle (▶ Fig. 15.14).

- The carbonyl group of urea (red) comes from carbon dioxide (which circulates in the blood as HCO_3^-).
- The two amino groups on urea (blue) come from ammonium ion (NH_4^+) and Asp.

Ammonia

Ammonium ion (NH_4^+) is produced via deamination reactions as amino acids are degraded (see ▶ Fig. 15.7, ▶ Fig. 15.8, ▶ Fig. 15.9, and ▶ Fig. 15.10). It must be kept at low levels because even slightly raised levels (hyperammonemia) are toxic to the CNS. The normal range of blood ammonia (NH_3) is 5 to 35 μM. However, it may reach levels as high as 1 mM under certain conditions, such as liver dysfunction, urea cycle disorders, and mitochondrial dysfunction.

Brain. In the brain, increased ammonia leads to pH imbalance. It also affects energy metabolism by depleting α-ketoglutarate (a TCA cycle intermediate) and by depleting levels of Glu, a neurotransmitter. Increased ammonia in astrocytes results in the formation of reactive oxygen species (ROS), mitochondrial dysfunction and brain edema.

- The brain removes excess ammonium ions as either Glu or Gln using the enzymes glutamate dehydrogenase and glutamine synthetase, respectively (▶ Fig. 15.13).
- The synthesis of Glu by reductive amination of α-ketoglutarate uses NADPH as the donor of reducing equivalents and is the preferred direction of the reaction in the brain.

Other tissues. Ammonia from other tissues ends up in the liver in the form of Glu, Gln and Ala because Glu and Gln transport ammonia from the brain to the liver, and Ala transports ammonia from muscle to the liver.

- In the liver (and kidneys), ammonium ion is released by the action of glutaminase, which converts Gln to Glu. The ammonium ion produced in the liver is directed to the urea cycle, but in the kidneys, it may be directly excreted in the urine.
- In the liver, Ala donates the amino group to α-ketoglutarate to form Glu. The ammonium ion in Glu is then released through the action of glutamate dehydrogenase during the

conversion of Glu to α-ketoglutarate. Subsequently, the ammonium ion is used in the urea cycle.

15.5.2 Urea Cycle Mechanism

The enzymes that catalyze the first two reactions of the urea cycle are located in the mitochondrial matrix, whereas the remaining three are present in the cytosol (▶ Fig. 15.14).

1. In the first mitochondrial step, ammonium ion (NH_4^+) generated from the deamination of Glu or Gln is condensed with bicarbonate to generate carbamoyl phosphate. This ligation reaction, which is catalyzed by carbamoyl phosphate synthetase-1 (CPS-1), requires the energy of hydrolysis of two ATP molecules. CPS-1 activity is absolutely dependent on the allosteric activator, N-acetylglutamate (NAG), which is produced from Glu and acetyl CoA by the action of NAG synthase also located in the mitochondria.
    - NAG synthase is activated allosterically by Arg.
    - A genetic defect in NAG synthase would have the same effect as a defect in CPS-1 and lead to hyperammonemia.
2. Carbamoyl phosphate is then transferred to the amino acid ornithine, by ornithine transcarbamoylase, to form citrulline. Citrulline is then transported out of the mitochondria by the citrulline transporter.
    - An X-linked recessive defect in ornithine transcarbamoylase manifests as orotic aciduria with hyperammonemia. Orotic aciduria develops as a result of elevated amounts of carbamoyl phosphate that enters the cytosol for use in the pyrimidine biosynthetic pathway (see **Fig. 16.7**).
3. In the cytosol, the enzyme argininosucccinate synthetase ligates Asp to citrulline to generate argininosuccinate. This reaction requires the hydrolysis of ATP to AMP and PP_i.
4. Argininosuccinate is then cleaved by argininosuccinate lyase to generate Arg and fumarate.
    - Fumarate, a TCA cycle intermediate, is recycled to Asp by the action of cytosolic fumarase, malate dehydrogenase, and aspartate aminotransferase.
5. Arg is then cleaved to ornithine and urea by the liver-specific enzyme, arginase.
    - Ornithine, which inhibits arginase, is transported back into mitochondria by the ornithine transporter to continue the urea cycle.

▶ Table 15.5 provides a summary of disorders associated with defects in key urea cycle enzymes.

Table 15.5 Defective urea cycle enzymes and their associated disorders

Defective enzyme	Inheritance	Disorder/Presentation
N-acetylglutamate synthetase (NAGS)	Autosomal recessive	Hyperammonemia
Carbamoyl phosphate synthetase I	Autosomal recessive	Hyperammonemia
Ornithine transcarbamoylase	X-linked recessive	Orotic aciduria
Argininosuccinate synthetase	Autosomal recessive	Citrullinemia
Argininosuccinate lyase	Autosomal recessive	Argininosuccinate aciduria
Arginase	Autosomal recessive	Slight hyperammonemia

IV

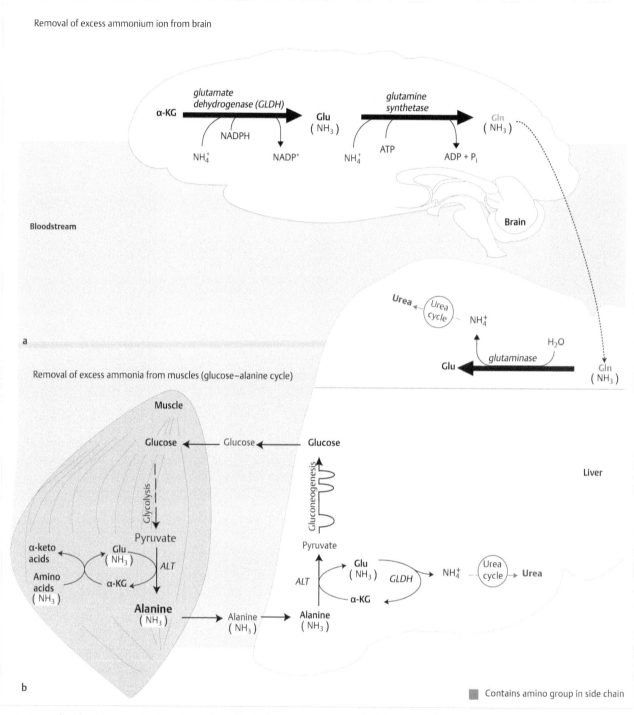

Removal of excess ammonium ion from brain

glutamate dehydrogenase (GLDH)

α-KG → Glu (NH₃)

NADPH

NH₄⁺ → NADP⁺

glutamine synthetase

Glu (NH₃) → Gln (NH₃)

ATP

NH₄⁺ → ADP + Pᵢ

Bloodstream

Brain

Urea ← Urea cycle ─ NH₄⁺

H₂O

Glu ← *glutaminase* ← Gln (NH₃)

a

Removal of excess ammonia from muscles (glucose–alanine cycle)

Muscle

Glucose ← Glucose ← Glucose

Glycolysis

Gluconeogenesis

Liver

Pyruvate

Pyruvate

α-keto acids ← Glu (NH₃) → ALT

Amino acids (NH₃) ← α-KG

ALT → Glu (NH₃) → GLDH → NH₄⁺ ─ Urea cycle → Urea

α-KG

Alanine (NH₃) → Alanine (NH₃) → Alanine (NH₃)

b

■ Contains amino group in side chain

Fig. 15.13 The glucose-alanine cycle and urea. (a) In the brain, excess ammonium (NH⁺₄) is removed as either Glu, or Gln, using the enzymes glutamate dehydrogenase and glutamine synthetase, respectively. Gln transports ammonia from the brain to the liver, where the action of glutaminase (which converts Gln to Glu) releases ammonium for conversion to urea via the urea cycle. **(b)** In extrahepatic tissues (e.g., muscle), the amino group from amino acids is transferred to α-ketoglutarate (α-KG), which generates Glu. Glu then transfers its amino group to pyruvate, which generates alanine. Ala is then transported to the liver (via the blood), where it carries out the reverse reaction and transfers its amino group to α-ketoglutarate to regenerate pyruvate and Glu. Deamination of this Glu by glutamate dehydrogenase (GLDH) releases ammonium, which is converted to urea via the urea cycle. The pyruvate that was regenerated in the liver is converted to glucose (via gluconeogenesis), which is sent to muscle cells (via the blood). The glucose-alanine cycle is reminiscent of the Cori cycle (see **Fig. 12.6**). The ammonia in parentheses are attached to the indicated amino acids. ADP, adenosine diphosphate; ATP, adenosine triphosphate; NADP⁺, nicotinamide adenine dinucleotide phosphate; NADPH, reduced form of nicotinamide adenine dinucleotide phosphate.

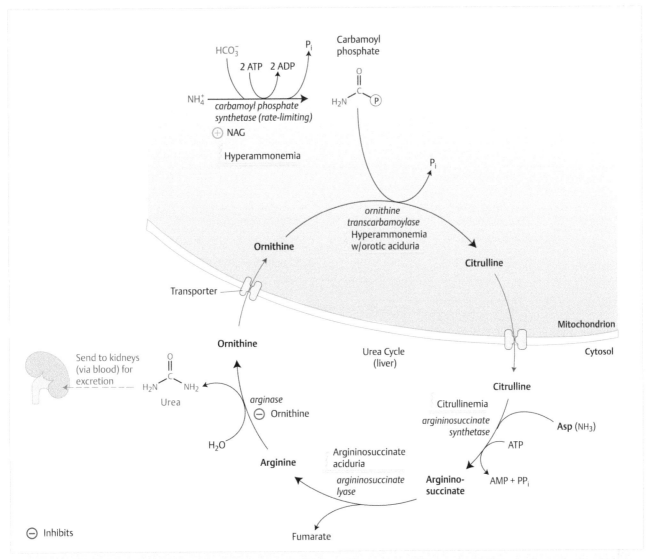

Fig. 15.14 Urea cycle. Nitrogen is not used to generate energy. It is eliminated (from amino acids and nucleotides) as urea. The urea cycle, which was the first cyclic pathway discovered by Sir Hans Krebs, consists of five steps. The first two steps occur in the mitochondrial matrix and the rest in the cytosol. Various disorders are associated with defects in urea cycle enzymes (▶ Table 15.5). ADP, adenosine diphosphate; ATP, adenosine triphosphate; NAG, N-acetylglutamate.

Therapeutics

Nitric oxide

Nitric oxide (NO) is an important gaseous signaling molecule synthesized from Arg by endothelial cells and phagocytes (monocytes, macrophages, and neutrophils) and neuronal cells. Biosynthesis of NO is catalyzed by NO synthase (NOS) and requires NADPH, O_2, and tetrahydrobiopterin (BH_4). Three isoforms of NOS have been identified. Neuronal cells express nNOS or NOSI, whereas phagocytic cells contain the inducible isoform iNOS or NOSII. Endothelial cells have eNOS or NOSIII. Characteristics of the NO generated by the three isoforms of NOS include the following:

- NO produced by nNOS may have functions as a messenger and as a modulator of neurotransmitter release.
- Cytokines induce iNOS in macrophages to produce large amounts of NO, which has antimicrobial effects in fighting infections.
- NO produced by eNOS serves to prevent vascular smooth muscle contraction and platelet aggregation by increasing Ca^{2+} influx and intracellular cGMP production.

Nitrodilators lower blood pressure through either spontaneous (e.g., nitroprusside) or enzyme-mediated (e.g., nitroglycerin, isosorbide dinitrate) release of NO and the resultant relaxation of smooth muscle. Nitrodilators are useful in the treatment of acute hypertensive emergencies.

IV

Creatine

Creatine is made from three amino acids, Gly, Arg, and Met. The guanidinium group of Arg is transferred to Gly to form guanidinoacetate, which is methylated by *S*-adenosylmethionine (SAM) to generate creatine. Creatine is phosphorylated by mitochondrial creatine kinase (CK), using ATP as a phosphodonor. Phosphocreatine serves as a storage form of energy in muscle, brain, and sperm. It can be used to quickly generate ATP from ADP using cytosolic CK. The presence of the cardioselective isoform of creatine kinase (CK-MB) in serum is diagnostic of myocardial infarction (MI). Serum CK-MB peaks at 10 to 24 hours after MI and returns to normal values in 2 to 3 days. A relative index value relating the mass of CK-MB to total enzyme activity ([mass of CK-MB (μg/L)/total CK activity (U/L)] × 100) > 3 when CK-MB mass is > 4 μg/L, is indicative of MI.

Hyperammonemia

Persistent hyperammonemia in newborns results from defects in any of the six enzymes (including NAG synthase) associated with urea cycle or in three distinct transporters (mitochondrial ornithine carrier, mitochondrial Asp/Glu carrier, and dibasic amino acid carrier). Defects in the mitochondrial enzymes lead to a more severe hyperammonemia than those in the cytosolic enzymes of the urea cycle. A defect in ornithine transcarbamoylase (OTC) causes a mitochondrial buildup of carbamoyl phosphate, which then spills out into the cytoplasm. It can be metabolized by the cytosolic pyrimidine synthetic pathway to the intermediate, orotic acid, which tends to accumulate and is excreted in the urine (orotic aciduria) of male patients. Management of the urea cycle defects involves limiting protein intake while ensuring adequate calorie consumption and the use of agents that can conjugate certain amino acids into excretable metabolites. For example, sodium benzoate combines with glycine to form hippuric acid, and phenylacetate can conjugate glutamine. In some cases, the diet may be supplemented with citrulline or arginine.

Ammonia toxicity

Excess ammonia, due to either a disorder of the urea cycle or liver failure, can have highly toxic effects on the brain and the CNS. Uncharged ammonia (NH_3), rather than the ammonium ion (NH_4^+), is the toxic agent due to its ability to traverse biological membranes. In addition to pH imbalance, ammonia causes a swelling of astrocytes in the brain, leading to cerebral edema and intracranial hypertension. The activity of the TCA cycle is inhibited due to a depletion of α-ketoglutarate. Postsynaptic excitatory potentials are inhibited, leading to a depression of CNS function. Depletion of Glu (due to its conversion to Gln) results in a disruption of its neurotransmitter activity. Ammonia also causes mitochondrial dysfunction.

Carbamoyl phosphate synthetase II (cytosolic)

The first and the rate-limiting step in *de novo* synthesis of pyrimidines is catalyzed by a cytosolic isoform of carbamoyl phosphate synthetase (CPS-II, see **Fig. 16.7**). Please note that this enzyme is different from the mitochondrial version (CPS-I) that initiates the urea cycle. CPS-II does not require *N*-acetylglutamate (NAG), but it is stimulated by phosphoribosyl pyrophosphate (PRPP) and inhibited by uridine triphosphate (UTP). Orotic acid is an intermediate in the pathway for synthesis of uridine monophosphate (UMP) from cytosolic carbamoyl phosphate. An autosomal recessive defect in UMP synthase can lead to an accumulation of orotic acid and result in orotic aciduria. However, unlike the case in ornithine transcarbamoylase deficiency, orotic aciduria due to defects in UMP synthase is not accompanied by hyperammonemia or a reduction in blood urea nitrogen (BUN) levels. In the case of a defect in ornithine transcarbamoylase of urea cycle, carbamoyl phosphate spills out of mitochondria into cytosol and since it has bypassed the rate-limiting step of CPS-II, drives the formation of downstream intermediates of pyrimidine biosynthetic pathway such as orotic acid.

Citrullinemia

Classical citrullinemia (type I) is the result of an autosomal recessive deficiency in argininosuccinate synthetase. Infants with type I citrullinemia develop hyperammonemia within a few days after birth with symptoms of lethargy, poor feeding, vomiting, and seizures. A less common type II citrullinemia with adult incidence is caused by a defect in a mitochondrial citrulline/ornithine transporter, called citrin. The type II disorder is mainly found in the Japanese population.

Urea cycle and high-protein diet

Urea production is increased by a high-protein diet and is decreased by a high-carbohydrate diet. Insulin and glucagon appear to play a role in urea production. About 20 to 30% of the urea produced is hydrolyzed in the gastrointestinal tract by bacterial urease and provides a source of ammonia nitrogen for gut bacteria and for possible salvage and reuse. High-protein diets appear to enhance both urea production and hydrolysis.

16 Nucleotide and Heme Metabolism

16.1 Nucleosides, Nucleotides, and Deoxynucleotides

Nucleosides and nucleotides, in both monomeric and polymeric arrangements, play central roles in cellular processes as cosubstrates in enzymatic reactions, activated carriers, regulatory agents, and, of course, components of RNA and DNA.

- Nucleosides are composed of a five-carbon sugar, ribose, attached to a heterocyclic base from either the purine or the pyrimidine families. The base is attached to the carbon 1' position (or anomeric carbon) of ribose on its "top" or β-face (▶ Fig. 16.1a).
- Nucleotides are nucleosides with one or more phosphates attached to the carbon 5' position of ribose on its "top" or β-face (▶ Fig. 16.1b).

- Deoxynuclosides and deoxynucleotides lack a 2'-hydroxyl (OH) group on the ribose ring (▶ Fig. 16.1c).

16.1.1 Purines and Pyrimidines

Nucleosides and nucleotides contain purine or pyrimidine bases. The purines possess two, fused, heterocyclic rings, whereas pyrimidines possess one heterocyclic ring (▶ Fig. 16.2).

Purines

There are four common purines that appear either in RNA and DNA or in the metabolic pathways involving these bases. They are guanine (Gua), adenine (Ade), hypoxanthine (Hyp),

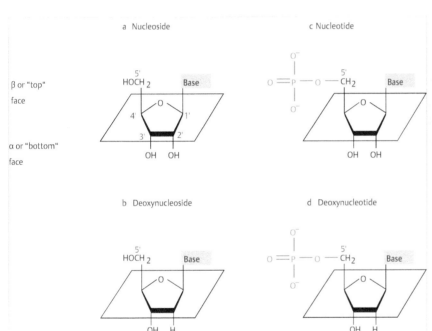

Fig. 16.1 Nucleoside, nucleotide, and deoxynucleotide structures and their numbering system. (a-d) The Haworth projections for the furanose form of D-ribose places the base at C-1′ and the hydroxylmethyl (CH_2OH) or $CH_2OPO_3^{2-}$ groups at C-4′ on the so-called top or β-face and the two hydroxyl groups at C-2′ (which is absent in a deoxynucleoside or a deoxynucleotide) and C-3′ on the bottom or α-face. C, carbon.

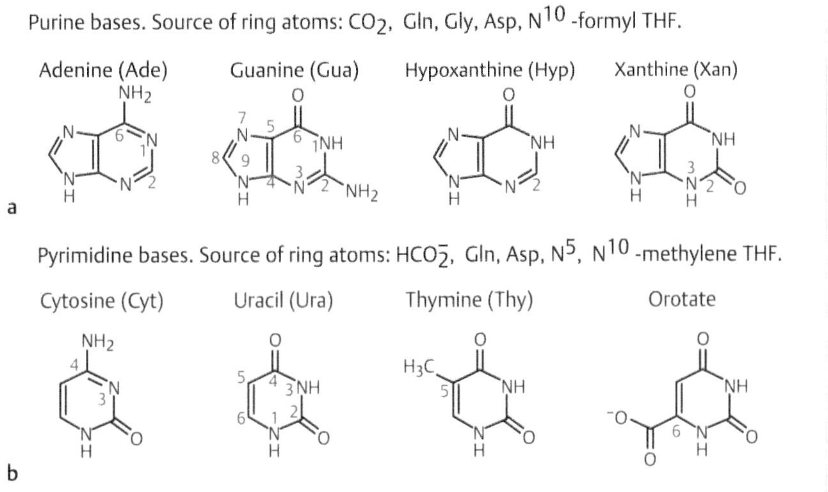

Purine bases. Source of ring atoms: CO_2, Gln, Gly, Asp, N^{10}-formyl THF.

Adenine (Ade)   Guanine (Gua)   Hypoxanthine (Hyp)   Xanthine (Xan)

Pyrimidine bases. Source of ring atoms: HCO_2^-, Gln, Asp, N^5, N^{10}-methylene THF.

Cytosine (Cyt)   Uracil (Ura)   Thymine (Thy)   Orotate

Fig. 16.2 Common purine and pyrimidine bases. (a) The common purines have two fused heterocyclic rings, four internal nitrogen atoms, and varying numbers of carbonyl groups. **(b)** The common pyrimidines have one heterocyclic ring, two internal nitrogen atoms, and varying numbers of carbonyl groups. Uracil and thymine differ only in that the latter possesses a methyl group. Uracil and orotate differ only in that the latter possesses a carboxylate (CO_2^-) group. Asp, aspartate; Gln, glutamine; Gly, glycine; THF, tetrahydrofolate.

Table 16.1 Purine and pyrimidine nucleosides and nucleotides: Common abbreviations and appearance in RNA and/or DNA

	Base (Abbreviation)	Nucleoside (Abbreviation)	Nucleotide* (Abbreviation)	Appear in
Purines	Adenine (Ade)	Adenosine (A)	AMP	DNA, RNA
	Guanine (Gua)	Guanosine (G)	GMP	DNA, RNA
	Hypoxanthine (Hyp)	Inosine (I)	IMP	tRNA
	Xanthine (Xan)	Xanthosine (X)	XMP	—
Pyrimidines	Cytosine (Cyt)	Cytidine (C)	CMP	DNA, RNA
	Uracil (Ura)	Uridine (U)	UMP	RNA
	Thymine (Thy)	Thymidine (T)	TMP	DNA

*Nucleotide-nucleoside monophosphate.

xanthine (Xan) (▶ Fig. 16.2a). The purine bases form a covalent bond to C-1′ of ribose via their N-9 nitrogen.

Nomenclature. The attachment of a ribose (or a deoxyribose) to a purine base results in a nucleoside with a name ending in "sine" (e.g., adenosine, guanosine).

- Addition of a 5′-monophosphate to a purine nucleoside produces a purine nucleotide with a name ending in "sine 5′-monophosphate." Diphosphates and triphosphates have names that end with the corresponding "sine 5′-diphosphate" and "sine 5′-triphosphate," respectively. The abbreviations for the bases and the corresponding nucleosides and nucleotides are summarized in ▶ Table 16.1.

Source of ribose and N, C, O, and H atoms. The ribose in purine nucleotides comes from the degradation of glucose 6-phosphate in the pentose phosphate pathway or from the diet. The atoms in the purine bases are supplied by CO_2; the amino acids Gln, Gly, and Asp; and a derivative of the vitamin folate, called N^{10}-formyltetrahydrofolate.

Use. Ade and Gua appear in both DNA and RNA. In DNA, they participate in hydrogen bonding (with Thy and Cyt, respectively), an essential stabilizing feature of the DNA double helix. The purine bases are also "flat" structures in which the π electrons are delocalized across the bicyclic structure. This allows them to provide additional stability to DNA via van der Waals stacking interactions.

Pyrimidines

There are four common pyrimidines that appear either in RNA and DNA or in the metabolic pathways involving these bases. They are uracil (Ura), thymine (Thy), cytosine (Cyt), and orotic acid or its salt, orotate. These common bases form a covalent bond to carbon 1′ of ribose through their N-1 nitrogen.

Therapeutics
"Sulfa" drugs
Antibacterial agents in the sulfonanilamide family ("sulfa" drugs) act as a competitive inhibitor of the bacterial enzyme that incorporates p-aminobenzoic acid (PABA) into folate. This inhibition disrupts purine biosynthesis and thereby DNA replication in bacteria. Because humans acquire folate as a vitamin from their diet, sulfa drugs selectively affect bacteria.

Nomenclature. The addition of ribose (or deoxyribose) to a pyrimidine base generates a nucleoside with a name ending in "dine" (e.g., cytidine, thymidine, uridine).

- The addition of a 5′-monophosphate to a pyrimidine nucleoside produces a pyrimidine nucleotide with a name ending in "dine 5′-monophosphate." Diphosphates and triphosphates have names that end with the corresponding "dine 5′-diphos-phate" and "dine 5′-triphosphate," respectively. The abbreviations for the bases and the corresponding nucleosides and nucleotides are summarized in ▶ Table 16.1.

Source of ribose, N, C, O, and H atoms. As with purine nucleotides, the ribose in pyrimidine nucleotides comes from the degradation of glucose 6-phosphate in the pentose phosphate pathway or from the diet. The carbon atoms in the pyrimidine bases are supplied by HCO_3^-, the amino acid, Asp, and another derivative of folate, N^5,N^{10}-methylenetetrahydrofolate. The nitrogen atoms come from the amino acids, Gln and Asp.

Therapeutics
Methotrexate
In humans, antineoplastic agents such as methotrexate target dihydrofolate reductase which converts dietary folate to the biologically active tetrahydrofolate in the liver. This inhibition disrupts DNA replication in rapidly dividing cancer cells by limiting the supply of purine nuclotides. Efficacy depends, in part, on selective drug uptake by cancer cells versus normal cells.

Use. The pyrimidine base Cyt appears in both DNA and RNA, Ura appears only in RNA, and Thy usually appears only in DNA (▶ Table 16.1) in mammals. Together with their purine counterparts, the pyrimidine bases in DNA participate in stabilizing hydrogen bonding. Because of their "flat" structures, their delocalized π electrons provide additional stability to via van der Waals stacking interactions.

Therapeutics
Pentose phosphate pathway
In humans, the pentose phosphate pathway produces ribose 5′-phosphate and NADPH. It operates in erythrocytes, liver, testes, mammary glands, and the adrenal cortex, all of which make use of NADPH to maintain a reducing environment (i.e., reduced form of glutathione) and to provide reducing power for the biosynthesis of fatty acids and steroids. In humans, the liver is the principal site of purine and pyrimidine synthesis and utilizes ribose 5′-phosphate and three of the five principal free amino acids in the liver—Asp, Gln, and Gly (but not Glu and Ala) —as starting materials.

16.1.2 Phosphate Groups

Nucleotides possess C-5' mono-, di-, or triphosphate groups attached to ribose via an ester bond. The phosphate groups are typically displayed in ionized form, reflecting the fact that the pK_a values for the phosphoryl groups are considerably less than physiological pH.

- Ester bonds in monophosphate nucleotides are hydrolyzed enzymatically to give nucleosides. The standard free energy ($\Delta G^{o\prime}$) for this hydrolysis is approximately -3.1 kcal/mol.
- Diphosphate and triphosphate nucleotides, as well as pyrophosphate (PP_i), possess "high-energy" phosphoanhydride bonds. Phosphoanhydride bonds are hydrolyzed with free energies that are considerably larger than that of the ester bond in monophosphate nucleotides.
- The $\Delta G^{o\prime}$ for the hydrolysis of adenosine triphosphate (ATP) to adenosine monophosphate (AMP) and PP_i is -10.9 kcal/mol, that for the hydrolysis of ATP to adenosine diphosphate (ADP) and P_i is -7.3 kcal/mol, and for the hydrolysis of PP_i to two P_i, $\Delta G^{o\prime}$ is -4.0 kcal/mol. (See **Fig. 8.3**.)

16.1.3 Deoxynucleotides

Because deoxyribonucleotides have greater chemical stability than ribonucleotides, they are utilized in DNA. Deoxynucleotides possess either purine (Ade or Gua) or pyrimidine bases (Cyt or Thy), and a 5'-phosphate group on a deoxyribose ring (see ▶ Fig. 16.1).

Nomenclature. The nomenclature for deoxynucleotides is identical to that of nucleotides except the prefix "deoxy" is inserted in the name. Thus, adenosine 5'-monophosphate (AMP) becomes deoxyadenosine 5'-monophosphate (dAMP); the small case "d" specifies the loss of the 2'-hydroxyl group.

Source. The reduction (removal) of the 2'-hydroxyl group in the ribose ring of nucleoside diphosphates (NDPs) to generate deoxynucleoside diphosphates (dNDPs) is catalyzed by the key enzyme ribonucleotide reductase. Key features of this enzyme and its reaction are as follows:

- The reduction requires the reduced form of nicotinamide adenine dinucleotide phosphate (NADPH), and the reducing power is transferred through a Cys-rich protein, thioredoxin, to the ribose.
- Ribonucleotide reductase possesses two allosteric sites, called the activity and specificity sites. The binding of a specific deoxynucleoside triphosphate (dNTP) at the specificity site dictates the selectivity for the catalytic site for synthesis of specific dNDPs and thereby balances the need for various purine and pyrimidine nucleotides. The activity site dictates whether ribonucleotide reductase is activated or inhibited; ATP or dATP in the activity site activates or inhibits the enzyme, respectively.
- Ribonucleotide reductase uses only NDPs as substrates and not NMPs or NTPs.

Foundations

Specific roles of nucleosides and nucleotides

Nucleotides such as ATP and guanosine triphosphate (GTP) are important cosubstrates in an array of enzymatic reactions.

Nucleotides/nucleosides are also components of several important molecules, including coenzyme A (CoA), flavin adenine dinucleotide (FAD), flavin mononucleotide (FMN), S-adenosyl methionine (SAM), 3'-phosphoadenosine-5'-phosphosulfate (PAPS), uridine diphosphate glucose (UDP-Glc), deoxyadenosylcobalamin (vitamin B_{12}) and nicotinamide adenine dinucleotides with and without the phosphate group at C-2' (NADPH and NADH). In addition, nucleotides such as cyclic adenosine and guanosine monophosphate (cAMP and cGMP) play roles in signal transduction as second messengers. Nucleotides can serve as stabilizing regulatory elements, such as the 7-methylguanosine 5'-triphosphate (m7GTP) cap at the 5' end of eukaryotic mRNA. ATP and adenosine serve as purinergic neurotransmitters.

Normal

Oxidation levels of purines

Catabolism involves oxidative processes whereby usually oxygen is added to a molecule to make it more polar. Adenine lacks oxygen, guanine and hypoxanthine each have one oxygen, xanthine has two oxygens, and uric acid has three oxygens. Thus, uric acid is the metabolic end point in the catabolism of purines and the most oxidized member of the common purines. It has an acidic hydrogen (attached to N-7 in ▶ Fig. 16.2a) and limited aqueous solubility. The limited solubility of urate is a factor that plays a key role in gout.

16.2 Degradation of Nucleotides

The degradation of dietary DNA and RNA, as well as internal processing, generates nucleoside monophosphates (NMPs) via a succession of enzymes (▶ Fig. 16.3):

- Ribonucleases and deoxyribonucleases convert RNA and DNA into short oligomers.
- Phosphodiesterases convert these oligomers to 3'- and 5'-NMPs or dNMPs.

These monomeric nucleotides are further degraded by the action of the following enzymes:

- Nucleotidases hydrolyze the phosphomonoesters and thereby convert these NMPs and dNMPs to nucleosides and deoxynucleosides, respectively.
- Nucleosidases remove the ribose group and thereby convert nucleosides and deoxynucleosides to pyrimidines and purines.

16.2.1 Catabolism of Purines

Dietary purines are largely converted to uric acid, which has limited water solubility. However, uric acid in plasma may play an important antioxidant role. The degradation of the purine nucleotides AMP, GMP, and inosine monophosphate (IMP) initially generates the nucleosides adenosine, guanosine, and inosine, respectively (▶ Fig. 16.4a). AMP or adenosine is further processed to IMP or inosine by AMP deaminase or adenosine

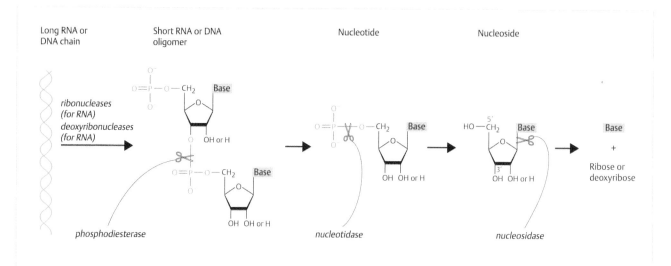

Fig. 16.3 Digestion of RNA and DNA. A succession of enzymes convert dietary RNA and DNA to their constituent parts: Ribonucleases and deoxyribonucleases respectively convert RNA and DNA to short oligomers; phosphodiesterases convert these oligomers to nucleoside monophosphates (NMPs) or deoxynucleoside monophosphates (dNMPs); nucleotidases hydrolyze the NMPs or dNMPs to nucleosides and deoxynucleosides; and nucleosidases convert nucleosides and deoxynucleosides to ribose or deoxyribose and the various bases.

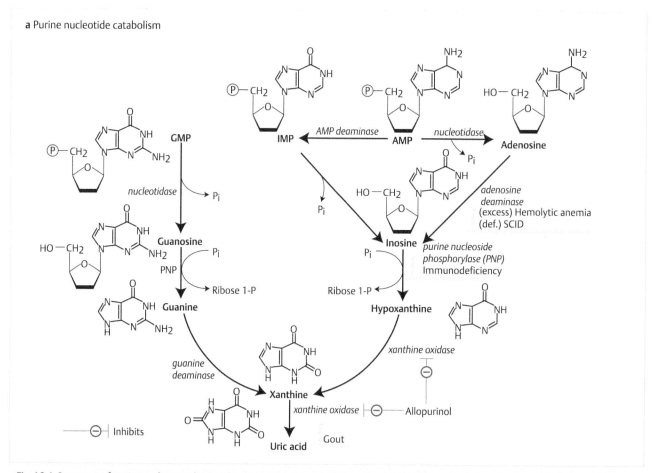

Fig. 16.4 Summary of purine and pyrimidine nucleotide catabolism. (a) Dephosphorylation of the nucleotides adenosine monophosphate (AMP), inosine monophosphate (IMP), and guanosine monophosphate (GMP) leads to the nucleosides adenosine, inosine, and guanosine, respectively. Deamination by adenosine deaminase or AMP deaminase converts the adenosine to inosine or AMP to IMP, respectively. Removal of the ribose on inosine and guanosine by purine nucleoside phosphorylase (PNP) generates the bases hypoxanthine and guanine, respectively. Further processing leads initially to xanthine and finally to uric acid. **Summary of purine and pyrimidine nucleotide catabolism.**

deaminase, respectively. The removal of the ribose (as ribose 1-phosphate) from the two nucleosides, inosine and guanosine by the enzyme, purine nucleoside phosphorylase (PNP), generates the bases, hypoxanthine (Hyp) and guanine (Gua), respectively, and these bases ultimately converge at xanthine, which is converted to uric acid. Three enzymes in purine catabolism bear detailed discussion:

- **Adenosine deaminase (ADA):** ADA plays an important role in purine metabolism by catalyzing the irreversible, hydrolytic deamination of adenosine (and 2-deoxyadenosine) to the nucleoside inosine.
  - ADA also plays an important role in adenosine homeostasis and modulates signaling by extracellular adenosine and so contributes indirectly to cellular signaling events.
  - Overproduction of ADA (an erythrocyte isoform) is one cause of hemolytic anemia (rare). The increased destruction of adenosine depletes adenine nucleotide pools and triggers premature red blood cell destruction.
  - Underproduction of ADA is associated with the second most common autosomal form of severe combined immunodeficiency (SCID) by severely reducing the lives of both T and B lymphocytes. It is thought that the accumulation of adenosine leads to a secondary accumulation of dATP, which could be toxic to the immune system.
- **Purine nucleoside phosphorylase (PNP):** PNP is responsible for the conversion of the nucleosides, inosine and guanosine, into their corresponding bases, hypoxanthine and guanine.
  - An autosomal recessive deficiency of PNP causes an immunodeficiency that is less severe than ADA-deficient SCID.
  - PNP deficiency mainly affects T cells.
- **Xanthine oxidase:** This biochemically unusual liver enzyme catalyzes the oxidation of hypoxanthine to xanthine and xanthine to uric acid. It has two flavin adenine dinucleotides (FADs), two Mo atoms (molybdopterin cofactors), and eight Fe atoms (ferredoxin iron-sulfur clusters) bound per enzymatic unit.
  - Xanthine oxidase is a target of drugs such as allopurinol and febuxostat used in the treatment of gout.

16.2.2 Catabolism of Pyrimidines

Dietary pyrimidines are converted to readily metabolized ketogenic or glucogenic water-soluble compounds such as malonyl coenzyme A (CoA), methylmalonyl CoA, and succinyl CoA. There is less convergence in pyrimidine base catabolism than in purine base catabolism (▶ Fig. 16.4b).

- The degradation of cytidine and uridine nucleotides initially generates the nucleosides uridine (U) and cytidine (C), as well as their deoxy analogues (dU and dC). Further processing converts C to U and dC to dU. Removal of the ribose or 2'-deoxyribose generates uracil, and its further degradation leads to the water-soluble ketogenic intermediate malonyl CoA.
- The degradation of thymidine nucleotides initially generates the nucleoside deoxythymidine (dT) (▶ Fig. 16.4b). Removal of the 2'-deoxyribose generates thymine, and further degradation of thymine leads to the water-soluble glucogenic intermediates methylmalonyl CoA and succinyl CoA.

Therapeutics
Severe combined immunodeficiency

SCID is an invariably fatal genetic disorder in which both "arms" (B cells and T cells) of the adaptive immune system are crippled. Young patients with this disorder are often males because the most common form of SCID is X-linked. Mutations affect the interleukin 2 receptor subunit gamma (IL2RG), necessary for the development and differentiation of T and B cells. These children are referred to as "bubble boys" because of their need to be completely protected from the environment. The ADA deficiency (the second most common form of SCID) is most pronounced in lymphocytes that have the highest levels of ADA activity. This deficiency leads to the accumulation of high levels of the nucleoside adenosine. Adenosine is subsequently converted to AMP and ADP by kinases and hence to dADP by ribonucleotide reductase and finally to dATP by still other kinases. The rising levels of dATP inhibit the activity site of ribonucleotide reductase that in turn blocks formation of all other dNDPs. The low levels of dNDPs and the corresponding dNTPs impair DNA synthesis and compromise the immune system by abolishing both T and B lymphocytes.

Therapeutics
Gout

Gout is a disorder characterized by high levels of uric acid in the blood resulting from overproduction of uric acid ("primary hyperuricemia"), as in the Lesch-Nyhan syndrome, or, more commonly, by poor excretion of uric acid ("secondary hyperuricemia"). Deposits of sodium urate in the joints of the extremities are exceedingly painful (gouty arthritis), and deposits in the kidneys can cause kidney damage. Diets rich in purines (e.g., beans, lentils, spinach) together with meat, seafood, and alcohol may trigger episodes of gout. Acidemia, in particular due to lactate accumulation, stimulates reabsorption of uric acid in the kidney via the urate transporter URAT1. Treatment for gout involves the use of drugs such as colchicine which decrease the movement of granulocytes to the affected areas and allopurinol and febuxostat which inhibits xanthine oxidase and increases the levels of the more soluble purines, hypoxanthine and guanine.

Normal
Uric acid levels as a diagnostic marker for gout

Serum uric acid levels are a diagnostic marker for gout. Normal serum urate levels are 4.0 to 8.6 mg/dL in adult males and 3.0 to 5.9 mg/dL in adult females. Urinary urate levels are normally < 750 mg/24 h. Serum urate levels > 9 mg/dL increase the risk of gout. Urinary urate levels are variable day to day and are most reliable when the patients are on a low purine diet.

IV

b Pyrimidine nucleotide catabolism

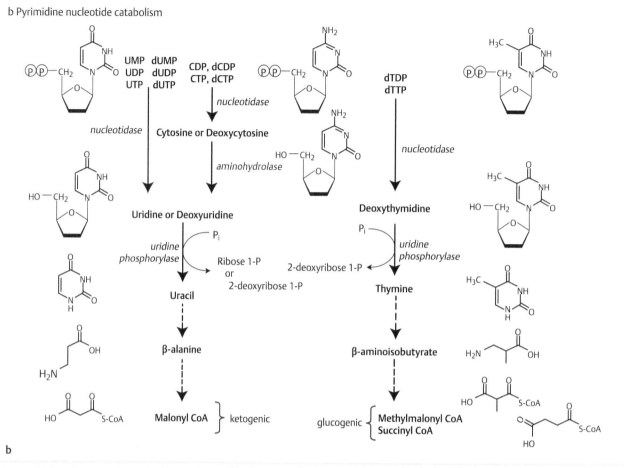

Fig. 16.4 (continued) (**b**) The catabolism of pyrimidines involves the removal of phosphate groups, a deamination in the case of cytosine or deoxycytosine, removal of the ribose or 2'-deoxyribose to generate uracil or thymine, and degradation of these pyrimidine rings to either ketogenic or glucogenic intermediates. CDP, cytidine diphosphate; CoA, coenzyme A; CTP, cytidine triphosphate; dCDP, deoxycytidine diphosphate; dCTP, deoxycytidine triphosphate; dTDP, deoxythymidine diphosphate; dTTP, deoxythymidine triphosphate; dUMP, deoxyuridine monophosphate; dUDP, deoxyuridine diphosphate; dUTP, deoxyuridine triphosphate; P_i, inorganic phosphate; SCID, severe combined immunodefciency; UDP, uridine diphosphate; UMP, uridine monophosphate; UTP, uridine triphosphate.

16.3 *De Novo* Synthesis of Nucleotides

16.3.1 *De Novo* Synthesis of Purines

The *de novo* synthesis of purine nucleotides occurs in the cytosol (principally in liver cells) and proceeds in the following four phases (▶ Fig. 16.5):

Phase I: Ribose 5-phosphate Activation

The *de novo* synthesis of purine nucleotides begins with ribose 5-phosphate, a metabolic product of the oxidative phase of the pentose phosphate pathway. Via a reaction that uses ATP, ribose 5-phosphate is converted to an "activated" form called 5-phospho-α-D-ribosyl-1-pyrophosphate (PRPP) by PRPP synthetase.
- This step is allosterically activated by phosphate levels (P_i levels signal cellular activity because of ATP consumption) and negatively regulated by the levels of the purine nucleotides GMP, AMP, and IMP.

Phase II: Conversion of PRPP into Phosphoribosylamine

The next, committed step in purine synthesis involves substitution of pyrophosphate with an amino group (NH₃) at C-1' of PRPP by glutamine:phosphoribosyl pyrophosphate amidotransferase. This reaction, which obtains the amino group from Gln, generates phosphoribosylamine (PRA).
- This step is allosterically and positively regulated by PRPP levels (feed-forward activation) and negatively regulated by the levels of the purine nucleotides GMP, AMP, and IMP.

Phase III: Construction of the Inosine Monophosphate, Branch Point Purine Ring

PRA enters a nine-step ring-constructing sequence of reactions that produce IMP. Key features of the ring-construction steps are as follows:
- All intermediates are phosphorylated (i.e., nucleotides) because the pathway carries the original phosphate group in ribose 5-phosphate.

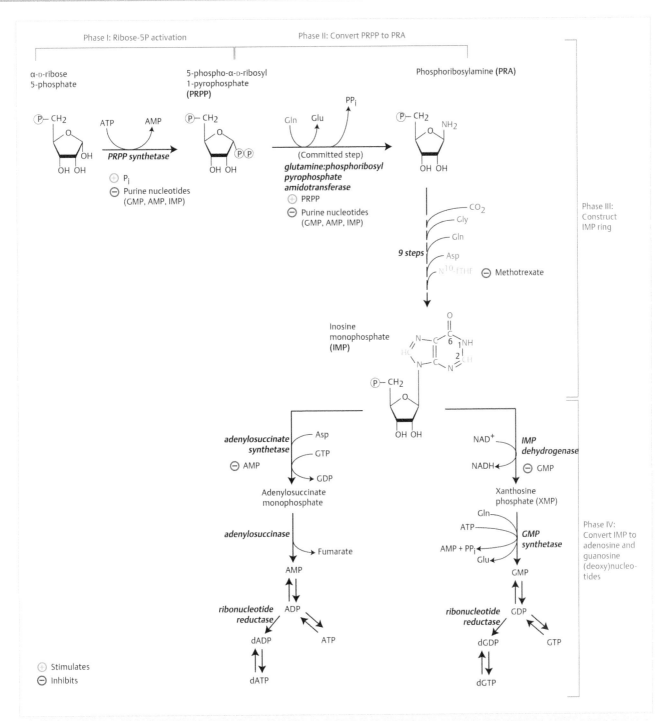

Fig. 16.5 Phases of the *de novo* synthesis of purine nucleotides and deoxynucleotides. Phase I: Substitution of pyrophosphate at C-1' of ribose 5-phosphate generates its activate form, 5-phospho-a-d-ribosyl-1-pyrophosphate (PRPP). Phase II: Conversion of PRPP to phosphoribosylamine (PRA) requires an amino group provided by glutamine (Gln). Phase III: The remaining atoms in the purine ring arise from CO_2, the amino acids glycine (Gly), Gln, and aspartate (Asp), and N^{10}-formyltetrahydrofolate (N^{10}-FTHF) derived from folate (vitamin B_9), which leads to the branch point intermediate inosine monophosphate (IMP). Further modifications of IMP provide the nucleoside and deoxynucleoside triphosphates for RNA and DNA synthesis, respectively. For instance, replacing the oxygen with an amino group from Asp at C-6 of IMP and adding a double bond between C-6 and N-1 gives adenosine monophosphate (AMP). Adding an amino group from Gln to C-2 gives guanosine monophosphate (GMP). Conversion of these nucleoside monophosphates to di- and triphosphates requires various kinases, and the reduction of the nucleoside diphosphates to deoxynucleoside diphosphates is catalyzed by ribonucleotide reductase. GMP, AMP, IMP, P_i, and PRPP exert control over the activity of various enzymes. Methotrexate inhibits dihydrofolate reductase, an enzyme essential for the conversion of dihydrofolate to tetrahydrofolate (see ▶ Fig. 16.8). Tetrahydrofolate is needed for the formation of N^{10}-formyltetrahydrofolate. ADP, adenosine diphosphate; GDP, guanosine diphosphate; Glu, glutamate; GTP, guanosine triphosphate; P_i, inorganic phosphate; PP_i, pyrophosphate.

IV

- The process consumes ATP (four equivalents) in reaching IMP, the branch point in the synthesis of purine nucleotides.
- Two carbons of the purine ring originate from the folate derivative N^{10}-formyltetrahydrofolate, one carbon originates from CO_2, and the remaining carbons and nitrogens come from the amino acids Gln, Gly, and Asp.
  - Dietary folate (vitamin B_9) is reduced in the liver to its active form, tetrahydrofolate (THF), by dihydrofolate reductase. THF accepts carbons from His and Gly/Ser and donates carbon atoms to purines, thymidine, and Met at various oxidation levels in biosynthetic processes.
  - The steps in the synthesis of purines and pyrimidines that utilize folates are the subject of drug interventions that either block folate synthesis in bacteria (e.g., "sulfa" drugs) or block the conversion of folate to THF in humans (e.g., methotrexate).

Phase IV: Conversion of Inosine Monophosphate into Adenosine and Guanosine nucleotides

IMP serves as a metabolic branch point for the synthesis of AMP and GMP. The important points to glean from ▸ Fig. 16.5 are as follows:

- AMP exerts negative allosteric control on adenylosuccinate synthetase at the same points regulated by IMP. GMP exerts negative allosteric control on IMP dehydrogenase at the same points regulated by IMP.
- The conversion of IMP to adenylosuccinate monophosphate and the subsequent elimination of fumarate leads to AMP. This sequence for the replacement of a carbonyl group with an amino group is reminiscent of a similar sequence in the urea cycle for the conversion of citrulline to arginosuccinate using Asp and the elimination of fumarate from arginosuccinate to give arginine (see **Fig. 15.14**).
- The conversion of IMP to xanthosine monophosphate (XMP) is an oxidation reaction requiring NAD^+. The subsequent activation by ATP and condensation with an amino group from Gln generates GMP.
- AMP and GMP exert a negative allosteric regulatory control on the synthesis of themselves. This helps to ensure the balance of these two nucleotide pools. That is, this allosteric control ensures that if AMP levels are high, the intermediate IMP is shuttled toward the formation of additional GMP.
- ATP and GTP are used in the synthesis of GMP and AMP, respectively. That is, a balance between the pools of the two principal purine nucleotides is maintained by consuming one

purine nucleotide triphosphate during the synthesis of the other.
- The conversion of the monophosphates AMP and GMP to the diphosphates ADP and GDP, respectively, requires a specific nucleoside monophosphate kinase for each monophosphate. Additionally, the conversion of either ADP or GDP to the corresponding triphosphates involves a broad-spectrum nucleoside diphosphate kinase. ATP is the phosphoryl group donor in all cases.

Deoxynucleotides. ADP and GDP undergo reduction to dADP or dGDP via a reaction catalyzed by ribonucleotide reductase (see ▸ Fig. 16.6). dADP and dGDP are then converted to deoxynucleoside triphosphates by kinases.

16.3.2 *De Novo* Synthesis of Pyrimidines

The *de novo* synthesis of pyrimidine nucleotides occurs in the cytosol and mitochondria (principally in liver cells) and proceeds in the following three phases (▸ Fig. 16.7):

Phase I: Fabrication of Pyrimidine Ring as Orotate

This phase requires the action of a cytosolic multifunctional enzyme that has three activities (carbamoyl phosphate synthetase II (CPS-II), aspartate transcarbamoylase, and dihydroorotase), and a nicotinamide adenine dinucleotide (NAD^+)-dependent mitochondrial enzyme called dihydroorotate dehydrogenase. The first three cytosolic and the single mitochondrial reactions of this phase are as follows:

- Ammonia from Gln is condensed with bicarbonate (HCO_3^-) and two ATP molecules to give carbamoyl phosphate.
- Carbamoyl phosphate is then condensed with Asp to generate carbamoyl aspartate.
- Carbamoyl aspartate cyclizes to give dihydroorotate, which enters the mitochondria.
- In the mitochondria, dihydroorotate is oxidized to orotate, which enters the cytosol.
  - In humans, the regulation of this pathway involves activation of CPS-II by PRPP and its inhibition by uridine triphosphate (UTP).
  - Elevated levels of mitochondrial carbamoyl phosphate (due to a defect in the ornithine transcarbamoylase (OTC) in the urea cycle) manifest as hyperammonemia with orotic aciduria. Orotic aciduria is the result of excess carbamoyl

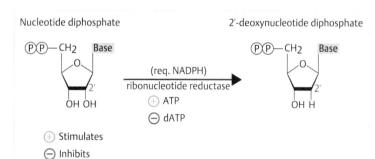

Nucleotide diphosphate   2'-deoxynucleotide diphosphate

(req. NADPH) ribonucleotide reductase
⊕ ATP
⊖ dATP

⊕ Stimulates
⊖ Inhibits

Fig. 16.6 Reduction of nucleoside diphosphates by ribonucleotide reductase. With adenosine triphosphate (ATP) in the activity site, ribonucleotide reductase catalyzes the reduction of the 2'-hydroxyl group in nucleoside diphosphates (NDPs) to generate 2'-deoxynucleoside diphosphates (dNDPs). dATP, deoxyadenosine triphosphate; NADPH, reduced form of nicotinamide adenine dinucleotide phosphate.

IV

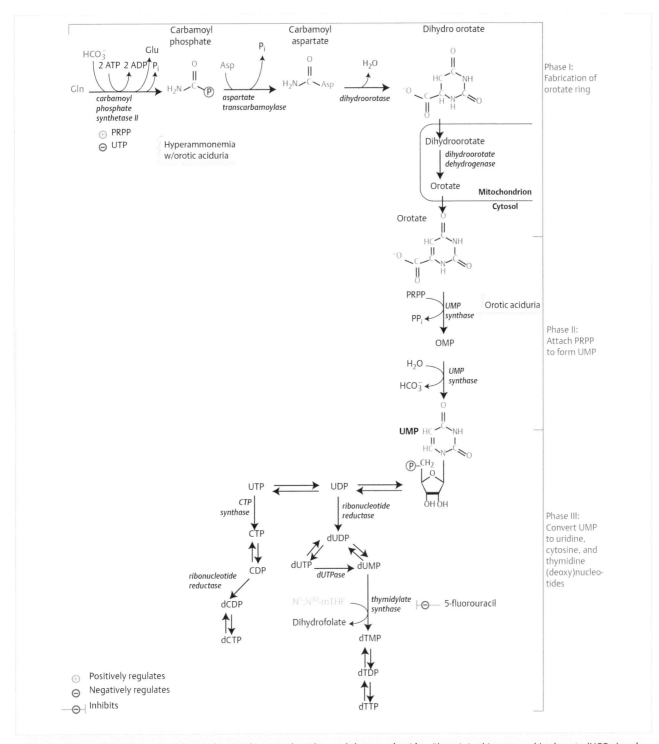

Fig. 16.7 Phases of the *de novo* synthesis of pyrimidines, nucleotides, and deoxynucleotides. Phase I: In this process, bicarbonate (HCO_3^-) and ammonia from glutamine (Gln) are activated in the presence of adenosine triphosphate (ATP) as carbamoyl phosphate. The latter is condensed with aspartate (Asp) and cyclized to give the prefabricated pyrimidine ring in dihydroorotate. A mitochondrial enzyme, dihydroorotate dehydrogenase, which requires NAD^+, oxidizes dihydroorotate to orotate. Phase II: A cytosolic enzyme, uridine monophosphate (UMP) synthase, attaches orotate to 5-phospho-a-d-ribosyl-1-pyrophosphate (PRPP) and catalyzes its decarboxylation to give UMP. Phase III: UMP undergoes phosphorylation to uridine diphosphate (UDP) and uridine triphosphate (UTP). UDP provides the platform for the generation of deoxythymidine triphosphate (dTTP), and UTP provides the platform for the production of cytidine triphosphate (CTP) and deoxycytidine triphosphate (dCTP). Elevated levels of carbamoyl phosphate (due to a defect in the urea cycle) manifest as hyperammonemia with orotic aciduria. On the other hand, orotic aciduria in the absence of hyperammonemia is caused by a defect in UMP synthase. PRPP, UTP, and 5-fuorouracil affect the activities of the indicated enzymes. CDP, cytidine diphosphate; dCDP, deoxycytidine diphosphate; OMP, orotidine monophosphate; PP_i, pyrophosphate; N^5,N^{10}-mTHF, N^5,N^{10}-methylenetetrahydrofolate.

phosphate spilling over into the cytoplasm (thereby bypassing the highly regulated CPS-II) and getting converted to orotic acid by pyrimidine biosynthesis enzymes.

Phase II: Attachment of Orotate to PRPP to Generate Uridine Monophosphate, the Branch Point Pyrimidine Ring

A bifunctional cytosolic enzyme, uridine monophosphate (UMP) synthase, attaches orotate to PRPP to give orotidine monophosphate (OMP), then decarboxylates OMP to generate UMP.

- A deficiency in UMP synthase is associated with hereditary orotic aciduria in which pyrimidines are lacking. The lack of pyrimidines inhibits erythropoiesis and results in a megaloblastic anemia. This condition is resistant to both folate and vitamin B_{12} supplementation.
- Orotic aciduria due to UMP synthase deficiency may be distinguished from that due to OTC deficiency as the former is associated with megaloblastic anemia while the latter is accompanied by hyperammonemia.
- Treatment is with uridine supplementation which restores UMP production as well as results in the inhibition of CPS-II by UTP, leading to a reduction in orotic acid production.

Phase III: Conversion of Uridine Monophosphate into Cytosine and Thymidine (Deoxy) nucleotides

UMP is sequentially phosphorylated by nucleoside monophosphate and diphosphate kinases to generate uridine diphosphate (UDP) and UTP. Both serve as key portals to the other needed pyrimidine nucleotides, as follows:

- UDP serves as a portal for the synthesis of the pyrimidine nucleotide deoxythymidine triphosphate (dTTP) needed for DNA synthesis.
  - UDP first undergoes reduction by ribonucleotide reductase to give dUDP. Various kinases and phosphatases interconvert dUTP, dUDP, and dUMP. One phosphatase,

dUTPase, is of particular importance in the conversion of dUTP to dUMP. Although energetically wasteful in the sense that dUDP is first converted to dUTP and then back to dUMP, it is thought that dUTPase keeps dUTP at low levels to prevent it from incorporating into DNA during replication.
  - dUMP in particular serves as the crucial bridge to the thymidine nucleotides. dUMP undergoes methylation by thymidylate synthase to give deoxythymidine monophosphate (dTMP). The source of the methyl group is N^5,N^{10}-methylenetetrahydrofolate, another member of the folate family. This unique methylation step in the *de novo* synthesis of nucleotides is a therapeutic target useful in disrupting DNA replication in rapidly dividing neoplastic cells by depriving them of dTTP (▶ Fig. 16.8).
- UTP, which itself is used in RNA synthesis, serves as a portal for the synthesis of the pyrimidine nucleotides cytidine triphosphate (CTP) and dCTP.
  - UTP undergoes an amination reaction by CTP synthetase to give CTP. This reaction requires ATP (to activate UTP) and Gln as a source of ammonia.
  - CTP is then converted to cytidine diphosphate (CDP), reduced by ribonucleotide reductase to dCDP, and phosphorylated to give dCTP.

▶ Table 16.2 provides a summary of the key features of the *de novo* synthesis of purines and pyrimidines.

Normal

CO_2 versus HCO_3^-

CO_2 and bicarbonate are interchangeable forms in aqueous media. The CO_2 gas may be considered as anhydrous carbonic acid (H_2CO_3). When CO_2 is dissolved in water, it is converted into carbonic acid, which can be deprotonated to bicarbonate (HCO_3^-).

$$CO_2 + H_2O \leftrightarrow H_2CO_3 \leftrightarrow H^+ + HCO_3^-$$

This reaction plays a role in the transport and excretion of CO_2. The hydration of CO_2 is normally a slow process, but red blood cells contain the enzyme carbonic anhydrase, which greatly enhances their rate of bicarbonate formation from CO_2.

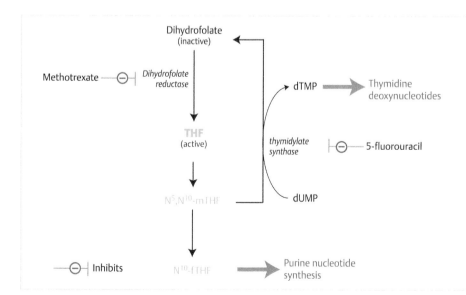

Fig. 16.8 Antineoplastic agents and folate derivatives. Dihydrofolate, the inactive form of folate, is converted to active tetrahydrofolate (THF) by dihydrofolate reductase. Methotrexate inhibits dihydrofolate reductase. 5-Fluorouracil (5-FU) is a "suicide" inhibitor of thymidylate synthase. Initial incorporation of 5-FU into the *de novo* synthesis pathway for pyrimidine nucleotides leads to fluorodeoxyuridine monophosphate (FdUMP). The fluoro substituent, however, prevents methylation by thymidylate synthase and thereby deprives neoplastic cells of deoxythymidine triphosphate (dTTP) necessary for cell division. N^5,N^{10}-mTHF, N^5,N^{10}-methylenetetrahydrofolate; N^{10}-fTHF, N^{10}-formyltetrahydrofolate.

Table 16.2 Comparison of features of *de novo* purine and pyrimidine synthesis

	Purine synthesis	Pyrimidine synthesis
General steps	Uses an activated ribose platform, PRPP, on which the base is constructed	Generates the base independently of ribose; the base is attached to PRPP late in synthesis
Subcellular location	Cytosol	Cytosol and mitochondria
Source of atoms for C, H, O, N	Gln, Gly, Asp, CO_2 (as HCO_3^-), N^{10}-formyl THF *Note:* N^{10}-formyl THF introduces two carbons into the purine ring	Gln, Asp, CO_2 (as HCO_3^-), N^5, N^{10}-methylene THF *Note:* N^5, N^{10}-methylene THF introduces a methyl group (CH_3) on the pyrimidine ring in dUMP, which generates dTMP
Energy requirements to generate branch point nucleotide	4 ATP to generate IMP	3 ATP to generate UMP
Uses nucleoside diphosphates as substrates for reduction to deoxynucleoside diphosphates	Yes	Yes It should be noted that the reduction of UDP to dUDP precedes the methylation of dUMP to dTMP necessary to provide dTTP required for DNA replication

Abbreviations: Asp, aspartate; ATP, adenosine triphosphate; d, deoxy; Gln, glutamine; Gly, glycine; IMP, inosine monophosphate; PRPP, 5-phospho-a-d-ribosyl-1-pyrophosphate; THF, tetrahydrofolate; TMP, thymidine monophosphate; TTP, thymidine triphosphate; UDP, uridine diphosphate; UMP, uridine monophosphate.

Therapeutics

Depriving cells of GMP and dGTP

The unique oxidation step in the conversion of IMP to XMP provides an opportunity for therapeutic intervention. The enzyme in this reaction, IMP dehydrogenase, is a target for drugs, such as the immunosuppressant mycophenolic acid, which disrupt DNA replication in B and T cells of the immune system by depriving these cells of adequate supplies of GMP and hence dGTP. Disruption of GMP synthesis is a useful strategy in drugs preventing graft rejection.

16.4 Salvage Pathways for Synthesis of Nucleotides

Although purine and pyrimidine nucleotides can be synthesized *de novo*, salvage pathways exist so that bases recovered through nucleotide turnover or digestion can be reincorporated into nucleotides. The salvage pathway normally dominates the *de novo* synthesis pathway as a source of purine nucleotides, particularly in nonhepatic tissues.

16.4.1 Purine Salvage Pathway

The bicyclic purine bases are salvaged and reconverted into nucleotides by two enzymes that catalyze the transfer of the base onto C-1' of PRPP—the activated form of ribose. In doing so, the N-9 of a purine base displaces the pyrophosphate (PP_i) in PRPP to regenerate a nucleoside monophosphate. There are two key enzymes involved (▶ Fig. 16.9):

1. **Adenine phosphoribosyltransferase (APRT):** This enzyme transfers adenine onto PRPP (with the removal of PP_i) to generate AMP.
   - Defects in APRT lead to renal lithiasis and the appearance of 2,8-dihydroxyadenine in the urine.

2. **Hypoxanthine-guanine phosphoribosyltransferase (HGPRT):** This enzyme transfers guanine or hypoxanthine onto PRPP (also with the loss of PP_i) to generate GMP or IMP, respectively (▶ Fig. 16.9). It is encoded by the *HPRT1* gene.
   - Defects in HGPRT lead to excess uric acid formation.
   - If there is less than 1.5% of normal HGPRT activity, Lesch-Nyhan syndrome (LNS) results with additional severe neurologic problems, including spastic cerebral palsy, choreoathetosis, and self-destructive biting (mostly fingers and lips) despite normal pain reception.
   - If there is more than 8% of normal HGPRT activity, Kelley-Seegmiller syndrome results with gout and kidney destruction and with only mild neurologic symptoms and a lack of self-destructive behavior.
   - Patients with 8–15% HGPRT activity have variant LNS with mild neurologic problems from clumsiness to motor dysfunction. Allopurinol can reduce the joint and kidney problems but has no effect on the neurologic ones.

16.4.2 Pyrimidine Salvage Pathway

Given the water solubility of the pyrimidine bases and their ready metabolism to glucogenic and ketogenic intermediates, the salvage pathway for pyrimidines has less clinical significance than that of purines. However, the pyrimidine salvage pathway allows for the use of recovered uracil and thymidine to generate uridine and deoxythymidine and their corresponding nucleotides. There are two types of enzymes that catalyze key steps in pyrimidine salvage:

1. **Phosphorylases:** These enzymes attach ribose 1-phosphate (or deoxyribose 1-phosphate) to the salvaged bases of uracil and thymine to generate the nucleosides uridine and deoxythymidine, respectively (▶ Fig. 16.9); inorganic phosphate (P_i) is displaced.

2. **Kinases:** A kinase catalyzes the phosphorylation of uridine to generate UMP, which can be converted to UTP. A specific kinase called thymidine kinase phosphorylates deoxythymidine to generate dTMP, which can be converted to dTTP.

IV

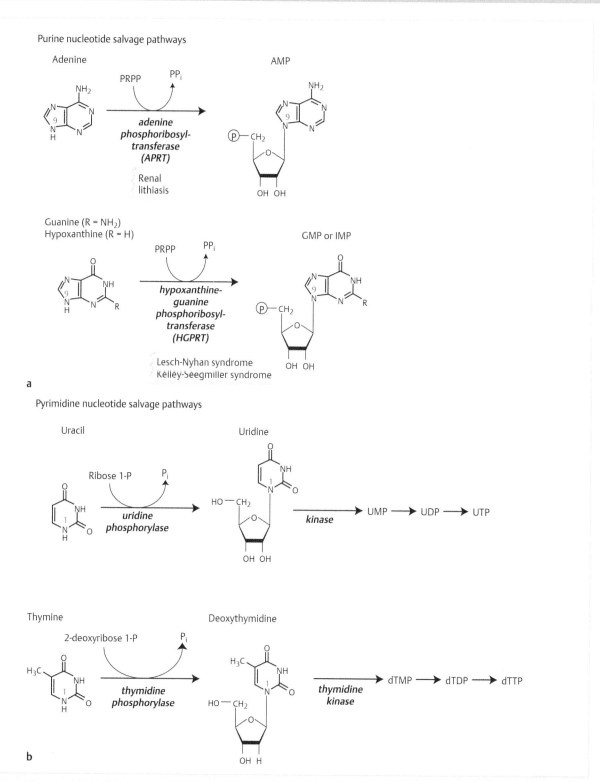

Fig. 16.9 Purine and pyrimidine salvage pathways. (a) Adenine phosphoribosyltransferase (APRT) and hypoxanthine-guanine phosphoribosyltransferase (HGPRT) are transferases in the purine salvage pathway that capture the purine bases adenine, guanine, and hypoxanthine and incorporate them into 5-phospho-a-D-ribosyl-1-pyrophosphate (PRPP) in a substitution reaction. This salvage mechanism converts free purine bases to the corresponding nucleotide monophosphates. A defect in APRT is associated with renal lithiasis, and defects in HGPRT associated with Lesch-Nyhan and Kelley-Seegmiller are syndromes. **(b)** Uracil and thymine, produced during digestion or other catabolic pathways, are salvaged by uridine phosphorylase or thymidine phosphorylase to generate the nucleosides uridine and deoxythymidine, respectively. Subsequent phosphorylations by kinases generate the nucleotides uridine triphosphate (UTP) and deoxythymidine triphosphate (dTTP). AMP, adenosine monophosphate; dTMP, deoxythymidine monophosphate; GMP, guanosine monophosphate; IMP, inosine mono-phosphate; P, phosphate; PPi, pyrophosphate; UDP, uridine diphosphate; UMP, uridine monophosphate.

Therapeutics
Lesch-Nyhan syndrome

Lesch-Nyhan syndrome results from a defect in the HGPRT enzyme in the purine salvage pathway and is a rare form of primary hyperuricemia (i.e., overproduction of uric acid). Patients afflicted with this disorder have hyperuricemia and hyperuricosuria (leading to gout), urate kidney stones, poor muscle control, mental retardation, and a tendency for self-mutilation. In a normal situation, the levels of IMP and GMP are maintained by de novo synthesis from PRPP and by the salvage pathway mediated by HGPRT. Excess purines, above levels normally needed, are processed by nucleotidases and nucleosidases that convert GMP and IMP to guanosine and inosine, respectively, and ultimately to uric acid. In these patients, however, defects in the purine salvage pathway lead to two consequences:

1. Because the circulating levels of hypoxanthine and guanine that are not used in the salvage pathway are higher than normal, they are shunted toward uric acid, leading to the observed hyperuricemia (six times normal levels) and hyperuricosuria.

2. Purine biosynthesis also proceeds at levels 200 times that in normal situations and undoubtedly underlies the problems associated with mental retardation and self-mutilation. The PRPP, which normally would have been used in the salvage pathway, is available for additional purine biosynthesis and also serves as an allosteric activator of the next enzyme in the purine synthesis pathway, namely, glutamine: phosphoribosyl pyrophosphate amidotransferase that generates PRA. The combination of more PRPP leading to additional PRA has a mass action effect on the synthesis of still more purines than are needed. Thus, the activation of glutamine:phosphoribosyl pyrophosphate amidotransferase by this excess PRPP is the underlying cause of the elevated levels of purines.

Therapeutics
Acyclovir

Thymidine kinase phosphorylates the nucleoside deoxythymidine (dT) to generate dTMP, using ATP as the phosphoryl donor. The antiviral agent acyclovir, which has a base that more closely resembles guanine than deoxythymidine, undergoes phosphorylation by viral thymidine kinase at a rate that exceeds that of cellular thymidine kinase. Thus, viral thymidine kinase rapidly converts acyclovir to its monophosphate, acyclo GMP. Other kinases subsequently convert acyclo GMP to acyclo GTP. The triphosphate of acyclovir is a surrogate for GTP and is incorporated into the DNA of rapidly dividing viral cells. Because the incorporated acyclovir lacks a $3'$-hydroxyl group, it leads to the termination of DNA replication. Acyclovir is used to promote healing of sores produced by varicella (chickenpox), herpes zoster (shingles), and genital herpes.

16.5 Heme

The presence of hemoglobin in red blood cells provides them with the means with which to transport oxygen. Hemoglobin is composed of four globular protein subunits, each of which is bound to an iron-containing heme prosthetic group (▸ Fig. 16.10a). Examination of the structure of heme reveals that it is composed of a heterocyclic porphyrin ring with iron bound to its center. Key features of porphyrin rings include the following:

- Their structures contain an alternating system of five-membered, nitrogen-containing rings connected by single-carbon "bridges" (▸ Fig. 16.10b). This characteristic structure appears in the heme groups of hemoglobin, myoglobin, and several cytochromes.
- They typically bind iron in the ferrous (Fe^{2+}) oxidation state. Thus, the active form of heme in hemoglobin has iron exclusively in the Fe^{2+} state and oxidation to the ferric (Fe^{3+}) state generates the inactive methemoglobin (MetHb).

16.5.1 Heme Synthesis

While many tissues are capable of heme synthesis, it occurs primarily in the liver and in erythroid cells of bone marrow because of the requirements to incorporate heme into cytochromes and hemoglobin. Defects in the biosynthesis of heme manifest as disorders called porphyrias (▸ Table 16.3). The hepatic porphyrias tend to be characterized by symptoms that are neurologic, whereas the erythropoietic porphyrias manifest primarily as deposition of porphyrin precursors in the skin, leading to photosensitivity. The former are classified as acute porphyrias and the latter as cutaneous porphyrias.

The complexity of intermediates in the eight-step biosynthesis of heme is best understood if the synthesis is considered as occurring in three location-based phases (▸ Fig. 16.11): (1) the single initiating mitochondrial step, (2) the four central cytosolic steps, and (3) the final three mitochondrial steps. In this sense, heme synthesis shares a similarity with the biosyntheses of pyrimidine nucleotides and urea (see Fig. 15.14 and Fig. 16.7) that also involve synthesis in two compartments.

Phase I (Mitochondrial): Generating ALA, the Basic Unit for Constructing Heme Rings

Glycine is condensed with succinyl CoA, and, with the loss of CO_2, generates δ-aminolevulinic acid (δ-ALA). (Succinyl CoA is produced in the mitochondria principally in the tricarboxylic acid cycle via anaplerotic reactions.) This condensation reaction is catalyzed by δ-aminolevulinic acid synthase (ALA synthase, ALAS), which occurs in two isoforms. ALAS1 is ubiquitously expressed, whereas ALAS2 is expressed only in erythroid precursor cells. The enzyme exhibits the following properties:

- It requires pyridoxal phosphate (vitamin B_6) as a cofactor.
- In the liver, it is inhibited by heme or its oxidized form, hemin (via feedback inhibition).
- Heme and glucose inhibit the transcription of *ALAS1*.
- The NH_2-terminal region of ALAS1 contains a mitochondrial targeting sequence. Binding of heme to this motif blocks its

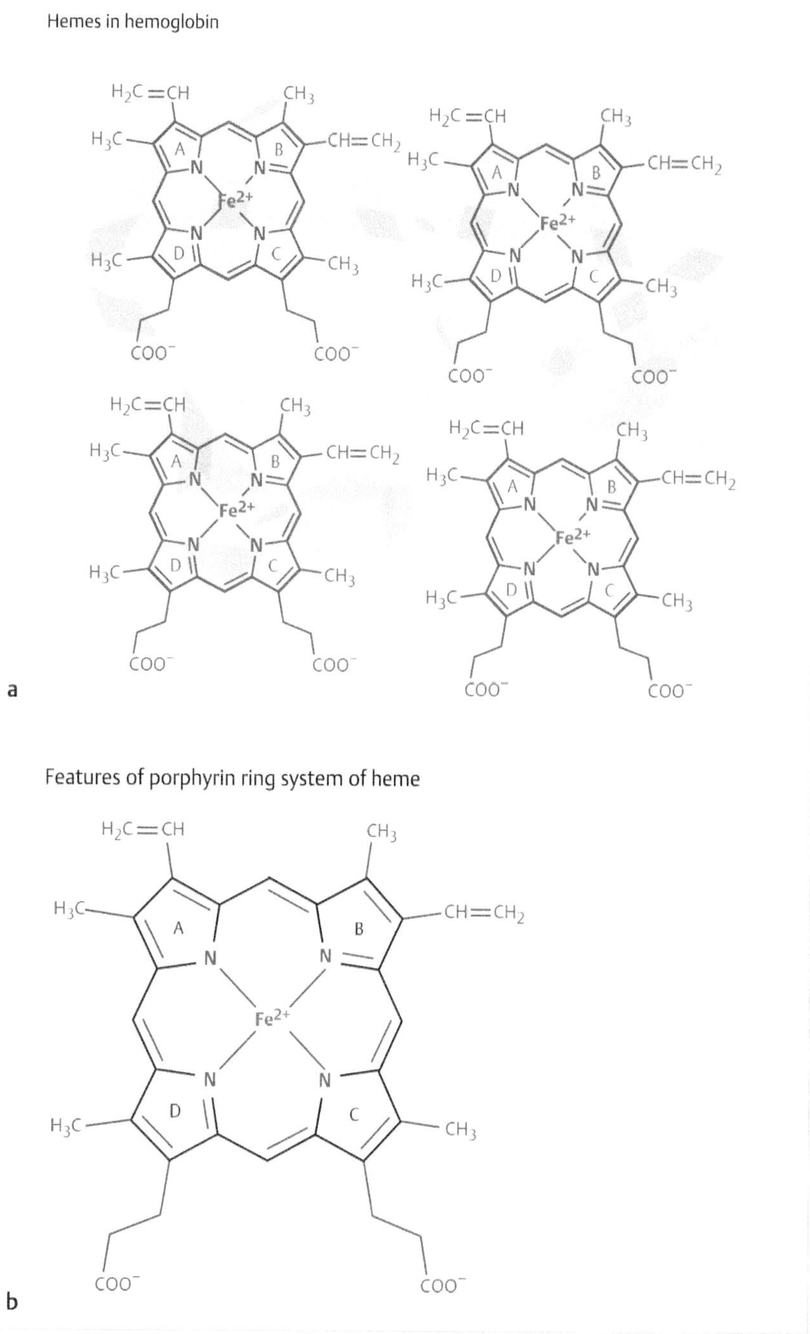

IV

Hemes in hemoglobin

Features of porphyrin ring system of heme

b

Fig. 16.10 Hemoglobin and the porphyrin structure of heme. (a) The four globular subunits of hemoglobin ($\alpha_2\beta_2$) each contain a heme group. **(b)** The porphyrin ring of heme is a tetrapyrrole made up of four 5-membered nitrogen-containing rings (called pyrroles) labeled A, B, C, and D. These pyrroles are connected by single-carbon "bridges."

import into mitochondria. Heme also enhances the decay of ALAS1 mRNA. In addition, binding of heme to certain regulatory motifs on ALAS1 promotes its degradation.

- In erythroid cells of bone marrow, ALAS2 synthesis is regulated at the translational level by cellular iron content.
  ○ The mRNA for ALAS2 contains an iron response element (IRE) sequence. When the cells are iron deficient, an iron-binding protein (cytosolic aconitase) binds to the IRE and prevents the translation of the message. When sufficient iron is present, aconitase binds to the iron instead of the IRE, thus allowing efficient translation. This mechanism ensures that ALA synthase is made only when sufficient iron is available for heme synthesis.

- The liver and erythroid enzymes are encoded by separate genes on chromosome 3 (*ALAS1*) and X-chromosome (*ALAS2*), respectively. Mutations in *ALAS2* cause X-linked sideroblastic anemia. A severe deficiency of pyridoxine (vitamin B_6) may also result in sideroblastic anemia as B_6 is a necessary coenzyme for ALAS.
- ALAS1 synthesis can be induced by many drugs metabolized by the liver (e.g., barbiturates). Induced ALAS1 may provide the heme necessary for cytochrome P-450 enzymes needed for drug metabolism.
- A carrier protein may function to exchange mitochondrial δ-ALA for cytosolic glycine across the inner mitochondrial membrane.

Table 16.3 Porphyrias

Defective Enzyme	Associated Porphyria	Inheritance and features	Type of porphyria
δ-ALA dehydratase	δ-ALA dehydratase deficiency porphyria	• Autosomal recessive • Acute attacks of abdominal pain and neuropathy	Hepatic/Acute
PBG deaminase (in liver)	Acute intermittent porphyria	• Autosomal dominant • Deficiency leads to excessive production of ALA and PBG • Periodic attacks of abdominal pain and neurologic dysfunction	Hepatic/Acute
Uroporphyrinogen III synthase (in erythrocytes)	Congenital erythropoietic porphyria	• Autosomal recessive • Deficiency leads to accumulation of uroporphyrinogen I and its red-colored, air oxidation product uroporphyrin I • Photosensitivity; red color in urine and teeth; hemolytic anemia	Erythropoietic/Cutaneous
Uroporphyrinogen decarboxylase	Porphyria cutanea tarda (PCT)	• Autosomal dominant • Deficiency leads to accumulation of uroporphyrinogen III, which converts to uroporphyrinogen I and its uroporphyrin oxidation products • *Most common porphyria in the United States*; photosensitivity resulting in vesicles and bullae on skin of exposed area; wine red–colored urine	Hepatoerythropoietic/Cutaneous
Coproporphyrinogen oxidase	Hereditary coproporphyria	• Autosomal dominant • Photosensitivity and neurovisceral symptoms (e.g., colic)	Hepatic/Mixed
Protoporphyrinogen IX oxidase	Variegate porphyria	• Autosomal dominant • Photosensitivity and neurologic symptoms and developmental delay in children	Hepatic/Mixed
Ferrochelatase	Erythropoietic protoporphyria	• Autosomal dominant • Photosensitivity with skin lesions after brief sun exposure. • Patients may have gallstones and mild liver dysfunction	Erythropoietic/Cutaneous

Abbreviations: ALA, δ-aminolevulinic acid; PBG, porphobilinogen.
Note: Acute and mixed porphyrias cause neurologic symptoms, whereas those that lead to the accumulation of cyclic tetrapyrroles (coproporphyrinogen III and beyond) result in photo-sensitivity and are classified as cutaneous pophyrias. Urine that turns dark or reddish on standing is seen with all porphyrias except ALA dehydratase deficiency porphyria.

Phase II (Cytosolic): Generation of the Small Pyrrole Ring and the Large Porphyrin Ring

Two molecules of δ-ALA are condensed to form porphobilinogen (PBG), a five-membered nitrogen-containing ring (a pyrrole) that is found in each of the four corners of a porphyrin ring. This cytosolic condensation reaction is catalyzed by a Zn-dependent enzyme, d-aminolevulinic acid dehydratase (δ-ALA dehydratase or porphobilinogen synthase).

• δ-ALA dehydratase is inhibited by heavy metal ions such as lead (Pb), which displaces the Zn atoms from δ-ALA dehydratase's active center.
• δ-ALA dehydratase deficiency porphyria is a rare autosomal recessive disorder.
• δ-ALA is neurotoxic and may account for many of the neurologic symptoms of lead poisoning.

Next, four PBGs are condensed by PBG deaminase (hydroxymethylbilane synthase), which leads to the assembly of hydroxymethylbilane—a linear porphyrin-ring precursor. Uroporphyrinogen III synthase then converts the linear precursor into uroporphyrinogen III—a cyclic porphyrin ring.

• Acute intermittent porphyria is an autosomal dominant disorder caused by mutations in the PBG deaminase gene. Over 200 such mutations have been identified. Despite the

dominant inheritance, a majority of the heterozygotes remain asymptomatic. Acute intermittent porphyria is the second most common form of the porphyrias with an incidence rate of 1 in 20,000.

• In the absence of adequate levels of uroporphyrinogen III synthase in erythrocyte precursors, hydroxymethylbilane can be nonenzymatically cyclized to a "symmetrical" isomer, uroporphyrinogen I and this isomer and other symmetric porphyrinogens accumulate (▶ Fig. 16.12). However, only the "unsymmetrical" form, uroporphyrinogen III, is a substrate for heme synthesis.
• Congenital erythropoietic porphyria is an autosomal recessive disorder caused by a deficiency in uroporphyrinogen III synthase.

The last cytosolic step involves the removal of four CO_2 molecules from the side-chain groups of uroporphyrinogen III to generate coproporphyrinogen III. This reaction is catalyzed by uroporphyrinogen decarboxylase.

• Porphyria cutanea tarda is an autosomal dominant disorder caused by a deficiency in uroporphyrinogen decarboxylase. This is the most common form of the porphyrias with an incidence rate of 1 in 10,000.

Coproporphyrinogen III is transported into the mitochondria with the aid of an ATP-binding cassette transporter, ABCB6.

IV

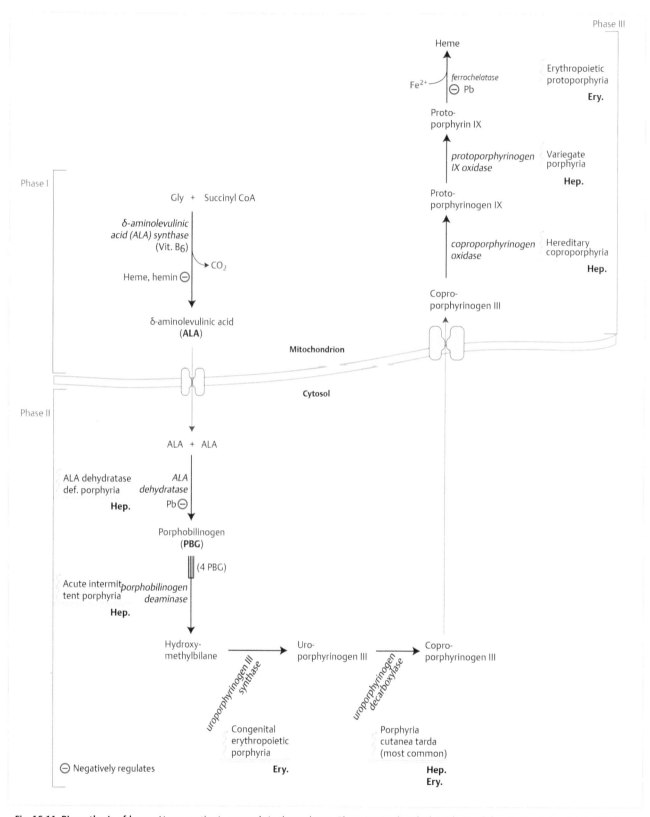

Fig. 16.11 Biosynthesis of heme. Heme synthesis proceeds in three phases. Phase I: mitochondrial synthesis of d-aminolevulinic acid (δ-ALA) from glycine (Gly) and succinyl coenzyme A (CoA). Phase II: cytosolic reactions involving the condensation of two δ-ALAs leading to porphobilinogen and then the use of four porphobilinogens to assemble the tetrapyrrole ring system of coproporphyrinogen III. Phase III: two oxidation reactions of coproporphyrinogen III to install the side-chain vinyl groups in protoporphyrinogen IX and introduce the fully conjugated ring system of protoporphyrin IX, again in the mitochondria. Installation of the ferrous ion Fe²⁺ by ferrochelatase gives heme. The defective enzymes associated with the acute hepatic (Hep.) porphyrias and the erythropoietic (Ery.) porphyrias are indicated.

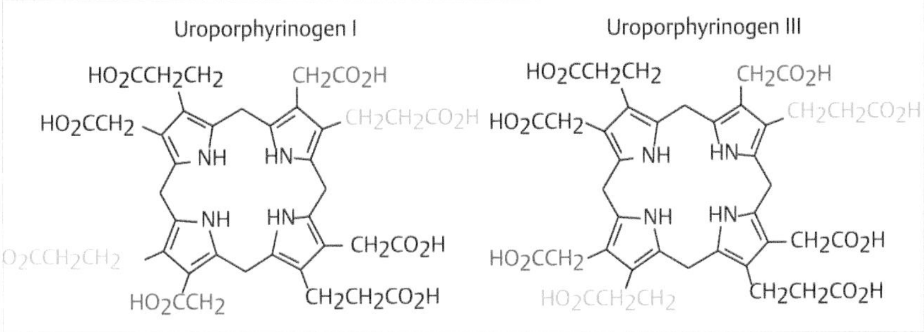

Fig. 16.12 Uroporphyrinogens I and III. Note the relative positions of the acetate (red) and propionate (green) side chains of the "symmetrical" uroporphyrinogen I and the "unsymmetrical" but desired uroporphyrinogen III.

Phase III (Mitochondrial)

The oxidation of coproporphyrinogen III (by coproporphyrinogen oxidase) modifies the side-chain groups to generate protoporphyrinogen IX. A second critical oxidation step (by protoporphyrinogen IX oxidase) converts protoporphyrinogen IX, which has eight partially conjugated double bonds, to protoporphyrin IX, which has 11 fully conjugated double bonds.

- It is this second oxidation step that converts the colorless porphyrin precursor (with "-ogen" suffixes) into the red-colored protoporphyrin IX.
  - Hereditary coproporphyria is an autosomal dominant disorder caused by a deficiency in coproporphyrinogen oxidase.
  - Variegate porphyria is an autosomal dominant disorder caused by a deficiency in protoporphyrinogen IX oxidase.

In the last step, protoporphyrin IX binds ferrous ions (Fe^{2+}) to form heme. This reaction is facilitated by ferrochelatase.

- Ferrous iron (Fe^{2+}) is imported into mitochondria from ferritin stores in the cytosol through the transporter mitoferrin (MFRN). Once imported, Fe^{2+} is stored in mitochondrial ferritin or incorporated into either protoporphyrin IX or Fe-S clusters.
  - Erythropoietic protoporphyria (EPP) is an autosomal dominant disorder caused by a deficiency in ferrochelatase. This is the third most common form of the porphyrias with an incidence rate of 1 in 60,000.
  - Lead poisoning also leads to an accumulation of protoporphyrin in erythrocytes.
  - Patients with EPP are prone to develop protoporphyrin gallstones.
  - Treatment for EPP includes administering β-carotene to quench porphyrin fluorescence and protect against photosensitivity, and cholestyramine (a nonabsorbable resin capable of binding protoporphyrin) to block the enterohepatic circulation of protoporphyrin, and bone marrow transplantation.

The various types of porphyrias are summarized in ▶ Table 16.3.

16.5.2 Heme Degradation

After red blood cells (RBCs) reach the end of their lifespan of ~120 days, they undergo phagocytosis by the cells of the reticuloendothelial system (e.g., spleen). In destroying RBCs, this system breaks down hemoglobin such that the globin portion is digested into its constituent amino acids, and the heme portion is removed for degradation. The degradation of heme in the reticuloendothelial system proceeds as follows (▶ Fig. 16.13).

Oxidation of Heme to Biliverdin

In the initial oxidation of heme to biliverdin, heme oxygenase catalyzes the removal of one of the "bridges" between two specific pyrrole rings as carbon monoxide (CO). This reaction requires oxygen and results in the following conversions:

- The synthesis of heme oxygenase can be induced up to 100-fold by heme, metals ions, and phenylhydrazine.
- The purple-colored heme is converted to the green-colored, "linear" biliverdin. (Associate bil*verd*in with *verde*, the Spanish word for *green*.)
- Fe^{2+} is removed as its oxidized form, Fe^{3+}.

Carbon monoxide competes well with oxygen for binding to hemoglobin, and under normal circumstances, ~ 1% of circulating hemoglobin contains carbon monoxide as a consequence of the normal degradation of heme.

Reductions of Biliverdin to Other Pigments

- Biliverdin undergoes an NADPH-mediated reduction to bilirubin (a red-orange pigment) by the enzyme biliverdin reductase. (Associate bili*rub*in with *red* as in *ruby*.)
- Bilirubin is transported by serum albumin to the liver, where UDP glucuronyl transferase conjugates bilirubin to glucuronic acid, which makes bilirubin monoglucuronide and then bilirubin diglucuronide. These reactions are the rate-limiting steps in the removal of bilirubin from the blood.
  - Unconjugated bilirubin is called indirect bilirubin, and glucuronic acid–conjugated bilirubin is called direct bilirubin. The more soluble, conjugated bilirubin diglucuronide is concentrated in the bile.
  - A deficiency in UDP-glucuronyl transferase is associated with Crigler-Najjar syndrome (< 10% residual activity) and Gilbert syndrome (25% residual activity).
  - Hepatic UDP-glucuronyl transferase activity is low at birth and lower still in pre-term infants. Such babies are prone to hyperbilirubinemia (neonatal jaundice), particularly if there is fetal-maternal blood group incompatibility.

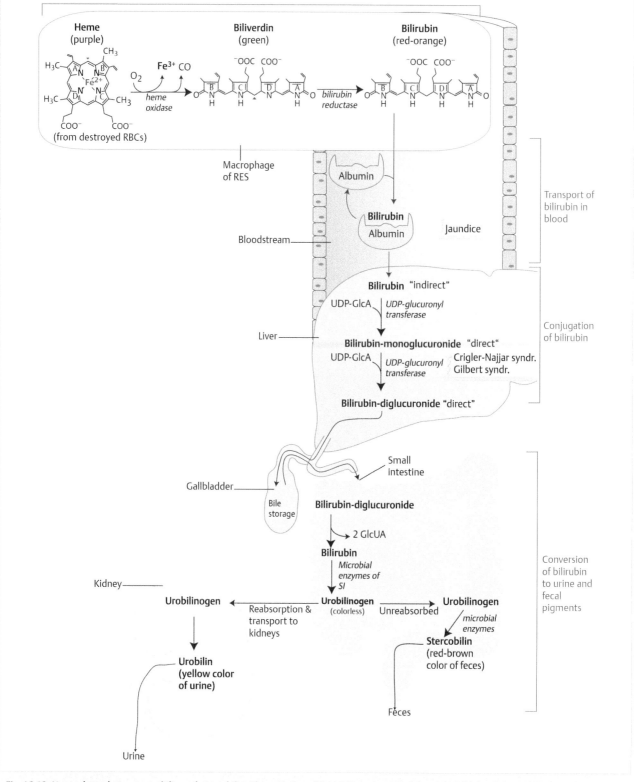

Fig. 16.13 Heme degradation to urobilin and stercobilin. The oxidation of heme liberates one of the carbon bridges (see red arrowhead) as carbon monoxide (CO), converts the ferrous ion (Fe²⁺) into ferric ion (Fe³⁺), and produces the green pigment biliverdin. Subsequent reduction of biliverdin produces the red-orange bilirubin that is conjugated in the liver, collected in bile, and secreted into the small intestine, where it undergoes microbial reduction to urobilinogen. Some urobilinogen is reabsorbed and processed by the kidneys to produce the yellow pigment urobilin, found in urine; some urobilinogen undergoes further microbial reduction to the red-brown pigment stercobilin, found in the feces. The uptake of bilirubin by the liver is not an energy-dependent process. However, the release of conjugated bilirubin into the biliary system is energy dependent. GlcA, glucuronic acid; RBCs, red blood cells; RES, reticuloendothelial system; SI, small intestine; UDP, uridine diphosphate.

Table 16.2 Differential diagnosis of jaundice based on serum/urine markers

Test	Prehepatic jaundice	Intrahepatic Jaundice	Posthepatic Jaundice
Serum direct bilirubin	normal	increased	increased
Serum ALT/AST	normal	increased	normal
Serum ALP	normal	normal	increased
Urine direct bilirubin	absent	present	present
Urine urobiliogen/urobilin	present	present	absent
Fecal stercobilin	present	present	absent

Abbreviations: ALT, alanine aminotransferase; AST, aspartate aminotransferase; ALP, alkaline phosphatase.

Bile secretion into the small intestine leads to the next stage of processing in which microbial enzymes reduce bilirubin to the colorless urobilinogen.

- Because urobilinogen is also lipophilic, it is reabsorbed, transported to the kidney, and oxidized to urobilin, the yellow pigment of the urine.
- The urobilinogen that is not reabsorbed is oxidized by microbial enzymes to stercobilin, the red-brown pigment of feces.

Hyperbilirubinemia (Jaundice)

Hyperbilirubinemia or jaundice is defined by elevated levels of bilirubin in the bloodstream. This condition may be classified as due to prehepatic, intrahepatic, or posthepatic disorders. Normal blood levels of conjugated (direct) bilirubin are 0.1 to 0.3 mg/dL, and those of unconjugated (indirect) bilirubin are 0.2 to 0.9 mg/dL.

Prehepatic: Increased production of unconjugated bilirubin. This can be due to several causes, including hemolytic anemias and internal hemorrhage. The capacity of liver to take up, conjugate, and excrete bilirubin is exceeded. Examples of conditions leading to unconjugated hyperbilirubinemia include glucose 6-phosphate dehydrogenase deficiency and neonatal jaundice due to incompatibility of fetal–maternal blood groups.

- Elevated blood levels of unconjugated (indirect) bilirubin
- Normal blood levels of conjugated (direct) bilirubin
- Normal serum alanine aminotransferase (ALT) (< 35 U/L) and aspartate aminotransferase (AST) (< 40 U/L)
- Urobilinogen is present in urine because the capacity of liver to conjugate and excrete bilirubin is not impaired. Bilirubin in bile is processed to urobilinogen in the small intestine.
- Bilirubin is absent in urine because there is no excess conjugated form in the bloodstream and because the unconjugated form is not excreted in urine.

Intrahepatic: Problems with the liver, which are reflected as deficiencies in bilirubin metabolism (e.g., reduced hepatocyte uptake, impaired conjugation of bilirubin, and reduced hepatocyte secretion of bilirubin). This condition is associated with increased levels of hepatic aminotransferases in serum. Some examples would be cirrhosis and viral hepatitis. Genetic deficiencies in the conjugating enzyme lead to Gilbert syndrome and Crigler-Najjar syndrome.

- Variable increases in conjugated and unconjugated bilirubin levels in the bloodstream, depending on whether the problem is pre- or post-conjugation
- Increased levels of serum ALT and AST

- Urobilinogen is present in urine because some bile and bilirubin still reach the small intestine.
- Conjugated bilirubin is detected in urine.

Posthepatic: Cholestasis (decreased bile flow) reflected as deficiencies in bilirubin excretion. (Obstruction can be located in the biliary tree either within the liver or in the bile duct.) Although serum AST and ALT are usually normal, the levels of serum alkaline phosphatase (ALP), a bile canalicular membrane enzyme, are elevated. Cholestasis may be caused by biliary obstruction (cholangiocarcinoma or stones in the common bile duct), infiltrative liver disease or space-occupying lesion (tumor, abscess, or granulomatous disease), or drugs (anabolic hormones, chlorpromazine, phenytoin).

- Elevated blood levels of conjugated bilirubin with much smaller increases in the unconjugated form
- Normal profile of hepatic AST and ALT in serum
- Elevated levels of the canalicular enzyme ALP in serum (normal is < 90 U/L)
- Conjugated bilirubin is present in urine due to its elevation in the bloodstream, and the urine is dark colored.
- Because bile is not reaching the small intestine bilirubin, no urobilinogen is formed. Therefore, there is no urobilinogen in urine and no stercobilin in the feces as well (dark urine, pale stools).

▶ Table 16.2 provides a summary of the differential diagnosis of the three types of jaundice based on serum and urine marker values.

Therapeutics

Direct and indirect bilirubin

Unconjugated bilirubin is fairly insoluble in aqueous media while bilirubin conjugated to glucuronate is relatively soluble. Soluble bilirubin reacts with Diazo reagent (p-diazobenzenesulfanilic acid) to produce a pink to reddish-purple product which absorbs light at 540 nm (direct bilirubin). Unconjugated bilirubin can be made soluble in the presence of 50% methanol and can then react with the Diazo reagent (indirect bilirubin). Therefore, treating equal aliquots of plasma or serum samples with the Diazo reagent in the presence and absence of methanol allows the measurement of total and direct bilirubin, respectively. The difference between the two values would yield indirect bilirubin (total – direct = indirect). An improvement to the assay involves replacing methanol with a solution of sodium acetate and caffeine-benzoate. Sodium acetate provides an alkaline pH and caffeine-benzoate accelerates the coupling of unconjugated bilirubin with the Diazo reagent, leading to the formation of a blue product that absorbs at 600 nm. Normal serum values in adults are 0.2 to 1.2 mg/dL for total bilirubin and 0.1 to 0.3 mg/dL for direct (conjugated) bilirubin. Total bilirubin levels in infants are in the range of 1 to 12 mg/dL with negligible amounts of direct bilirubin.

Therapeutics
Cyanide poisoning

In the case of cyanide poisoning, one treatment involves limited oxidation of heme (Fe^{2+}) to hemin (Fe^{3+}), which scavenges for cyanide ions. In the United States, the standard cyanide antidote kit first uses a small inhaled dose of amyl nitrite, followed by intravenous sodium nitrite, followed by intravenous sodium thiosulfate. The nitrites oxidize some of the hemoglobin (Hb) from the ferrous state to the ferric state, thereby converting it into methemoglobin (MetHb). Treatment with nitrites is not innocuous because MetHb cannot carry oxygen. The abundant MetHB competes with the more critical cytochrome-c oxidase for binding to cyanide, and in binding to MetHb, cyanide forms cyanmethemoglobin. It is crucial to protect cytochrome-c needed for oxidative phosphorylation and sacrificing a small amount of Hb to achieve this end is a worthwhile albeit dangerous strategy. In the last step of the cyanide poisoning protocol, the intravenous sodium thiosulfate reacts with the cyanmethemoglobin, yielding thiocyanate, sulfite, and MetHb. The thiocyanate is excreted. A recently approved treatment for cyanide prisoning in the U.S. is hydroxocobolamin (Cyanokit, Meridian Medical Technologies) which complexes cyanide to form cyanocobalamin. Cyanocobalamin can be excreted in the urine.

Therapeutics
Lead poisoning

ALA dehydratase is inhibited by heavy metal ions, and this inhibition causes the anemia seen in patients with lead poisoning. This inhibition leads to an increase in δ-aminolevulinic acid (ALA) in the blood, and given its chemical resemblance to the neurotransmitter, γ-aminobutyric acid (GABA), ALA may account for the psychoses that accompany lead poisoning. Lead also interferes with ferrochelatase, the last step in heme biosynthesis, causing an accumulation of protoporphyrin in erythrocytes.

Therapeutics
Congenital erythropoietic porphyria

Congenital erythropoietic porphyria results from a deficiency of uroporphyrinogen III cosynthase. Key intermediates are diverted to the nonfunctional uroporphyrinogen I isomer that produces a red color in the urine, red fluorescence of the teeth, premature destruction of erythrocytes, and skin photosensitivity.

Therapeutics
Color changes in bruises

A bruise or contusion is a type of hematoma due to pooling of blood caused by damage to capillaries. Cleanup of the lesion by macrophages leads to degradation of hemoglobin sequentially to heme, biliverdin, and bilirubin. The released iron may be trapped as hemosiderin. Heme is red in color, whereas biliverdin is green, bilirubin is reddish yellow, and hemosiderin is reddish brown. The formation of these degradation products explains the color changes in bruises as they heal.

Therapeutics
Neonatal jaundice

Physiological jaundice in newborns is due to low levels of conjugating enzyme (UDP-glucuronyl transferase) at birth. At birth, serum total bilirubin levels of term infants are ~1 mg/dL. Three days after birth bilirubin levels increase to 10 to 12 mg/dL, and after 7 to 10 days they usually return to normal. Either hemolysis due to blood group incompatibility or liver dysfunction can cause pathological jaundice. Premature birth exacerbates physiological jaundice. Excess unconjugated bilirubin (> 15 mg/dL) can diffuse into basal ganglia, causing toxic encephalopathy (kernicterus). Babies are placed under blue fluorescent light to allow photochemical conversion of bilirubin to more polar (water-soluble) isomers. A recent treatment is intramuscular administration of tin-mesoporphyrin (SnMP, 4.5 mg/kg). SnMP is a potent inhibitor of heme oxygenase.

Therapeutics
UDP-glucuronyl transferase–related disorders

Crigler-Najjar syndrome results from a deficiency of UDP-glucuronyl transferase. Type 1 results from a complete absence of the gene with severe hyperbilirubinemia that accumulates in the brain of affected newborns and that causes a form of encephalopathy called kernicterus. Therapy includes transfusions in the immediate neonatal period, phototherapy, heme oxygenase inhibitors to reduce transient worsening of hyperbilirubinemia (although the effect decreases over time), oral calcium phosphate and carbonate to form complexes with bilirubin in the gut, and liver transplantation prior to the onset of brain damage and before phototherapy becomes ineffective at a later age. Type II is a benign form of this disorder resulting from a mutation that causes a partial deficiency of the gene (it is also known as Arias syndrome). Gilbert syndrome is a relatively common, benign disorder (affecting 2 to 10% of the population) that results from decreased activity (25%) of UDP-glucuronyl transferase. Serum total bilirubin is almost always < 6 mg/dL but may increase with fasting, stress, or alcohol consumption.

Therapeutics

Hemin and therapy

Hemin (Panhematin, BDI Pharma, Columbia, SC) is an iron-containing porphyrin consisting of protoporphyrin IX containing a ferric (Fe^{3+}) ion bound by a chloride ligand. It is beneficial in treating acute intermittent porphyria, which is caused by a defective porphobilinogen deaminase. Hemin, a heme-like molecule, inhibits ALA synthase to prevent the buildup of ALA.

Foundations

Iron transport and storage

Iron that is acquired from the diet is transported in the bloodstream via transferrin and stored as ferritin in the liver and spleen. Excess iron is stored as hemosiderin.

Foundations

Globin synthesis

Several mechanisms regulate not only heme synthesis but also the corresponding protein, globin, needed for hemoglobin. In reticulocytes (immature erythrocytes), heme stimulates the synthesis of globin via a mechanism in which rising heme levels inhibit a kinase, called heme-regulated inhibitor (HRI). This inhibition blocks the phosphorylation of an initiation factor eIF2 and allows eIF2 to participate in translation initiation.

Therapeutics

Hepatitis

Hepatitis, which is sometimes caused by viral infections, is an inflammation of the liver that leads to hepatic dysfunction. It causes an increased level of conjugated and unconjugated bilirubin. When there is a high level of conjugated bilirubin in the blood, it accumulates in the skin and the sclera of the eyes, causing yellow coloration. It also may spill over into the urine, causing the urine to be tea colored.

Therapeutics

Celebrity porphyrias

King George III (1738 to 1820), who ruled Great Britain during the time of the American Revolution, suffered from intermittent episodes of abdominal pain and delirium, and his symptoms included port-colored urine, hallucinations, and convulsions. A recent chemical analysis of his hair sample suggested chronic arsenic poisoning. Coupled with the known symptoms, a retrospective diagnosis of acute intermittent porphyria or variegate porphyria has been suggested, and the agent that triggered the periodic psychotic episodes could have been arsenic, a contaminant in medicines routinely administered to the king. Other celebrities that are suspected of suffering from porphyrias are King George IV, Queen Anne, and Vincent van Gogh, among others.

Review Questions: Metabolism

1. Inosine 5′-monophosphate (IMP) is the initial product of purine nucleotide anabolism. Which nucleotides are subsequently synthesized from IMP, each in two enzymatic steps?

A	AMP and GMP
B	AMP and OMP
C	dATP and dGTP
D	UTP and CTP
E	XMP and CMP

   A) Row A
   B) Row B
   C) Row C
   D) Row D
   E) Row E

2. 5-Phospho- α- D-ribosyl 1-pyrophosphate (PRPP) appears in the biosynthesis of both purine and pyrimidine nucleotides. Which among the following compounds are required for purine ring synthesis?
   A) Glycine, glutamine, carbon dioxide, aspartate and formyl tetrahydrofolate.
   B) Aspartate, glutamine and carbon dioxide.
   C) Aspartate, ammonia and carbon dioxide.
   D) Aspartate, ammonia and glycine.
   E) Crabamoyl phossphate and ammonia

3. Which of the following statements about gout is correct?
   A) Gout is a defect in pyrimidine nucleotide metabolism.
   B) Gout is characterized by high levels of uric acid in the blood.
   C) Gout is characterized by high levels of xanthine in the blood.
   D) Gout is treatable with the bacteriostatic antimicrobial chloramphenicol.
   E) Gout is the result of a defect in one specific enzyme in 90% or more of all cases.

4. What types of hyperbilirubinemia are produced by Gilbert syndrome and cholestasis?
   A) Row A
   B) Row B
   C) Row C
   D) Row D

	Gilbert Syndrome	Cholestasis
A.	Conjugated	Conjugated
B.	Unconjugated	Unconjugated
C.	Conjugated	Unconjugated
D.	Unconjugated	Conjugated

5. Which of the following enzymes would be found in the cytoplasmic fraction after differential centrifugation of homogenized liver cells?

A) Porphobilinogen (PBG) deaminase
B) δ-Aminolevulinic acid (δ-ALA) synthase
C) Protoporphyrinogen oxidase
D) Ferrochelatase
E) Coproporphyrinogen oxidase

6. A 55-year-old homeless woman presents to the clinic with complaints of fatigue and dyspnea on exertion. Laboratory examinations reveals microcytic anemia. The physician suspects that the woman is lacking nutrients that are essential for heme synthesis. Which of the following vitamins provides a cofactor for the initiation of porphyrin biosynthesis?
A) Thiamine
B) Riboflavin
C) Pyridoxine
D) Methylcobalamin
E) Cholecalciferol

7. The rate-limiting step of the metabolic pathway that synthesizes glucose *de novo* from noncarbohydrate precursors is:
(ADP, adenosine diphosphte; ATP, adenosine triphosphate; BP, bisphosphate; P, phosphate; Pi, inorganic phosphate)
A) $ATP + Pyruvate + HCO_3^- \rightarrow Oxaloacetate + ADP + P_i$
B) $Fructose\ 6\text{-}P + ATP \rightarrow Fructose\ 1,6\text{-}BP + ADP$
C) $Glucose\ 6\text{-}P + H_2O \rightarrow Glucose + P_i$
D) $Fructose\ 1,6\text{-}BP + H_2O \rightarrow Fructose\ 6\text{-}P + P_i$
E) $3\text{-}Phosphoglycerate + ATP \rightarrow 1,3\text{-}Bisphosphoglycerate + ADP$

8. Because the breakdown of glycosaminoglycans is noted as a critical consequence of inflammation in inflammatory bowel disease, some researchers wanted to conduct a pilot study on the effects of administering a modified sugar component of glycosaminoglycans to pediatric patients afflicted with Crohn disease. The component, which was obtained through enzymatic degradation of crab shell chitin and is not negatively charged at physiological pH, could be
A) Iduronate (IdoA)
B) N-acetylneuraminic acid (NANA)
C) N-acetylglucosamine (GlcNAc)
D) Glucuronate (GlcA)
E) N-acetylgalactosamine-6-sulfate (GalNAc-S)

9. A patient in the end stage of cancer shows muscle and adipose tissue wasting (cachexia) in a routine exam. Following up on this finding, a reduced glucose tolerance combined with insulin resistance is diagnosed. Increased concentrations of which of the following hormones may be responsible for this complication?
A) Glucagon
B) Insulin
C) Progesterone
D) Thyroid hormone
E) Cortisol

10. Metastasis of cancers is aided by overexpression of glycoproteins containing a nine-carbon acid found at the nonreducing ends of the oligosaccharide side chains. The high density of negative charges on these glycoproteins that aids cell dispersion is due to:

A) Hyaluronic acid
B) N-acetylneuraminic acid
C) Iduronic acid
D) Glucuronic acid
E) Gluconic acid

11. A 10-year-old boy is admitted to the hospital for weakness in his arms and legs. This had intensified over the past 2 weeks from frequent falls to quadriplegia. The patient was unable to communicate or eat, his face was masklike, but his bladder and bowel worked normally. On exam, dermatitis, an inflamed tongue, hypotonia, and exaggerated reflexes were noted with ankle clonus (continuous involuntary twitching of foot triggered by dorsiflexion). Blood tests were noncontributory, and magnetic resonance imaging (MRI) revealed focal lesions in the basal ganglia. Questioning of the parents revealed that the boy had received one raw egg every other day for "extra nutrition." This patient requires substitution with which vitamin?[1]
A) Thiamine
B) Riboflavin
C) Cobalamin
D) Folic acid
E) Biotin

12. A young woman is fleeing from a civil war. Together with other people from her village, she is trying to reach the safety of a refugee camp in a neighboring country on foot. She has not eaten for 3 days. Which of her organs will maintain her blood glucose level?
A) Muscle
B) Adipose tissue
C) Intestine
D) Liver
E) Brain

13. Which of the following enzymes is involved in the conversion of amino acid nitrogen into a compound that directly provide the urea nitrogen?
A) Pyruvate dehydrogenase
B) Asparaginase
C) Fumarase
D) Aspartate aminotransferase (AST)
E) Glutamine synthetase

14. Which of the following enzymes can utilize ammonia for the synthesis of the α–amino group of an amino acid?
A) Glutamate dehydrogenase
B) Arginase
C) Carbamoyl phosphate synthetase -I
D) Intestinal urease
E) Glutaminase

15. The enzyme enteropeptidase is important in the intestinal digestion of dietary proteins because it converts
A) pepsinogen to pepsin
B) proelastase to elastase
C) trypsinogen to trypsin
D) procarboxypeptidase B to carboxypeptidase B
E) chymotrypsinogen to chymotrypsin

16. A 26-year-old man is attempting to improve his performance as an amateur weightlifter. To this end, he

purchases a bottle of lysine supplements at a health food store because he has heard this will help build muscle tissue. To speed his progress in training, he takes 10 times the amount of lysine recommended on the container. After 4 weeks, he presents to his physician with skin rashes, intestinal discomfort, and general lethargy. After learning of the lysine supplements, his physician notes that the symptoms may be due to negative nitrogen balance. An elevated level of BUN (blood urea nitrogen) supports this diagnosis. The excess intake of lysine was likely impairing the intestinal absorption of

A) proline
B) arginine, histidine
C) phenylalanine, tyrosine
D) aspartate, glutamate
E) serine, alanine

17. Glutamate dehydrogenase carries out the oxidative deamination of glutamate in liver mitochondria. The products of this reaction are:

A) glutamate, NH_4^+, NADH
B) α-ketoglutarate, NH_4^+, NAD +
C) α-ketoglutarate, NH_4^+, NADH
D) α-ketoglutarate, NH_4^+, ATP
E) α-ketoglutarate, NH_4^+, $NADP^+$

18. Metabolism of aromatic amino acids involves the following pathways. Which choice matches the conditions with the correct enzymatic deficiencies (numbered 1 through 5 in the table shown below)?

	1	2	3	4	5
A.	Alkaptonuria	Tyrosinemia type II	Tyrosinemia type III	Phenylketonuria (PKU)	Albinism
B.	Phenylketonuria	Tyrosinemia type II	Homocystinuria	Albinism	Alkaptonuria
C.	Phenylketonuria	Tyrosinemia type II	Tyrosinemia type III	Alkaptonuria	Albinism
D.	Phenylketonuria	Nonclassical PKU	Tyrosinemia type III	Alkaptonuria	Albinism
E.	Phenylketonuria	Maple syrup urine disease	Tyrosinemia type III	Alkaptonuria	Albinism

A) Row A
B) Row B
C) Row C
D) Row D
E) Row E

19. The shift in the equilibrium of the glutamate dehydrogenase reaction toward the formation of glutamate when the cells are in ammonia toxicity state will deplete the brain cells of which important metabolic intermediate?

A) Thiamine pyrophosphate
B) α-Ketoglutarate
C) ADP
D) Flavin nucleotides
E) NAD^+

20. Lack of functional ABC-type membrane transporter (ABCD1) causes adrenoleukodystrophy, a rare disease that

became famous because of the film Lorenzo's Oil. Patients with adrenoleukodystrophy cannot degrade VLCFAs. The defect is most likely located at:

A) mitochondria
B) lysosomes
C) golgi complex
D) peroxisomes
E) endosomes

21. In a research project studying diabetic complications, juvenile female Wistar rats were injected with streptozotocin, a substance that selectively destroys the β cells in the islets of Langerhans in the pancreas. In the following weeks, the rats developed polydipsia, polyuria (producing half their body weight in urine every day) and wasting of adipose tissue and muscles. When tested with a urine nitroprusside dipstick, the urine tested negative for ketone bodies. The fatty acids contained in the lost adipose tissue were likely converted into

A) glucose
B) acetone
C) acetoacetate
D) β-hydroxybutyrate
E) glycogen

22. A 25-year-old medical student had a breakfast with eggs, bacon, and bread with cheese. She realizes she just had a fat rich meal. Which among the following is correct regarding fat metabolism in the body?

A) Long- chain fatty acids enter mitochondria via the malate shuttle for degradation.
B) The product of fatty acid synthase is stearic acid (C18:0).
C) 129 ATP molecules can be generated by the complete oxidation of one molecule of palmitate (C16:0).
D) The CoA derivatives of long -chain fatty acids (> 12 C atoms) can enter mitochondria by diffusion.
E) In phospholipids, the 2-position of glycerol is usually occupied by a saturated fatty acid with 16 to 18 C atoms.

23. Several lipases are involved in the storage and retrieval of fat in adipocytes. They include capillary lipoprotein lipase (LPL) and hormone-sensitive lipase (HSL). How would these lipases respond to a heavy but balanced meal?

A) Row A
B) Row B
C) Row C
D) Row D
E) Row E

	LPL	HSL
A.	Expression ↑	Activity ↑
B.	Expression ↑	Activity ↓
C.	Activity ↑	Activity ↓
D.	Activity ↓	Activity ↑
E.	Activity ↑	Expression ↓

24. Which readily available intermediate of glycolysis is used as a direct precursor for the synthesis of the glycerol moiety of triacylglycerols?

A) Pyruvate

B) 3-Phosphoglycerate

C) Glycerol 3-phosphate

D) Phosphoenolpyruvate

E) Dihydroxyacetone phosphate

25. Which of the following processes would you expect to be more active in the liver in the fasting than the fed state?

A) Carnitine palmitoyl transferase-I (CPT-I)

B) ATP: citrate lyase.

C) Acetyl CoA carboxylase.

D) HMG CoA Reductase.

E) Fatty acid synthase

26. Which among the following statements best describes a ganglioside?

A) A source of second messenger in signal transduction mechanism.

B) Contains choline.

C) Contains phosphate groups.

D) A signifcant source of energy to the cells.

E) Contains sialic acid.

27. A newborn is diagnosed with 17α-hydroxylase deficiency. Further laboratory studies may reflect increased levels of:

A) Testosterone

B) Cortisol

C) Estradiol

D) Progesterone

E) Androstenedione

28. A drug that helps sequester bile acids in the intestine and is prescribed to patients with hypercholesterolemia is:

A) Cholestyramine

B) Allopurinol

C) Atorvastatin

D) Methotrexate

E) Aspirin

29. Which of the following enzymes is involved in the conversion of progesterone to testosterone?

A) 5α-Reductase

B) 17,20-Lyase

C) 11β-Hydroxylase

D) Aromatase

E) 21- Hydroxylase

30. Excess free cholesterol within the hepatic cell may lead to

A) activation of the enzyme, HMG CoA reductase.

B) decreased production of bile acids by the liver.

C) inactivation of acyl CoA: cholesterol acyltransferase.

D) activation of lipoprotein lipase.

E) reduction in the number of LDL receptors on the cell membrane.

31. The tissue site of synthesis for chylomicrons is

A) pancreatic cells.

B) enterocytes.

C) hepatocytes.

D) adipocytes.

E) muscle cells.

32. Which of the following intermediates of cholesterol biosynthesis serves as a direct side chain?

A) Mevalonic acid

B) HMG CoA

C) Squalene

D) Lanosterol

E) Isopentenyl pyrophosphate

33. A 6-year-old boy was referred to a pediatric surgeon for evaluation and treatment of lip lacerations. The parents reported that from infancy, the child had been quiet and did not respond to many stimuli. Cerebral palsy and mental retardation were not noted. His condition remained unchanged until the age of 2 years, when he aggressively started biting his thumb and fingers. The child appeared in the clinic with his hands wrapped with bandages, and once these were removed, it was apparent that there was self-mutilating behavior that extended well beyond just lip damage. Laboratory: megaloblastic anemia, hyperuricemia, hyperuricosuria. Which of the following enzymes is most likely to be deficient in this child?[2]

A) Adenine phosphoribosyltransferase (APRT)

B) Adenosine deaminase (ADA)

C) Hypoxanthine-guanine phosphoribosyl transferase (HGPRT)

D) 5-Phosphoribosyl-1-pyrophosphate (PRPP) synthetase

E) Xanthine oxidase

34. A 31-year-old man presents to his physician with a "tight sensation" in his thighs and calves, which is aggravated by exertion. He runs long distances whenever his job as land surveyor allows. The sensation of tightness does not change with posture; it has increased over the past 30 months. During that time, he has lost 7 kg (15.4 lb) in weight. His own and his family's medical history are noncontributory. Vital signs and electrocardiogram (EKG) are normal. Further examinations reveal small crystals in the pingueculae of the eye and sluggish tendon reflexes but no other abnormality. On an ergometer, the patient performs to Olympic standard, with aching in the legs developing after 15 minutes. Electromyography (EMG) shows myopathy with normal nerve conduction. Routine blood, cerebrospinal fluid (CSF), and urine tests are all normal except for persistently low uric acid levels and slightly raised creatine kinase. Further investigation reveals hypoxanthineuria and xanthinuria. Biopsy of the gastrocnemius muscle shows rodlike aggregates of rhomboidal crystals in electron microscopy (EM). Which enzyme is most likely defective in this patient?[3]

A) Adenosine deaminase (ADA)

B) Adenosine phosphoribosyltransferase (APRT)

C) Guanine deaminase (GDA)

D) 3-Phosphoribosyl-1-pyrophosphate (PRPP) synthetase

E) Xanthine oxidase

35. A newborn girl is transferred to the neonatal intensive care unit for severe nonspherocytic hemolytic anemia and jaundice. She was born by cesarean section at week 30 as the fourth child to a first-cousin couple; none of her older siblings had survived. She was given two exchange transfusions on her first day and phototherapy for 8 days. She was maintained with monthly red blood cell (RBC) transfusions until a splenectomy was performed at age 3. From then on, transfusions were required only rarely, usually after infections. Her mental development was normal, physical development was delayed. She is now 12

years old. The jaundice of this patient is due to increased plasma concentrations of which of the following compounds?[4,5]

A) Direct bilirubin
B) Indirect bilirubin
C) δ-Bilirubin
D) Biliverdin
E) Lumirubin

36. A 3-year-old child was brought to the local emergency room by her mother because of abdominal pain, diarrhea, vomiting, difficulty walking, and reduced visual acuity. She was found to be dehydrated, and a complete blood count (CBC) revealed microcytic, hypochromic anemia. Her mother indicated that they lived in a poorly maintained older apartment building and that her daughter had pica. X-ray revealed opaque areas consistent with paint chips in her digestive tract, and her bones had areas of increased density. The patient recovered on whole bowel irrigation; three-drug chelation therapy with British anti-Lewisite, calcium disodium EDTA, and oral succimer; and Zn supplementation. In this type of poisoning, the encephalopathy is caused by elevated levels of

A) δ-aminolevulinic acid (δ-ALA)
B) porphobilinogen (PBG)
C) hydroxymethylbilane
D) uroporphyrinogen (UROGEN)
E) coproporphyrinogen (COPROGEN)

37. You are on a group hiking tour in South Tirol (Europe). You had a brilliant if slightly strenuous day out and a nice group dinner in the hotel, consisting of ricotta cheese and spinach-filled potato dumplings with tossed salad and fried eggs, accompanied by a local red wine. Two hours later you are called to one of your companions, who is feeling sick. You find an elderly lady, pale, clammy, in obvious distress. She is complaining about abdominal pain, vomiting, belching, diarrhea, and flatulence. After arranging transport to a local polyclinic, you find that temperature, vital signs, EKG, serum analysis, chest and abdominal X-ray, and ultrasound are normal. What is the most likely diagnosis?

A) Acute myocardial infarction
B) Appendicitis
C) Overexertion
D) Foodborne illness
E) Lactose intolerance

38. A 2-year-old girl is transferred to the metabolic unit of a state pediatric hospital because of failure to thrive and severe fasting hypoglycemia with neurological sequelae. A physical exam reveals hepatomegaly. Laboratory: hyperlipidemia and impaired liver and kidney function. A transcutaneous liver biopsy reveals the accumulation of excessive amounts of glycogen. The most likely diagnosis is

A) Conn syndrome
B) Adrenoleukodystrophy (ALD)
C) Von Gierke disease
D) Alzheimer disease
E) Dubin-Johnson syndrome

39. A 2-week-old boy is brought to a family doctor because of lethargy, feeding difficulties, frequent vomiting, and yellow

skin. He has been exclusively breast-fed. Physical exam reveals jaundice, cataracts, hepatomegaly, and edema. Laboratory: galactosuria, aminoaciduria, albuminuria, hypoglycemia, elevated serum bilirubin (direct + indirect), and liver enzymes. Ultrasound: enlarged fatty liver. The cataract is caused by which of the following compounds?

A) Galactitol
B) Erythritol
C) Xylitol
D) Mannitol
E) Sorbitol

40. A 6-month-old boy is brought to a pediatric unit because he fails to gain weight and has become increasingly weak to the point that he can no longer breast-feed. He is the second son of a healthy Caucasian couple, born by normal vaginal delivery after an uneventful pregnancy. Results of routine pediatric investigations after birth were unremarkable. Physical exam reveals mild cyanosis, shallow respiration, moderate hepatomegaly, an unusually large tongue (macroglossia), and generalized muscular flaccidity. Laboratory: complete blood count (CBC), electrolytes, glucose, blood urea nitrogen (BUN), and creatinine are all normal, but creatine kinase 2 (CK2) and alanine aminotransferase (ALT) are high. Chest X-ray and echocardiogram show extreme cardiomegaly with outflow tract obstruction and congestive heart failure. Muscle and liver biopsy show intracytoplasmic and lysosomal glycogen accumulation. The most likely diagnosis is

A) von Gierke disease
B) Pompe disease
C) Cori disease
D) Andersen disease
E) Fanconi-Bickel syndrome

41. A 1-year-old girl is brought to a family physician because of concerns about her development. She had an uncomplicated birth in a developing country at term. The mother reports that her daughter is not achieving normal milestones for a baby of her age. She also reports an unusual "mousy" odor of her urine and some hypopigmentation of skin and hair. On exam, the girl shows muscle hypotonia and microcephaly. To the physician's surprise, a test for phenylalanine hydroxylase activity comes back normal. Her metabolic deficiency might also affect the synthesis of which of the following hormones?

A) Serotonin
B) Thyroxine
C) Calcitriol
D) Pregnenolone
E) Progesterone

42. A 2-year-old boy presents to his physician with nystagmus, photosensitivity, and a failure to thrive. Laboratory tests reveal that serum concentrations of amino acids are unremarkable, but levels of neutral amino acids in the urine are elevated. The patient is diagnosed with Hartnup disease. Daily supplementation of which of these compounds would alleviate the severity of symptoms of this disorder?

A) Tetrahydrobiopterin
B) Folic acid

C) Nicotinic acid

D) Vitamin B$_6$

E) Serotonin

43. A 14-year-old boy was diagnosed with acute lymphocytic leukemia (ALL). Researchers have shown that ALL cells cannot produce a particular amino acid (which is normally nonessential), and thus must take it up from circulation. Based on these findings, the prescribed treatment for ALL includes administration of a bacterially purified enzyme that depletes circulating levels of this ALL essential amino acid by converting it to aspartate. What is the enzyme that is administered, and which particular amino acid serum levels must be measured to determine efficacy of the enzyme?

A) Aspartate aminotransferase (AST), glutamate

B) Asparagine synthetase, glutamine

C) Argininosuccinate lyase, arginine

D) Asparaginase, asparagine

E) Glutaminase, glutamine

44. A 6-month-old male infant is admitted to the emergency room with vomiting, lethargy, and irritability. Diagnostic tests reveal plasma ammonia levels of 200 µM. The mother reveals that one of her male siblings died in infancy after a similar episode, although she herself has never had such an episode. Based on the high ammonium levels and the family history, the physician suspects that the patient has a deficiency in ornithine transcarbamoylase (OTC), an X-linked disorder. To test this diagnosis, the physician orders additional tests on levels of particular metabolites in the blood plasma and urine. High levels of which of the following metabolites would support the diagnosis of OTC deficiency?

A) Orotic acid

B) Citrulline

C) Fumarate

D) Arginine

E) Urea

45. A mother brought her 2-year-old daughter to the emergency room with the concern her child may have accidentally overdosed on acetaminophen earlier in the day. The child presents with nausea and abdominal pain. Treatment includes administration of a particular amino acid derivative to the patient. The rationale is that the acetaminophen has depleted the body's supply of glutathione, an important detoxifying agent, and the amino acid derivative will serve to replenish the levels of glutathione. The amino acid derivative administered was:

A) N-acetylglutamate

B) N-acetylcysteine

C) S-adenosylmethionine

D) 5-hydroxytryptophan

E) dihydroxyphenylalanine

46. A 4-month-old female infant was rushed to the emergency room with grand mal seizures. She was the second child of nonconsanguineous parents, born by normal vaginal delivery after a 38-week unremarkable pregnancy. Her birthweight was 7.5 lb (3.4 kg). From the beginning, she was a poor feeder. Laboratory investigations showed blood

glucose 1.4 mM (25 mg/dL), 134 pM (1.8 U/dL) plasma insulin, 108 pM C-peptide, with normal serum cortisol (381 nM). Her serum hydroxybutyrylcarnitine concentration was elevated both when fed and when fasted. There were no ketones in her urine. She was maintained with frequent feeds of glucose polymer, which kept her blood glucose between 3.0 and 4.5 mM.

The activity of which of the following enzymes should be measured?

A) Short-chain 3-hydroxyacyl CoA dehydrogenase

B) Medium-chain acyl CoA dehydrogenase

C) Long-chain enoyl CoA hydratase

D) Electron-transferring flavoprotein (ETF): ubiquinone reductase

E) Fatty acyl CoA synthetase

47. A 50-year-old woman was brought to her family physician because of muscle weakness, loss of balance and coordination, and possibly dementia. Family history: two maternal uncles with adrenoleukodystrophy (ALD). Laboratory: elevated VLCFAs in serum, leucocytosis (34× 109/L), and cytosine insertion in codon 515 of one of the ABCD1 genes. She developed Addison disease at age 14 and spastic paraparesis at age 25 with cognitive deficits. The most likely diagnosis is

A) ALD

B) Adrenomyeloneuropathy (AMN)

C) adult Refsum disease

D) rhizomelic chondrodysplasia punctata

E) cerebrohepatorenal (Zellweger) syndrome

48. A 3-year-old boy was brought to a pediatric hospital because of abdominal pain. Parents reported that the child had had a distended abdomen since a few months after birth and that he was less active than most of his peers. There had been two episodes of bronchitis in the last year. Physical exam: eupnoic, normal breath sounds, 98% oxygen saturation. Lung function was at the lower end of the normal range, but the patient had difficulties following the instructions. Hypotonia and hepatosplenomegaly were noted 3 and 2 cm below the costal margin, respectively. Weight was at the 75th percentile, height at the 25th. Laboratory: complete blood count (CBC), erythrocyte sedimentation rate (ESR), partial thromboplastin time (PTT), ferritin, and C-reactive protein were normal. Liver enzymes, cholesterol, angiotensin-converting enzyme (ACE), and LDL were elevated, high-density lipoprotein (HDL) was low. Tuberculin skin test, sweat chloride test, and serological tests for various pathogens were all negative. Chest X-ray showed diffuse interstitial lung infiltrates with a nodular pattern, CT showed interstitial opacities with a reticular pattern in all lobes but no adenopathy. Foam cells (sphingolipid-laden macrophages) were found in bronchoalveolar lavage fluid and bone marrow biopsy. The activity of which of the following enzymes should be checked to get a definitive diagnosis?[6]

A) α-Galactosidase

B) Sphingomyelinase

C) Hexosaminidas B

D) Hexosamidase A

E) Glucocerebrosidase

49. A 32-year-old woman is brought to the emergency department in premature labor. Despite the best efforts of the medical team, she gives birth to a son 4 weeks early; he is immediately taken to the neonatal intensive care unit for observation. Initial examination reveals a mild heart murmur but an otherwise healthy child, considering the circumstances. Within 3 hours he becomes tachycardic and shows signs of dyspnea. A chest X-ray and echocardiogram show a substantial patent (open) ductus arteriosus (PDA), with increased blood flow to the lungs. The ductus arteriosus is a small blood vessel that connects the pulmonary artery to the aortic arch during fetal development. It allows blood from the right ventricle to bypass the nonfunctioning lungs and mix with oxygenated blood leaving the left ventricle. Prostaglandins, specifically PGE_1, are responsible for the patency of the ductus arteriosus. Which of the following medications would be best suited to treat this condition?
A) Propranolol (antagonist of β_1 and β_2-adrenergic receptors)
B) Indomethacin (nonselective COX-1/COX-2 inhibitor)
C) Alprostadil (prostaglandin E_1)
D) Spironolactone (a steroidal antimineralocorticoid agent)
E) Albuterol (agonist of β_2-adrenergic receptors)

50. A 26-year-old Hispanic woman visits her ob-gyn during the ninth week of her pregnancy. During the course of her physical exam, the patient mentions that she is particularly concerned about the pregnancy because she's had two prior miscarriages. It was further revealed that her mother and older sister had been diagnosed with systemic lupus erythematosus in their early 30 s. In addition to routine blood work, the physician orders a test for the presence of an antibody against a particular phospholipid. The presence of this antibody is often indicative of an autoimmune disorder that can cause a hypercoagulable state. What are the components of the lipid against which the antibodies are produced?
A) Glycerol, phosphate, fatty acid chain, amino alcohol
B) Ceramide, phosphate, choline
C) Glycerol, phosphate, fatty acid chain
D) Diphosphatidylglycerol, fatty acid chains

51. A 55-year-old man is suffering from Cushing disease. What would you expect to find on laboratory analysis of his blood?
A) Increased serum cortisol
B) Increased plasma glutamine
C) Increased serum androgens
D) Decreased serum dihydrotestosterone
E) Increased serum phenylalanine

52. A 10-year-old boy is brought to the emergency room with an apparent fracture of the right femur; an X-ray confirms the injury. He tells the staff that the injury occurred during a soccer game when he took a rough tackle while playing the ball. He also mentions that over the past several months, several of his joints have hurt after exercising and that he gets fatigued quite easily. Upon further questioning, he complains of polyuria and polydipsia. Initial blood chemistry shows elevated levels of calcium and low levels of phosphorus and vitamin D_3. Which of the following best explains the patient's symptoms?

A) Primary hyperparathyroidism
B) Sarcoidosis
C) Paget disease
D) Rhabdomyolysis

53. Lovastatin exerts its hypolipidemic effect by inhibiting
A) Cranitine palmitoyl transferaseII(CPTII)
B) HMG CoA reductase
C) Hormone sensitive lipase
D) Acetyl CoA acetyltransferase
E) Pyruvate dehydrogenase

54. A 13-year-old boy is referred to a cardiologist for dyspnea and chest pain after exertion. He is the son of a first-cousin couple; both parents have hypercholesterolemia; two of his cousins are also affected. His father had just undergone a triple bypass operation at age 39. The boy has been on atorvastatin and cholestyramine since age 4. Physical exam reveals yellowish lipid-laden bumps under the skin (xanthoma and xanthelasma). Angiography shows a 60% stenosis of the left coronary and a 50% stenosis of the left anterior descending arteries. The total serum cholesterol is 19.2 mM (750 mg/dL). The boy undergoes a bypass operation and could leave the hospital after a 3-day uneventful recovery. Which lipoprotein accumulates in the blood of this patient?[6]
A) Chylomicrons
B) High-density lipoprotein (HDL)
C) Intermediate-density lipoprotein (IDL)
D) Low-density lipoprotein (LDL)
E) Very-low-density lipoprotein (VLDL)

55. Which of the following compounds serves as a precursor to the pyrimidine nucleotides containing either ribose or deoxyribose?
A) Cytidine monophosphate (CMP)
B) Deoxyuridine monophosphate (dUMP)
C) Glycine
D) Inosine monophosphate (IMP)
E) Uridine monophosphate (UMP)

56. Methotrexate disrupts the *de novo* biosynthesis of thymidylate by preventing the addition of carbon atoms originating from which form of tetrahydrofolate (THF)?
A) N^{10}-formyl-THF
B) N^5-methyl-THF
C) N^5, N^{10}-methylene-THF
D) N^5-formimino-THF
E) N^5, N^{10}-methenyl-THF

57. A scientist adds ^{15}N-labeled uroporphyrinogen III to a human bone marrow cell system. ^{15}N, a stable isotope of nitrogen that can be distinguished from the common ^{14}N in a mass spectrometer, is located in the four pyrrole rings of uroporphyrinogen III. She subsequently isolates and analyzes the intermediates in the heme biosynthetic pathway that have incorporated 15N. Which of the following compounds do you expect to have incorporated the label?
A) δ-Aminolevulinic acid (δ-ALA)
B) Porphobilinogen (PBG)
C) Protoporphyrin IX

IV

D) Uroporphyrinogen I

E) Hydroxymethylbilane

58. A 4-week old boy is transferred to a Children's hospital with severe jaundice that appeared at birth and has been worsening ever since. The infant is the first child of a healthy Jewish couple; pregnancy and vaginal delivery were unremarkable. He is of average height and weight for his age, in no acute distress, but shows marked jaundice and slight hepatomegaly. Lab results: complete blood count (CBC) normal, indirect bilirubin high, fecal urobilinogen low. What is the most likely diagnosis?

A) Crigler-Najjar syndrome

B) Neonatal jaundice

C) Dubin-Johnson syndrome

D) Rotor (-Manahan-Florentin) syndrome

E) Glucose-6-phosphate dehydrogenase (G6PD) deficiency

59. Which among the following events is involved in the breakdown of muscle glycogen to glucose -1-phopshate in response to increased epinephrine?

A) Decrease in cytosolic Ca^{2+}

B) Activation of Aldolase

C) Inhibition of adenylyl cyclase

D) Conversion of inactive phosphorylase to active phosphorylase

E) Conversion of glycogen synthase to glycogen synthase

60. A 15-year-old girl is running away from a perceived attack to survive. Which of the following enzymes in her muscle is inactivated by phosphorylation?

A) Glycogen phosphorylase

B) Phosphorylase kinase

C) Glycogen synthase

D) Branching enzyme

E) Debranching enzyme

61. The immediate products of oxidation of one mole of glucose 6-phosphate through the oxidative portion of the pentose phosphate pathway are

A) two moles of NADH, one mole of ribulose 5-phosphate, and one mole of CO_2.

B) two moles of $NADP^+$, one mole of ribulose 5-phosphate, and one mole of CO_2.

C) two moles of NADPH, one mole of xylulose 5-phosphate, and one mole of CO_2.

D) two moles of NADPH, one mole of ribulose 5-phosphate, and one mole of CO_2.

E) one mole of fructose 6-phosphate and five moles of CO_2.

62. In glucose 6-phosphate dehydrogenase deficiency, increased red blood cell lysis is ultimately due to

A) problems with ATP production in mitochondria.

B) a deficiency in the ability to carry out glycolysis.

C) increased leakage of K^+ ions into the cells.

D) increased sensitivity to malaria parasites.

E) the inability of the cell to maintain normal levels of NADPH.

63. The carbon skeletons of which of the following amino acids can be utilized in the synthesis of both glucose and ketone bodies?

A) Glutamate and glutamine

B) Methionine and cysteine

C) Aspartate and asparagine

D) Leucine and lysine

E) Tyrosine and threonine

64. The infantile form of Parkinson disease is due to the defects in tyrosine hydroxylase. Such patients may show low levels of:

A) Serotonin

B) Dopamine

C) Heme

D) Glutathione

E) γ-aminobutyric acid (GABA)

65. Which of the following statements about the glucose-alanine cycle is correct?

A) It serves to carry amino groups from skeletal muscle to the liver.

B) It requires the participation of glycogenesis in the liver.

C) It provides the liver with glucose made by the muscle.

D) It requires the participation of oxidative deamination reactions in both the skeletal muscle and the liver.

E) It results from the conversion of alanine to pyruvate in the muscle and pyruvate to alanine in the liver.

66. Certain amino acids can increase the concentration of blood glucose because their carbon chain can be converted into:

A) acetoacetyl CoA

B) acetone

C) oxaloacetate

D) acetyl CoA

E) α-keto acids

67. Many intracellular proteins in our bodies are targeted for degradation by

A) the phosphorylation of mannose residues.

B) the covalent attachment of a polyubiquitin chain.

C) proteolysis by trypsin and chymotrypsin.

D) proteolysis by pepsin at low pH.

E) transport to ribosomes.

68. A pharmaceutical company is testing a new drug acting on acetyl CoA carboxylase (ACC). The Western blot below shows the drug's effect on ACC in a native gel electrophoresis of homogenized cells exposed to insulin, with and without the drug. Actin was used as loading control, that is, to ensure that the same amount of proteins was used in all experiments. Given the results of the experiment, what is the effect of the presence of the drug?

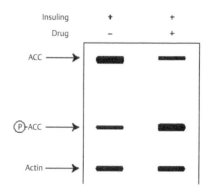

	Predominant ACC structure	Fatty acid synthesis
A.	Multimer	Stimulated
B.	Multimer	Inhibited
C.	Dimer	Stimulated
D.	Dimer	Inhibited
E.	Multimer	Stimulated

A) Row A
B) Row B
C) Row C
D) Row D
E) Row E

69. Which of the following is a property of acetyl CoA carboxylase (ACC), the rate limiting enzyme for *de novo* fatty acid synthesis in the body?
A) It converts acetyl CoA into cholesterol.
B) It is activated by cAMP mediated phosphorylation.
C) It is a multienzyme complex.
D) It is inactivated by citrate.
E) It requires biotin as a cofactor.

70. Which compound is the donor of the transferred group in the conversion of phosphatidylethanolamine to phosphatidylcholine?
A) N^5, N^{10} -Methylene tetrahydrofolate (methylene-THF)
B) S-Adenosylmethionine (SAM)
C) 3'-Phosphoadenosyl-5'-phosphosulphate (PAPS)
D) Acyl CoA
E) Uridine diphosphate N-acetyl glucosamine (UDP-GlcNAc)

71. If vascular endothelia are damaged by atherosclerosis, their ability to produce prostaglandin I2 (PGI^2, prostacyclin) is reduced. In this situation, low-dose acetylsalicylate (aspirin) is prescribed to inhibit the production of which eicosanoid no longer kept in check by the PGI^2?
A) PGD_2
B) PGE_2
C) $PGF_{2\alpha}$
D) PGH_2
E) TXA_2

72. β-Oxidation of an odd-chain fatty acid produces several two-carbon and one three-carbon molecules. The latter enters the TCA cycle in the form of which compound?
A) Citrate
B) Isocitrate
C) α-Ketoglutarate
D) Succinyl CoA
E) Malate

73. A 10-month-old boy was referred to a tertiary care hospital for chronic, intractable diarrhea. He was the child of first-degree consanguineous parents of Middle Eastern descent. Physical exam revealed moderate growth retardation, a distended abdomen, and normal neurologic function. Lab results: steatorrhea, hypocholesterolemia, and chylomicrons absent even after fatty meal. Ultrasound revealed moderate hepatomegaly, and X-ray showed reduced bone mineralization. An initial diagnosis of chylomicron retention (Anderson) disease was confirmed

by endoscopy (which showed the typical "frosting" of the mucosa) and duodenal biopsy, which showed fat-loaded enterocytes and a lack of SAR1B expression. SAR1B protein is a component of the coat protein complex II (COPII) required for endoplasmic reticulum (ER) → Golgi transport. The patient was maintained on a fat-free diet and supplemented with fat-soluble vitamins.
Which of the following fatty acids need to be supplemented in his diet?
A) Oleic acid (C18:1)
B) α-Linolenic acid (C18:3)
C) Palmitic acid (C16:0)
D) Docosahexaenoic acid (DHA, C22:6)
E) Eicosapentaenoic acid (EPA, C20:5)

74. In a study on bile acid metabolism, researchers have separated bile acids by thin layer chromatography (see image below). Unfortunately, they have no reference compounds available; they must therefore identify each spot by chemical analysis. Spot #3 contains carbon, oxygen, hydrogen, sulfur, and nitrogen. For each sulfur atom, the compound contains five oxygen atoms. (Rf, retention factor.)
Which of the following bile acids would give this elemental analysis?
A) Glycocholic acid
B) Taurocholic acid
C) Taurolithocholic acid
D) Lithocholic acid
E) Chenodeoxycholic acid

75. With a deficiency in 21-hydroxylase, which of the following compounds could accumulate in the adrenal cortex?
A) Progesterone
B) Aldosterone
C) Deoxycorticosterone
D) Cortisol
E) 11-Deoxycortisol

76. Which of the following best describes lipoprotein lipase (LPL)?
A) It requires co-lipase for its activity.
B) It mobilizes fat in adipose tissue.
C) It is a cytoplasmic enzyme.
D) It hydrolyzes triacylglycerols of plasma lipoproteins.
E) Its defect may lead to Familial Hypercholesterolemia.

77. During an overnight fast, the triacylglycerols are mainly packaged and released into the bloodstream as:
A) LDL
B) HDL
C) VLDL
D) Chylomicrons
E) Bile salts

78. A 40-year-old man visits his family doctor because of a chronic, recurrent rash on sun-exposed parts of his body. He has noticed that recurrence coincides with alcohol intake. His urine turns dark if left standing. Physical exam reveals vesicles and bullae on sun-exposed areas; skin in these sites is friable with whitish plaques (milia). Hypertrichosis and hyperpigmentation of the face are noted. Laboratory: urine is fluorescent, the uroporphyrin level is up markedly. Also,

IV

serum iron, transferrin, and aminotransferases are increased. Skin biopsy reveals iron deposits, intense porphyrin fluorescence, and long, thin cytoplasmic inclusions. The patient is most likely suffering from which disease?
A) Porphobilinogen synthase (PBGS) porphyria
B) Acute intermittent porphyria
C) Congenital erythropoietic porphyria
D) Porphyria cutanea tarda
E) Porphyria variegata

79. Unconjugated bilirubin is
A) elevated in neonatal hyperbilirubinemia.
B) usually found in the gallbladder.
C) normally excreted in the urine.
D) water-soluble.
E) conjugated by intestinal bacteria.

80. Which of the following processes is involved in purine nucleotide metabolism?
A) Purine catabolism yields water soluble products.
B) Ribonucleotide reductase converts nucleoside triphosphates into deoxynucleoside triphosphates.
C) The purine base is assembled on the activated sugar framework.
D) Orotidine 5' monophosphate (OMP) serves as the branch point for the synthesis of other purine nucleotides.
E) The committed step in the *de novo* synthesis of purine nucleotides is catalyzed by carbamoyl phosphate synthetase II.

81. A professional runner is at the 20 km mark of a marathon. Which of the following enzymes of glycogen metabolism or regulation will be phosphorylated and active in his body at this time?
A) Glycogen synthase kinase 3 (GSK-3)
B) Glycogen synthase
C) Phsophorylase kinase
D) Debranching enzyme

82. While reviewing carbohydrate content for his class exam, a medical student makes the following five statements about gluconeogenesis that he thinks the study group should know. A classmate, however, disagrees with one of his statements. Which would it be?
A) Glucose can be synthesized from noncarbohydrate precursors.
B) Gluconeogenesis is not a reversal of glycolysis.
C) Gluconeogenesis and glycolysis are reciprocally regulated.
D) Lactate and alanine formed by contracting muscle are converted into glucose in muscle.
E) Six high-energy phosphate bonds are spent in synthesizing one molecule of glucose from pyruvate.

83. A 7-year-old girl is presented to a pediatric unit for weakness in her upper limbs. She is the first child of a third-degree consanguineous marriage; perinatal and neonatal history was unremarkable. At 5 months of age, she suffered from an infection during which hepatomegaly and a few hypoglycemic seizures were documented. Liver and muscle enzymes were elevated in her serum. Anthropometric measurements (e.g., height and weight) are at the fifth percentile. A physical exam

reveals the liver 7 cm below the costal margin, as well as mild weakness in the distal muscles with normal tendon reflexes. Liver and muscle biopsies reveal large amounts of glycogen with short outer branches. Which enzyme is most likely to be defective?[7]
A) Glycogen synthase
B) Amylo-1,6-glucosidase (debranching enzyme)
C) Glucose 6-phosphatase
D) Phosphoglucomutase
E) UDP-glucose pyrophosphorylase

84. Glycogen storage disease type Ia (von Gierke disease) is often associated with hyperuricemia and joint pain. How does hyperuricemia develop from the inability to convert glucose 6-phosphate to glucose?
Statement 1: Increased levels of glucose 6-phosphate can spill into the hexose monophosphate shunt, leading to increased levels of ribose 5-phosphate for increased purine synthesis.
Statement 2: Increased levels of glucose 6-phosphate can spill into the hexose monophosphate shunt, leading to increased levels of NADPH for increased purine synthesis.
Statement 3: Elevated levels of lactate resulting from inhibition of pyruvate dehydrogenase compete with uric acid for excretion by the kidneys.
Statement 4: Hypoglycemia resulting from impaired gluconeogenesis and glycogenolysis results in a high glucagon:insulin ratio, which increases the rate of purine degradation.
A) Statement 1 only
B) Statement 2 only
C) Statements 1 and 3
D) Statements 2 and 4
E) All statements are correct

85. The product of which of the following enzymes regenerates the antioxidant required to neutralize reactive oxygen species such as hydrogen peroxide (H_2O_2) in the red blood cells?
A) Pyruvate kinase
B) Glyceraldehyde 3-phosphate dehydrogenase (GAPDH)
C) Lactate dehydrogenase (LDH)
D) Glucose 6-phosphate dehydrogenase
E) Glucose 6-phosphate isomerase

86. A genetic defect in N-acetyl glutamate (NAG) synthase may lead to:
A) orotic aciduria
B) hyperammonemia
C) megaloblastic anemia
D) citrullinemia
E) argininoosuccinic aciduria

87. The coenzyme involved in transaminations and many other amino acid transformations is derived from which of the following?
A) Niacin
B) Pyridoxine
C) Flavins
D) Thiamine
E) Vitamin B_{12}

IV

88. In maple syrup urine disease (now called branched-chain aminoaciduria), the defective metabolic step involves
A) oxidative decarboxylation.
B) an amino acid transaminase.
C) methionine deficiency in the diet.
D) an amino acid hydroxylase.
E) fixation of amino groups to carbon skeletons.

89. Which among the following conversion reactions will be defective in patients with B_{12} deficiency?
A) Argininosuccinate to fumarate and arginine
B) Homocysteine to cystathionine
C) Phenylalanine to tyrosine
D) Citrulline and aspartate to arginosuccinate
E) Methylmalonyl CoA to succinyl CoA

90. Non-steady-state kinetics is used to elucidate the reaction mechanism of enzymes. The figure below shows the principle of one of the methods used: quenched flow. A ram, driven at a constant rate by a stepper motor, drives enzyme and substrate solution into a mixer. Inside the mixer, the input and output lines meet at an offset, resulting in highly turbulent flow that ensures mixing of the reactants in less than 1 ms. The reaction mix then flows through an aging tube into a sampling vial with boiling denaturant, which stops the reaction instantly. The experiment is repeated several times; each time a known length is cut off the aging tube, so that shorter and shorter contact times result. Finally, the collected samples are analyzed. In an investigation of fatty acid synthase, malonyl CoA labeled with ^{14}C in the methylene (-CH_2-) group was used as a substrate. Acetyl CoA, NADPH, and a buffer were also present. Analysis was by autoradiography of a thin-layer chromatogram of the samples. The major fatty acids at each aging tube length are identified as a black horizontal line in each column. At 20 cm aging tube length, how many NADPHs have been used to synthesize one molecule of the major fatty acid product?
A) 4
B) 6
C) 8
D) 10
E) 12

91. Aspirin is an irreversible inhibitor of cyclooxygenase enzyme and covalently modifies the enyme by:
A) methylation
B) carboxylation
C) decarboxylation
D) acetylation
E) oxidation

92. Which among the following biochemical processes do you expect to increase in a patient experiencing stress from severe injuries?
A) PEPCK induction by cortisol.
B) Glycogen synthase activation by insulin.
C) FAS induction by insulin.
D) CPT-I inhibition by malonyl CoA.
E) HSL inhibition by insulin

93. Metabolic adjustment to diabetes mellitus type 1 is similar to that of long-term starvation in that there is a decrease in which of the following?
A) Ketone body levels in the blood
B) Production of glucose
C) Fatty acid synthesis
D) Utilization of ketone bodies by the brain
E) Protein breakdown

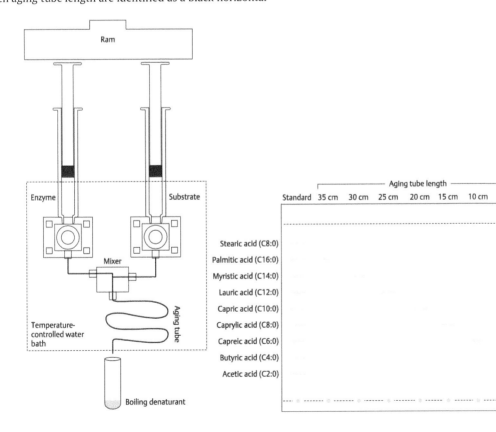

94. Excessive alcohol consumption can lead to an elevation in plasma triglycerides by which of the following mechanisms?
A) A rise in plasma low-density lipoprotein (LDL) levels
B) A rise in plasma high-density lipoprotein (HDL) levels
C) Inhibition of nutrient oxidation
D) Stimulation of the carnitine shuttle
E) Inhibition of acetyl CoA carboxylase

95. Quantitatively, the major way for cholesterol to be eliminated from the body is by biliary excretion after conversion to which of the following?
A) Bilirubin
B) Bile acids
C) Bile pigments
D) Cholesterol ester
E) LDL

96. Which compound is an intermediate in the cholesterol synthesis pathway and immediately convertible to cholecalciferol by ultraviolet (UV) light?
A) Squalene
B) Lanosterol
C) 7-Dehydrocholesterol
D) Calcitriol
E) Farnesyl pyrophosphate

97. By binding bile acids, cholestyramine prevents their enterohepatic circulation and promotes their removal with feces. How would the body respond to such loss of bile acids?
A) Inhibition of 7α-hydroxylase
B) Inhibition of lipoprotein lipase (LPL)
C) Inhibition of lecithin:cholesterol acyltransferase (LCAT)
D) Increased LDL receptor expression
E) Increased intestinal cholesterol absorption

98. A 29-year-old man with rheumatoid arthritis entered the hospital in renal failure. Further tests revealed hyperuricemia and an asymptomatic renal insufficiency with creatinine clearance that was 60% of normal values. The patient's renal damage was presumably caused by the formation of uric acid crystals in the nephrons. Given this information, which of the following diagnoses is not consistent with this patient's condition?
A) A deficiency of hypoxanthine guanine phosphoribosyltransferase (HGPRT)
B) An exceptionally active isoform of xanthine oxidase
C) An overactive isoform of carbamoyl phosphate synthetase I
D) An overactive isoform of phosphoribosyl pyrophosphate (PRPP) synthetase
E) Overconsumption of purine-rich foods and dehydration

99. An 18-year-old male patient comes to his family physician complaining of pain and muscle cramps during even moderate exercise. Physical exam reveals no hepato-, spleno-, or cardiomegaly, and an electrocardiogram reading is normal. There is no fasting hypoglycemia, glucose intolerance, hyperlipidemia, or ketosis. After exercise on an ergospirometer, a blood sample is taken that does not show lactic acidosis but does show increased creatine kinase 3

and myoglobin. The most likely diagnosis is which of the following?
A) von Gierke disease (glycogen storage disease Ia [GSD Ia])
B) Pompe disease (GSD II)
C) Cori-Forbe disease (GSD IIIa)
D) McArdle disease (GSD V)
E) Hers disease (GSD VI)

100. A 16-year-old boy presents to his physician with renal colic brought on by the presence of kidney stones (renal calculi). Laboratory tests show a positive nitroprusside urine test. The patient is diagnosed with cystinuria. The sulfur atoms in the precipitating amino acid have their origin from which other amino acid?
A) Threonine
B) Serine
C) Tryptophan
D) Methionine
E) Citrulline

101. A pharmaceutical company is developing a new drug that inhibits fatty acid synthesis in obese (body mass index [BMI] > 30) patients. The drug is supposed to prevent the insulin-dependent activation of the key regulated enzyme of fatty acid synthesis. To check the efficacy of drug candidates in cell cultures, the inhibition of which of the following enzymes would serve as a suitable marker?
A) Long-chain acyl CoA dehydrogenase (LCAD)
B) Protein phosphatase
C) Glycogen phosphorylase
D) Adenylyl cyclase
E) Protein kinase A (PKA)

102. Which of the following heme degradation step is defective in patients with Crigler-Najjar syndrome?
A) Conversion of biliverdin to bilirubin
B) Conversion of bilirubin to bilirubin diglucuronide
C) Conversion of bilirubin to stercobilinogen
D) Conversion of bilirubin to urobilinogen
E) Conversion of heme to biliverdin

103. An 8-year old girl presents with the following symptoms: onset of osteoporosis, ectopia lentis (lens detachment), and mild mental retardation. The patient was diagnosed with homocystinuria. A treatment regimen was prescribed that included dietary restriction of a particular essential amino acid and dietary supplements of vitamin B_{12}, B_6 and folic acid. Which amino acid was restricted, and what biosynthetic reaction would be affected by the vitamin supplements?
A) Methionine; enhance the conversion of homocysteine to methionine
B) Cysteine; enhance the conversion of homocysteine to cysteine
C) Glycine; enhance the conversion of serine to glycine
D) Serine; inhibit the conversion of serine to glycine
E) Cysteine; increase the absorption of cystine

104. A 6-week-old boy is brought in for a postmortem examination after sudden infant death. He had one healthy sibling; another had died from sudden infant death syndrome (SIDS) 8 days after birth. The child was born by emergency cesarean section when the mother showed hypertension, proteinuria, jaundice, elevated liver enzymes, low serum albumin, abdominal pain, lethargy, and decreased fetal movements at week 35. The operation was complicated by profuse bleeding of the mother, which led to anoxic encephalopathy and coma. Birth weight, height, and head circumference of the boy were at the 3rd percentile. He had to be placed on a respirator and was given surfactant. On the third day, newborn screening revealed elevated levels of long-chain acylcarnitines, 3-OH acylcarnitines, and dicarboxylic acids in serum and urine. Free carnitine in serum was low. The infant was maintained on intravenous glucose and a formula with increased medium-chain fatty acids until his death. Autopsy revealed heart ventricular hypertrophy, jaundice, and an enlarged, fatty liver. The child most likely had a defect in which enzyme?

A) Thiokinase
B) Carnitine palmitoyltransferase I (CPT-I)
C) Mitochondrial trifunctional protein (TFP)
D) 3,5–2,4-dienoyl CoA isomerase
E) Long-chain acyl CoA dehydrogenase (LCAD)

105. A lack of LDL receptors will probably result in which of the following?
A) a low level of plasma LDL
B) a low activity of hepatic 3-hydroxy-3-methylglutaryl (HMG) CoA reductase
C) a decrease in plasma cholesterol
D) a decrease in endocytosis of LDL
E) an increase in the activity of hepatic acyl CoA: cholesterol acyl transferase (ACAT)

106. A 15-year-old girl is stranded without food on an island for about three days. What do you think will be the predominant fate of pyruvate in her body?
A) Aerobic glycolysis
B) Enter TCA cycle for complete oxidation into CO_2 and water
C) Conversion into oxaloacetate to synthesize glucose
D) Redox reaction coupling with ATP production
E) Synthesis of biologically important compounds

IV

Answers and Explanations: Metabolism

1. A AMP (adenosine monophosphate) and GMP (guanosine monophosphate) are the purine nucleoside monophosphates synthesized from IMP in two enzymatic steps.

B Although AMP is a purine nucleotide that can be made from IMP, Orotidine 5′-monophosphate (OMP) is an intermediate in the synthesis of the pyrimidine UMP (uridine monophosphate).

C IMP can be converted to AMP and GMP in two enzymatic steps. Conversion of IMP into dATP (deoxyadenosine triphosphate) and dGTP (deoxyguanosine triphosphate) requires phosphorylation to the NDP (nucleoside diphosphate), reduction to dNDP (deoxy–NDP), and then phosphorylation to dNTP (deoxynucleoside triphosphate)—five steps in total.

D UTP (uridine triphosphate) and CTP (cytidine triphosphate) are pyrimidine nucleotides; therefore, they cannot be made from the purine IMP.

E XMP (xanthosine monophosphate) is produced from IMP in a single reaction, as an intermediate in the synthesis of GMP. CMP is a pyrimidine and cannot be made from the purine IMP.

2. A Glycine, glutamine, carbon dioxide, aspartate and formyl tetrahydrofolate each contribute at least one carbon or nitrogen to the purine ring.

B, C, D Aspartate, glutamine and carbon dioxide each contributes at least one carbon or nitrogen to the pyrimidine ring.

E Carbamoyl phosphate and ammonia are required for urea synthesis.

3. B Gout is the result of either an overproduction of uric acid or, more commonly, its underexcretion.

A Gout is the result of high concentrations of uric acid, a product of purine (not pyrimidine) nucleotide metabolism.

C Gout is caused by high levels of uric acid rather than xanthine. One of the major drugs against gout, allopurinol, works by preventing the oxidation of xanthine to uric acid.

D Gout is not caused by a bacterial infection but by the accumulation of a metabolite. Antibiotics therefore are not a suitable treatment.

E Gout is not the result of a defect in one specific enzyme in the majority of cases. Approximately 12% of the cases of gout are caused by diets high in meat and alcohol and low in fiber. The low-fiber content allows long contact time of chyme with intestinal nucleases and phosphatases, which produce nucleosides from the DNA in meat. These are absorbed by enterocytes and either passed into the bloodstream or directly turned into uric acid. Alcohol consumption leads to acidemia, and this increases uric acid reabsorption in the kidney via the urate transporter, URAT1. The combined result is an acute gout attack a few hours after the nutritional indiscretion.

4. D (A, B, and C are incorrect.) Gilbert syndrome produces an elevated level of unconjugated bilirubin in the bloodstream, as a result of the reduced activity of the enzyme uridine diphosphate (UDP) –glucuronyltransferase, which conjugates bilirubin and some other lipophilic molecules with glucuronic acid. Mild jaundice may appear under conditions of exertion, stress, fasting, and infections, but the condition is otherwise usually asymptomatic. Cholestasis is any condition in which the flow of bile from the liver is blocked and will lead to an elevated blood level of conjugated bilirubin.

5. A Of the enzymes listed, only the PBG deaminase is located in the cytosol. This enzyme condenses four porphobilinogen pyrrole rings into a linear hydroxymethylbilane. The other enzymes are found in mitochondria.

B δ-ALA synthase is located in mitochondria.

C Protoporphyrinogen oxidase is found in mitochondria.

D Ferrochelatase is located in mitochondria.

E Coproporphyrinogen oxidase is found in mitochondria.

6. C The first step in the synthesis of heme is performed by δ-ALA synthase, an enzyme that requires the coenzyme, pyridoxal phosphate, the active form of pyridoxine (vitamin B_6). δ-ALA synthase condenses glycine and succinyl coenzyme A (CoA) to generate δ-aminolevulinic acid with the loss of CO_2. Remember: Reactions modifying amino acids usually require pyridoxine (vitamin B_6).

A Thiamine is not required by δ-ALA synthase, the enzyme that carries out the first step of heme synthesis. Thiamine is required for oxidative decarboxylations where the remaining molecule is transferred onto CoA and for transketolase.

B Riboflavin is not required by δ-ALA synthase, which catalyzes the first step of heme synthesis. Riboflavin is used to make flavin adenine dinucleotide (FAD) and flavin mononucleotide (FMN) for oxidoreductases.

D Methylcobalamin is not required by δ-ALA synthase, which carries out the first step of heme synthesis. Only two enzymes in the human body require vitamin B_{12}: methylmalonyl CoA mutase and methionine synthase.

E Cholecalciferol is not required by δ-ALA synthase, which catalyzes the first step of heme synthesis. Cholecalciferol (vitamin D_3) is the precursor for calcitriol, which regulates the homeostasis of Ca^{2+}, PO_4^{3-}, and Mg^{2+} and acts as a paracrine hormone regulating the immune system.

7. D The rate-limiting step of gluconeogenesis (the pathway that synthesizes glucose *de novo* from noncarbohydrate precursors) is catalyzed by fructose 1,6-bisphosphatase. It is a phosphatase that hydrolyzes a phosphate group (Pi) from the carbon 1 position of fructose 1,6-bisphosphate, thus generating fructose 6-phosphate.

A Although this reaction is catalyzed by a gluconeogenic (glucogenic) enzyme, pyruvate carboxylase, it is not the rate-limiting step of gluconeogenesis.

B This is a phosphorylation reaction performed by phosphofructokinase-1, the rate-limiting enzyme of glycolysis, not gluconeogenesis.

C This dephosphorylation reaction is performed by a gluconeogenic (glucogenic) enzyme, glucose 6-phosphatase; however, it is not the rate-limiting enzyme of gluconeogenesis.

E This phosphorylation reaction is catalyzed by phosphoglycerate kinase, an enzyme that is common to both glycolysis and gluconeogenesis. Remember: Rate-limiting reactions are usually committed (irreversible) steps.

8. C N-acetylglucosamine (GlcNAc) does not have acidic groups and hence no negative charges at neutral pH. GlcNAc is a major component of mucopolysaccharides (glycosaminoglycans) in the extracellular matrix and in glycoproteins. It is also used to posttranslationally modify proteins on serine or threonine residues to regulate their activity.

A Iduronic acid at physiological pH will be ionized to iduronate and have a negative charge. Iduronate, for example, does occur in heparan sulfate.

B N-acetylneuraminic acid (NANA) occurs in sphingolipids, specifically gangliosides. It is not found in glycosaminoglycans. In addition, at neutral pH this molecule will be ionized and have a negative charge.

D Glucuronate is the salt of glucuronic acid (glucose with the sixth carbon oxidized to a carboxylic acid group) and is negatively charged at neutral pH.

E N-acetylgalactosamine, like the corresponding glucose derivate, occurs in glycosaminoglycans. Sulfate groups may be added to both, either as an ester on the sixth carbon or on the amino group. Those sulfate groups, however, have a negative charge.

9. E Overproduction of cortisol commonly leads to wasting in terminally ill patients. Cortisol is a hormone of chronic stress; it initiates the conversion of long-term energy stores (protein and fat) into more easily accessible short-term stores (glucose, glycogen). It also counteracts insulin to keep blood [glucose] high for use in an emergency (hence the observed insulin resistance marked by high blood glucose despite high insulin levels). The ineffectiveness of insulin and the overproduction of cortisol lead to reduced glucose tolerance, i.e., high blood glucose concentrations after dietary glucose uptake. Anything that leads to relaxation can be used to reduce the inappropriate cortisol production (e.g., music, massage, laughing, crying, moderate exercise, and sexual activity).

A Glucagon is not overproduced in stressful situations; its production in the pancreas is controlled strictly by blood [glucose].

B Insulin is not overproduced in stressful situations; its production in the pancreas is controlled strictly by blood [glucose]. It is the response of peripheral tissues to insulin that may be reduced in chronic stress.

C Progesterone is a steroid hormone that is one of the treatment options for cachexia because it stimulates appetite and promotes weight gain. Progesterone does not contribute to insulin resistance.

D Thyroid hormones are not overproduced under conditions of chronic stress.

10. B N-acetylneuraminic acid (NANA), whose nine carbon atoms come from mannose and pyruvate, is the most common sialic acid in mammals. It is located at the nonreducing (outer) end of N-linked sugar trees in glycoproteins and in gangliosides (glycolipids).

A Hyaluronic acid is a polysaccharide consisting of alternating D-glucuronic acid and D- N-acetylglucosamine molecules. It is found in cartilage, synovial fluid, and skin.

C Iduronic acid (IdoA) is a six-carbon molecule, distinguished from glucuronic acid by the position of the COO-group on C-5. It occurs in glycosaminoglycans such as heparin, heparan sulfate, and dermatan sulfate.

D Glucuronic acid is a six-carbon molecule derived from glucose by oxidation of C-6 to a carboxylic acid group. It is used to conjugate lipophilic substances such as bilirubin to make them more water soluble.

E Gluconic acid is a six-carbon molecule obtained from glucose by oxidizing the aldehyde group on C-1 to a carboxylic acid group. Its salts (gluconates) are widely distributed in nature. Ca-gluconate is used to treat osteoporosis and as a gel for hydrofluoric acid burns (forming insoluble CaF^2). In food processing, gluconates are used as buffers ("acid regulators").

11. E Egg whites contain the protein avidin, which forms a very strong association with biotin. Biotin bound in this man-

IV

ner cannot be absorbed in the intestine, leading to biotin deficiency. Uncooked avidin cannot be digested by the proteases of our alimentary system, but cooking renders it harmless.

A Thiamine (vitamin B_1) deficiency leads to beriberi, characterized by neuropathy, confusion, convulsions, nausea, muscle wasting, tachycardia, and heart hypertrophy, with or without edema.

B Riboflavin (vitamin B_2) deficiency leads to ariboflavinosis, which is characterized by inflammation of the mouth and tongue, seborrheic dermatitis, confusion, and normocytic anemia. Because the symptoms are unspecific, a definitive diagnosis requires measurement of erythrocyte glutathione reductase activity with and without added riboflavin.

C Cobalamin (vitamin B_{12}) deficiency results in megaloblastic anemia and demyelinization. Typically, patients are elderly and suffer from an autoimmune gastritis, which prevents production of intrinsic factor and hence cobalamin uptake.

D Folic acid (vitamin B_9) deficiency presents with megaloblastic anemia. In a developing fetus, it can cause problems with neural tube formation.

12. D Intestinal content will provide glucose for ~ 4 hours after the last meal, and then liver glycogen stores last until ~ 16 to 20 hours after the last meal. From then on, the only source of glucose is gluconeogenesis from lactate and amino acids (from muscle) and glycerol (from adipose tissue), which is performed mainly in the liver.

A Muscle does not have glucose-6-phosphatase, the enzyme required to release glucose into the bloodstream. In addition, after 3 days without a meal but with high physical activity, the muscle glycogen stores are likely to be depleted.

B Adipose tissue can release fatty acids and glycerol but not glucose into the bloodstream. Thus, adipose tissue will provide most of the energy for the body but not the glucose required for erythrocyte, brain, and kidney function.

C Intestinal content supplies glucose for ~ 4 hours after the last meal.

E Brain critically depends on a supply of glucose but cannot produce it.

13. D AST leads to the production of aspartate through a transamination reaction. Aspartate feeds into the urea cycle, and its nitrogen atom is incorporated into urea.

A Pyruvate dehydrogenase functions in converting pyruvate to acetyl CoA and does not function in the urea cycle.

B Asparginase converts asparagine into aspartate and ammonium. Although this enzyme results in free ammonium, this is not the major mechanism in which ammonium enters into the urea cycle. Rather, deamination of glutamate by glutamate dehydrogenase and glutamine by glutaminase in hepatocytes is the major source of ammonium that enters the urea cycle.

C In this case, fumarase is the enzyme that does not function in converting nitrogen atoms into the urea molecule. Fumarase converts fumarate to malate. This reaction is important in the conversion of fumarate produced from the urea cycle to the TCA cycle. However, fumarate is not a nitrogen-containing molecule.

E Glutamine synthetase catalyzes the synthesis of glutamine from glutamate and ammonium ions. The reaction is important in converting ammonium ions in extrahepatic tissues into a

nontoxic form for transport to the liver. Glutaminase converts glutamine to glutamate and ammonium ions. Glutamine transported to the liver undergoes this reaction, and the ammonium ion can enter the urea cycle. Significantly, glutamine synthetase and glutaminase function in maintaining the acid–base balance in the kidneys.

14. A Glutamate dehydrogenase can, under conditions of abundant energy, react ammonium ion (NH_4^+) with α-ketoglutarate to form glutamate. Subsequently, the amino group of glutamate can be transferred to an α-keto acid to form its corresponding amino acid (i.e., transamination of pyruvate to alanine). Aminotransferases and their associated pyridoxal phosphate cofactor catalyze the transamination reactions.

B The urea cycle is not reversible. Although arginine is formed in the urea cycle by arginase, its α-amino group does not originate from reactions catalyzed in the urea cycle.

C Carbamoyl phosphate is formed in the mitochondria of hepatocytes through the action of carbamoyl phosphate synthetase I. Once formed, the carbamoyl phosphate is conjugated with ornithine to form citrulline in the urea cycle. Carbamoyl phosphate is not used in incorporation of amino groups of amino acids.

D Intestinal ammonia arises from bacteria that deaminate amino acids. Intestinal bacteria also produce urease, which degrades urea in the intestine to free ammonia. However, the incorporation of amino groups into nonessential amino acids is not dependent on ammonia produced in the intestine.

E The amide group in the glutamine side chain is used as a nitrogen donor in several important reactions, including amidation of the side chain of aspartate to form asparagine. Glutamine is also converted to glutamate and NH_4^+ by glutaminase. However, glutamine is not required in the synthesis of the α-amino groups of amino acids.

15. C Enteropeptidase, found on the membranes of cells of the intestinal mucosa, makes the initial conversion of trypsinogen to trypsin. Trypsin then converts the other zymogens to their active forms. These reactions occur at neutral pH values.

A Pepsin is released as the inactive zymogen, pepsinogen, into the stomach from gastric chief cells in the stomach. Under the low pH values (pH 2 to 3) in the stomach, pepsinogen is converted to the active pepsin through autocatalysis.

B The zymogen, proelastase, is converted to its active form, elastase, upon cleavage by trypsin (not enteropeptidase).

D The zymogen, procarboxypeptidase B, is converted to its active form, carboxypeptidase B, upon cleavage by trypsin (not enteropeptidase).

E The zymogen, chymotrypsinogen, is converted to its active form, chymotrypsin, upon cleavage by trypsin (not enteropeptidase).

16. B Arginine, histidine, and lysine are all basic amino acids. They will compete with one another for the same transport mechanisms.

A Proline is transported into intestinal cells via transport systems specific for this amino acid. As such, the basic lysine will not be competing with proline for the same transport systems.

C Phenylalanine and tyrosine enter into intestinal cells via transport systems that bind large, neutral amino acids. As such, the basic lysine will not be competing with the aforementioned amino acids for the same transport systems.

D Aspartate and glutamate enter into intestinal cells via a transport system that selectively binds acidic amino acids. As such, the basic lysine will not be competing with the aforementioned amino acids for the same transport systems.

E Serine and alanine enter intestinal cells via transport systems that selectively bind small, neutral amino acids. As such, the basic lysine will not be competing with the aforementioned amino acids for the same transport systems.

17. **C** Glutamate dehydrogenase, operating in the catabolic direction, yields NH_4^+, the reduced form of nicotinamide adenine dinucleotide (NADH), and α-ketoglutarate as products. The cofactor for oxidative deamination of glutamate is NAD^+, which is reduced to NADH during the reaction. The NADH produced can be used as reducing agent during ATP synthesis.

A Glutamate is the substrate, not the product, in this oxidative deamination reaction.

B NAD^+ is the cofactor used for oxidative deamination and is reduced to NADH during the reaction.

D ATP is not a product of oxidative deamination of glutamate. ATP and GTP are allosteric effectors of glutamate dehydrogenase. In conditions of low ATP levels and high ADP levels, glutamate dehydrogenase will oxidatively deaminate glutamate to yield NADH reducing equivalents, which in turn can be used in ATP synthesis.

E $NADP^+$ is not a product of the oxidative deamination of glutamate. However, the reduced form of nicotinamide adenine dinucleotide phosphate (NADPH) is oxidized to $NADP^+$ in the reverse reaction (i.e., the reductive amination of α-ketoglutarate to yield glutamate).

18. **C** (A, B, D, E are incorrect) Phenylketonuria (PKU) is caused by a block in the hydroxylation of phenylalanine, by phenylalanine hydroxylase (1), to form tyrosine. Tyrosinemia type II results from a deficiency in tyrosine aminotransferase (2), which catalyzes the conversion of tyrosine to rho-hydroxy-phenylpyruvate. Tyrosinemia type III is a block in the oxidation of rho-hydroxyphenylpyruvate, by rho-hydroxyphenylpyruvate oxidase (3), to homogentisic acid. Alkaptonuria results from an accumulation of homogentisic acid due to a block in the formation of maleylacetoacetate by homogentisate oxidase (4). Last, albinism results from a defect in tyrosinase (5), an enzyme that catalyzes the conversion of tyrosine to melanin.

19. **B** (C, E) The shift in the equilibrium of the glutamate dehydrogenase reaction toward the formation of glutamate will yield glutamate and the oxidized form of nicotinamide adenine dinucleotide (NAD^+) as products, depleting cells of α-ketoglutarate.

A Thiamine pyrophosphate is a cofactor for several enzymes, including pyruvate dehydrogenase and α-ketoglutarate dehydrogenase. It is not required for glutamate formation.

D Flavin nucleotides are used as cofactors in oxidation-reduction reactions. They are not required for glutamate formation.

20. **D** Very long chain fatty acids (VLCFAs, ≥ 22 C atoms) like cerotic acid (hexacosanoic acid, C26:0) have to be shortened to ≤ 20 C atoms in the peroxisomes before they can be catabolized in the mitochondria. Entry into peroxisomes is via an ABC-type membrane transporter, ABCD1 (or adrenoleukodystrophy

protein, ALDP), which is encoded on the X chromosome and is lacking in patients with adrenoleukodystrophy. Patients with adrenoleukodystrophy cannot degrade VLCFAs.

A Only the CoA derivatives of short-chain and medium-chain fatty acids (< 12 C atoms) can enter mitochondria by diffusion. Long-chain fatty acids require the carnitine shuttle. VLCFAs such as cerotic acid have to be shortened in peroxisomes first before they can enter mitochondria.

B Long-chain fatty acids enter mitochondria via the carnitine shuttle for degradation. VLCFAs such as cerotic acid have to be shortened in peroxisomes first before they can enter mitochondria.

C In phospholipids, the 1-position of glycerol is usually occupied by a saturated fatty acid with 16 to 18 C atoms. The fatty acids in the 2-position are usually 18 to 22 C atoms in length and unsaturated. VLCFAs are found in sphingolipids.

E The product of fatty acid synthase is palmitate (C16:0).

21. **D** Under the conditions of diabetic ketoacidosis, the liver has an excess of NADH and therefore reduces acetoacetate, the primary ketone body, to β-hydroxybutyrate. Thus, the ratio of acetoacetate:β-hydroxybutyrate, which is normally ~1:1, changes to 1:10 in ketoacidosis. Urine test sticks for ketone bodies contain nitroprusside sodium, a compound that gives a cherry red complex with ketones. Because β-hydroxybutyrate does not have a ketone group (even though it is called a ketone body!), it cannot be detected by this test. Thus, in the one situation where knowledge of the ketone bodies in urine is clinically most necessary, this test is likely to give a false-negative result. Use of β-hydroxybutyrate dehydrogenase test strips with blood will give the correct result.

A There is no net glucose synthesis from fatty acids in humans because the β-oxidation of even chain fatty acids leads to acetyl CoA whose two carbons are released as CO_2 in the TCA cycle. Thus, there is no carbon left from which glucose can be made.

B Acetone would give a weak positive reaction with the test sticks. Also, because of its volatility, most of it is breathed out rather than excreted into urine.

C Acetoacetate would not only give a positive reaction with the test stick but is actually the compound detected by them.

E Because there is no net synthesis of glucose from fatty acids, glycogen cannot be made from fatty acids either.

22. **C** Using the conventional P:O ratios of 3 ATP for $NADH + H^+$ and 2 ATP for $FADH_2$, we get the following:

Reaction	Number of ATPs
Activation of fatty acid to acyl CoA	-02 ATP
Oxidation of 7 $FADH_2$ (2 ATP each)	(7x 2) = +14 ATP
Oxidation of 7 NADH (3 ATP each)	(7x 3) = +21 ATP
Oxidation of 8 Acetyl CoA (12 ATP each)	(8x 12) = +96ATP
Net Gain	+129ATP

A Long-chain fatty acids enter mitochondria via the carnitine shuttle for degradation and not malate shuttle.

B The product of fatty acid synthase is palmitate (C16:0).

IV

D Only the CoA derivatives of short-chain and medium-chain fatty acids (< 12 C atoms) can enter mitochondria by diffusion. Long-chain fatty acids require the carnitine shuttle.

E In phospholipids, the 1-position of glycerol is usually occupied by a saturated fatty acid with 16 to 18 C atoms. The fatty acids in the 2-position are usually 18 to 22 C atoms in length and unsaturated.

23. B (A, C, D, and E are incorrect.) Capillary lipoprotein lipase cleaves fats in chylomicrons and very-low-density lipoproteins (VLDL) into fatty acids and 2-monoacylglycerol for uptake into muscle, heart, mammary gland, and adipose tissue. Insulin increases the expression of capillary LPL. Insulin acts through a cellular signaling cascade and hence cannot influence the activity of preformed extracellular enzymes. HSL, which cleaves mainly triacylglycerol to diacylglycerol and a fatty acid, is involved in the mobilization of fat from adipocytes. HSL's activity is reduced by insulin via dephosphorylation. This makes physiological sense because insulin is a satiety hormone that stimulates storage of nutrients rather than their mobilization.

24. E Dihydroxyacetone phosphate (DHAP) is reduced to glycerol-3-phosphate in mitochondria of hepatocytes and adipocytes by glycerol-3-phosphate dehydrogenase and then acylated to produce lysophosphatidic acid.

A Pyruvate is not a direct precursor of the glycerol moiety of triacylglycerols.

B 3-Phosphoglycerate is not a direct precursor of the glycerol moiety of triacylglycerols.

C Glycerol-3-phosphate does serve as a precursor for the glycerol moiety of triacylglycerols; however, it is not an intermediate of glycolysis.

D Phosphoenolpyruvate is not a direct precursor of the glycerol moiety of triacylglycerols.

25. A Glucagon in the fasting state stimulates the production of cAMP in hepatocytes, which stimulates protein kinase A (PKA). PKA phosphorylates and inactivates acetyl CoA carboxylase, thereby reducing its product malonyl CoA, thus activating CPT-1, the rate limiting enzyme for fatty acid oxidation.

B ATP:citrate lyase helps to shuttle acetyl units from mitochondria into cytoplasm for the synthesis of fatty acids. Its activity is stimulated by glucose and insulin, levels of both of which would be low in the fasting state.

C The activity of acetyl CoA carboxylase is suppressed by glucagon, a hormone whose levels rise during the fasting state.

A Glucagon in the fasting state stimulates the production of cAMP in hepatocytes, which stimulates protein kinase A (PKA). PKA phosphorylates and inactivates HMG CoA Reductase., the rate limiting enzyme for *de novo* cholesterol synthesis in the liver.

E Fatty acid synthase complex is induced by insulin, a hormone whose levels are low in the fasting state.

26. E Gangliosides are defined as globosides (sphingosine, fatty acid, and sugars) with sialic acid side groups on the sugar tree. In mammals, the most common sialic acid is N-acetylneuraminic acid (NANA).

A Phosphatidylinositol is composed of diacylglycerophosphate with inositol bound to the phosphate group. Phosphatidyl inositol bis phosphate is a source of IP3, a second messenger in signal transduction mechanism.

B Choline is an amino alcohol typically found esterified to the phosphate group of glycerophospholipids and sphingomyelin.

C Gangliosides are made up of sphingosine, a fatty acid chain, and sugar groups. They do not contain phosphate groups.

D They are important as cell membrane components and serve as a binding site for toxins. They do not serve as a source of energy for the cells.

27. D Progesterone is produced from pregnenolone and does not require 17α-hydroxylase activity. The additional steroid hormones that can be produced in the absence of 17α-hydroxylase are pregnenolone, deoxycorticosterone, and corticosterone.

A Testosterone synthesis requires the activity of 17α-hydroxylase; therefore, its levels would be reduced when this enzyme is deficient.

B Cortisol synthesis requires the activity of 17α-hydroxylase; therefore, its levels would be reduced when this enzyme is deficient.

C Estradiol synthesis requires the activity of 17α-hydroxylase; therefore, its levels would be reduced when this enzyme is deficient.

E Androstenedione synthesis requires the activity of 17α-hydroxylase; therefore, its levels would be reduced when this enzyme is deficient.

28. A Cholestyramine is a strong anion exchanger that binds bile acids in the intestine and prevents their enterohepatic cycling. They are then excreted from the body with the stool. This releases feedback inhibition at the committed step of bile acid synthesis, 7α-hydroxylase, a CYP-450 monooxygenase at the hepatocytes' endoplasmic reticulum. Thus, more cholesterol is converted to bile acids, reducing hypercholesterolemia.

B Allopurinol is xanthine oxidase inhibitor and is prescribed to patients with hyperuricemia.

C Atorvastatin would inhibit HMG CoA reductase and is not a bile sequestrant.

D Methotrexate inhibits dihydrofolate reductase and is a chemotherapeutic agent.

29. B Progesterone conversion to testosterone involves hydroxylation by 17α-hydroxylase, removal of the side chain by 17,20-lyase (aka 17,20-desmolase), and reduction of the keto group in position 17 to the corresponding alcohol by 17-β-hydroxysteroid dehydrogenase.

A 5α-Reductase converts testosterone into dihydrotestosterone.

C 11β-Hydroxylase introduces a hydroxyl group into 11-deoxycorticosterone and 11-deoxycortisol, converting them into corticosterone and cortisol, respectively.

D Aromatase converts the 19-carbon androgens androstenedione and testosterone into the 18-carbon estrogens estrone and estradiol, respectively, by removing C-19 and introducing additional double bonds into the first ring of the steroid system.

E 21- Hydroxylase converts progesterone into deoxycorticosterone.

30. E Excess free cholesterol within the cell leads to a reduction in the number of LDL receptors on cell membranes and would reduce the endocytosis of LDL, causing an accumulation of LDL in circulation. Excess cholesterol would decrease the processing of the transcription factor, SREBP2, and cause decreased expression of LDL receptors.

A, B Excess free cholesterol within the cell leads to idecreased expression of HMG CoA reductase again through decreased processing of SREBP2. Bile acids are produced from cholesterol; and would be high.

C Excess free cholesterol within the cell leads to the activation of acyl CoA: cholesterol acyltransferase (ACAT) for storage of excess cholesterol as cholesterol ester.

D Capillary lipoprotein lipase cleaves fats in chylomicrons and very-low-density lipoproteins (VLDL) into fatty acids and 2-monoacylglycerol for uptake into muscle, heart, mammary gland, and adipose tissue and not modulated by hepatic cholesterol pool.

31. B (A) In the enterocytes of the small intestine, fatty acids and monoacylglycerols are absorbed and then converted back into triacylglycerols, packed into chylomicrons at the endoplasmic reticulum, and released into the lymphatics.

C Hepatocytes can synthesize fats and cholesterol, but those are packed into VLDL rather than into chylomicrons.

D Triacylglycerols synthesized by adipocytes are stored in fat droplets (not packaged into chylomicrons).

E Muscle cells do not release lipoproteins (e.g., chylomicrons) into the bloodstream, and they do not even store dietary fat.

32. E Isopentenyl pyrophosphate, a 5-carbon building block of all prenyl compounds, serves as the substrate for synthesis of the decaprenyl sidechain of Coenzyme Q (ubiquinone). Myalgia in some patients treated with statins (HMGCoA reductase inhibitor) may be due to reduced production of isopentenyl pyrophosphate and its product, ubiquinone.

A, B, C, D HMG CoA reductase in the committed step of isoprenoid synthesis. The enzyme converts HMG CoA to mevalonate. Neither of these intermeduiates serve as a direct prenyl side chain.

33. C This patient has Lesch-Nyhan syndrome (LNS) resulting from a deficiency of HGPRT. HGPRT is required to recycle the purines hypoxanthine and guanine by attaching PRPP to them. A deficiency in HGPRT leads first to excess production of uric acid, resulting in kidney destruction and gout. This is treatable with allopurinol, an inhibitor of xanthine oxidase. Second, it interferes with vitamin B_{12} metabolism, resulting in megaloblastic anemia.

A APRT deficiency leads to excess formation of insoluble 2,8-dihydroxyadenine (DHA), which causes kidney stones (renal lithiasis). There are no mental derangements. There are two forms of this disease: in type I there is no functional enzyme; in type II the deficiency can be overcome *in vitro* by increased PRPP. Both types can be present to a varying degree, so that onset can be anywhere from 5 months to adulthood. The disease is diagnosed from elevated adenine levels in urine and low or absent enzyme activity in red cells. Treatment is with a purine-restricted diet and allopurinol. The disease is rare except in Japan.

B ADA-SCID (15% of all cases) is an autosomal recessive disorder (Chr 20) due to ADA deficiency. In this disease adenine nucleotides cannot be broken down, which leads to a 100-fold increase in the concentration of dATP, which in turn downregulates ribonucleotide reductase. As a consequence, there are not enough other dNTPs to support cell division, leading to a lack of both T and B cells. For unknown reasons, production of red blood cells is not affected. The patients have to be kept in reverse isolation ("bubble babies") because they cannot fight infections. They can be maintained with enzyme replacement therapy using PEGylated ADA, but bone marrow transplantation is currently the only long-term curative treatment available. X-SCID, which is more prevalent (45% of all cases), is due to a deficiency of the common gamma subunit (γc) of T cell growth factor receptor. Common, because it is a component of several cytokine receptors on lymphocytes.

D PRPP synthetase deficiency can lead to X-linked recessive Charcot -Marie -Tooth disease 5 (CMTX5, optic atrophy, deafness, and polyneuropathy) or, in complete absence, to Arts syndrome (mental retardation, early-onset hypotonia, ataxia, delayed motor development, hearing impairment, optic atrophy, immune deficiency). Because the absence of PRPP synthetase prevents nucleotide synthesis, there is no hyperuricemia. In addition, the self-destructive biting described in the case is pathognomonic (characteristic of another disease). Superactivity of PRPP synthetase leads to hyperuricemia and gout and, in severe cases, sensorineuronal deafness. PRPP synthetase is encoded on the X chromosome.

E A deficiency in xanthine oxidase would prevent the synthesis of uric acid and lead to xanthinuria.

34. E Xanthine oxidase is deficient in this patient. Xanthine oxidase converts hypoxanthine (from inosine) to xanthine and subsequently converts xanthine to uric acid in the purine degradation pathway. Xanthine is also produced from guanine by the enzyme guanine deaminase (guanase). A deficiency of xanthine oxidase leads to abnormal levels of hypoxanthine and xanthine in urine and blood. Because xanthine cannot be converted to uric acid, laboratory investigations will show hypouricemia. Usually, patients present with xanthine kidney stones in middle or advanced age, but the high physical activity of the patient here led to precipitation in the muscle. Treatment is symptomatic with high fluid intake and a low purine diet.

A ADA deficiency leads to ADA–SCID. Patients present in early infancy with high infection rates and may have to be kept in reverse isolation ("bubble babies") until a bone marrow transplant can be performed.

B Patients with APRT deficiency present with kidney stones consisting of 2,8-dihydroxyadenine because the salvage of adenine is impossible. This patient has no accumulation of that compound.

C GDA converts guanine to xanthine and ammonia. No genetic defects have been reported for this enzyme.

D A complete defect in PRPP synthetase would be incompatible with life because no nucleotides could be made. There are patients whose PRPP synthetase does not react normally to feedback inhibition. The increased [PRPP] activates glutamine:phosphoribosyl pyrophosphate amidotransferase, the rate-limiting enzyme of purine synthesis. These patients make excessive amounts of purines and hence present with gout.

35. B "Indirect" bilirubin is unconjugated and has a very low solubility in water. Therefore, it is transported in plasma bound to serum albumin; once the binding capacity of albumin (40

IV

μM) is exceeded, bilirubin precipitates in the sclera, skin (jaundice), and basal ganglia (kernicterus). The attribute "indirect" refers to the fact that bilirubin bound to albumin can be detected in the laboratory only after solubilization with methanol. The hemolysis in this patient results in high amounts of hemoglobin that are converted to bilirubin, which overwhelms the capacity of the immature liver to perform the conjugation of each bilirubin molecule with two molecules of glucuronic acid.

A "Direct" or conjugated bilirubin (bilirubin diglucuronide) is a compound that is reasonably soluble in water and eliminated with bile unless there are posthepatic problems. In this patient, the high amounts of bilirubin produced from hemolyzed erythrocytes overwhelm the capacity of the patient's immature liver to perform the conjugation; hence unconjugated bilirubin accumulates and causes jaundice.

C δ-Bilirubin is bilirubin covalently bound to albumin; it contributes only a few percent of the total bilirubin in plasma and has no medical significance.

D Biliverdin is a blue-green compound that occurs in the catabolic pathway from hemoglobin to bilirubin. It does not cause jaundice (the word jaundice is derived from French jaune = yellow).

E Lumirubin is one of the products formed from bilirubin during phototherapy. Because it is much more water soluble than bilirubin, it can be eliminated with urine, resolving the jaundice.

36. A The patient is suffering from lead (Pb) poisoning caused by ingestion of paint chips from an older building. Ingested Pb replaces a Zn ion from the catalytic center of δ-ALA dehydratase, leading to the accumulation of δ-ALA, which then acts as a γ-aminobutyric acid (GABA)-agonist and also leads to the formation of reactive oxygen species. In addition, the lack of heme removes the inhibition of δ-ALA synthase, further increasing the concentration of δ-ALA. The results are neuropsychiatric and neurovisceral symptoms, which can be very confusing to an emergency room physician. For example, the patient may present with all the signs and symptoms of acute abdomen, but neither imaging studies nor exploratory surgery would find any problems there. Lack of heme leads to microcytic, hypochromic anemia. Removal of Pb by chelating agents is aided by "flushing" chemically bound Pb with Zn. Before they were forbidden in the United States (1977), Pb-based pigments like white lead and chrome yellow were widely used and may still be found in older buildings in poor neighborhoods. Lead plumbate–based paints were used as a primer to protect iron from corrosion.

B, C, D, and E Pb poisoning affects heme synthesis by inhibiting δ-ALA dehydratase and ferrochelatase, leading to elevated levels of δ-ALA.

37. E All other causes are excluded by the patient's presentation and by the exam results. The signs and symptoms fit those of someone who is lactose intolerant. Lactose-intolerant patients usually know about the problems they get when ingesting lactose and will avoid doing so. Problems arise when their food is prepared by others, and milk products "hide." In this case, the dumplings turned out to contain ricotta cheese. Advising the preparer of special dietary needs unfortunately does not always prevent these problems.

A The patient's presentation does not fit an acute myocardial infarction. In addition, EKG and serum analysis were normal.

B An inflamed appendix would have shown up on physical exam and ultrasound.

C Although one might suspect that an elderly patient may have been overtaxed during a group hiking tour, the patient's presentation does not fit overexertion.

D Food poisoning with bacteria or virus has incubation periods of one to several days, during which the pathogens multiply. In addition, when several people eat the same meal, but only one falls sick, food poisoning is improbable even when one of the components of the meal (here, spinach) is a common cause of such problems. Chemical food poisoning would be unlikely because, first, other people who shared the meal stayed healthy, and, second, there were no items consumed that are commonly associated with such problems (wild mushrooms, plants, or seafood).

38. C This patient has von Gierke disease (glycogen storage disease Ia), marked by the accumulation of glycogen in the liver and hepatomegaly. It is caused by a defect of glucose-6-phosphatase in the liver endoplasmic reticulum. As a result, the liver cannot release glucose into the bloodstream to keep blood glucose concentrations constant during fasting, for example, at night. This affects the organs that rely on glucose for their catabolic needs (brain, erythrocyte, kidney). At the same time, high concentrations of glucose-6-phosphate in hepatocytes stimulate glycogen synthesis, leading to glycogen accumulation and hepatomegaly.

A This patient does not have Conn syndrome because it is caused by the overproduction of aldosterone, usually either because of adrenal hyperplasia or adrenal carcinoma, and marked by hypernatremia, hypokalemia, and metabolic alkalosis.

B This patient does not have ALD because it is caused by a defect in the ABCD1 transport ATPase, which transports CoA esters of VLCFAs (> 20 carbons) from the cytosol into the peroxisome, where they have to be shortened enough that mitochondrial β-oxidation can break them down completely. Accumulation of VLCFAs in the brain and adrenals of patients with ALD leads to loss of neurologic functions and Addison disease.

D Alzheimer disease is caused by the accumulation of misfolded proteins (amyloid) in neuritic plaques in the brain. This is caused by a mutation in the gene for amyloid precursor protein (APP), which predisposes APP breakdown products to amyloid formation. Note also that the patient is only 2 years old; early-onset Alzheimer disease is usually diagnosed around age 40.

E Dubin-Johnson syndrome is caused by a defect in the canalicular multiple organic anion transporter (cMOAT, Mrp2, ABCC2) and leads to the accumulation of conjugated (direct) bilirubin, which can no longer be exported from the hepatocytes into the bile. This is a benign condition that usually does not require treatment. However, during pregnancy or after oral contraceptives, jaundice may occur. The latter are contraindicated in these patients.

39. A The child is suffering from galactokinase deficiency, an enzyme that phosphorylates galactose in order for it to be metabolized further for use in glycolysis. As a consequence, accumulating galactose is reduced by aldose reductase to the sugar alcohol galactitol, which causes osmotic swelling of the eye lens and membrane damage. In addition, the depletion of NADPH prevents detoxification of reactive oxygen species. Both effects lead to cataract formation, which is reversible if galactose is withheld from the diet early enough (remember that milk sugar [lactose] is a disaccharide of galactose and glucose). Unfortunately, this is not true for the brain damage caused by galactosemia. This makes early detection of the disease essential, and newborn screening is mandatory in many jurisdictions.

B Erythritol is a four-carbon sugar alcohol used as an artificial sweetener. Because little of it is metabolized, it adds little energy to food. It also does not promote tooth decay. Because it is absorbed in the small intestine and then excreted in urine, it causes less flatulence than other sugar alcohols. Erythritol is not linked to cataract formation.

C Xylitol is used as a sweetener because it has a low glycemic index, does not promote tooth decay, and has a somewhat lower energy content than sucrose with about the same sweetness. Unlike many sweeteners, it does not have a bad aftertaste. The only disadvantage is flatulence after excess consumption. Xylitol is not linked to cataract formation.

D Mannitol is a sugar alcohol used as energy storage by some microorganisms and plants. In medicine, it is used to treat head trauma and kidney failure, as a primer for the heart–lung machine, and to make the blood–brain barrier permeable for drugs. The inhaled solid may be useful for the treatment of cystic fibrosis by osmotically liquefying mucus. Mannitol is also used as a low glycemic index, tooth-friendly sweetener, although it is only about half as sweet as sucrose and in high doses causes flatulence. Mannitol is not linked to cataract formation.

E Sorbitol is the sugar alcohol corresponding to glucose. It occurs naturally in many fruits and is converted to fructose in our body. It is used as a sweetener in tooth paste and mouthwash and as a laxative. In uncontrolled diabetics, some glucose is converted to sorbitol, leading to lens and nerve damage. However, this patient is not suffering from diabetes.

40. B The accumulation of glycogen in the lysosomes indicates that the acid maltase enzyme is defective; therefore, this patient has Pompe disease.

A The accumulation of glycogen in the lysosomes shows that the acid maltase is defective. In von Gierke disease (glycogen storage disease Ia) the glucose-6-phosphatase in the endoplasmic reticulum (ER) is defective so that the liver cannot release glucose into the bloodstream. This results in fasting hypoglycemia, hyperlipidemia, and damage to liver and kidney. A defect in the transport protein that moves glucose-6-phosphate from the cytosol into the ER (glycogen storage disease Ib) has similar consequences.

C The accumulation of glycogen in lysosomes shows that the acid maltase is defective. In Cori disease (glycogen storage disease IIIa) the debranching enzyme in liver and muscle is defective. This leads to fasting hypoglycemia and to the accumulation of abnormal glycogen in liver, heart, and skeletal muscle (hepato- and cardiomegaly, myopathy). In glycogen storage disease IIIb only the liver enzyme is affected.

D The accumulation of glycogen in lysosomes shows that the acid maltase is defective. In Andersen disease, the branching enzyme is defective, which leads to the accumulation of unbranched, insoluble glycogen in the liver. The resulting liver cirrhosis leads to death by age 5 unless a transplant is performed.

E The accumulation of glycogen in lysosomes shows that the acid maltase is defective. In Fanconi-Bickel syndrome, the glucose transporter GLUT2 is defective. This leads to decreased uptake/release of glucose and galactose by liver. Decreased glucose sensing in the pancreas and reuptake in the renal tubules lead to prandial hyperglycemia, increased sugar excretion in urine, and ketoacidosis. There is damage to liver, bone, kidney, and pancreas.

41. A The patient is suffering from a rare form of phenylketonuria (PKU) caused by a deficiency of dihydrobiopterin reductase. This affects phenylalanine, tyrosine, and tryptophan hydroxylases, and hence the conversion of phenylalanine to tyrosine, tyrosine to dopa, and tryptophan to serotonin.

B Thyroxine is formed by the iodination of tyrosine in thyroglobulin via a reaction catalyzed by thyroperoxidase. This does not require dihydrobiopterin reductase, which is defective in this patient.

C Calcitriol is produced not only by the kidneys to regulate Ca_2^+ metabolism but also as a paracrine hormone, for example, in the immune system. The hydroxylation of calcidiol to calcitriol does not require dihydrobiopterin reductase, which is defective in this patient.

D Conversion of cholesterol to pregnenolone by desmolase does not require dihydrobiopterin reductase, which is defective in this patient.

E Conversion of pregnenolone to progesterone does not require dihydrobiopterin reductase, which is defective in this patient.

42. C The reabsorption of the neutral amino acid tryptophan in the kidneys is defective in Hartnup disease. Tryptophan is a significant source of niacin in the body. Nicotinamide-containing molecules such as NAD^+ and $NADP^+$ are synthesized from tryptophan. Thus, treatment involves supplementation with nicotinic acid.

A Tetrahydrobiopterin is a coenzyme for several enzymes, including the aromatic amino acid hydroxylases. Levels of tetrahydrobiopterin are not affected by Hartnup disease.

B Folic acid is converted into tetrahydrofolate, which functions in various one-carbon transfer reactions. The levels of tetrahydrofolate are not affected by Hartnup disease.

D Vitamin B_6 and its derivatives are important coenzymes in several enzymes, including those that catalyze transaminations and decarboxylations in amino acid metabolism. The levels of vitamin B_6 are not affected by Hartnup disease.

E Tryptophan is also a precursor for serotonin. Dietary supplements of serotonin will not alleviate the deficiency in nicotinamide that occurs in Hartnup disease.

43. D Administration (typically by intravenous injections) of asparaginase is used for the treatment of ALL because it depletes blood plasma levels of asparagine, an amino acid that cannot be synthesized by ALL cells. Asparagine levels must be monitored to determine if the enzyme is depleting blood plasma levels of asparagine.

A AST interconverts aspartate and oxaloacetate. This enzyme will not affect blood plasma levels of asparagine.

Further, the levels of glutamate are not indicative of asparaginase activity.

B Asparagine synthetase leads to the synthesis of asparagine from aspartate. This would increase, rather than decrease, blood plasma levels of asparagine. Further, levels of glutamine would not be indicative of asparaginase activity.

C Argininosuccinate lyase is a urea cycle enzyme that converts argininosuccinate to fumarate and arginine. Further, arginine levels are not affected by asparaginase activity.

E Glutaminase converts glutamine to glutamate plus ammonium. Following transport of glutamine from extrahepatic tissues to the liver, this enzyme plays a role in breaking down glutamine. The ammonium produced then enters the urea cycle. Additionally, glutaminase is important in maintaining the acid–base balance in the kidneys. However, glutaminase activity will not reduce blood plasma levels of asparagine. Further, the blood plasma levels of glutamine are not diagnostic of asparaginase activity.

44. A A deficiency in OTC results in a buildup of carbamoyl phosphate in the mitochondria of hepatocytes. The excess carbamoyl phosphate diffuses into the cytosol, where it can be converted to orotic acid in the pyrimidine biosynthetic pathway. The amount of carbamoyl phosphate generated by CPS I in mitochondria is much greater than that by CPS II in cytosol. This excess carbamoyl phosphate spills over into the cytoplasm and bypasses the normal rate-limiting step of CPS II. The increased flux through the pyrimidine synthetic pathway causes orotate accumulation because UMP synthase cannot handle all the orotate being produced. High levels of orotic acid in the urine, combined with hyperammonemia, are characteristic of OTC deficiency.

B OTC catalyzes the conjugation of carbamoyl phosphate with ornithine to produce citrulline. A deficiency in OTC would therefore result in low levels of citrulline. A low blood plasma level of citrulline is also diagnostic of OTC deficiency.

C Fumarate is produced in the urea cycle upon the hydrolysis of argininosuccinate. Although the levels of fumarate produced by the urea cycle are reduced in OTC deficiency, the levels of fumarate are not used as a diagnostic of this condition because fumarate can be rapidly converted to malate. Subsequently, malate can be transported into the mitochondrial matrix and enter the TCA cycle.

D Oxaloacetate does contribute indirectly to the urea cycle because it is the precursor for aspartate through a transamination reaction. Aspartate subsequently enters the urea cycle and combines with citrulline to form argininosuccinate. In OTC deficiency, the levels of citrulline are not sufficient for this reaction to occur. The levels of oxaloacetate are not used as a diagnostic of OTC deficiency because oxaloacetate will instead be used in the TCA cycle or for synthesis of glucose.

E OTC deficiency will lead to a block in production of urea.

45. B N-Acetylcysteine (NAC) is used to treat acetaminophen poisoning. The major toxic metabolite of acetaminophen is N-acetyl- p-benzoquinone imine (NAPQI), which is normally detoxified in the liver by glutathione. An overdose of acetaminophen depletes glutathione levels. Glutathione is a tripeptide consisting of glutamate, cysteine, and glycine. Cysteine and glycine are linked through a normal peptide bond, whereas glutamate is linked to cysteine by linkage between the amino group

of cysteine and the side-chain γ-carboxylate group of glutamate. Administration of NAC facilitates synthesis of glutathione because the level of cysteine is the limiting factor in glutathione production.

A N-Acetylglutamate (NAG) is the allosteric activator of carbamoyl phosphate synthetase I, the enzyme that catalyzes the rate-limiting step in the urea cycle. NAG is synthesized in the liver from glutamate and acetyl CoA by the enzyme N-acetylglutamate synthase. It does not play a role in glutathione synthesis.

C S-Adenosylmethionine (SAM) is an important coenzyme that serves as the methyl group donor in a variety of methyl transfer reactions. Synthesis of glutathione does not require SAM.

D 5-Hydroxytryptophan (5HT) is produced from tryptophan by the enzyme tryptophan 5-monooxygenase (tryptophan hydroxylase). The product 5HT can then be converted to serotonin through a decarboxylation reaction.

E Dihydroxyphenylalanine (DOPA) is produced from tyrosine by the enzyme tyrosine hydroxylase. DOPA can be converted to dopamine, which in successive steps can be converted to norepinephrine and epinephrine.

46. A Because hydroxybutyrylcarnitine accumulates, the enzyme handling short-chain hydroxyacyl CoA in β-oxidation must be defective. Note that the carnitine palmitoyltransferase II reaction is reversed because β-oxidation is blocked. This provides a way for the body to excrete some fatty acid derivatives via the kidney.

B C Because a metabolite of short-chain fatty acid oxidation accumulates, the problem is not with enzymes that metabolize medium chain or long chain fatty acids.

D A defect in this enzyme would block the oxidation of all fatty acids by preventing the reoxidation of $FADH_2$.

E If fatty acyl CoA synthetase were defective, no acyl CoA and hence no carnitine derivatives could be formed.

47. B AMN can be caused when a female carries one X chromosome with a defect in the ABCD transporter. In males, who have only one X chromosome (hemizygote), this defect usually would cause ALD, although the less severe AMN is observed too, even in the family of patients with ALD (i.e., same mutation).

A Adrenoleukodystrophy is an X-linked recessive disease; affected females have not been described.

C Adult Refsum disease is caused by a deficiency of phytanic acid metabolism; if phytanic acid (found in ruminant and fish fat from the breakdown of chlorophyll) is withheld, patients can develop normally.

D Rhizomelic chondrodysplasia punctata is a defect in plasmalogen biosynthesis due to defects in key enzymes (GNPAT or AGPS). Characteristic are the short proximal long bones (the opposite is mesomelic, in which the distal long bones are affected), coupled with severe psychomotor retardation, cataract, and facial dysmorphism. Patients do not survive for more than 1 year.

E Cerebrohepatorenal syndrome (Zellweger syndrome) is caused by the total absence of peroxisomes. Patients die during the first half-year of life.

IV

48. **B** The signs and laboratory values are consistent with Niemann-Pick disease. This is a lysosomal storage disease caused by the inability to break down sphingomyelin to ceramide by removal of phosphocholine. Characteristic of both Niemann-Pick and Gaucher disease is the presence of sphingolipid-laden macrophages (foam cells), but in morbus Gaucher there is bone involvement. Hepatosplenomegaly and mental retardation (which can be diagnosed only from age 6 onward) are other signs in both diseases.

A α-Galactosidase is defective in Fabry disease, which presents with problems of bone, skin, heart, and eye, but not with hepatomegaly or foam cells.

C Hexosaminidase B deficiency (together with that of hexosaminidase A) is associated with Sandhoff disease.

D Hexosaminidase A deficiency causes Tay-Sachs disease; patients have mental retardation with seizures and paralysis. Destruction of ganglion cells in the retina leads to a cherry red macula surrounded by a white field. There is neither hepatosplenomegaly nor foam cells.

E Glucocerebrosidae deficiency causes Gauchers disease; macrophages become engorged with glucocerebroside. The "crumpled tissue paper" appearance of the cytoplasm of the Gaucher cell is caused by enlarged elongated lysosomes filled with glucocerebroside.

49. **B** The physical problems this child is having can be directly attributed to the PDA. Because prostaglandins, specifically PGE_1, are responsible for the patency of the ductus arteriosus, the use of medications that block their synthesis can be used to help achieve a faster closure. Indomethacin is a nonselective inhibitor of both the COX-1 and COX-2 enzymes that mediate key steps in prostaglandin synthesis, and it has been successfully used to treat PDA in preterm infants.

A Propranolol is a sympatholytic antagonist of both the $β_1$- and $β_2$-adrenergic receptors. Sympatholytic agents inhibit the postganglionic functioning of the sympathetic nervous system and are often used as antihypertensive and antianxiety medications. Hypertension in neonates is rare, although it is much more common in high-risk infants. Although hypertension can be a long-term symptom of a PDA, treatment with β-blockers is not warranted at this time.

C Alprostadil is the pharmaceutical name for prostaglandin E_1; therefore, giving this medication would only exacerbate the problem. It is, however, an important perinatal medication. Alprostadil is often used when a child is born with a congenital heart defect that does not allow for proper circulation to occur, such as in transposition of the great arteries. In this case, the only way for oxygenated and deoxygenated blood to mix is through the ductus arteriosus. PGE_1 can be given to delay closure of the ductus arteriosus until the defect can be corrected surgically.

D Spironolactone is a steroidal antimineralocorticoid agent, commonly used as a diuretic and antihypertensive agent. It is in the class of drugs known as potassium-sparing diuretics and acts as a competitive antagonist of the aldosterone receptor. Although the use of diuretic agents may be expected to help relieve the developing pulmonary edema, their use is not indicated for this condition and will not address the primary issue.

E Albuterol is a short-acting agonist of the $β_2$-adrenergic receptor typically used to alleviate bronchospasm in diseases such as asthma and chronic obstructive pulmonary disease (COPD). It works by relaxing the smooth muscles that surround the airway, causing dilation of the bronchi and bronchioles. Although the patient shows signs of dyspnea, it is not caused by a constricted airway; therefore, albuterol would not be of much use.

50. **D** The physician is looking for antibodies raised against cardiolipin, an important component of the inner mitochondrial membrane. Cardiolipin is a type of glycerophospholipid, more specifically a diphosphatidylglycerol lipid, and therefore contains glycerol, phosphate, and fatty acid chains (typically 18-carbon alkyl chains with two unsaturated bonds). The autoimmune disorder in which antibodies are raised against cardiolipin is called antiphospholipid syndrome, or Hughes syndrome. Other common complications of this disorder are thrombosis, thromboembolism, stillbirth, preterm delivery, and preeclampsia. It is most commonly treated with anticoagulants such as low-dose aspirin and heparin.

A The components glycerol, phosphate, fatty acid, and amino alcohol make up a subclass of glycerophospholipids called phosphatidyl alcohols. Included in this group are phosphatidylcholine, phosphatidylserine, and phosphatidylethanolamine. These phospholipids are the most abundant in human tissues, comprising a majority of cellular membranes.

B The components ceramide, phosphate, and choline make up the lipid sphingomyelin. This lipid represents roughly 85% of all sphingolipids found in the body. It is typically found in cell membranes, especially in many neural axons where it is a major component of the myelin sheath.

C The components glycerol, phosphate, and a fatty acid comprise the basic structure of phosphatidic acid, a vital cellular lipid that acts as the biosynthetic precursor of all acylglycerol derivatives found in the cell.

51. **A** Cushing disease is caused by an adrenocorticotropic hormone (ACTH)–producing adenoma of the pituitary. It is the most common cause of Cushing syndrome and marked by elevated cortisol concentrations because of an overactive adrenal gland. Other forms of secondary hypercortisolism (Cushing syndrome) include corticotropin-releasing hormone (CRH)–producing tumors in the hypothalamus and tumors in the adrenal cortex. Sometimes tumors in other organs start producing ACTH (ectopic Cushing syndrome, e.g., in small-cell lung cancer). Temporarily increased cortisol may also be found during stress.

B In urea cycle disorders, the levels of glutamine and alanine in the plasma will increase. Glutamine and alanine are the major amino acids used to transport nitrogen from extrahepatic tissues to the liver. Alanine is transported from muscle tissue to the liver through the glucose-alanine cycle. Glutamine is formed in extrahepatic tissues by the activity of glutamine synthetase.

C In Cushing disease, the concentration of cortisol would be increased because of an ACTH-producing adenoma of the pituitary. Increased androgens would be found, for example, in congenital adrenal hyperplasia, caused by deficient 21-hydroxylase or 11β-hydroxylase. This prevents the synthesis of cortisol and aldosterone from progesterone; instead, progesterone is converted into androgens.

D In Cushing disease, the concentration of cortisol would be increased because of an ACTH-producing adenoma of the pituitary. Decreased dihydrotestosterone (DHT) is seen in 5α-reductase isoform 2 deficiency. Because DHT is required for virilization in utero, newborns with this condition present with ambiguous genitalia. Virilization occurs around puberty, when extragonadal isoform 1 produces enough DHT ("penis-at-12 syndrome").

E Phenylketonuria (PKU) is caused by a block in the hydroxylation of phenylalanine by phenylalanine hydroxylase, leading to high serum phenylalanine levels.

52. A Primary hyperparathyroidism is often the outcome of the excessive secretion of parathyroid hormone (PTH) from the parathyroid gland. Such secretions are often caused by a parathyroid adenoma and can lead to the observed hypercalcemia, hypophosphatemia and low vitamin D$_3$. Elevated PTH leads to the activation of osteoclasts, which begin to break down bone; weakening the bones as fibrous tissue replaces their calcified support structures. The patient's polyuria and polydipsia are secondary to the hypercalcemia.

B Sarcoidosis is a systemic, granulomatous inflammatory disease that can affect virtually every organ system in the body. Common symptoms are vague and can include general fatigue unchanged by sleep, aches and pains, arthritis, and shortness of breath, among others. Vitamin D production is often dysregulated, causing symptoms of hypervitaminosis D (with accompanying low D$_3$ levels). Calcium levels are typically not affected because normal compensation mechanisms are in place (i.e., a normally functioning parathyroid gland).

C Paget disease is a chronic, localized bone disorder that affects bone remodeling (i.e., it typically affects only one or a few bones). It results from overactive osteoclast activity, followed by compensatory osteoblast activity. New pagetic bone is structurally disordered, often leading to an increase in deformities and fractures. Its absolute etiology is unknown, although evidence of genetic factors and viral infection exist. Although no two people are affected the same way by this disease, common symptoms include arthritis, bone pain, elevated alkaline phosphatase, and hypercalcemia if many bones are affected. A diagnosis of Paget disease in this patient is not likely due to the constellation of other symptoms that are not associated with the disease.

D Rhabdomyolysis is a serious condition stemming from the breakdown of muscle fiber as a result of direct or indirect muscle injury. Upon breakdown, the muscle fibers release their contents into the bloodstream, leading to complications such as kidney failure and in some cases death. Symptoms of rhabdomyolysis can include muscle pain, tenderness, or weakness. An imbalance in electrolytes may also result from the release of muscle components into the bloodstream, leading to headache, nausea, vomiting, arrhythmias, and, in extreme cases, coma.

53. B Lovastatin is a member of a family of compounds called statins that inhibit the first committed step in cholesterol synthesis catalyzed by HMG CoA reductase. Statins are often prescribed together with lifestyle changes and cholestyramine to lower serum cholesterol levels.

A Lovastatin does not inhibit β-oxidation. The regulated step of β-oxidation is the carnitine shuttle, which transports activated fatty acids into mitochondria and its enzyme, carnitine

palmitoyl transferase-I (CPT-I) is inhibited by malonyl CoA (the substrate for fatty acid synthesis).

C Fats stored in adipocytes are mobilized by the combined action of various lipases including hormone sensitive lipase, none of which is inhibited by lovastatin.

D Ketone bodies have several uses in our body. Apart from being the precursors of cholesterol and other isoprenoids, they also serve as an energy source for heart, skeletal muscle, and, in starvation, even the brain. Inhibiting their synthesis would probably lead to increased glucose consumption and hence a life-threatening hypoglycemia. Lovastatin does not inhibit acetyl CoA acetyltransferase.

E Pyruvate dehydrogenase is the link between glycolysis and the TCA cycle. It is inhibited by NADH and acetyl CoA (endproduct inhibition) and by enzymatic phosphorylation.

54. D The patient is suffering from homozygous familial hypercholesterolemia (FH), caused by an autosomal dominant mutation in the gene for the LDL receptor. In ~ 50% of these cases, no receptor is detectable at all. In the remaining cases, the receptor is either nonglycosylated, cannot interact with LDL, or cannot bind clathrin. Heterozygous patients have a 25-fold increased risk of suffering an acute myocardial infarction (AMI) before age 60, whereas homozygous patients suffer from severe atherosclerosis from childhood on. Cholesterol levels in these patients are elevated not only because cholesterol from the liver is not removed in the periphery but also because, in the absence of usable cholesterol from the liver, peripheral cells start to make their own cholesterol (lack of inhibition of HMG CoA reductase). Treatment is by reducing dietary cholesterol, blocking cholesterol synthesis with statins, and lowering enterohepatic cycling of bile acids with cholestyramine, and by monthly removal of plasma LDL on a dextran sulfate matrix (Liposorber, Kaneka Pharma America).

A Chylomicrons are elevated in familial hyperlipoproteinemia type I, caused by mutations in the gene for lipoprotein lipase. The autosomal recessive disease results in attacks of abdominal pain, hepatosplenomegaly, eruptive xanthomas, and milky plasma. Hyperlipidemia vanishes after a few days of fat-free diet. There may be some haplo-insufficiency, but patients in that case are only mildly affected.

B Hyperalphalipoproteinemia (excess production of "good" cholesterol, HDL, caused by a defect in the genes for either cholesterol ester transfer protein or apolipoprotein C-III). Clinically, these individuals impress with the absence of atherosclerosis and longer life expectancy. Mental and physical development is normal. Inheritance seems to be autosomal dominant with significant environmental influence.

C There are no diseases that affect specifically only IDL. However, type III hyperlipoproteinemia, caused by a mutation in the gene for apolipoprotein E, affects the uptake of chylomicrons, VLDL, IDL, and LDL. This leads to an increased risk for atherosclerosis; however, this also requires the presence of (unknown) environmental risk factors. There are several other, rarer, proteins whose mutations have a similar effect.

E There are no diseases that affect specifically only VLDL. However, type III hyperlipoproteinemia, caused by a mutation in the gene for apolipoprotein E, affects the uptake of chylomicrons, VLDL, IDL, and LDL. This leads to an increased risk for atherosclerosis; however, this also requires the presence of (unknown) environmental risk factors. There are several other, rarer, proteins whose mutations have a similar effect.

55. E UMP, made by decarboxylation of orotate, is the precursor for the other pyrimidine nucleotides.

A CMP cannot be converted to other pyrimidines.

B dUMP can only contribute to the production of deoxyuridine and deoxythymidine nucleotides.

C Glycine is utilized in the synthesis of purines. It plays no role in the synthesis of pyrimidines.

D IMP is a purine, and all other purines are derived from it. It plays no role in pyrimidine synthesis.

56. C Methotrexate competitively inhibits dihydrofolate reductase and thereby prevents the activation of folate to THF. Methyl group transfer in pyrimidine anabolism occurs at the monophosphate level; that is, dUMP is converted to deoxythymidine monophosphate (dTMP) by thymidylate synthase, using N^5, N^{10}-methylene-THF.

A N^{10}-formyl-THF is utilized in purine synthesis. In pyrimidine synthesis, N^5, N^{10}-methylene-THF adds a methylene group to dUMP (not UMP), to generate dTMP.

B N^5-methyl-THF is a substrate of methionine synthase, not nucleotide synthesis. In pyrimidine synthesis, a methyl group is added from N^5, N^{10}-methylene-THF to dUMP (not dUDP) to generate dTMP.

D N^5-formimino-THF is produced by histidine degradation and has to be converted to N^5, N^{10}-methylene-THF before it is added to dUMP (not dUDP) to make dTMP.

E N^5, N^{10}-methenyl-THF is an intermediate of the conversion of N^5-formimino-THF from His degradation to N^5, N^{10}-methylene-THF. The latter adds a methyl group to dUMP to generate dTMP.

57. C The downstream intermediate in the pathway from uroporphyrinogen III to heme is protoporphyrin IX. All the other intermediates are upstream of uroporphyrinogen III. A δ-ALA is the first intermediate of heme synthesis. Because the reactions leading from δ-ALA to uroporphyrinogen III are irreversible, there is no way for labeled nitrogen from uroporphyrinogen III to appear in δ-ALA. Note that the breakdown of heme leads to derivatives of bilirubin that are excreted in either feces or urine, so no recycling is possible.

B PBG is the second intermediate of heme synthesis. Because the reactions leading from PBG to uroporphyrinogen III are irreversible, there is no way for labeled nitrogen from uroporphyrinogen III to appear in PBG. Note that the breakdown of heme leads to derivatives of bilirubin that are excreted in either feces or urine, so no recycling is possible.

D Uroporphyrinogen I is not an intermediate of heme synthesis; rather, it is produced instead of uroporphyrinogen III by a spontaneous reaction from hydroxymethylbilane if uroporphyrinogen III synthase is defective, as in congenital erythropoietic porphyria. Because the reaction leading from hydroxymethylbilane to uroporphyrinogen III is irreversible, there is no way for labeled nitrogen form uroporphyrinogen III to appear in uroporphyrinogen I.

E Hydroxymethylbilane is the precursor of uroporphyrinogen III, and the reaction is irreversible. Therefore, labeled nitrogen from uroporphyrinogen III cannot appear in hydroxymethylbilane.

58. A The observed unconjugated or indirect hyperbilirubinemia points to the inability of the liver to conjugate bilirubin which can be caused by UDP-glucuronyl transferase deficiency, hepatitis or cirrhosis. Given the patient's age (4 weeks), it is probably Crigler-Najjar II with some remaining transferase activity. The patient might benefit from phenobarbital treatment to induce the expression of the glucuronyl transferase.

B Physiological neonatal jaundice leads to elevated serum levels of unconjugated bilirubin that occurs in the first days of life when the liver is too immature to handle all of the bilirubin delivered to it. The indirect hyperbirubinemia in newborns usually resolves by 2 weeks after birth. Persistence of high levels of unconjugated serum bilirubin in the patient excludes this diagnosis.

C Dubin-Johnson syndrome is caused by a defective protein, which transports conjugated (direct) bilirubin from the hepatocytes into the bile. This would lead to some direct hyperbilirubinemia but usually does not require treatment. Dark pigments are observed in histological examination of hepatocytes.

D Rotor (-Manahan-Florentin) syndrome is also caused by a defective protein, which transports conjugated (direct) bilirubin from the hepatocytes into the bile. This would lead to some (direct) hyperbilirubinemia but usually does not require treatment. This disease has only been described in the Philippines; it is similar to Dubin-Johnson syndrome except that no dark pigment is formed in the liver.

E A hemolytic crisis caused by G6PD deficiency, for instance, would also cause elevated levels of unconjugated bilirubin, as bilirubin is delivered to the liver at a rate faster than what the liver can handle. However, the CBC would be abnormal because G6PD deficiency is associated with hemolytic anemia.

59. D (C) Epinephrine in muscle acts via β-adrenergic receptors that activate adenylyl cyclase and hence stimulate the production of cyclic adenosine monophosphate (cAMP). The latter then triggers a protein kinase–mediated cascade that eventually phosphorylates phosphorylase, converting it to the active form, leading to glycogenolysis.

A Muscle has β-adrenergic receptors that use cAMP as a second messenger and not Ca_2^+. Also, cytosolic Ca_2^+ levels are usually elevated under conditions of muscle glycogenolysis.

B Aldolase is an enzyme in glycolysis, the breakdown of glucose. It does not influence the rate of glycogenolysis, the breakdown of glycogen.

E Glycogenolysis is the breakdown of glycogen to glucose 1-phosphate via the action of glycogen phosphorylase-a. Glycogen synthase catalyzes the opposite process, the synthesis of glycogen.

60. C Glycogen synthase is inactivated through phosphorylation by protein kinase A (PKA) in response to glucagon (in liver) and epinephrine (in liver and muscle).

A Epinephrine, a "fight or flight" hormone released by adrenal gland during periods of acute stress promotes the degradation of glycogen in both liver and muscle tissue via a signaling cascade (ie., GPCR→Gs activation→Adenylyl cyclase (AC) activation→↑c AMP →Protein kinase A (PKA) activation. Glycogen phosphorylase is activated through phosphorylation by phosphorylase kinase in response to glucagon (in liver) and epinephrine (in liver and muscle).

IV

B Phosphorylase kinase is activated via phosphorylation by PKA. In turn, phosphorylase kinase phosphorylates and thereby activates glycogen phosphorylase, stimulating the breakdown of glycogen to glucose in liver (under the influence of glucagon) and in both liver and muscle (under the influence of epinephrine). Remember that glucagon and epinephrine mobilize nutrients by phosphorylation, whereas insulin activates storage by dephosphorylation.

D Branching enzyme activity is allosterically regulated by substances that indicate high energy (e.g., citrate, adenosine triphosphate [ATP], glucose 6-phosphate), but not by modification. Because branch points are introduced every 12 to 14 glucose residues in glycogen by transfer of a growing chain from an α–1,4 to an α–1,6 position, regulation can occur at the glycogen synthase level.

E Debranching enzyme activity in cells is much lower than the activity of the glycogen phosphorylase. Because the debranching enzyme works only on the limit branch left by glycogen phosphorylase, separate regulation of the activity of debranching enzyme is not necessary.

61. D The products of the oxidative branch include two NADPH plus the removal of carbon-1 of the glucose 6-phosphate as CO_2, yielding the pentose, ribulose 5-phosphate. The latter, a ketose, is then converted to the corresponding aldose, ribose 5-phosphate. Thus, the main products of the pentose-phosphate pathway in mammals are NADPH as the reducing agent for both anabolic processes and protection against reactive oxygen species, and ribose 5-phosphate for nucleotide biosynthesis.

A The oxidative pentose phosphate pathway reduces $NADP^+$, not NAD^+. The resulting $NADPH + H^+$ is required to protect cells against reactive oxygen species and as a reducing agent in some biosynthetic pathways. The other products are ribulose 5-phosphate and CO_2.

B Oxidation of glucose in the pentose phosphate pathway leads to reduced $NADP^+$, that is, $NADPH + H^+$. Remember that oxidation and reduction are always coupled (redox reaction). The other products are ribulose 5-phosphate and CO_2.

C Xylulose 5-phosphate is an intermediate in the nonoxidative part of the pentose phosphate pathway, which is used to convert 2 six-carbon sugars (fructose 6-phosphate) and 1 three-carbon sugar (glyceraldehyde 3-phosphate) into 3 five-carbon sugars (ribulose 5-phosphate). Ribose 5-phosphate is required for nucleotide synthesis.

E The oxidative portion of the pentose phosphate pathway produces two NADPH, one CO_2, and one ribulose 5-phosphate.

62. E NADPH is required by glutathione reductase to convert oxidized glutathione (GSSG) back to two reduced glutathiones (2 GSH). It is generated by the oxidative branch of the pentose phosphate pathway, the only source of NADPH in erythrocytes. Glucose 6-phosphate dehydrogenase is the first reaction in this pathway. In the absence of NADPH, red cells are subject to the formation of Heinz bodies and hemolysis, resulting in Heinz body anemia. An anemic crisis in these patients is usually the result of ingestion of compounds that lead to increased formation of reactive oxygen species. Those can be contained in food (e.g., fava beans), or they may be prescribed as pharmaceuticals (e.g., the three As: antipyretics, antibiotics, and antimalarials).

A Mammalian erythrocytes (red blood cells) do not have mitochondria.

B Glucose 6-phosphate dehydrogenase is not an enzyme of glycolysis, but of the pentose phosphate pathway. Indeed, since glycolysis is the only energy source of erythrocytes, its failure would be incompatible with life.

C Animal cells have high K^+ and low Na^+ inside, compared with the surrounding medium. K^+ therefore cannot leak into these cells.

D Heterozygotes with glucose 6-phosphate dehydrogenase deficiency (i.e., females, as glucose 6-phosphate dehydrogenase is encoded on the X chromosome) are resistant to the blood-stage of malaria because their erythrocytes are affected just enough to bring their average life span below the time required for the malaria parasite to complete its development in them. That is the reason that this mutation is endemic in malaria-infested regions.

63. E Tyrosine and threonine are known to have both glucogenic and ketogenic properties because they are both degraded to products that can be used in the synthesis of glucose and ketone bodies. The glucogenic products of tyrosine and threonine are fumarate and succinyl coenzyme A (succinyl CoA), respectively. The ketogenic products are acetyl CoA and acetoacetate.

A Glutamate and glutamine are glucogenic amino acids, as they are metabolized to α-ketoglutarate. Entry of α-ketoglutarate into the tricarboxylic acid (TCA) cycle leads to the production of oxaloacetate, which can then enter into the gluconeogenesis pathway.

B Methionine and cysteine are glucogenic amino acids, as they are metabolized to products that can be used to synthesize glucose. Methionine and cysteine are metabolized to succinyl CoA and pyruvate, respectively.

C Aspartate and asparagine are glucogenic amino acids, as they are metabolized to oxaloacetate, which is used to synthesize glucose.

D Leucine and lysine are classified as ketogenic amino acids only because they are metabolized to acetyl CoA and acetoacetate. These metabolites are used to synthesize ketone bodies, but not glucose.

64. B Dopamine is derived from dihydroxphenylalanine (dopa), an oxidative product of tyrosine. Tyrosine, in turn, is formed from phenylalanine.

A Cysteine is a sulfur-containing amino acid. It is a conditionally essential amino acid, provided there are sufficient levels of methionine in the diet. Cysteine is important in the synthesis of glutathione, an important detoxifying agent.

C Glycine is a nonessential amino acid. It serves as a precursor in purine and heme biosyntheses.

D Tryptophan is a precursor in the synthesis of serotonin, another neurohormone. It is not involved in the synthesis of dopamine.

E Glutamate plays a central role in amino acid metabolism, via transamination and oxidative deamination reactions. In addition to this role, glutamate is the precursor to γ-aminobutyric acid (GABA), an inhibitory neurotransmitter. It does not play a role in dopamine synthesis.

65. **A** This is a correct statement regarding the glucose-alanine cycle. Alanine, produced from the transamination of pyruvate, serves as the major transporter of amino groups from skeletal muscle to the liver.

B This is an incorrect statement regarding the glucose-alanine cycle. As stated above, upon transamination of alanine to pyruvate, the pyruvate is utilized in gluconeogenesis in the liver to produce glucose. The glucose, in turn, is transported through the blood to the working muscle, rather than being used to synthesize glycogen.

C This is an incorrect statement regarding the glucose-alanine cycle. Muscle cannot release glucose into the bloodstream because it lacks glucose 6-phosphatase.

D This is an incorrect statement regarding the glucose-alanine cycle. The reversible transamination reaction that interconverts alanine and pyruvate are the key reactions in the glucose-alanine cycle. In the working muscle, pyruvate is preferentially transaminated to alanine, whereas the reverse reaction occurs preferentially in the liver, with alanine being deaminated to form pyruvate.

E This is an incorrect statement regarding the glucose-alanine cycle. In the muscle, pyruvate is converted to alanine. The alanine is transported through the blood to the liver, where it is converted to pyruvate. In the liver, the pyruvate is used in gluconeogenesis, and the resulting glucose is transported to the skeletal muscle to be used in glycolysis.

66. **C** The TCA cycle intermediate, oxaloacetate, can be diverted from the TCA cycle to initiate gluconeogenesis. The carbon atoms of other TCA cycle intermediates that are incorporated into oxaloacetate are also important in gluconeogenesis.

B Acetone is not used in the synthesis of glucose.

D, A Amino acids that can be converted to acetyl CoA and derivatives are referred to as ketogenic because they can be used in the synthesis of ketone bodies.

E Many amino acids undergo transamination reactions to form their corresponding α-keto acids. However, not all of the α-keto acids are converted to compounds that can be used in gluconeogenesis.

67. **B** Proteins that have been covalently linked to a chain of at least four ubiquitin polypeptides are targeted to the proteasome for degradation. Proteins targeted for degradation include those that are damaged or that function at only specific times during the cell cycle.

A Phosphorylation of mannose residues targets N-glycosylated proteins in the golgi complex to lysosomes but not for degradation.

C Trypsin and chymotrypsin are used in the degradation of dietary protein. They are released from the pancreas and transported to the intestines as inactive zymogens. Following activation of these endopeptidases in the intestines, trypsin and chymotrypsin cleave peptide bonds at specific sites. They do not function in the intracellular degradation of proteins.

D Pepsin is released from gastric chief cells in the stomach as the inactive zymogen pepsinogen. Pepsinogen is autoactivated to pepsin in the low pH of the stomach following food intake. Pepsin cleaves dietary protein at specific sites, with the resulting peptide fragments being released into the intestines for further proteolysis by the activated pancreatic proteases. Pepsin does not function in the intracellular degradation of proteins.

E The ribosome functions in protein synthesis, not degradation.

68. **D** (A, B, C, E) ACC exists in two forms–as an inactive phosphorylated dimer and as an active dephosphorylated multimer. Insulin activates ACC by stimulating its dephosphorylation by a protein phosphatase. If the cell has a high enough energy status (indicated by elevated citrate and glucose concentrations), dephosphorylated ACC will oligomerize into the active form. This multimer (with ~10 monomers) moves more slowly through the gel. The band is therefore closer to the start of the gel. In the presence of the drug, the enzyme is converted to a phosphorylated inactive dimer which moves further into the gel during electrophoresis. Because the drug prevents the activation of ACC by insulin, it will inhibit fatty acid synthesis. Drugs that inhibit fatty acid synthesis are used not only for preventing weight gain, but also as anticancer drugs. Cancer cells divide frequently and require phospholipids to make the new membranes.

69. **E** Carboxylases use biotin as a cofactor, which is formed by the reaction of biotin with the ε-amino group of a lysine residue in the enzyme.

A ACC coverts acetyl CoA into malonyl CoA.

B, D ACC exists as a dephosphorylated active multimer and a phosphorylated inactive dimer. Insulin and citrate promote multimer formation and glucagon promotes dimer formation.

C Fatty acid synthase complex, an enzyme for the synthesis of palmitic acid in the body is a multi enzyme complex and not ACC.

70. **B** The phospholipids in question are phosphatidylcholine (PC, outer membrane) and phosphatidylethanolamine (PE, inner membrane). PE is converted to PC by transferring three methyl groups from SAM onto the primary amino group, forming a quaternary amino group.

A Methylene-THF is used to transfer a methyl group onto dUMP to make dTMP for DNA synthesis. It is not involved in the remodeling of phospholipids.

C PAPS is an activated form of sulfuric acid that can form sulfate esters with xenobiotics for increased water solubility and with the sugar residues in mucopolysaccharides to increase water- and ion-binding capacity. PAPS is not involved in phospholipid remodeling.

D Acyl CoA is the activated form of fatty acids. Although it is used to make the phosphatidic acid from which both phospholipids in question are derived, it is not involved in the remodeling of phospholipids.

E UDP-GlcNAc is the activated form of GlcNAc and used to transfer this sugar derivative onto the sugar trees of glycoproteins and mucopolysaccharides. It is not involved in phospholipid remodeling.

71. **E** Thromboxane A_2 (TXA_2) is produced by platelets; it stimulates their aggregation and the constriction of blood vessels and bronchi via a decrease of intracellular cAMP. If the balance between TXA_2 and PGI_2 production is disturbed, pathologies will develop. Examples include vascular complications in diabetes mellitus type 2 and atherosclerosis.

A PGD_2 is involved in bronchoconstriction and sleep induction. Antagonists are used to treat asthma.

B PGE_2 is involved in bronchodilation and vasodilation (similar to PGI_2). In the stomach, it inhibits H^+ secretion and stimulates the production of mucins. It stimulates lipolysis in adipose tissue, and it is involved in inflammation and fever. Its antagonist is $PGF_2\alpha$, not PGI_2.

C PGF_2^{α} is the antagonist of PGE_2, not PGI_2. It leads to constriction of the blood vessels, bronchi, and uterus (the latter is clinically used).

D PGH_2 is an intermediate in the synthetic pathway of eicosanoids.

72. D β-Oxidation of an odd-chain fatty acid gives several molecules of acetyl CoA and one molecule of propionyl CoA. Propionyl CoA. Isocitrate is also produced from the amino acids threonine, methionine, valine, and isoleucine. It is converted into succinyl CoA via propionyl CoA carboxylase (biotin-dependent), methylmalonyl CoA racemase, and methylmalonyl CoA mutase (vitamin B_{12}–dependent). Failure of the latter reaction leads to methylmalonic aciduria, either because of the inability to activate vitamin B_{12} (which manifests as acidosis and anemia) or because of a defect in the enzyme itself (which manifests as acidosis only). A defect in propionyl CoA carboxylase leads to propionic acidemia with ketoacidosis and protein intolerance.

A β-Oxidation of an odd-chain fatty acid gives several molecules of acetyl CoA and one molecule of propionyl CoA. Citrate is produced from acetyl CoA, not from propionyl CoA.

B β-Oxidation of an odd-chain fatty acid gives several molecules of acetyl CoA and one molecule of propionyl CoA. Isocitrate is produced from acetyl CoA via citrate, not from propionyl CoA.

C β-Oxidation of an odd-chain fatty acid gives several molecules of acetyl CoA and one molecule of propionyl CoA. α-Ketoglutarate is a metabolite formed from acetyl CoA via citrate and isocitrate.

E β-Oxidation of an odd-chain fatty acid gives several molecules of acetyl CoA and one molecule of propionyl CoA. Malate is eventually formed from both, but it is the entry point of neither.

73. B Of all the fatty acids mentioned, only α-linolenic acid is essential. It shares this property with linoleic acid (C18:2). Even the much-hyped ω-3-fatty acids DHA and EPA can be made from α-linolenic acid, even though a moderate supply in the diet is probably helpful. Chylomicron retention (Anderson) disease is usually caused by the inability to make SAR1B protein. Thus, dietary fats accumulate in the enterocytes rather than being exported as chylomicrons. SAR1B is also expressed in liver, muscle, and brain, explaining the hepatomegaly, cardiomyopathy, and ophthalmic and neuronal problems in these patients, all of which are usually mild if essential fatty acids and fat-soluble vitamins are supplied.

A Oleic acid is not an essential fatty acid; it can be made from palmitic acid by elongation to stearate and desaturation. Only α-linolenic and linoleic acid (C18:2) are essential in humans.

C Palmitic acid is not an essential fatty acid. It is the first endogenous fatty acid synthesized by fatty acid synthase.

D DHA is not an essential fatty acid; it can be made from α-linolenic acid by successive elongation and desaturation. Only α-linolenic and linoleic acid (C18:2) are essential in humans.

E EPA is not an essential fatty acid; it can be made from α-linolenic acid by successive elongation and desaturation. Only α-linolenic and linoleic acid (C18:2) are essential in humans.

74. C The presence of sulfur and nitrogen in a bile acid indicates that compound #3 must be a taurine conjugate. Taurolithocholic acid has five oxygens per sulfur (i.e., a hydroxyl group in position 3, a keto group in position 24, and three oxygens attached to sulfur).

A Glycocholic acid does not contain sulfur.

B Taurocholic has three hydroxyl groups, a keto group, and three oxygens attached to sulfur, for a total of seven oxygens per sulfur.

D Lithocholic acid lacks nitrogen and sulfur.

E Chenodeoxycholic acid lacks nitrogen and sulfur.

75. A (B, C, D, E incorrect.) 21-Hydroxylase converts progesterone into deoxycorticosterone and 17-hydroxyprogesterone into 11-deoxycortisol. In an enzyme deficiency, the substrate (and its precursors) accumulates, whereas the product (and its metabolites) is deficient. Conversion of progesterone to adrenal androgens is also elevated.

76. D LPL is required to hydrolyze triacylglycerols of chylomicrons (dietary fat) and very low-density lipoproteins (VLDL containing fat synthesized by the liver). LPL is synthesized by adipocytes and muscle cells and secreted into the interstitium. From there it diffuses into the capillaries, where it is bound to the heparan sulfate on the luminal surface of the enterocyte. This leads to dimerization and activation of the enzyme.

A Diet contains lipids. In the intestines, lipids are digested by pancreatic lipase, which requires colipase and cholic acid for activity.

B Mobilization of fat in adipose tissue during starvation or exercise is performed by the concerted action of adipose tissue triglyceride lipase, hormone-sensitive lipase, and monoacylglycerol lipase.

C Lipoproteins occur in the blood plasma, not the cytoplasm.

E Familial Hypercholesterolemia results from defects in functional LDL receptors.

77. C During an overnight fast, the triacylglycerols are packaged and released from the liver into the bloodstream as VLDL.

E Bile salt is ionized form of bile acid stored in the gall bladder and released with bile into the intestine. It aids in lipid absorption. Fat-soluble vitamin absorption also requires functioning lipid absorption, including pancreatic lipase and bile salts from the liver. If either of these cannot reach the intestines (e.g., due to blockage of the common bile duct), no fat-soluble vitamins can be absorbed.

B HDL mediates reverse transfer of cholesterol and is triglyceride poor.

D After a fat rich meal, the triacylglycerols are mainly packaged and released from intestinal mucosal cells into lymphatic and then bloodstream as chylomicrons than after overnight fast.

A LDL are enriched in cholesterol and are main carriers of cholesterol than triglycerides in the blood. LDL is not released by the liver but is produced in circulation from the metabolism of VLDL.

78. D Accumulation of uroporphyrinogen points to a defect in uroporphyrinogen decarboxylase. Uroporphyrin can form by spontaneous oxidation, causing the urine's fluorescence and dark color. The disease has autosomal dominant inheritance, but with incomplete penetrance. Any liver damage, for example, caused by alcohol consumption, makes it worse. In a case like this, one would also expect pink fluorescence of the teeth when illuminated with a Wood lamp.

A PBGS porphyria (also known as Doss porphyria) affects the second step of heme synthesis, the conversion of δ-aminolevulinic acid (δ-ALA) to porphobilinogen (PBG). The accumulating δ-ALA causes acute porphyria with neurovisceral symptoms, rather than a chronic porphyria with cutaneous symptoms. PBG cannot be converted to a protoporphyrin by a spontaneous reaction; therefore, there will be no red, fluorescent urine, even after exposure to air and sunlight.

B Acute intermittent porphyria is caused by a deficiency of PBG desaminase, the enzyme that converts PBG, an individual five-membered ring to hydroxymethylbilane (a chain of five-membered rings). The accumulating PBG causes an acute porphyria with neurovisceral symptoms, rather than a chronic porphyria with cutaneous symptoms. PBG cannot be converted to a porphyrin by a spontaneous reaction; therefore, there will be no red, fluorescent urine, even after exposure to air and sunlight.

C Congenital erythropoietic porphyria is caused by a deficiency of uroporphyrinogen III synthase, the enzyme that converts hydroxymethylbilane into uroporphyrinogen III. The patient has elevated uroporphyrinogen levels in the urine, indicating that this enzyme is working. However, in feces, it is coproporphyrin I, rather than coproporphyrin III, that is slightly increased. This indicates that accumulating hydroxymethylbilane is converted to uroporphyrinogen I and coproporphyrinogen I spontaneously. Therefore, the block must be in uroporphyrinogen decarboxylase.

E Porphyria variegata is caused by a deficiency of protoporphyrinogen oxidase, which converts protoporphyrinogen IX into protoporphyrin IX. Therefore, in this disease protoporphyrinogen IX would accumulate rather than uroporphyrinogen I. Variegate porphyria also has a mixture of neurovisceral and cutaneous symptoms.

79. **A** Bilirubin is normally conjugated with two molecules of glucuronic acid to make it more water-soluble. In situations where the liver is unable to perform this reaction in a timely fashion, unconjugated bilirubin accumulates until the binding capacity of albumin is exceeded, and the bilirubin precipitates in skin, sclera (hallmarks of jaundice), and basal ganglia (a marker of kernicterus). The latter leads to severe brain damage. Unconjugated hyperbilirubinemia is seen in liver damage (cirrhosis, hepatitis, neonatal hyperbilirubinemia) or (together with conjugated bilirubin) when an unusually high amount of bilirubin is produced (e.g., in hemolytic disease of the newborn or hemolytic anemia).

B Excretion of bilirubin into the bile occurs only after conjugation.

C Unconjugated bilirubin is too tightly bound to albumin for it to be excreted by the kidneys. Urobilin (not bilirubin) is found in urine. It is produced when gut bacteria convert conjugated bilirubin into urobilinogen, which is taken up into the bloodstream and part of it delivered to kidneys. Urobilinogen gets further oxidized to urobilin in the bladder before excretion.

D Bilirubin is not water-soluble. Its polar groups form intramolecular hydrogen bonds and are therefore no longer able to form intermolecular bonds with surrounding water. Conjugation with glucuronic acid breaks the intramolecular interactions and adds the highly hydrophilic sugar acids.

E Bacteria can deconjugate bilirubin glucuronides but do not conjugate free bilirubin.

80. **C** The purine base is assembled on the 5-phosphoribosyl-1-pyrophosphate (PRPP) framework, building first the five-membered and then the six-membered ring. Closure of this second ring leads to IMP, which serves as the starting material to make GMP and AMP.

A Pyrimidine catabolism yields water soluble products not purine catabolism.

B Ribonucleotide reductase converts nucleoside diphosphates into deoxy nucleoside diiphosphates.

D OMP is an intermediate of pyrimidine, not purine, biosynthesis.

E The committed step in the *de novo* synthesis of pyrimidine nucleotides is catalyzed by carbamoyl phosphate synthetase II and not purine, biosynthesis.

81. **C** (A, B) In this metabolic situation, the liver will supply glucose from its glycogen stores into the bloodstream to keep blood glucose levels up against a high muscular demand. (Note that the depletion of liver glycogen stores, known by runners as "hitting the wall" occurs after ~30 km.) Protein kinase A (PKA) will be active as a consequence of high glucagon levels and will phosphorylate phosphorylase kinase into the active form. This, in turn, switches on glycogen phosphorylase by serine phosphorylation, ensuring the breakdown of glycogen to glucose 1-phosphate. Plasma insulin will be low, and hence also the activity of protein kinase B (PKB). Thus, GSK-3 will not be phosphorylated, but is subject to dephosphorylation by protein phosphatase 1. Consequently, GSK-3 will be in the active, unphosphorylated form. It will in turn phosphorylate, and hence inactivate, glycogen synthase. The high cyclic adenosine monophosphate (cAMP) concentrations in the liver cells will also allosterically activate glucose 6-phosphastase and release glucose from the cell.

D Debranching enzyme activity in cells is much lower than the activity of the glycogen phosphorylase. Because the debranching enzyme works only on the limit branch left by glycogen phosphorylase, separate regulation of the activity of debranching enzyme is not necessary.

82. **D** It is the job of the liver to maintain the blood glucose level. To do so, the liver will remove sugar from the blood after a meal and store it as glycogen. During fasting, the liver breaks down the glycogen. If the latter is insufficient, the liver also performs gluconeogenesis from amino acids (muscle protein) and glycerol (adipose tissue triglyceride). In addition, the liver (not muscle) regenerates glucose from the lactate that is produced. Muscle cannot regenerate glucose from lactate because this process requires ATP, which, under anaerobic conditions, could only be produced by converting sugar to lactate (i.e., via an energy-wasting cycle). Instead, either lactate itself or alanine is sent to the liver for processing.

A This is a correct statement because glucose can be synthesized from noncarbohydrate precursors such as amino acids or glycerol.

B This statement is correct because gluconeogenesis and glycolysis share many (but not all) steps that are easily reversible. The irreversible steps of glycolysis, however, have to be circumvented: pyruvate kinase (which produces one ATP) by pyruvate carboxylase and phosphoenolpyruvate carboxykinase (which uses one ATP and one guanosine triphosphate [GTP], respectively), phosphofructokinase by fructose 1,6-bisphosphatase (i.e., the ATP invested in the kinase reaction is not regenerated) and hexokinase by glucose 6-phosphatase. Thus, gluconeogenesis requires more energy-rich phosphates than glycolysis produces.

C This statement is correct because gluconeogenesis and glycolysis share many steps that are easily reversible, and they have to be reciprocally regulated to avoid wasting the cell's energy.

E This statement is correct because ATP is required for pyruvate carboxylase (one each for two pyruvates), pyruvate carboxykinase (one GTP each for two oxaloacetates; GTP and ATP are energetically equivalent), and phosphoglycerate kinase (one each for two phosphoglycerates).

83. B The debranching enzyme breaks down the 1 → 6 branch points of glycogen. A defective debranching enzyme leads to incomplete removal of the branch points. This results in cardiomegaly, muscle weakness, fasting hypoglycemia, dyslipidemia, and eventually cardiomyopathy (Cori disease, glycogenolysis, GSD III). It is managed by ketogenic diet (i.e., high-fat, low-carbohydrate, adequate protein diet) with frequent meals.

A A defective glycogen synthase (GSD 0) would result in a lack of glycogen, rather than its accumulation.

C Glucose 6-phosphatase is required in the liver to remove the phosphate group from glucose 6-phosphate, forming glucose that can be released into the bloodstream. Deficiency in this enzyme (GSD Ia, von Gierke disease) results in glycogen accumulation in liver (not in muscle), severe fasting hypoglycemia and hyperlipidemia, causing severe liver and kidney damage.

D Phosphoglucomutase interconverts glucose 1-phosphate and glucose 6-phosphate. A deficiency of this enzyme is exceedingly rare (one case described) and is associated with exercise intolerance up to rhabdomyolysis.

E UDP-glucose pyrophosphorylase converts glucose 1-phosphate to UDP-glucose for synthesis of glycogen and glycosylation. There are no known human diseases caused by defects in this enzyme.

84. C Statement 1 is correct because increased levels of glucose-6-phosphate can indeed spill into the hexose monophosphate shunt, leading to increased levels of purine synthesis, which will eventually call for increased levels of purine degradation, which will yield high levels of uric acid.

Statement 3 is correct. Increased levels of lactate result largely from chronic hypoglycemia, which activates fatty acid oxidation. Acetyl CoA resulting from fatty acid degradation inhibits pyruvate dehydrogenase. With pyruvate dehydrogenase inhibited, pyruvate levels increase, leading to lactate formation. Organic anions such as pyruvate and lactate get reabsorbed in the kidneys via the SLC5A8 transporter (via symport with Na +) and are then exchanged for urate via URAT1.

A, B, D, E Statement 2 is incorrect. Although the hexose monophosphate shunt does produce NADPH, NADPH is not consumed in the synthesis of the purines AMP and GMP. Statement 4 is incorrect. A high glucagon:insulin ratio does not increase the rate of purine degradation.

85. D The erythrocyte does not have mitochondria; its metabolism is largely limited to glycolysis and the pentose phosphate pathway. The products of the former are ATP and lactate; the latter produces NADPH plus intermediates of glycolysis (glyceraldehyde 3-phosphate and fructose 6-phosphate). NADPH is used to regenerate reduced glutathione (GSH) via the reaction $GSSG + NADPH + H^+ \rightleftharpoons 2\ GSH + NADP^+$ and protect the erythrocyte from oxidative damage. A lack of NADPH (e.g., in glucose 6-phosphate dehydrogenase deficiency) leads to Heinz body anemia.

A Pyruvate kinase catalyzes the reaction: phosphoenolpyruvate $+$ ADP $\rightarrow$ pyruvate $+$ ATP. This reaction does not produce any reducing equivalents.

B GAPDH catalyzes the reaction: $GAP + P_{i\ +\ NAD+} \rightleftharpoons$ 1,3-bisphosphoglycerate $+$ NADH $+$ H^+. NADH cannot be used to protect cells from oxidative damage; this requires NADPH.

C LDH catalyzes the reaction: pyruvate $+$ NADH $+$ $H^+ \rightleftharpoons$ lactate $+$ NAD$^+$. It is required during anaerobic glycolysis to regenerate NAD$^+$. Even if it were running in reverse, the resulting NADH could not be used to protect cells from oxidative damage; this requires NADPH.

E Glucose 6-phosphate isomerase converts glucose 6-phosphate to fructose 6-phosphate in glycolysis. No reducing equivalents are produced in this reaction.

86. B (C) Ammonium ion (NH_4^+) generated from the deamination of glutamate or glutamine is condensed with bicarbonate to generate carbamoyl phosphate in the mitochondria. This ligation reaction is catalyzed by carbamoyl phosphate synthetase I (CPS-I). CPS-I activity is absolutely dependent on the allosteric activator, N-acetyl glutamate (NAG). NAG is produced by NAG synthase also located in the mitochondria. A genetic defect in N-acetyl glutamate (NAG) synthase will have the same effect as a defect in CPS-I and lead to hyperammonemia.

A A genetic defect in ornithine transcarbomylase, another mitochondrial enzyme of urea cycle may lead to orotic aciduria and hyperammonemia.

D A genetic defect in argininoosuccinate synthetase, a cytosolic enzyme of urea cycle may lead to citrullinemia and hyperammonemia.

E A genetic defect in argininoosuccinate lyase, another cytosolic enzyme of urea cycle may lead to arginosuccinic aciduria and hyperammonemia.

87. B The cofactor for transaminases is pyridoxal phosphate, which is derived from pyridoxine (vitamin B_6). Pyridoxal phosphate is covalently bound to the active site of aminotransferases. The cofactor acts as an intermediate acceptor of the amino group, forming pyridoxamine phosphate. In the reverse reaction, pyridoxamine phosphate reforms pyridoxal phosphate upon transfer of the amino group to an α-keto acid substrate.

A Niacin (vitamin B_3) is a precursor in the synthesis of nicotinamide adenine dinucleotide. NAD$^+$/NADH and the phosphory-

IV

lated NADP+/NADPH redox pairs are used primarily as cofactors in oxidation-reduction reactions. Transamination reactions do not involve a change in redox state and thus do not require these cofactors.

C Flavin adenine dinucleotide (FAD) and flavin mononucleotide (FMN) function as cofactors in oxidation-reduction reactions.

D Phosphorylated forms of thiamine include thiamine pyrophosphate (TPP). TPP is an important cofactor for enzymes in the TCA cycle, including pyruvate dehydrogenase and α-ketoglutarate dehydrogenase. In both of these reactions, the substrates are decarboxylated and conjugated with CoA.

E Vitamin B_{12} is a cofactor for enzymes that catalyze two notable reactions: the conversion of homocysteine to methionine (by homocysteine methyltransferase), in which N^5-methyl-THF is converted to THF, and the conversion of methylmalonyl CoA to succinyl CoA (by methylmalonyl CoA mutase).

88. A Defective oxidative decarboxylation of the α-keto acids that are produced from the branched-chain amino acids (isoleucine, leucine, and valine) is the cause of maple syrup urine disease. This defective metabolic step leads to the accumulation of the branched-chain keto acid by-products in blood and urine. The mixture of these ketones in urine has the odor of maple syrup. The treatment for maple syrup urine disease is to restrict dietary intake of the essential branched-chain amino acids. A significant challenge of this treatment is to provide sufficient amounts of these amino acids for protein synthesis, while restricting metabolism of the amino acids to prevent accumulation of these amino acids and their α-keto acid byproducts.

B The first step in the catabolism of branched-chain amino acids is a transamination reaction to form their respective α-keto acids. This step is fully functional in maple syrup urine disease. It is the subsequent metabolic step, oxidative decarboxylation of the branched-chain α-keto acids, that is defective.

C Methionine is not involved in maple syrup urine disease.

D Amino acid hydroxylases include the aromatic amino acid hydroxylases, such as phenylalanine hydroxylase. A deficiency in phenylalanine hydroxylase results in phenylketonuria (PKU), which leads to an accumulation of phenylalanine and its α-keto acid by-products. Analogous to the treatment for maple syrup urine disease, PKU is treated by restricting the dietary intake of the essential amino acid phenylalanine.

E Fixation of amino groups to carbon skeletons may occur through transamination reactions. However, maple syrup urine disease occurs through a defect in the decarboxylation of the α-keto acid carbon skeleton of the branched-chain amino acids. Removal of the amino group is not affected in this metabolic disorder.

89. E Methylmalonyl CoA is converted to succinyl CoA by methylmalonyl CoA mutase that requires B_{12} (Cobalamin). Methylmalonyl CoA is formed in the metabolic pathway of several amino acids, including isoleucine, valine, threonine, and methionine (as well as from the degradation of odd-chain fatty acids). A deficiency in methylmalonyl CoA mutase results in the metabolic disorder methylmalonic acidemia.

A Argininosuccinate is hydrolyzed to fumarate and arginine in a single step in the urea cycle. This reaction is catalyzed by argininosuccinate lyase and doesnot require B_{12}.

B Cystathionine β-synthase catalyzes the formation of cystathionine. Cystathionine β-synthase requires pyridoxal phosphate (derived from pyridoxine, B_6). A deficiency in cystathionine β-synthase results in homocystinuria.

C Phenylalanine to tyrosine conversion reaction requires tetrahydrobiopterin and not B_{12}.

D In the urea cycle, citrulline combines with aspartate to form argininosuccinate and doesnot require B_{12}.

90. C (A, B, D, E) At 20 cm aging tube length, the major fatty acid produced is capric acid (C10:0). To make this compound, fatty acid synthase uses one molecule of acetyl CoA, four molecules of malonyl CoA, and eight molecules of NADPH.

91. A (B, C, D, E) Acetylsalicylic acid (aspirin) is an irreversible inhibitor of cyclo oxygenase enzyme and covalently modifies the enzyme's protein structure by acetylating a serine residue in the active site. Aspirin inactivates cyclooxygenase-1 (COX-1) and thus prevents the synthesis of prostaglandins. At the same time, it switches cyclooxygenase-2 (COX-2) activity from making (proinflammatory) prostaglandins from ω-6 fatty acids to (antiinflammatory) resolvins and protectins from ω-3 fatty acids. The latter effect is not shown by other nonsteroidal antiinflammatory drugs (NSAIDs).

92. A (D) Cortisol is a hormone of stress. The transcription of PEP carboxykinase is induced by cortisol. It initiates the conversion of long-term energy stores (protein and fat) into more easily accessible short-term stores (glucose, glycogen). It also counteracts insulin to keep blood [glucose] high for use in an emergency (hence the observed insulin resistance marked by high blood glucose despite high insulin levels). The ineffectiveness of insulin and the overproduction of cortisol lead to reduced glucose tolerance, i.e., high blood glucose concentrations after dietary glucose uptake. Anything that leads to relaxation can be used to reduce the inappropriate cortisol production (e.g., music, massage, laughing, crying, moderate exercise, and sexual activity).

B, C, E Insulin is not overproduced in stressful situations; its production in the pancreas is controlled strictly by blood [glucose]. It is the response of peripheral tissues to insulin that may be reduced in chronic stress.

93. C In diabetes mellitus type 1, fatty acid wasting is seen. Fatty acid synthesis occurs in the fed state, which is signaled by insulin.

A Plasma ketone bodies are increased in diabetes mellitus type 1, where a life-threatening ketoacidosis can occur if the patient is not treated with regular insulin.

B Although blood levels of glucose are increased in type 1 diabetics, the insulin deficiency in their tissues leads to a lack of glucose and hence increased gluconeogenesis.

D Brain's utilization of ketone bodies is normally limited by the rate at which these compounds cross the blood–brain barrier. This rate increases when the ketone body concentration increases (as seen in both diabetes mellitus 1 and starvation).

E Although blood levels of glucose are increased in type 1 diabetics, the insulin deficiency in their tissues leads to a lack of glucose and hence increased gluconeogenesis. The starting materials for gluconeogenesis are amino acids from body protein and glycerol from fat.

IV

94. C Alcohol is treated by the liver as a xenobiotic and removed as rapidly as possible. Oxidation of alcohol leads to reducing equivalents (NADH) and acetyl CoA. If the energy contained in these molecules is not required, ketone bodies and fatty acids will be synthesized. This "high-energy" state will also reduce the catabolism of other nutrients: citrate inhibits phosphofructokinase-1 (PFK-1), and malonyl CoA inhibits the carnitine shuttle. Gluconeogenesis is blocked by the high NADH:NAD$^+$ ratio. (If liver glycogen stores are depleted, hypoglycemia is possible.)

A LDL is used to transport triglycerides and cholesterol from the liver to peripheral tissues. Although excessive alcohol consumption will lead to a rise in LDL, this is a consequence rather than the cause of increased fatty acid synthesis.

B HDL ("good cholesterol") is required to return lipids and cholesterol from the peripheral tissues to the liver. Its production is not stimulated by alcohol.

D The carnitine shuttle is required to transport medium- and long-chain fatty acids into mitochondria; it is the rate-limiting step in their degradation. Stimulation of the carnitine shuttle would therefore increase fatty acid breakdown and reduce plasma lipids.

E Acetyl CoA carboxylase is the rate-limiting enzyme in fatty acid synthesis. Its inhibition would therefore reduce plasma lipids.

95. B Although metabolites of steroid hormones are excreted (as well as a little cholesterol itself), bile acids are the major end product of cholesterol metabolism. About 10 g/d of bile acids are secreted into bile, but 9.4 g/d are reabsorbed and undergo enterohepatic circulation. Cholestyramine (polystyrene resin with attached quaternary amino groups) binds bile acids in the gut and prevents their reabsorption. This causes increased conversion of cholesterol into bile acids and hence lowered serum cholesterol levels.

A Bilirubin is produced from heme, not cholesterol.

C Bile pigments is produced from heme, not cholesterol.

D Cholesterol esters are made from cholesterol and acyl CoA in the intestine and the liver and then packed into chylomicrons and LDL, respectively. The cholesterol esters are less soluble in membranes than cholesterol itself and therefore safer to transport and store. The cholesterol content of membranes needs to be tightly controlled. Cholesterol esters are not excreted into bile.

E LDL is a product of VLDL via IDL in circulation. It transports lipid and cholesterol to peripheral tissues. It is not excreted into bile.

96. C 7-Dehydrocholesterol is the 5,7-diene that is cleaved between carbon 9 and carbon 10 by UV light to form cholecalciferol (vitamin D$_3$). Further UV exposure would lead to inactive compounds such as lumisterol and tachysterol, which is why one cannot overdose on vitamin D by sun exposure. 7-Dehydrocholesterol is the immediate precursor of cholesterol and cholecalciferol.

A Squalene is an intermediate of the cholesterol synthesis pathway but cannot be converted to cholecalciferol by UV light.

B Lanosterol is an intermediate of the cholesterol synthesis pathway but cannot be converted to cholecalciferol by UV light.

D Calcitriol, the active form of vitamin D (a hormone), is not an intermediate of the cholesterol synthesis pathway and is produced from cholecalciferol (D$_3$, calciol, found in animals) or ergocalciferol (D$_2$, found in fungi and yeast).

E Farnesyl pyrophosphate is an intermediate of the cholesterol synthesis pathway but cannot be converted to cholecalciferol by UV light.

97. D (A) Cholestyramine is a polystyrene resin with quaternary groups attached. By binding bile acids, cholestyramine prevents their enterohepatic circulation and promotes their removal with feces. This causes the liver to convert more cholesterol to new bile salts which lowers the plasma cholesterol level. In order to meet the increased need for cholesterol, the liver upregulates receptor-mediated endocytosis of LDL.

B Cholestyramine binds to bile acids and is not involved in the inhibition of LPL.

C Cholestyramine binds to bile acids and is not involved in the inhibition of LCAT.

E Cholestyramine binds to bile acids and is not involved in intestinal cholesterol absorption.

98. C This is an incorrect statement. Carbamoyl phosphate synthetase I (CPS-I) is a mitochondrial enzyme that catalyzes the formation of carbomyl phosphate from NH4$^+$ and HCO$_3^-$ in the urea cycle. Its hyperactivity would not lead to hyperuricemia. In contrast, hyperuricemia would result from an increase in xanthine oxidase and PRPP synthetase activity, dehydration, and overconsumption of purines (secondary gout), or a decrease in HGPRT activity (Kelley-Seegmiller syndrome).

A This is a correct statement. The patient's condition could be caused by a reduction in the activity of HGPRT, that is, Kelley-Seegmiller syndrome. A complete deficiency of HGPRT would lead to Lesch-Nyhan syndrome, which is characterized by not only hyperuricemia, but also mental retardation, choreoathetosis (irregular and abnormal body movements), and the pathognomic self-destructive chewing down of lips, fingers, and toes. The neurologic problems are not treatable with allopurinol and therefore not caused by excess uric acid. Lesch-Nyhan syndrome is a rare disease in clinical practice, with a frequency of one in 380,000; however, in board exams its prevalence is near 100%.

B This is a correct statement. Exceptionally active xanthine oxidase would lead to hyperuricemia. However, this is very rare.

D This is a correct statement. An overactive PRPP synthetase that does not respond to feedback inhibition leads to hyperuricemia and gout; in severe cases, sensorineural deafness may also be found. The condition is X-linked recessive.

E This is a correct statement. Overconsumption of purine-rich foods (i.e., meat), especially in combination with alcohol, is the most common cause of hyperuricemia and gout. Males are more sensitive than females. Nucleic acids are degraded to nucleotides by nucleases in the intestine. If the diet is high in fiber (plant-based), most of the nucleotides are removed with feces. If the diet is meat-based, the chyme stays in the digestive tract longer, and nucleotides are dephosphorylated to nucleosides. These are absorbed by enterocytes and either transported to the bloodstream or directly converted to uric acid. This results in an acute gout attack a few hours after the nutritional indiscretion. Alcohol leads to blood acidification, which stimulates urate reabsorption in the kidney via the urate-anion transporter 1 (URAT1).

99. D McArdle disease is caused by a defect in muscle phosphorylase; the muscle cannot utilize stored glycogen, which accumulates in the muscle cells. During exercise, muscle suffers from fuel deprivation, which can lead to rhabdomyolysis with release of creatine kinase and myoglobin. The latter can lead to kidney damage. In this disease, only skeletal muscle, but not liver and heart, are affected (note that a normal heart does not store much glycogen). The prognosis is good; the patient should avoid strenuous exercise or have glucose beforehand.

A von Gierke disease is caused by a defect of glucose 6-phosphatase defect in the endoplasmic reticulum, which prevents the liver from releasing glucose to prevent hypoglycemia. This results in fasting hypoglycemia (which is treated with uncooked starch as an evening meal), hyperlipidemia, and gout. In this patient, the liver is not affected.

B Pompe disease is caused by a defect in acid maltase that breaks down glycogen in lysosomes. In effect, this is a lysosomal storage disease that leads to cardiomegaly and usually death before age 3.

C Cori disease is caused by a defect of the debranching enzyme in both muscle and liver. This leads to fasting hypoglycemia, hepatomegaly, cardiomyopathy, growth retardation, and progressive myopathy. Thus, liver, heart, and muscle would be affected. In this patient, only his muscles were affected.

E Hers disease is caused by a defect in liver phosphorylase; the liver cannot break down glycogen to keep the blood glucose constant. This leads to fasting hypoglycemia, ketosis and hepatomegaly. In this patient, the liver was not affected.

100. D Cystinuria is marked by renal calculi formed from the amino acid cystine, whose structure is composed of two cysteine amino acids linked via a disulfide bond. The sulfur atoms in cysteine are derived from methionine via homocysteine.

A Threonine is not a sulfur-containing amino acid, but rather contains a hydroxyl group in its side chain. It is not a precursor in the synthesis of cysteine.

B Although serine is a precursor to cysteine, it is not a sulfur-containing amino acid. Rather, its side chain contains a hydroxyl group, similar to threonine.

C Cysteine is not derived from tryptophan. Tryptophan is an aromatic amino acid with a nitrogen-containing indole group in its side chain, and it does not contain any sulfur atoms.

E Citrulline is not a precursor in the synthesis of cysteine. Citrulline is an intermediate in the urea cycle and is not a sulfur-containing amino acid.

101. B The key regulated enzyme of fatty acid synthesis is acetyl CoA carboxylase (ACC), the enzyme that converts acetyl CoA into malonyl CoA. ACC exists as a dephosphorylated active multimer and a phosphorylated inactive dimer. This interconversion between the phosphorylated and dephosphorylated forms is catalyzed by AMP–activated protein kinase (AMPK) and a Glu/Mg^{2+} –activated protein phosphatase. Therefore, inhibition of the latter (which would prevent the dephosphorylation and activation of ACC) is a suitable indicator of drug efficacy. AMPK is indirectly activated by glucagon and protein phosphatase appears to be activated by insulin. Insulin promotes multimer formation and glucagon promotes dimer formation.

A LCAD is involved in the β-oxidation of fatty acids, not their synthesis.

C Glycogen phosphorylase is involved in the degradation of glycogen. It is not a regulator of ACC.

D, E Adenylyl cyclase and PKA are generally active under hunger conditions when stored energy reserves are mobilized rather than created.

102. B Crigler-Najjar syndrome type I is a rare disorder of heme degradation (~0.6 to 1.0 per million live births) in which UDP glucuronyl transferase activity cannot be detected in hepatic tissue. Thus, the conversion of bilirubin to bilirubin diglucuronide (conjugated, or "direct" bilirubin) is impaired. Prior to the availability of phototherapy, these children died of kernicterus (i.e., bilirubin encephalopathy) or survived until early adulthood with clear neurologic impairment. Today, therapy includes transfusions in the immediate neonatal period, phototherapy, heme oxygenase inhibitors to reduce transient worsening of hyperbilirubinemia (although the effect decreases over time), oral calcium phosphate and carbonate to form complexes with bilirubin in the gut, and liver transplantation prior to the onset of brain damage and before phototherapy becomes ineffective at a later age. Crigler-Najjar syndrome type II is a milder form, with ~10% of normal glucuronyl transferase activity. These cases can be managed by induction of the transferase with barbitone. Even milder is Gilbert syndrome, where ~30% of the enzyme activity is preserved. About 3 to 10% of the population has this condition, which is benign and does not require treatment. Patients are diagnosed usually in the second decade of their life from a mild jaundice in stress situations (e.g., infections).

A Biliverdin is a blue-green compound and reasonably water-soluble because the methenyl groups between the rings prevent the formation of intramolecular hydrogen bonds. Increased levels may be seen in liver failure, but the main problem then will be bilirubin, not biliverdin. In mammals, biliverdin is reduced to bilirubin, whose hydrophobicity allows for transport across the placenta from fetal into the maternal circulation. Bilirubin also acts as an antioxidant.

C, D Urobilinogen, stercobilinogen, and stercobilin are produced from bilirubin by intestinal bacteria. Bilirubin is conjugated in the liver; the diglucuronide is excreted into bile and enters the intestine. Intestinal bacteria then perform the removal of the glucuronic acid residues and the oxidation to the brown pigment of stool, or stercobilin. The absence of this brown color can be seen when bile flow is restricted by a bile stone or a cancer of the pancreas head. The urine will then be darker, as more direct bilirubin is present.

E Heme is converted to biliverdin by ring opening (the only reaction in our body that produces carbon monoxide) and the removal of iron. This reaction is performed by heme oxygenase, which has an inducible (HMOX-1) and a constitutive (HMOX-2) isoform. HMOX-1 deficiency is a very rare disorder leading to growth retardation, hepatomegaly, asplenia (absent or abnormal spleen), and hemolytic anemia with hematuria.

103. A Homocystinuria occurs due to a block in the biosynthetic pathway from homocysteine to either cysteine or methionine. This results in a buildup of excess blood plasma levels of homocysteine, and in homocystinuria. As methionine is a precursor to homocysteine (through the production and utilization of S-adenosylmethionine), restricting the dietary levels of methionine reduces homocysteine levels. The B$_{12}$ sup-

IV

plement enhances the conversion of homocysteine to methionine because this reaction, which uses a folic acid derivative, is catalyzed by homocysteine methyltransferase. This enzyme requires cobalamin, a vitamin B_{12}–derived cofactor, for its activity. Supplementation with B_6 would lower homocysteine by increasing its conversion to cysteine. It is recommended that dietary restriction of methionine and vitamin supplements be used together in the treatment of homocystinuria. The levels of the essential amino acid methionine in the diet should be relatively low so that methionine will be used preferentially in protein synthesis, and the vitamin supplements will be useful in prompting the rapid conversion of homocysteine (once it is formed) to methionine and cysteine, to prevent the excess buildup of homocysteine.

B Cysteine is normally a conditionally essential amino acid. Because its biosynthesis is blocked in homocystinuria, it becomes an essential amino acid. Adequate levels of dietary cysteine are necessary in homocystinuria. The conversion of homocysteine to cysteine is blocked in homocystinuria by a genetic defect in cystathionine β-synthase.

C Glycine is a nonessential amino acid, and its levels are not affected by homocystinuria. Affecting the conversion of serine to glycine by serine hydroxymethyltransferase (which requires the vitamin B_6–derived coenzyme pyridoxal phosphate) will not alleviate the symptoms of homocystinuria.

D Serine is a nonessential amino acid, and although it is a precursor to cysteine, its levels are not affected by homocystinuria. Affecting the conversion of serine to glycine by serine hydroxymethyltransferase (which requires the vitamin B_6–derived coenzyme pyridoxal phosphate) will not affect the symptoms of homocystinuria.

E As stated above, cysteine becomes an essential amino acid in homocystinuria. Vitamin supplements will not affect the absorption of cystine, a dipeptide generated from the cross-linking of two cysteine molecules through their sulfhydryl-containing side chains. Faulty absorption of cystine occurs in cystinuria, which is a genetic defect in amino acid absorption. Cystinuria and homocystinuria are unrelated diseases.

104. C Mitochondrial TFP contains the enoyl CoA hydratase, hydroxyacyl CoA dehydrogenase, and thiolase for long-chain (C13–20) fatty acids. Its deficiency leads to liver degeneration to fetal liver failure in the worst cases. In addition, this disease in a fetus leads to acute fatty liver of pregnancy and HELLP syndrome (hemolysis, elevated liver enzymes, low platelets) in the mother. Intrauterine growth restriction often necessitates cesarean section. Prognosis for the baby depends on how many of the three reactions of the protein are affected and on the remaining activity. Three clinical forms are distinguished: neonatal (often ending in SIDS), infantile (Reye-syndrome like), and adolescent onset (skeletal myopathy). Prognosis for the mother depends mostly on timely diagnosis of the problem.

A Thiokinase is the enzyme required to activate fatty acids to acyl CoA for β-oxidation. Because the infant had acyl carnitines and 3-OH acylcarnitines in his blood, this enzyme activity appears to be normal.

B CPT-I is a protein on the outer mitochondrial membrane that converts acyl CoA into acyl carnitine for shuttling into mitochondria. In the blood of the patient, acyl carnitines were found; so, the transferase must have been functional. Note that in defects of β-oxidation, the excess acyl CoA derivatives that accumulate are converted back to the corresponding carnitine derivatives by CPT-II (on the inner mitochondrial matrix) for excretion; hence the appearance of 3-OH acylcarnitines in the blood of the patient.

D 3,5–2,4-dienoyl CoA isomerase converts 3,5,8-trienoyl CoA (a product of a minor side reaction of the β-oxidation of unsaturated fatty acids) into 2,4,8-trienoyl CoA for further metabolism. No deficiencies have been reported.

E Because long-chain 3-OH acylcarnitines were found in the blood of the patient, both the acyl CoA dehydrogenase and the enoyl CoA hydratase must be functional. Note that the accumulating 3-OH acyl CoA made the carnitine palmitoyltransferase II run in reverse, producing the corresponding carnitine derivatives. Those can be excreted with urine.

105. D The lack of LDL receptors will prevent receptor-mediated endocytosis of LDL in peripheral tissues. The resulting cellular cholesterol deficiency will increase the synthesis of cholesterol. Both the increased peripheral synthesis of cholesterol and the lack of its removal will increase serum cholesterol concentration and lead to familial hypercholesterolemia.

A If peripheral tissues cannot absorb LDL from the blood, its serum concentration must increase, not decrease.

B HMG CoA reductase catalyzes the committed step of cholesterol synthesis. Its activity is highly regulated. If cells are unable to meet their cholesterol needs by receptor-mediated endocytosis of LDL, the activity of this enzyme will increase.

C The main function of LDL is to transport cholesterol made in the liver to peripheral tissue. If LDL is not removed from the blood by receptor-mediated endocytosis in those tissues, then its concentration in the blood, and hence that of cholesterol, will increase. In addition, if cells are unable to meet their cholesterol needs by receptor-mediated endocytosis of LDL (or chylomicrons for dietary cholesterol), their own synthesis of cholesterol will increase, contributing to the problem.

E ACAT is present in the liver to make cholesterol esters for lipoproteins and in peripheral cells to convert excess cholesterol into hydrophobic esters that can be stored in droplets. The latter is necessary, as the cholesterol content of the cell membrane needs to be tightly controlled. If cells cannot obtain liver-produced cholesterol by receptor-mediated endocytosis of LDL, there will be little excess cholesterol to process in this manner.

106. C Under glucose deprived conditions, as in the above case, pyruvate is converted into oxaloacetate, which is then preferentially used to synthesize glucose.

A, B, D, E Fate of pyruvate under aerobic-fed conditions.

References

[1] Adhisivam B, Mahto D, Mahadevan S. Biotin responsive limb weakness. Indian Pediatr. 2007; 44(3):228–230

[2] Kale, Shah, Hallikerimath. J Indian Soc Pedod Prev Dent. 2008; 26:11–13

[3] Chalmers RA, Johnson M, Pallis C, Watts RW. Xanthinuria with myopathy (with some observations on the renal handling of oxypurines in the disease). Q J Med. 1969; 38(152):493–512

[4] Diez A, Gilsanz F, Martinez J, Pérez-Benavente S, Meza NW, Bautista JM. Life-threatening nonspherocytic hemolytic anemia in a patient with a null mutation in the PKLR gene and no compensatory PKM gene expression. Blood. 2005; 106(5):1851–1856

[5] Schröter W, Gahr M, Wonneberger B. [Pyrivate kinase deficiency. II. Biochemical studies (author's transl)]. Monatsschr Kinderheilkd. 1977; 125(7):713–719

[6] Bonetto G, Scarpa M, Carraro S, Baraldi E. A 3-year-old child with abdominal pain and fever. Eur Respir J. 2005; 26(5):974–977

[7] Sujatha J, Amithkumar IV, Lathaa B. Prenatal diagnosis of glycogen storage disorder type III. Indian Pediatr. 2010; 47(4):354–355

IV

Part V

Genetics and Cell Cycle

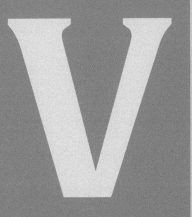

17 DNA Replication and Repair

17.1 Deoxyribonucleic Acid

Deoxyribonucleic acid (DNA) is found in the nucleus and mitochondria of animal cells. It encodes the genetic makeup of most organisms and is thus considered to be the central molecule of life. The central dogma of molecular biology states that genetic information flows from DNA to ribonucleic acid (RNA) to protein via three phases (▶ Fig. 17.1):

1. **Replication:** To ensure that the genetic information is transferred from parent to offspring, DNA is faithfully replicated in each subsequent generation of a cell or organism.
2. **Transcription:** The genetic information carried by DNA is transcribed into RNA.
3. **Translation:** The information carried in messenger RNA (mRNA) is translated into proteins, which carry out the work necessary to sustain life.

The central dogma of molecular biology holds true for most organisms, but exceptions are found in certain viruses (retroviruses) where the genetic material is RNA rather than DNA. Replication of this viral RNA in a host cell occurs via a DNA intermediate. One of the proteins encoded by the viral genome reverse transcriptase is an RNA-dependent DNA polymerase that reverse transcribes viral RNA into DNA, which then integrates into the host genome.

Although every cell in the body of a multicellular organism (e.g., humans) contains the complete genetic information carried by DNA, only a part of this code (particular genes) can be expressed (transcribed) in any given cell. There are some genes, however, that are expressed in all cells. Differences in gene expression patterns lead to the differentiation of certain cells into distinct organs and tissues capable of specialized function.

17.1.1 DNA Structure

DNA's structure consists of a polymer of deoxyribonucleotide units that have the following features:

- A 5′-phospho-2′-deoxyribose linked to one of the two purine bases (adenine and guanine) and two pyrimidine bases (cytosine and thymine) (▶ Fig. 17.2a).

- The deoxynucleotides are linked to each other via a phosphodiester bond formed between the 3′-hydroxyl group of one deoxynucleotide and the 5′-phosphate group of the succeeding deoxynucleotide (▶ Fig. 17.2b).

Foundations

Nucleic acid bases and nucleosides

Nucleic acid bases are the purines, adenine (Ade) and guanine (Gua), and the pyrimidines, thymine (Thy), uracil (Ura), and cytosine (Cyt). When these bases are attached to a sugar group (e.g., ribose or deoxyribose), they become nucleosides and are referred to as adenosine (A), guanosine (G), thymidine (T), uridine (U), and cytidine (C).

DNA Double Helix

DNA is typically in the form of a double helix that contains two strands of polydeoxyribonucleotides held together by noncovalent interactions between purine and pyrimidine bases. The two strands are arranged in opposite orientations (antiparallel), such that one strand runs in the 5′ → 3′ direction, whereas the other runs in the 3′ → 5′ direction (▶ Fig. 17.3a). Key features of double-stranded DNA are as follows:

1. **Complementary base pairing:** Whereas the sugar phosphates provide the structural backbone and give DNA its negative charge, the bases in the interior link the two strands together via base pairing between adenine and thymine, and a guanine base and cytosine (▶ Fig. 17.3a, b). As a result, when the sequence of nucleotides in one strand of DNA is known, the sequence of the complementary strand can be easily deduced.

- According to Chargaff's rule, in any given sample of double-stranded DNA, the number of adenines equals that of thymines, and the number of guanines equals that of cytosines.
- Complementary base pairing occurs by hydrogen bonding: adenine and thymine are linked by two hydrogen bonds, whereas three such bonds are present between guanine and cytosine (▶ Fig. 17.3a, b).
- Base pairing can be disrupted (melted) and DNA strands separated (denatured) by heat or alkaline pH. DNA that has

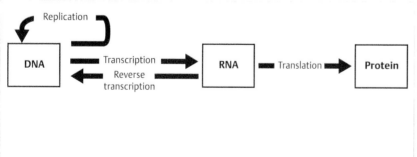

Fig. 17.1 Central dogma. Genetic information flows from DNA to RNA to protein. DNA carries the blueprint of the genetic map, and its replication ensures the transfer of genetic information from parent to offspring. The information carried in DNA is transcribed into RNA and finally translated into proteins. Only messenger RNA (mRNA), which represents a small fraction of a cell's total RNA population, is translated into protein. Some viruses with RNA genomes can transcribe RNA into DNA via a process known as reverse transcription.

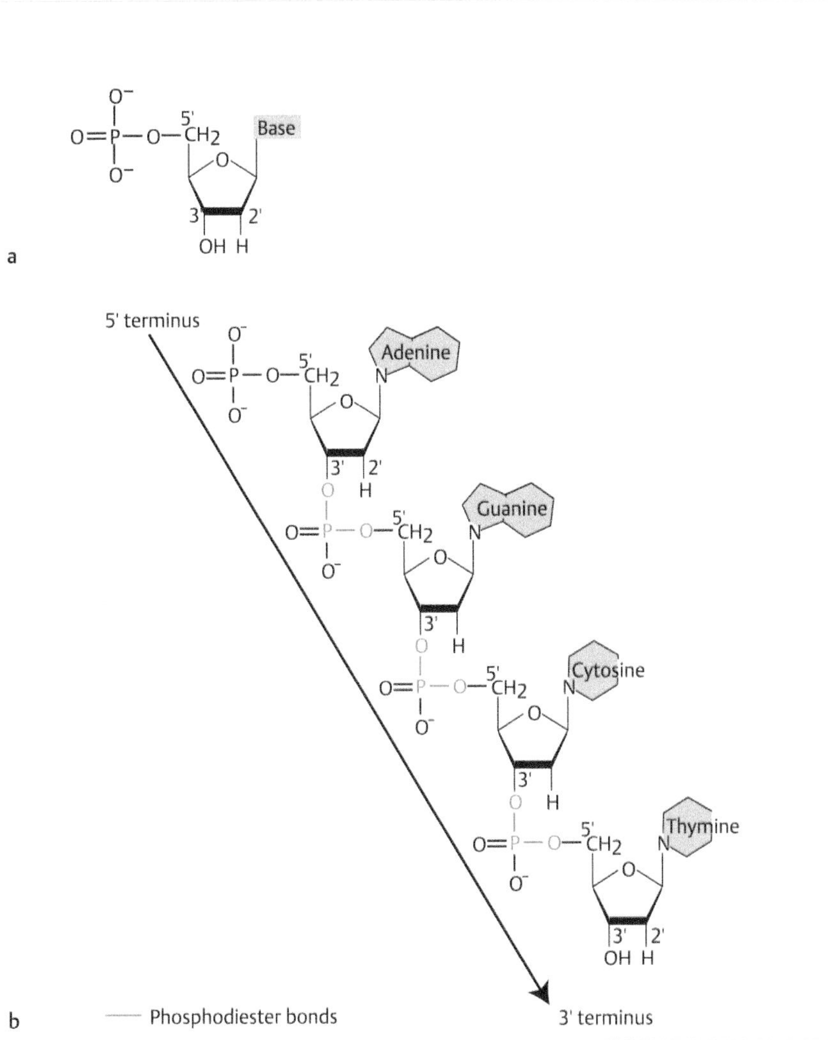

Fig. 17.2 DNA composition and structure. (a) An example of the general structure of a 5'-phospho-2'-deoxyribose unit. (b) DNA is typically represented in the 5' to 3' direction. The 3'-OH group of a nucleotide is connected in a phosphodiester linkage to the 5'-phosphate of the next nucleotide. Thus, every DNA strand has a phosphate residue at the 5' terminus and a free hydroxyl group at the 3' terminus.

V

a high GC content requires a higher melting temperature than DNA with a high AT content due to the greater number of hydrogen bonds in GC base pairs.

- Other noncovalent mechanisms such as base stacking, hydrophobic interactions, and van der Waals forces contribute to the stability of double-helical DNA.

2. **DNA forms:** The double helix is present mostly in the B form, although two other forms, the A form and the Z form, are known.

- In the B form of DNA (as described by Watson and Crick), the two strands wind about each other in a right-handed manner with 10 base pairs in a complete turn of the helix. Each turn contains a major and a minor groove (▶ Fig. 17.3b). Intercalation of DNA by planar molecules occurs at such grooves.
- Compared with the B form, the A form is more compact and contains 11 bases per turn in a right-handed helix. RNA-DNA hybrids assume the A form.
- The Z form is a left-handed helix containing only a single groove corresponding to the minor groove of the B form. The Z form is thinner and more elongated than the B form and occurs transiently in genes being actively transcribed.

17.1.2 DNA Packaging

If the DNA of a single human cell were stretched out in a single linear chain, it would extend nearly 2 m in length. Because the diameter of the nucleus of a typical human cell is $\sim 5 \times 10^{-8}$ m, DNA has to be compressed a great deal to fit into the nucleus yet still be accessible for replication.

The human genome is packaged into chromatin, a protein-DNA structure that can be relatively open and accessible or highly compact and inaccessible. Metaphase chromosomes are the most compact form of chromatin, as seen in the characteristic x-shaped structures examined in karyotyping. Each diploid human cell has 46 chromosomes. Compression of DNA involves the following:

1. **Chromatin formation:** DNA is supercoiled and wrapped around histones, which are abundant, small, basic (lysine- and arginine-rich) nuclear proteins (▶ Fig. 17.4a and ▶ Fig. 17.4b). The energy for the coiling of DNA is provided by electrostatic interactions between the positively charged histones and the negatively charged DNA.

- DNA is wrapped around pairs of four histones (H_2A, H_2B, H_3, and H_4) to produce a structure called a nucleosome that contains 147 base pairs of DNA.

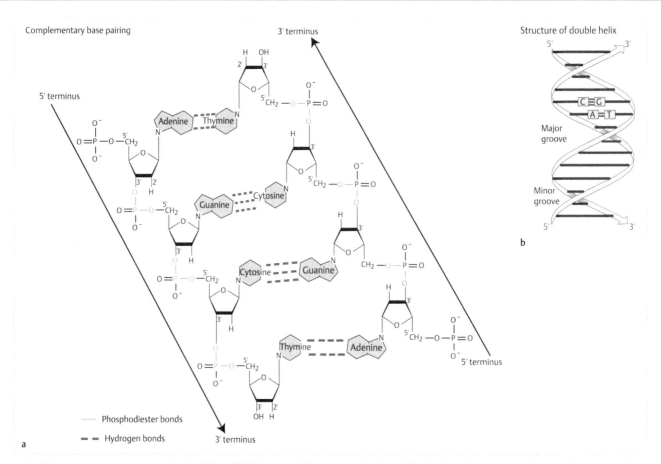

Complementary base pairing

5' terminus

3' terminus

Structure of double helix

Major groove

Minor groove

Phosphodiester bonds

Hydrogen bonds

3' terminus

a

b

Fig. 17.3 Complementary base pairing in DNA and DNA forms. (a) The two strands of the DNA double helix are arranged antiparallel to each other. Base pairing occurs between a purine (double-ring) and a pyrimidine (single-ring) by the formation of noncovalent hydrogen bonds. Adenine and thymine are linked by two hydrogen bonds, whereas guanine and cytosine are linked by three such bonds. **(b)** As a result, the two antiparallel strands typically create a B-form, right-handed double helix with the hydrophobic bases in the interior and the hydrophilic sugar phosphate backbone exposed to the aqueous exterior. The major and minor grooves of one complete turn of the helix are indicated.

The linker DNA between neighboring nucleosomes is approximately 50 base pairs long, of which about 20 base pairs are bound by histone H_1 (▶ Fig. 17.4c). This organization gives the DNA the look of beads on a string and is also known as 10-nm fiber.

- Nucleosomes are further packaged into 30-nm fibers (▶ Fig. 17.4d) and ultimately into chromatin (▶ Fig. 17.4e).
- During the nondividing phase of the cell cycle (i.e., the interphase: G_1, G_0, S, G_2), loosely packed, easily accessible chromatin (euchromatin, 10-nm fiber) is transcriptionally active, whereas highly condensed chromatin (heterochromatin, 30-nm fiber) is transcriptionally inactive.

2. **Metaphase chromosome formation:** The structure of chromatin is altered during the cell cycle such that it condenses into chromosomes when the cell divides—that is, during the mitotic (M) phase of the cell cycle (▶ Fig. 17.4f). This occurs to prevent physical damage to the DNA as the

chromosomes are separated and transferred to daughter cells.

Normal
Stem cells

There are two types of stem cells: embryonic and adult. Embryonic stem cells are derived from the embryo and are pluripotent (i.e., they are capable of becoming any cell type in the body). In contrast, adult stem cells are thought of as undifferentiated cells that generate cell types in the tissues in which they reside (e.g., hematopoietic stem cells will produce blood cells only). Stem cells differentiate into specialized cells in stages. These stages involve multiple factors that combine to produce epigenetic markers in the cell's DNA that restrict DNA expression and thus the type of cell that the stem cell will differentiate into. This DNA expression can be passed on to daughter cells through cell division, or daughter cells can retain their status as a stem cell and are therefore capable of long-term renewal.

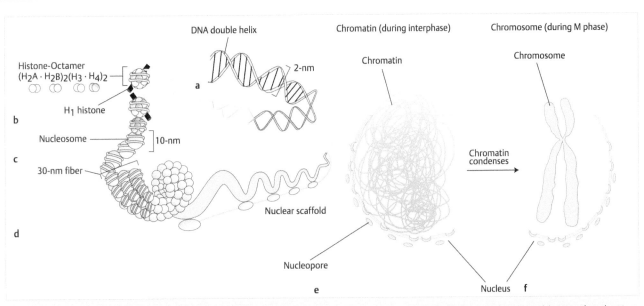

Fig. 17.4 Packaging of eukaryotic DNA. DNA double helix (**a**) wrapped around pairs of four histones (**b**) form nucleosomes (**c**). Note that the H_1 histone is attached to linker DNA. Nucleosomes are further packaged into 30-nm fibers (**d**) and ultimately into chromatin (**e**). When cells divide (M phase), chromatin condenses further into chromosomes (**f**).

Normal

Mosaicism

Mosaicism is a condition in which cells from an individual who has developed from a single fertilized egg have different genotypes. It is caused by an error in cell division early in embryonic life. The percentage of normal to abnormal cells determines the severity of the resulting disease, its symptoms, and its treatment. Individuals with a high percentage of mosaicism will present similarly to the typical (nonmosaic) form of the disease. It can be diagnosed by chromosomal or microarray analysis. Examples of this condition include mosaic Down syndrome, where there is trisomy of chromosome 21 in a percentage of cells; Klinefelter syndrome, where some cells are normal (46XY), and some have an extra X chromosome (47XXY); and Turner syndrome, where some cells are normal (46XX), and some have one X chromosome missing (45XO).

Normal

Uniparental disomy

Uniparental disomy (UPD) is a phenomenon when an individual receives two copies of a chromosome or part of a chromosome from one parent and no copies from the other parent. It may occur as a random error in meiosis during the formation of egg or sperm cells, or it may occur in early fetal development. It is often asymptomatic because the individual has at least one copy of each gene. However, if UPD occurs in imprinted genes, there may be delayed development, mental retardation, and other medical issues. The most well-known syndrome caused by UPD is Prader-Willi syndrome, which involves the imprinting gene on the long arm of chromosome 15. Dysfunction of this gene leads to uncontrolled eating and obesity.

Normal

Quantitation of DNA by its optical absorption

Nucleic acids absorb ultraviolet (UV) light maximally at a wavelength of 260 nm, whereas proteins absorb maximally at 280 nm and polysaccharides at 230 nm. Differences (sometimes subtle) in the absorption of UV light can distinguish among single- and double-stranded DNA, single-stranded RNA, proteins, and polysaccharides. Pure double-stranded DNA (50 µg/mL) has an absorbance (optical density [OD]) of 1.0, and the ratio of its absorbance at 260 nm to that at 280 nm (260/280 ratio) is 1.8. Single-stranded DNA has higher absorbance than double-stranded DNA, and this feature (hyperchromicity) is made use of to monitor the denaturation of DNA in response to temperature and to determine the melting point of a sample of DNA. Pure RNA (40 µg/mL) has an OD of 1.0 and a 260/280 ratio of 2.0.

Normal

Nomenclature of bases

The building block of DNA is a deoxyribonucleotide (▶ Fig. 17.2A), which is composed of 2-deoxyribose with a base (a purine or a pyrimidine) attached at the 1′ position and a phosphate attached at the 5′ position. Remember that a base plus a (deoxy)ribose yields a (deoxy)ribonucleoside (see **Fig. 16.1**). Thus, a (deoxy)ribonucleotide is a (deoxy)ribonucleoside with one to three phosphate groups.

V

Normal

RNA

While DNA is made of deoxyribonucleotides, the building block of RNA is a ribonucleotide (see **Fig. 16.1**). The 2'C of ribose in RNA has an OH group, while that in DNA does not.

Normal

Mitochondrial DNA

Human mitochondrial DNA (mtDNA) is a circular, double-stranded molecule of 16,569 bp that is maternally inherited. It is present in most cells at 100 to 10,000 copies/cell and replicates independently of chromosomal DNA. mtDNA codes for 2 ribosomal RNAs (rRNAs), 22 transfer RNAs (tRNAs), and 13 proteins that function in oxidative phosphorylation (see Chapter 11). There are virtually no redundant sequences in mtDNA and no repair mechanisms to detect and fix errors made during its replication. Thus, mutations can affect mitochondrial gene expression and oxidative phosphorylation. The inherited mitochondrial diseases (see ▸ Table 11.3), which are passed on only by mothers, include the following:

- Leber hereditary optic neuropathy (LHON): due to mutations in genes that encode the subunits of complex I. This results in a less active complex I, which presents as acute loss of vision in early adulthood.
- Myoclonic epilepsy and ragged red fibers (MERRF): caused by a mutation in the gene for the tRNA for lysine, which disrupts the synthesis of cytochrome-c oxidase. Patients with this condition display myoclonus (involuntary muscle spasms), myopathy (muscle disease), lack of coordinated muscle movement (ataxia), and seizures.
- Mitochondrial encephalopathy, lactic acidosis, and stroke-like activity (MELAS): due to a mutation in the tRNA gene for leucine, which disrupts the synthesis of complex I and cytochrome-c oxidase. Because this affects the nervous system and muscle functions, patients with this disorder present with a host of symptoms that include severe headaches, seizures, vomiting, and hemiparesis (muscle weakness on one side of the body).

Normal

Modes of inheritance

Autosomal dominant conditions are exhibited in individuals with just one copy of a mutant allele in one of the 22 autosomes (non-sex-determining chromosomes), the other copy being normal. It affects males and females equally, and any offspring have a 50% chance of inheriting the mutant allele. Autosomal recessive conditions manifest only when an individual has two copies of the mutant allele. If just one mutant allele is present, the individual is a carrier of the mutation but does not develop the associated condition. Females and males are affected equally. If two carriers of the mutation procreate, their child will have a 25% chance of being unaffected, a 25% chance of being affected, and a 50% chance of being an unaffected carrier. X-linked recessive conditions do not manifest in the presence of a normal copy of the gene.

Such conditions are always expressed in males because they have only one copy of each X chromosome. Women are rarely affected but can be if they have two copies of the mutant allele or random X-inactivation of the X chromosome with the normal allele during development leaves a relevant tissue vulnerable. Because the mutation is on the X chromosome, there is no father-to-son transmission, but there may be a transmission from father to daughter, or mother to daughter, or mother to son. X-linked dominant conditions dictate that, where the mutation is in the father's X chromosome, all of his daughters will express the condition (father-to-son transmission is not possible). Children of a mother with such condition have a 50% chance of inheriting the mutant allele.

Normal

Genomic imprinting

Normal Mendelian inheritance dictates that we receive an active copy of each gene from each of our parents. However, in genomic imprinting, certain genes are expressed only from the mother or the father. Imprinted alleles are silenced such that the gene is expressed only from the nonimprinted allele of the mother or father. Imprinting is an epigenetic process that involves the methylation and histone modification of egg or sperm cells during their formation while the genetic sequence is unchanged. Imprinting is duplicated in all somatic cells. Only a few genes are imprinted, but dysfunction of these genes leads to genetic defects such as Prader-Willi syndrome.

Normal

Heteroplasmy

Heteroplasmy is the presence of more than one type of mitochondrial DNA (some normal type and some mutant type) within a cell or organism. Symptoms usually do not develop until adulthood because these mutant mitochondrial alleles must undergo many cell divisions before a sufficient number of mutant copies are present to cause symptoms (e.g., in LHON, visual problems are not experienced until adulthood).

17.2 DNA Replication

High-fidelity (low-error) replication of DNA is necessary for the accurate transmission of genetic information from parent to off-spring. Errors in replication lead to mutations or changes in the genome and are associated with several clinical disorders. This section focuses on DNA replication in eukaryotic systems, which is somewhat more complex and involves more players than that in prokaryotic systems (▸ Table 17.1).

Eukaryotic DNA replication has the following features:

1. **DNA replication is semiconservative.** This involves the independent replication of each parental DNA strand so that the resulting two DNA molecules each contain one parental strand and one newly synthesized daughter strand (▸ Fig. 17.5a).

Table 17.1 Enzymes involved in eukaryotic DNA replication

Enzyme	Function
Helicase	Unwinds DNA helix
Topoisomerase	Relieves overwound supercoils (called DNA gyrase in bacteria)
Single-stranded DNA-binding protein	Binds the single-stranded DNA that has been separated
DNA polymerase α (in complex with primase)	Synthesizes RNA-DNA primer
DNA polymerases δ and ε	Synthesize new DNA chain in the 5′ →3′ direction (DNA Pol III in prokaryotes)
Flap endonuclease 1 (FEN1)	Removes RNA primers (DNA Pol I in prokaryotes)
DNA polymerase δ	Fills in gaps (DNA Pol I in prokaryotes)
DNA ligase	Seals nicks

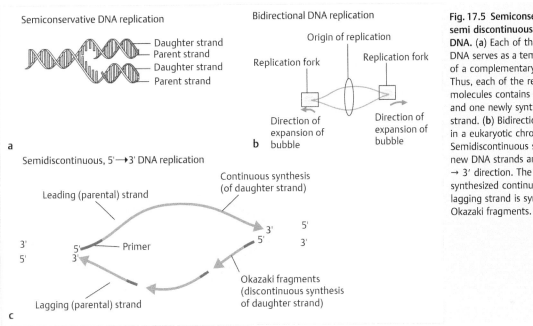

Fig. 17.5 Semiconservative, bidirectional, semi discontinuous 5′ → 3′ synthesis of DNA. (a) Each of the parental strands of DNA serves as a template for the synthesis of a complementary daughter strand. Thus, each of the replicated DNA molecules contains one parental strand and one newly synthesized daughter strand. **(b)** Bidirectional replication of DNA in a eukaryotic chromosome. **(c)** Semidiscontinuous synthesis of DNA. Both new DNA strands are synthesized in the 5′ → 3′ direction. The leading strand is synthesized continuously, whereas the lagging strand is synthesized in short Okazaki fragments.

2. **DNA replication is bidirectional.** Replication in eukaryotes starts at many points along the linear DNA double helix. These points are called origins of replication. The circular chromosome of prokaryotic organisms, however, contains a single origin of replication. Replication is preceded by unwinding and separation of the two strands, which forms a replication bubble. As DNA strands replicate, the bubbles expand in both directions simultaneously, giving rise to the bidirectional description of DNA replication (▶ Fig. 17.5b).
   - The two expanding ends of a replication bubble are called replication forks.

3. **DNA is synthesized in the 5′ →3′ direction and is semidiscontinuous.** The DNA strand being synthesized grows in the 5′ →3′ direction because each new nucleotide is successively added to the free 3′-OH of the preceding nucleotide. Given that the two strands of DNA are antiparallel, the synthesis of daughter strands occurs in a semidiscontinuous manner, as follows (▶ Fig. 17.5c):
   - Continuous synthesis: Synthesis of one daughter strand occurs continuously in the 5′ →3′ direction–that is, in the same direction as the movement of the replication fork. This strand is referred to as the leading strand.

   - Discontinuous synthesis: Synthesis of the other daughter strand occurs discontinuously in the 5′ →3′ direction in short fragments of ~ 200 nucleotides in eukaryotic cells (~ 1500 nucleotides in prokaryotic cells). These fragments are called Okazaki fragments. The discontinuous strand is referred to as the lagging strand.

17.2.1 Stages of DNA Replication

Parental DNA Strand Separation

The parental strands of the DNA helix must be separated in order for the synthesis of complementary daughter strands to occur. The separation of the two strands of the DNA is catalyzed and maintained through the cooperative efforts of three key DNA-binding proteins (▶ Fig. 17.6):

1. **Helicase:** This enzyme is found at replication forks where it unwinds the DNA helix by disrupting the hydrogen bonds between complementary nucleotides. As a consequence, though, the region of DNA ahead of the replication fork twists and becomes overwound and supercoiled.

2. **Topoisomerase:** This enzyme is bound to DNA just ahead of the replication fork. It relieves the overwound supercoils by

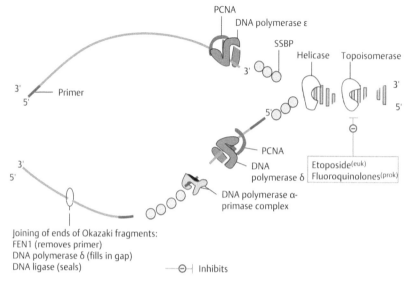

Fig. 17.6 **DNA synthesis requires a template and a primer.** (a) DNA polymerase cannot initiate DNA synthesis without a primer. It extends a preexisting oligonucleotide primer by adding new nucleotides to the 3'end. The template strand is read by the polymerase in the 3'→5' direction, but the complementary nucleotides are added to the primer in the 5'→3' direction. DNA polymerases are kept bound to the template with the aid of the sliding clamp proliferating cell nuclear antigen (PCNA). DNA helicase melts the hydrogen bonds and unwinds the DNA. Topoisomerases relieve the supercoils ahead of the replication fork. DNA polymerase a synthesizes the short RNA primers. Single-stranded DNA-binding proteins keep the template strands separated. SSBP, single-stranded DNA-binding proteins. (b) The polymerase uses free nucleotide triphosphates (NTPs) as substrates. The free 3'-OH group of the primer attacks the a-phosphate of the incoming NTP, thereby releasing the terminal two phosphates as pyrophosphate (PP$_i$). Subsequent hydrolysis of the pyrophosphate drives the reaction forward.

introducing and sealing nicks within the phosphate backbone.
- There are two types of topoisomerases. Type I enzymes cleave only one strand of DNA whereas type II topoisomerases cleave both strands to generate a staggered double-strand break. The topoisomerase II in bacteria is called DNA gyrase.
- Etoposide is an inhibitor of eukaryotic topoisomerase II, and fluoroquinolones such as ciprofoxacin and levofoxacin inhibit bacterial DNA gyrase.

3. **Single-stranded DNA-binding proteins (SSBPs):** These proteins bind to the separated DNA strands to prevent them from reannealing.

DNA Synthesis/Chain Elongation

Synthesis of new DNA chains is performed by a family of enzymes called DNA polymerases. DNA polymerase cannot initiate DNA synthesis by joining two individual deoxynucleotides. Rather, it extends from an RNA primer. Several enzymes are involved in this stage of replication (▶ Fig. 17.6).

1. **DNA polymerase α and primase:** Primase synthesizes an RNA primer that is 7 to 10 ribonucleotides long and is extended with ~ 25 nucleotides of DNA by DNA polymerase α. The resulting RNA-DNA primer is complementary to a segment of the parental strand. Synthesis of the leading strand requires a single primer, whereas that of the lagging strand requires a primer for each Okazaki fragment.
2. **DNA polymerases δ and ε:** These enzymes, in complex with the sliding clamp protein, proliferating cell nuclear antigen (PCNA), extend the primer by adding deoxyribonucleotides to the free 3′-OH of preceding nucleotides and elongates the new chain in the 5′ → 3′ direction. (In prokaryotes, elongation of a new DNA chain is performed by DNA polymerase III.)
- Individual nucleoside triphosphates act as substrates. During the formation of the phosphodiester bond, the two terminal phosphates are removed as pyrophosphate. The hydrolysis of pyrophosphate into inorganic phosphate provides the energy for the addition of each deoxynucleotide (▶ Fig. 17.6b).
- The choice of nucleotide to be added is determined by the sequence of the template strand, which is read by the polymerase in the 3′→5′ direction.
- The fidelity of DNA replication is extremely high, with an overall error rate of one in 440,000 nucleotides. Such fidelity is achieved by the ability of DNA polymerases (e.g., polymerase δ and polymerase ε) to proofread and correct any errors in base pairing. If an error is made, the polymerases use their built-in 3′→5′ exonuclease activity to excise the incorrect nucleotide and replace it with the correct one.
- PCNA keeps the polymerase associated with the template throughout the replication process.
- Polymerase ε appears to be involved in leading strand synthesis, whereas polymerase δ directs the synthesis of Okazaki fragments in the lagging strand.
- Nucleoside analogs such as arabinosylcytosine (AraC) inhibit chain elongation.
3. **DNA polymerase δ, FEN1, and DNA ligase:** DNA polymerase δ extends the RNA primers in the lagging strand in the 5′→3′

direction. When it reaches the next Okazaki fragment, it continues the extension, displacing the RNA primer as a flap. Flap endonuclease 1 (FEN1), either alone or in combination with another endonuclease, DNA2, removes the RNA primer. DNA ligase then seals the nick between adjacent Okazaki fragments. In prokaryotes, DNA polymerase I alone catalyzes the removal of the primer and fills in the resulting gap.
- Recent evidence suggests that the primary remover of RNA primers in mammalian cells is FEN1 rather than RNase H.

17.2.2 Telomeres and Telomerase

The ends of linear chromosomes in eukaryotes are capped and protected by special structures called telomeres. They are composed of thousands of hexameric repeats of the noncoding DNA sequence (TTAGGG), complexed to an array of proteins. Lagging strands of replicated telomeres undergo shortening after the removal of the last RNA primer from the 5′ ends during each successive cycle of cell division. The gap cannot be filled in due to the lack of a primer. Such shortening limits the number of times cells can divide as the loss of telomeres triggers programmed cell death (apoptosis). A class of enzymes called telomerases use their built-in RNA template to fill in these hexameric repeat sequences at the shortened 5′ end of chromosomal DNA (▶ Fig. 17.7). Telomerases, which are reverse transcriptases, have the following characteristics:
- They are ribonucleoproteins that contain a covalently bound CA-rich short RNA sequence that serves as a built-in RNA template.
- Germ line and stem cells express telomerase. However, somatic cells (i.e., most cells in the body) no longer express telomerase, which results in a limit on the number of times these cells can divide (~50 divisions, replicative senescence).
- Reactivation of telomerase expression in tumor cells contributes to continued cell division. Researchers are investigating telomerases not only as a target for cancer chemotherapy but also as a mechanism to counter aging in somatic cells.

Foundations
Prokaryotic DNA polymerases
Prokaryotic cells have similar if fewer, DNA replicative enzymes as eukaryotic cells. For instance, primase is the prokaryotic equivalent to DNA polymerase α (which synthesizes the RNA primers). DNA polymerase III is the prokaryotic equivalent to DNA polymerases δ and ε (which synthesize the DNA strand in the 5′→3′ direction). Gyrase is the prokaryotic equivalent to topoisomerase II (which relieves overwound supercoils). DNA polymerase I is the prokaryotic equivalent to DNA polymerase δ and FEN1 (which remove the RNA primer and fill the resulting gaps).

Normal
Heat-stable DNA polymerases
Bacteria adapted to growth at high temperatures express enzymes that can function at those temperatures. A heat-stable DNA polymerase isolated from one such organism

V

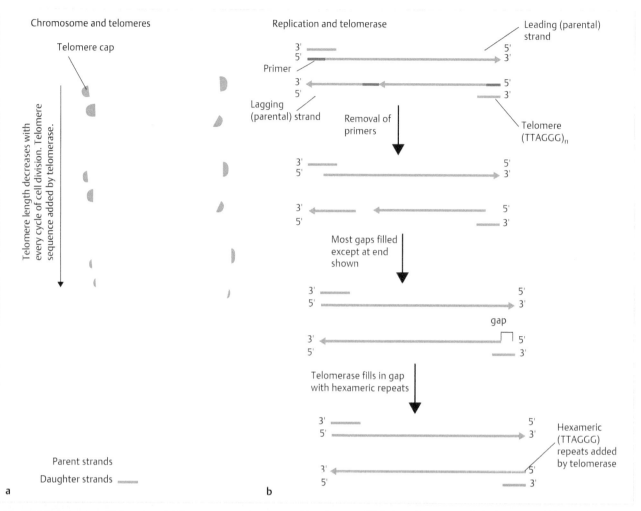

Fig. 17.7 Telomeres and telomerase. (a) Chromosome ends are capped by telomeres. **(b)** A class of enzymes called telomerase add hexameric repeat sequences (TTAGGG) to the ends of chromosomes to form the telomere caps. Telomerases are ribonucleoproteins that contain a built-in RNA template. For the sake of simplicity, the gap at the 5′-end of just one daughter strand is shown.

helped advance the molecular biological technique of polymerase chain reaction (PCR; see **Fig. 21.5**). *Taq* DNA polymerase from *Thermus aquaticus* is isolated from the hot springs of Yellowstone National Park. Its optimal activity occurs around 70 °C and is stable up to 100 °C.

Foundations

Polymerase chain reaction

Polymerase chain reaction (see **Fig. 21.5**) is a remarkably simple and rapid *in vitro* technique to synthesize up to 10^9 copies of a sequence of DNA in just a few hours. The key to the process is the use of a heat-stable DNA polymerase (e.g., *Taq* DNA polymerase). Short primers complementary to the 3′-ends of each strand of the target sequence (20 to 35 nucleotides) are extended by this polymerase in a series of 20 to 30 cycles, each consisting of a DNA denaturation phase, a primer annealing phase, and a primer extension phase.

Foundations

Reverse transcriptase

Retroviruses such as human immunodeficiency virus (HIV) and human T-lymphotropic virus (HTLV) contain single-stranded RNA genomes and utilize a DNA intermediate during their replication. This is achieved by the activity of a virally encoded RNA-dependent DNA polymerase called reverse transcriptase. Reverse transcriptase uses RNA as the template to first synthesize a complementary DNA strand, and then a second DNA strand complementary to the first. The double-stranded proviral DNA is then integrated into the host genome. When the virus is ready to replicate, the host's cellular machinery is utilized to transcribe the proviral DNA into the viral RNA genome.

Therapeutics

Nucleoside analog inhibitors of DNA synthesis

Because DNA synthesis involves the formation of $3' \rightarrow 5'$ phosphodiester bonds, nucleoside analogs that lack the 3'-OH group act as drugs that inhibit DNA replication. Such nucleosides need to be converted to dNTPs before they can act as inhibitors of DNA polymerase. Examples include arabinosylcytosine (ara-C, cytarabine), acycloguanosine (acyclovir), and azidothymidine (AZT). Ara-C contains the sugar arabinose and is converted by animal cells into ara-CTP, a potent competitive inhibitor of DNA polymerase. Ara-C is used in the treatment of leukemia. A herpesvirus-encoded thymidine kinase catalyzes the initial phosphorylation of acyclovir, and the host's enzymes convert the monophosphate into a triphosphate. AZT is used in HIV therapy because the drug is taken up by HIV-infected cells and after activation is utilized by viral reverse transcriptase (a sloppy RNA-dependent DNA polymerase). Both acyclovir and AZT lack a 3'-OH group and therefore arrest viral DNA synthesis by acting as chain terminators.

Therapeutics

Topoisomerase inhibitors

Etoposide is an inhibitor of eukaryotic topoisomerase II, which causes double-stranded breaks in supercoiled DNA. Etoposide is used to treat small-cell lung cancer, testicular cancer, acute nonlymphocytic leukemia, and malignant lymphoma. Topoisomerase inhibitors are also first-line agents for the treatment of neuroblastoma and retinoblastoma (in combination with other agents) and may be used for refractory leukemias. Fluoroquinolone antibiotics (e.g., ciprofloxacin and levofloxacin) are potent inhibitors of DNA gyrase (bacterial topoisomerase II). They are used to treat complicated infections of the genitourinary tract, as well as abdominal, respiratory, skin, and soft tissue infections that are resistant to other agents and gram-negative bone infections. Ciprofloxacin is also the first-line defense against anthrax. Fluoroquinolones are also effective against pathogens such as *Legionella*, *Klebsiella*, and *Mycoplasma*. Drug resistance to quinolones is an increasing problem, and we are now up to the third generation of fluoroquinolones.

Therapeutics

Bleomycin

Bleomycin is a mixture of complex glycopeptides that causes strand breakage of DNA by producing reactive oxygen species. It is unusual in that it produces very little bone marrow depression. It is administered intravenously and is enzymatically inactivated in several tissues (toxicity occurs in tissues with low inactivating activity, e.g., lungs and skin). Fifty percent is excreted unchanged in the urine. Bleomycin is used to treat Hodgkin and non-Hodgkin lymphomas, testicular cancer, and squamous cell carcinomas of the head, neck, nasopharynx, penis, vulva, and cervix.

Therapeutics

Trinucleotide repeat disorders

Although the hexameric repeats found in telomeres are good for cells, the presence of abnormal amounts of certain trinucleotide repeat sequences is associated with disorders known as trinucleotide repeat expansion diseases. For instance:

- Friedreich ataxia, in which progressive damage to the sensory neurons leads to deffective movement and speech, is marked by > 100 GAA repeats in the gene for the mitochondrial protein frataxin.
- Fragile X syndrome, characterized by intellectual disability, autism, and a loss of working memory, is marked by > 230 CGG repeats in the X-linked gene that encodes the fragile X mental retardation protein (FMR1).
- Huntington disease is marked by > 39 CAG repeats in the gene that encodes the huntingtin protein. Patients with this disease suffer from declines in cognition, psychiatric problems, lack of coordination, and abnormal involuntary movements.
- Myotonic dystrophy (DM1, Steinert disease) is marked by > 50 CTG repeats in the gene that encodes the dystrophia myotonica protein kinase. Patients have pain and progressive weakness in the lower extremities, as well as in the hand, face, and neck muscles.

17.3 DNA Damage and Mutations

The base, sugar, and phosphate groups of DNA are chemically reactive, and many physical and chemical agents are capable of interacting with, and damaging, DNA, including the following:

- **Physical agents:** These include ionizing radiation, which possesses enough energy to displace electrons from atoms, and nonionizing radiation, which does not. The main sources of ionizing radiation exposure for most people are related to medical imaging, such as X-rays and computed tomographic (CT) scans.
- **Chemical agents:** These include compounds that react with functional groups on DNA and others that intercalate between its stacked bases. Chemical agents that can cause permanent, heritable changes to DNA are termed mutagens. Most mutagens are also carcinogens because the mutations they cause can lead to the development of cancer.

Mutations involve the substitution, insertion, or deletion of one or more nucleotides from DNA. Germline mutations are changes in the DNA sequence that are passed on to subsequent generations. Somatic mutations are changes in the DNA of differentiated cells that are not passed on to subsequent generations.

Categories of single-nucleotide (point) mutations include the following:

- **Transitions:** These occur when a purine is substituted for a purine or a pyrimidine for another pyrimidine.
- **Transversions:** These occur when a purine is substituted for a pyrimidine and vice versa.
- **Insertions:** These occur when one or more nucleotides are added to DNA.
- **Deletions:** These occur when one or more nucleotides are removed from DNA.

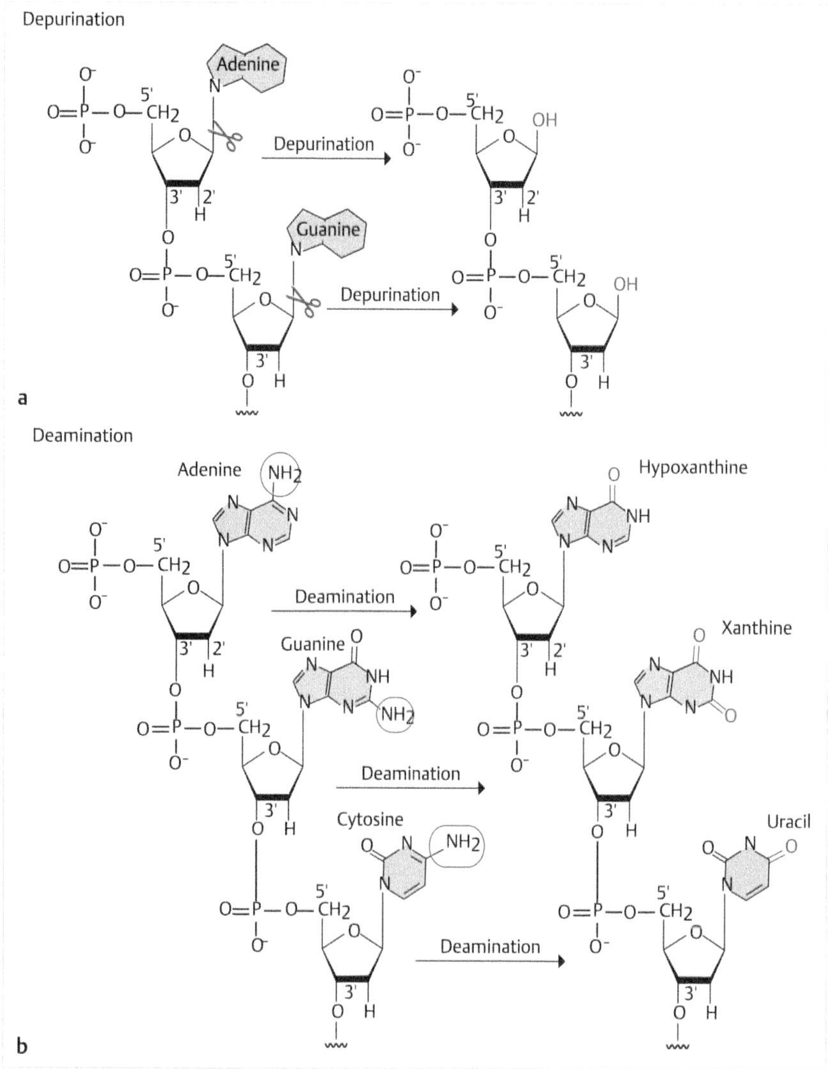

Depurination

a

Deamination

b

Fig. 17.8 Spontaneous damage by endogenous agents. (a) Depurination of adenosine and guanosine via removal of their bases. Depurination occurs via the hydrolysis of the N-glycosyl linkage, giving rise to an abasic (apurinic) site in the DNA strand. (b) Deamination of the bases adenine, guanine, and cytosine respectively generates hypoxanthine, xanthine, and uracil.

17.3.1 Types of DNA Damage

Spontaneous Damage by Endogenous Agents

Chromosomal DNA undergoes thousands of spontaneous changes daily as a result of damage due to hydrolysis, oxidation, and unregulated methylation. All the components of DNA, such as its base, sugar, and phosphate, can be altered by damaging agents. The following are two examples of frequently occurring spontaneous damage:

1. **Depurination:** The purine base (adenine or guanine) is removed from the nucleotide via hydrolysis of the N-glycosidic bond between the base and the deoxyribose group. This generates an apurinic (AP) or abasic site in the DNA strand (▶ Fig. 17.8a).
2. **Deamination:** The amino group of purine or pyrimidine base is hydrolyzed such that adenine is converted to hypoxanthine, guanine is converted to xanthine, and cytosine is converted to uracil, which forms an unnatural deoxyuridine (dU) (▶ Fig. 17.8b).

Radiation-Induced DNA Damage

Ionizing radiation (e.g., X-rays), and the resulting reactive oxygen species (e.g., superoxide, hydrogen peroxide and hydroxyl radical), can induce the following changes in DNA (▶ Fig. 17.9a):

- Forty to sixty chemically distinct base damages
- Direct strand breaks
- DNA–protein cross-links

Nonionizing radiation such as UV light (e.g., UV-B) damages DNA by inducing the formation of a covalent linkage between adjacent pyrimidine bases. This results in two major photoproducts that are toxic, mutagenic, and carcinogenic (▶ Fig. 17.9b):

1. Pyrimidine cyclobutane dimers (more common)
2. 6–4 covalent linkage of two pyrimidines
   - The characteristic mutations of these photoproducts are present in the *TP53* gene in cells from patients with sunlight exposure and are associated with basal and squamous cell carcinomas.

DNA Damage by Chemical Agents

Chemical agents that cause DNA damage may be broadly classified into two groups:

1. **Agents that require metabolic activation.** Examples of this class of agents include benzo(a)pyrene and aflatoxin B1. These compounds are bioactivated by hepatic cytochrome

V

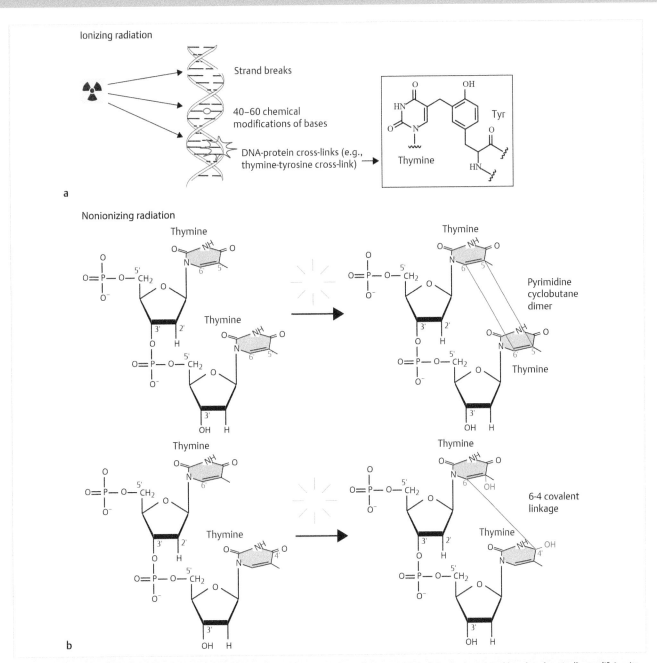

Fig. 17.9 Radiation-induced DNA damage. (a) Ionizing radiation (e.g., X-ray) can damage DNA by introducing strand breaks, chemically modifying its bases, or creating cross-links between DNA and protein. **(b)** Nonionizing radiation (e.g., UV light) damages DNA by triggering the formation of pyrimidine cyclobutane dimers or 6–4 linkages between two pyrimidines.

P-450 enzymes into benzo(a)pyrene-7,8-diol-9,10-epoxide (BPDE) and aflatoxin B1-epoxide, respectively, before they interact with DNA.

- Benzo(a)pyrene is present in many combustion products, such as cigarette smoke, automobile exhaust, and charred meats. The bioactive BPDE forms a bulky adduct with the exocyclic amino group of guanines in the DNA. Such adducts prevent both replication and gene expression (▶ Fig. 17.10a).
- Inhibition of expression of tumor suppressor genes (see Fig. 20.4) such as p53 is thought to be the mechanism by which BPDE acts as a carcinogen.

2. **Agents that act directly to modify DNA.** These include cross-linking agents (which form cross-links between bases in the same DNA strand or between two complementary DNA strands) alkylating agents (which induce a wide variety of methylated base changes and even alkylation of phosphodiesters into phosphotriesters), and intercalating agents (which insert between stacked bases of the DNA double helix, causing some unwinding of the helix and separation of base pairs). The following are examples of each (▶ Fig. 17.10b):
- Cross-linking agents: Nitrogen mustard, cisplatin, mitomycin C, and carmustine, which are well-known cancer chemotherapeutic agents

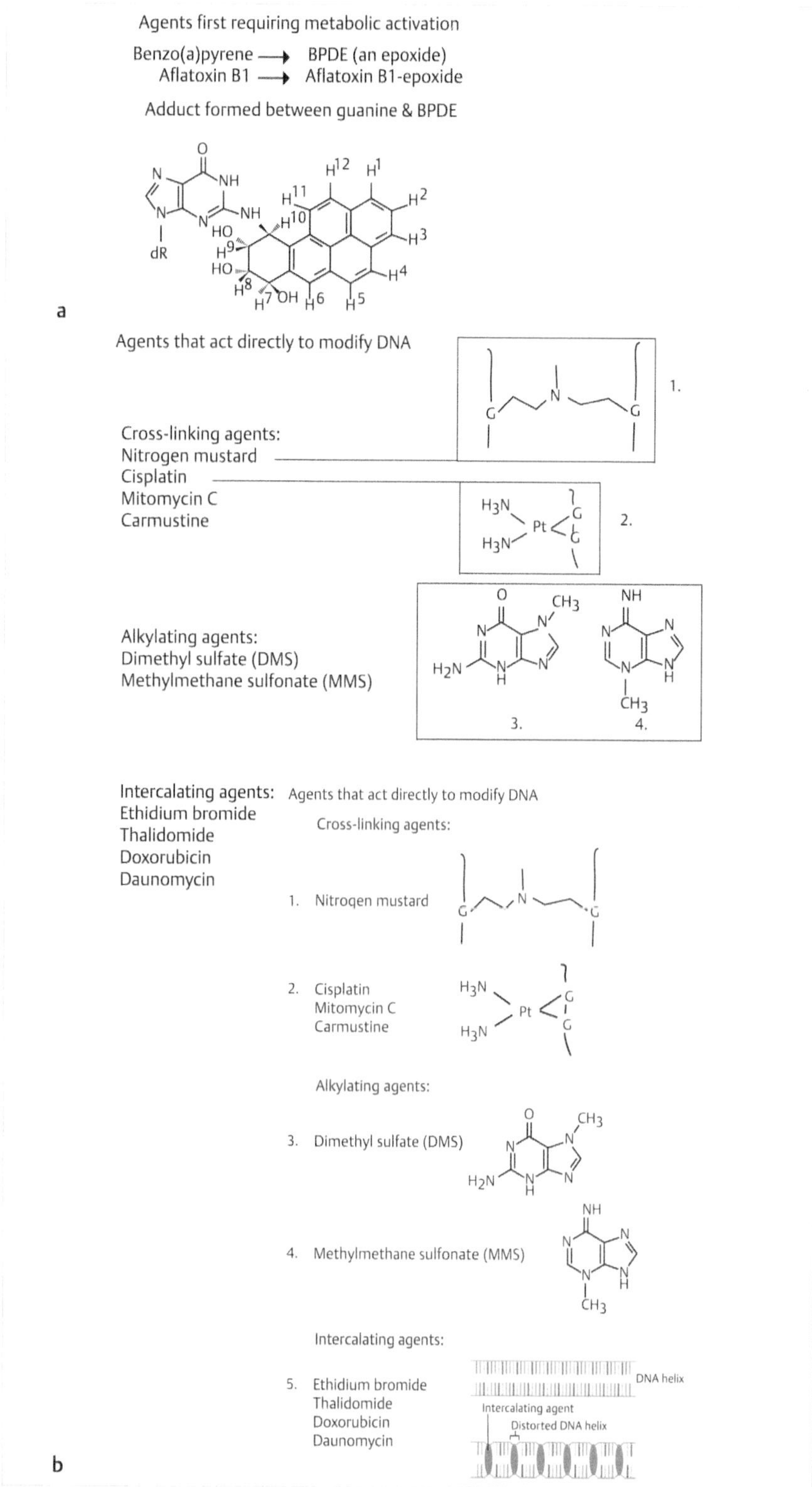

Agents first requiring metabolic activation

Benzo(a)pyrene ⟶ BPDE (an epoxide)
Aflatoxin B1 ⟶ Aflatoxin B1-epoxide

Adduct formed between guanine & BPDE

a

Agents that act directly to modify DNA

Cross-linking agents:
Nitrogen mustard
Cisplatin
Mitomycin C
Carmustine

1.

2.

Alkylating agents:
Dimethyl sulfate (DMS)
Methylmethane sulfonate (MMS)

3.   4.

Intercalating agents:
Ethidium bromide
Thalidomide
Doxorubicin
Daunomycin

Agents that act directly to modify DNA

Cross-linking agents:

1. Nitrogen mustard

2. Cisplatin
   Mitomycin C
   Carmustine

Alkylating agents:

3. Dimethyl sulfate (DMS)

4. Methylmethane sulfonate (MMS)

Intercalating agents:

5. Ethidium bromide
   Thalidomide
   Doxorubicin
   Daunomycin

DNA helix

Intercalating agent
Distorted DNA helix

b

Fig. 17.10 Damage by chemical agents. (a) Benzo(a)pyrene and aflatoxin B1 are agents that first require metabolic activation before they can damage DNA. The 9,10-epoxide group of the bioactive benzo(a)pyrene-7,8-diol-9,10-epoxide (BPDE) reacts with the exocyclic amino group of guanine in DNA to form an adduct that blocks transcription, dR, deoxyribose. **(b)** Direct-acting chemical agents that damage DNA include the cross-linking agents, nitrogen mustard and cisplatin. They form cross-links between guanine (G) bases between two complementary DNA strands (1) or in the same strand (2). These compounds act as antitumor drugs by blocking DNA replication. Alkylating agents such as dimethyl sulfate (DMS) and methylmethanesulfonate (MMS) cause cytotoxic methylation of bases in the DNA. Frequent products include 7-methylguanine (3) and 3-methyladenine (4). Agents such as ethidium bromide insert themselves between the stacked bases of the DNA (5) and distort the double helix.

- Alkylating agents: Dimethyl sulfate (DMS) and methylmethane sulfonate (MMS). Frequent products of alkylation are 7-methylguanine (nonmutagenic) and 3-methyladenine (toxic) (▶ Fig. 17.10b-3, -4).
- Intercalating agents: Ethidium bromide, thalidomide, and anthracycline antibiotics, such as doxorubicin and daunomycin. They are mutagenic and interfere with

replication, repair processes, and transcription. The anthracyclines are also known to interfere with the action of topoisomerase II and cause strand breaks. When such agents insert themselves between stacked bases in double stranded DNA, they cause a distortion of the double helix (Fig. 17.10b-5).

Foundations

Cisplatin

Cisplatin is a drug that consists of a complex of inorganic platinum ions. It acts by forming DNA cross-links, which prevents DNA replication and transcription. It is administered intravenously; binds to plasma proteins (90%); is concentrated in the liver, kidneys, intestine, and ovaries; and is excreted in urine. It is used to treat solid tumors, especially testicular, ovarian, and bladder cancer.

Therapeutics

Chromosomal mutations

Chromosomal mutations involve large segments of DNA, often encompassing millions of base pairs. They are classified into four types: inversion, deletion, duplication, and translocation. In inversion, a segment of chromosomal DNA is present in its reverse orientation; in deletion, a segment is lost; in duplication, a segment is copied, resulting in amplification of genes contained in that region. Translocation occurs when two different chromosomes exchange segments of their DNA. Translocation can be either balanced (where there is no net gain or loss of genetic material) or unbalanced (where there is either a gain or a loss of genetic material).

Therapeutics

Gene amplification

Gene amplification or duplication is an increase in the number of copies of a gene with potential for an increase in the RNA and protein coded by that gene. It may be caused by an error in homologous recombination, retrotransposition, or duplication of the entire chromosome. Errors in homologous recombination and duplication of the entire chromosome are caused by "unequal crossing over" during meiosis in homologous chromosomes. Retrotransposition occurs when reverse transcribed mature RNA is integrated into DNA at random sites in a genome. This rarely results in the expression of full-length coding sequences. Gene amplification is thought to play a critical role in evolution because duplicated genes are free from selective pressure and can, therefore, accumulate mutations faster than their single-gene counterparts.
The amplification of oncogenes is also one of the mechanisms by which cancer can propagate; amplification of the multidrug resistant (MDR) gene is one of the processes by which cancer cells develop resistance to chemotherapeutic drugs.

Foundations

Transposons

Transposons (so-called jumping genes) are mobile sequences of DNA that are able to change position within the genome of a single cell. This may occur via a "copy and paste" method via RNA intermediates (type I transposons) or via a "cut and paste" method that is mediated by transposase enzymes (type II transposons). Transposons are mutagenic for the following reasons: they are very likely to damage active genes into which they have inserted, the gap they leave in the original DNA sequence may be incorrectly repaired, and they may cause incorrect chromosomal pairing during meiosis and mitosis, resulting in unequal crossing over with subsequent chromosomal duplication. An example of a disease caused by transposons is hemophilia A, where transposon L1 inserted into the factor VIII gene renders factor VIII ineffective. In humans, type I or retrotransposons comprise the bulk (>90%) of total transposons, which account for nearly half of the genome.

Therapeutics

Cytotoxic versus cytostatic agents

Cytotoxic agents kill cells, whereas cytostatic agents merely prevent their proliferation. Cytostatic drugs tend to be more specific than cytotoxic drugs and exhibit fewer side effects. Thus, a cytostatic drug may not shrink a tumor, but it may prevent its growth and block metastasis. Many cytotoxic agents used in cancer chemotherapy (e.g., alkylating agents, cisplatin, topoisomerase inhibitors) induce apoptosis through DNA damage. Often such agents are effective only in cells having active DNA synthesis (S phase of the cell cycle). On the other hand, microtubule-targeting drugs such as paclitaxel and vincristine arrest cells in mitosis and are characterized as cytostatic. It should be noted that many drugs may act as cytostatic agents at low doses and as cytotoxic agents at higher doses.

Foundations

McCann-Ames test

The McCann-Ames test (popularly known as the Ames test) is an assay to detect chemicals that induce mutations in DNA. The assay employs a strain of *Salmonella typhimurium* that is dependent on exogenous histidine for its growth due to a genetic defect in the *His* operon. Chemicals are tested for their ability to induce the reversion of the auxotrophs to histidine-independent growth. Use of additional bacterial strains that have defects in DNA repair machinery, that have lost their lipopolysaccharide coats, or that express an antibiotic-resistant plasmid improves the range and sensitivity of the test.

The Ames test may be used to identify both mutagens and carcinogens. A mutagen is defined as a physical or chemical agent that can cause an alteration in the DNA sequence. Most of the time, such alterations are repaired or, when not repaired, induce apoptosis of the affected cell. A carcinogen is defined as an agent that can cause cancer. Although many carcinogens are mutagenic, some may induce cancer by interfering with metabolic or signaling pathways. A limitation of the Ames test is that it may yield a false-negative if the test chemical needs metabolic activation (e.g., benzo(a)pyrene) to become mutagenic. The test includes the option of adding a rat liver extract to simulate mammalian metabolism. The Ames test is one of the required initial screens in the testing of all new drugs.

V

V

Foundations

Reactive oxygen species

Reactive oxygen species (ROS), or free radicals, are chemically reactive molecules containing oxygen (e.g., superoxide and hydrogen peroxide). They are highly reactive due to their valence shell electrons. ROS are normal endogenous molecules that are generated by the partial reduction of oxygen in the electron transport chain. They play an important role in immune defense and platelet chemotaxis. However, most of the effects of ROS are deleterious to the cell and occur when their numbers are significantly increased as a result of exposure to ionizing radiation, for example. ROS may damage the cell in several ways: they may damage DNA; they may oxidize amino acids in proteins; they may oxidize fatty acids in lipids; or they may inactivate certain enzymes by oxidation of their cofactors.

Foundations

Mutations versus single-nucleotide polymorphisms

A mutation is an uncommon alteration in the DNA sequence, whereas a single-nucleotide polymorphism (SNP) is a commonly inherited change in a single base pair that occurs in at least 1% of the population. SNPs are used as markers in the mapping of genomes and in identifying genetic changes that lead to certain traits. In the human genome, SNPs occur once every 1000 to 2000 nucleotides. Occasionally, a polymorphism may be associated with (or increase an individual's susceptibility to) disease. Examples include polymorphisms of factor VII, apolipoprotein E (apoE) and cholesterol ester transfer protein (CETP).

Normal

p53

The normally labile tumor suppressor protein and transcription factor p53 is stabilized by DNA damage (e.g., due to exposure to UV radiation or reactive oxygen species), as well as other conditions (e.g., osmotic shock and oncogene expression). As p53 accumulates, it undergoes a conformational change due to phosphorylation of its N-terminal domain, which activates it. Active p53 induces the expression of several genes involved in DNA repair, cell cycle arrest, and induction of apoptosis. Therefore, p53 has been called the guardian of the genome. The gene encoding p53 is frequently mutated in human cancers. A common polymorphism in codon 72 of the *TP53* gene, which results in the replacement of an arginine with a proline, appears to be associated with susceptibility toward several types of cancer. While humans have two copies of the *TP53* gene, elephants have 40 copies, although 38 are retrogenes (variant sequence but functional). Following DNA damage, elephant cells undergo apoptosis at 3–5 times the rate of human cells. This fact may partially explain why elephants appear to have a 5-fold lower incidence of cancer than humans even though an elephant has 100 times the body mass of a human.

17.4 DNA Repair Mechanisms

Cells employ multiple repair mechanisms to maintain the integrity of the genetic information carried in chromosomal DNA. The basis for these repair mechanisms is the fact that, unless both strands of DNA are simultaneously damaged, the information from the undamaged strand may be used to repair the damaged complementary strand. If the DNA damage is not repaired, then several deleterious consequences may result, such as impaired cellular function, apoptosis, mutations, and genetic (chromosomic) instability leading to cancer (▶ Fig. 17.11).

The following are some well-known repair mechanisms (▶ Table 17.2):

1. **Direct repair**. This mechanism enzymatically reverses or repairs some types of DNA damage, as follows:
   - Cyclobutane pyrimidine dimers generated by UV light can be enzymatically separated with the aid of visible light. A photodependent enzyme called DNA photolyase binds to the dimers, and by absorbing light at the wavelength of 370 nm, it is activated to catalyze the breakage of bonds between adjacent pyrimidines in a process termed photo-reactivation ε. While this mechanism operates in a wide variety of organisms ranging from bacteria to plants to animals, it does not work in humans and other placental animals.
   - O^6-Methylguanine is mutagenic because it base pairs with T rather than C. The enzyme methylguanine methyltransferase (MGMT) transfers the methyl group from guanine to a cysteine on itself, thus directly reversing the damage (▶ Fig. 17.12a).

2. **Base excision repair (BER)**. Single-base mismatches and small, nondistorting alterations are repaired by this mechanism (▶ Fig. 17.12b). Examples include uracil, 8-oxoguanine, 3-methyladenine, and abasic sites. In this mechanism, a family of enzymes called DNA glycosylases are utilized because they have the ability to "flip out" the DNA bases to detect a single damaged base.
   - Once an altered base is detected, the enzyme then hydrolyzes the *N*-glycosidic linkage to remove the altered base, leaving an abasic site.
   - This AP site is recognized by an AP endonuclease, which cuts the phosphodiester linkage. The deoxyribose phosphate is removed by an AP lyase.
   - The single strand break (SSB) is recognized by Poly ADP-ribose polymerase (PARP-1) which is activated by binding to the break site. PARP-1 builds a branched polymer of ADP-ribose on itself which recruits DNA polymerase β, X-ray cross-complementing protein-1 (XRCC1) and the associated DNA ligase III (▶ Fig. 17.12b).
   - PARP-1 dissociates and DNA polymerase β and DNA ligase then replace the excised base and seal the nick, respectively, to complete the repair.

3. **Nucleotide excision repair (NER)**. This mechanism is used to repair chemical adducts that alter or distort the normal shape of DNA in the local area of the chemical damage. For example, damage due to UV light–induced pyrimidine dimers, BPDE-guanine adducts, and cisplatin adducts are repaired by this mechanism (▶ Fig. 17.12c).
   - Once the distortion in DNA is detected by recognition proteins in the NER complex, the double strand is

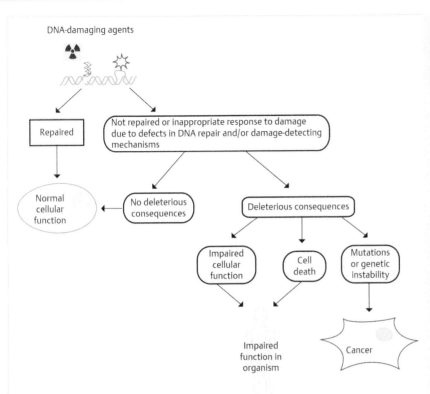

Fig. 17.11 Potential biological outcomes of DNA damage. Unrepaired DNA damage can lead to deleterious consequences, such as impaired cellular function, programmed cell death, and mutations that lead to cancer.

Table 17.2 DNA repair mechanisms

Repair mechanism	Types of damage repaired	Enzymes/Mechanism Involved/Associated disorder
1. Direct repair (enzymatic repair)	• Pyrimidine dimers • O^6-methylguanine	• DNA photolyase • Methylguanine methyltransferase
2. Base excision repair (BER)	Single-base mismatches, nondistorting alterations (e.g., depurination)	DNA glycolases, AP endonuclease, AP lyase (of DNA polymerase β), DNA polymerase β, DNA ligase III, poly ADP-ribose polymerase (PARP-1), XRCC1
3. Nucleotide excision repair (NER)	Chemical adducts that distort DNA (e.g., pyrimidine dimers, BPDE-guanine adducts, cisplatin adducts)	NER protein complex, DNA polymerase ε, DNA ligase Xeroderma pigmentosum
4. Transcription-coupled repair (TCR)	Stalled RNA polymerase during transcription (not replication)	ERCC-8 (CSA), ERCC-6 (CSB) Cockayne syndrome
5. Mismatch excision repair (MER)	Mismatched base in daughter strand	MER complex (MSH2, MSH6, MLH1 and PMS2), helicase/endonuclease, DNA polymerase δ, DNA ligase Hereditary nonpolyposis colorectal cancers
6. Recombination repair	Double-strand breaks, interstrand cross-linking	
• nonhomologous end joining (NHEJ)		• Damaged ends filled in and joined; some base pairs may be missing. Multiple proteins and enzymes including DNA ligase
• homologous recombination		• Exonucleases, DNA polymerase, MER system. Damaged duplex repair using information on undamaged homologous duplex *BRCA1/2* breast cancer
7. Translesion synthesis (bypass synthesis)	Unrepaired thymine dimers or apurini AP sites	DNA polymerases η and ζ (reduced-fidelity polymerases)

Abbreviations: AP, apurinic; XRCC1, X-ray cross-complementing protein-1; BPDE, benzo(a)pyrene-7,8-diol-9,10-epoxide; BRCA, breast cancer susceptibility gene.

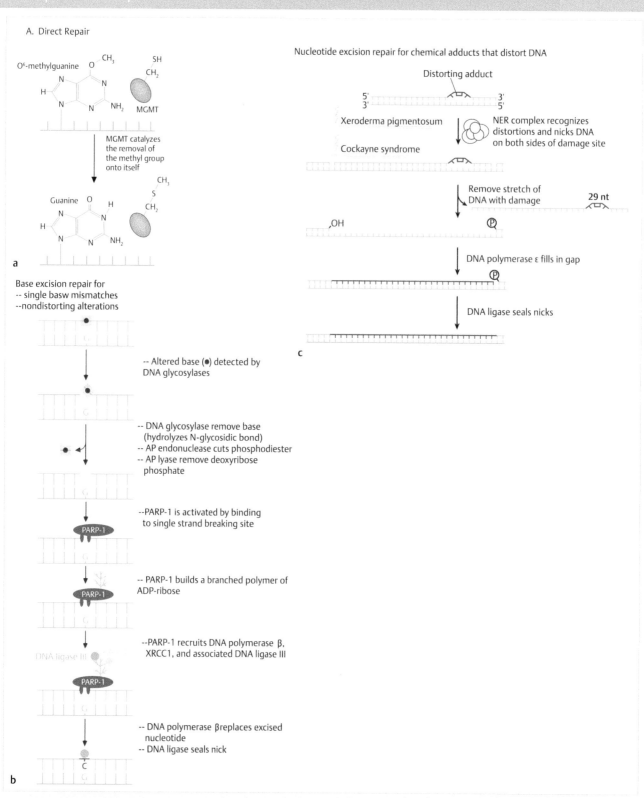

Fig. 17.12 Photoreactivation, base excision repair (BER), and nucleotide excision repair (NER) mechanisms. (a) O⁶-Methylaion of guanine can be reversed by methylguanine methyltransferase (MGMT) which transfers the methyl group onto a cysteine in the active site. **(b)** In BER, the altered or mismatched base is detected, cut out, and replaced by a variety of enzymes. Poly ADP-ribose polymerase (PARP-1) plays a vital role in the recognition of single strand breaks which occur during this repair process. **(c)** In NER, two cuts are made in the damaged strand on either side of the alteration, and a nucleotide (nt) stretch of sequence containing the damage is removed. The gap is then filled in by DNA polymerase e (polymerase I in prokaryotes), and the nick is sealed by DNA ligase. Individuals with xeroderma pigmentosum have defects in several proteins of the NER complex. AP, apurinic; MER, mismatch excision repair.

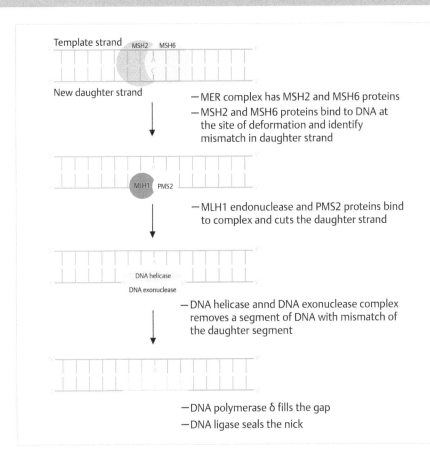

Template strand   MSH2   MSH6

New daughter strand

— MER complex has MSH2 and MSH6 proteins
— MSH2 and MSH6 proteins bind to DNA at
  the site of deformation and identify
  mismatch in daughter strand

MLH1 PMS2

— MLH1 endonuclease and PMS2 proteins bind
  to complex and cuts the daughter strand

DNA helicase

DNA exonuclease

— DNA helicase annd DNA exonuclease complex
  removes a segment of DNA with mismatch of
  the daughter segment

— DNA polymerase δ fills the gap
— DNA ligase seals the nick

Fig. 17.13 Mismatch excision repair (MER). MER complex (containing MSH2 and MSH6 proteins) binds to DNA at the site of mismatch and distinguishes between the parent and daughter strands. MLH1 endonuclease and PMS2 protein then bind to the lesion and the daughter strand is cut. With the help of a helicase, an exonuclease then removes nucleotides surrounding the mismatch from the daughter strand. The resultant gap is repaired by polymerase δ and DNA ligase.

unwound, and a nick is made on either side of the damage. A stretch of nucleotides (29 in the case of humans and 13 in the case of *Escherichia coli*) containing the damage is removed.
- DNA polymerase ε (polymerase I in the case of *E. coli*) then fills in the gap using the undamaged strand as the template, and the nick is then sealed by DNA ligase.
- Individuals with xeroderma pigmentosum have defects in several proteins of the NER complex.

4. **Transcription-coupled repair (TCR).** TCR is a type of NER that is initiated when RNA polymerase stalls at a lesion in the DNA template strand during transcription. In eukaryotes, TCR proteins called ERCC-6 and ERCC-8 recognize the stalled RNA polymerase and recruit other repair proteins.
- Defects in genes encoding ERCC-6 and ERCC-8 lead to Cockayne syndrome, which is associated with severe growth defects. Unlike xeroderma pigmentosum, patients with Cockayne syndrome do not exhibit pigmentary skin changes.

5. **Mismatch excision repair (MER).** In spite of the high fidelity of DNA polymerases, a wrong nucleotide occasionally gets inserted into the newly synthesized daughter strand. Such mismatches are repaired by the MER system, although it is unclear how the daughter strand is recognized in humans. (In bacteria, the daughter strand is undermethylated compared with the parent strand.) See ▶ Fig. 17.13.
- The MER complex containing MSH2 and MSH6 proteins binds to DNA at the deformation induced by the mismatch and appears to distinguish between the parent and

daughter strands to identify the mismatch in the daughter strand.
- The MLH1 endonuclease along with PMS2 protein then binds to the complex and cuts the daughter strand. A DNA helicase/exonuclease complex removes a segment of DNA containing the mismatch from the daughter strand. Polymerase δ fills in the gap, and DNA ligase seals the nick.
- Individuals with defective proteins of the MER complex have increased susceptibility to hereditary nonpolyposis colorectal cancers (also known as Lynch syndrome).

6. **Recombination repair.** When DNA undergoes double-strand breaks or interstrand cross-linking–as happens with ionizing radiation or certain antitumor agents–the damage cannot be repaired by the mechanisms described so far because no template is available to supply the missing information. Such double-strand breaks are recognized by the ATM (ataxia telangiectasia mutated) and ATR (AT and Rad3 related) kinases and then repaired by one of the two recombination mechanisms.
- *Nonhomologous end joining (NHEJ):* In this process the damaged segment is not replaced. Instead, the ends are polished by the removal of several overhanging nucleotides and the blunt ends are simply joined together by a DNA ligase, which repairs the double-strand break, but several base pairs at the site of the lesion would be missing (▶ Fig. 17.14a). Occasionally, broken ends from different chromosomes may be joined together by NHEJ, leading to chromosomal translocation. While NHEJ is the preferred mechanism for the repair of double-strand breaks, particularly during the interphase in humans, it should be noted that it is error-prone.

Nonhomologous end joining (NHEJ)

Homologous recombination

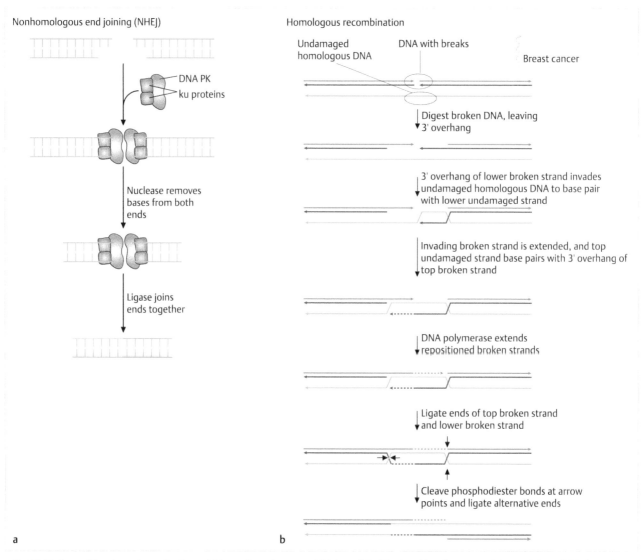

a

b

Fig. 17.14 Recombinant repair mechanisms. (a) In nonhomologous end joining of double-strand breaks, a complex containing a DNA-dependent protein kinase (PK) and Ku proteins binds to the ends of the double-strand break. Nucleases then remove several bases from both ends, and DNA ligase joins together the newly formed ends. **(b)** In homologous recombination, the pink duplex has a double-strand break, whereas the homologous blue duplex is intact. Exonucleases first digest the broken ends to generate 3′overhang regions. One of the pink single strands invades the intact duplex (with the help of Rad51 protein [RecA in bacteria]) and base pairs with its complementary intact strand and displaces the other blue strand. The invading strand is then extended by DNA polymerase. The displaced blue strand then base pairs with the other pink 3′overhang. The 3′ends are further extended until they reach the point of the original 5′ends generated at the beginning. The 3′and 5′ends are now ligated to generate a Holliday junction. The strands are then cut at the points indicated by arrows, and the alternative ends are ligated to generate two recombinant DNA sequences with double-strand breaks repaired.

- *Homologous recombination:* This method is used to repair double-strand breaks that occur after DNA has replicated but before cell division (G$_2$ phase) so that the replicated DNA helices are close together. The genetic information from the undamaged duplex is used to repair the damaged duplex (▶ Fig. 17.14b).
  - Initially, the broken ends are converted to have single-stranded 3′ overhangs by exonucleases that trim back one of the strands.
  - The single-stranded region then "invades" the good copy of its homologous DNA duplex and base pairs with the complementary strand.

- The 3′ end of the invading strand is then extended by DNA polymerase until the displaced parental strand from the good copy starts to base pair with the other 3′ overhang of the copy being repaired, which is then extended by DNA polymerase.
- The new 3′ ends generated by DNA synthesis are ligated to the 5′ ends originally generated by exonuclease digestion. The resulting duplexes with crossover points are called Holliday structures.
- The sequences are cleaved at the crossover points followed by ligation of appropriate ends to generate two recombinant DNA sequences. Each sequence contains sections of one parental DNA duplex on one side of the

break and the other parental duplex on the other side. At the initial break point, the DNA exists as a heteroduplex with one strand from each parent.

- Any base pair mismatches are repaired by the MER system.
- It should be noted that the breast cancer susceptibility genes (*BRCA1* and *BRCA2*) associated with hereditary breast cancer encode proteins that facilitate homologous recombination.
- Defects in the *BLM* gene, which encodes a DNA helicase involved in homologous recombination repair, lead to Bloom syndrome. Affected people have short stature, increased sensitivity to sun light and a greatly increased risk of cancer.

7. **Translesion synthesis.** This mechanism is also called bypass synthesis and utilizes DNA polymerases such as polymerase ξ and polymerase η. These are less stringent than polymerase δ, and they lack proofreading capability:

- DNA polymerase η incorporates A (which happens to be the correct base) opposite thymine dimers. However, the reduced fidelity of such polymerases also means that they incorporate incorrect nucleotides at a higher frequency, leading to mutations.

Therapeutics
Hereditary nonpolyposis colorectal cancer

Individuals with inherited mutations in one of the alleles of genes in the MER complex (*MSH2, MSH6, MLH1, PMS2*) have an increased susceptibility to hereditary nonpolyposis colorectal cancer (HNPCC, Lynch syndrome). While colon cancer is the most common result, cancers of other tissues such as endometrium, ovary, small intestine, brain and skin are also seen. Another susceptibility gene for HNPCC is *EPCAM*. Although *EPCAM* is not a DNA repair gene, it is located adjacent to *MSH2* gene on Chr 2. Certain *EPCAM* gene mutations cause the *MSH2* gene to be turned off.

Therapeutics
Xeroderma pigmentosum

Many of the proteins in the human NER complex were identified by studying the defects in the repair process in cultured cells obtained from individuals with an inherited disease called xeroderma pigmentosum (XP). The skin of people with this disease is extremely sensitive to direct sunlight, and they are prone to developing melanomas and squamous cell carcinomas. The UV component of sunlight often causes cyclobutane thymine dimers to form in the DNA. These dimers can be easily repaired in normal individuals by

NER. However, those with defects in various XP proteins (XP-A through XP-G) in the NER complex exhibit the disease.

Therapeutics
Cockayne syndrome

Cockayne syndrome is a rare autosomal recessive, congenital disorder. The mutant genes involved are *ERCC6* and *ERCC8*. These genes code for the ERCC-6 (CSB) and ERCC-8 (CSA) proteins, respectively, that are involved in TCR of DNA. If DNA is not repaired, then cell dysfunction and cell death may occur. Cockayne syndrome is characterized by developmental and neurologic delay, photosensitivity (abnormal sensitivity to sunlight), and progeria (premature aging). There are also commonly hearing loss and eye abnormalities (e.g., pigmentary retinopathy). Death usually occurs within the first 2 decades of life. Mutations in *ERCC8* and *ERCC6* genes lead to Cockayne syndrome types A and B, respectively. Type B accounts for 70% of the cases of Cockayne syndrome.

Therapeutics
Bloom syndrome

Bloom syndrome is the result of mutations in BLM helicase which plays an important role in homologous recombination during the early stages of cell division. Individuals with Bloom syndrome rarely exceed a height of 5 ft, develop skin rashes on sun exposure and have an increased risk of cancer and infections. Men with Bloom syndrome are infertile, and women reach an early menopause.

Therapeutics
BRCA mutations and breast cancer

BRCA1 (breast cancer susceptibility gene 1) and *BRCA2* (breast cancer susceptibility gene 2) are tumor suppressor genes. Mutations of these genes cause a fivefold increase in a woman's risk of developing breast and/or ovarian cancer before she reaches menopause. Men with mutations of these genes also have an increased risk of developing breast cancer. Mutations in *BRCA1* are also associated with a higher risk of developing cervical, uterine, pancreatic, and colon cancer in women and pancreatic, testicular, and early prostate cancer in men (although these are more often caused by *BRCA2* mutations). *BRCA2* mutations also increase the risk of developing melanoma and pancreatic, stomach, gallbladder, and bile duct cancer in women.

18 Transcription

18.1 Ribonucleic Acid

18.1.1 Structure and Function

Ribonucleic acid (RNA) is mainly a single-stranded polymer of ribonucleotides, each of which consists of a base (purine or pyrimidine), a pentose sugar, and a phosphate. Unlike DNA, which contains 2'-deoxyribose, the five-carbon sugar in RNA is ribose. Although RNA does contain cytosine, its second main pyrimidine is uracil. Just as in DNA, the ribonucleotides in RNA are linked by 3'-5' phosphodiester bonds (▶ Fig. 18.1). Following are some notable chemical and structural features of RNA:

- RNA is inherently more unstable than DNA due to nucleophilic attack by the reactive 2'-OH group on the 3'-5' phosphodiester linkage, particularly under basic conditions. One mechanism that cells employ to stabilize RNA is to extensively methylate the 2'-OH groups.
- Even though most RNA is technically single-stranded, it tends to have areas of complementary sequence that loop back on themselves, creating double-stranded regions.
- RNA is capable of folding into complex three-dimensional structures that exhibit secondary and tertiary structure.

The synthesis and metabolism of RNA are critical for life because RNA plays an important role in the central dogma (see **Fig. 17.1**) as the intermediary in gene expression–that is, the transfer of genetic information from DNA to a functional products such as proteins and certain types of RNA. Derangement in the regulation of the transcriptional process contributes to multiple diseases, including cancer. Additionally,

- several viruses, such as polio and influenza, and retroviruses, such as HIV, contain RNA genomes.
- some RNA molecules are catalytically active (ribozymes) just like enzymes.
- the mechanism of action of many drugs and toxins involves targeting the synthesis and function of RNA.

18.1.2 Types of RNA

Almost all RNA is synthesized (transcribed) from a cellular DNA template by DNA-dependent RNA polymerases. Therefore, RNA is complementary to a portion of a cell's DNA. A small fraction of RNA, however, is made in a template-independent fashion (e.g., 3' termini of mature tRNAs or the poly(A) tails of mature

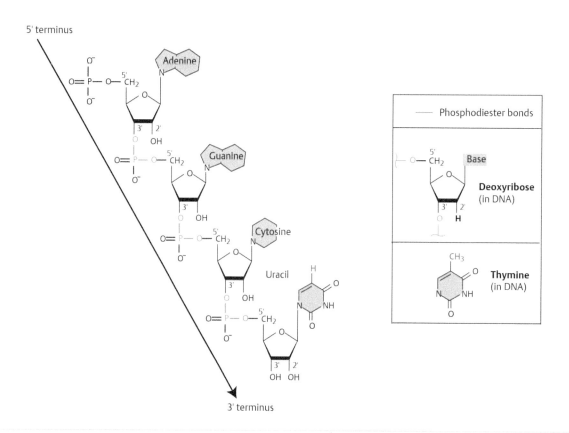

Fig. 18.1 Primary structure of RNA. RNA is a polyribonucleotide in which the individual nucleotides are linked by 3'-5' phosphodiester bonds. The sugar group in RNA is ribose (rather than DNA's deoxyribose, which lacks an OH group at its 2'carbon). Although RNA contains the bases adenine, guanine, and cytosine, the second major pyrimidine in RNA is uracil rather than thymine as in DNA. Nucleophilic attack by the 2'-OH group onto the phosphodiester linkage leads to accelerated hydrolysis of the backbone, particularly under basic conditions, making RNA less stable than DNA.

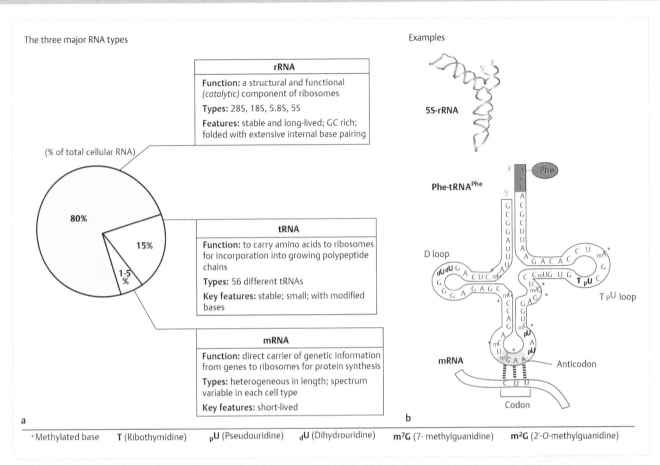

The three major RNA types

rRNA

Function: a structural and functional (*catalytic*) component of ribosomes

Types: 28S, 18S, 5.8S, 5S

Features: stable and long-lived; GC rich; folded with extensive internal base pairing

(% of total cellular RNA)

80%

15%

1-5 %

tRNA

Function: to carry amino acids to ribosomes for incorporation into growing polypeptide chains

Types: 56 different tRNAs

Key features: stable; small; with modified bases

mRNA

Function: direct carrier of genetic information from genes to ribosomes for protein synthesis

Types: heterogeneous in length; spectrum variable in each cell type

Key features: short-lived

Examples

5S-rRNA

Phe-tRNA^Phe

D loop

T pU loop

mRNA

Anticodon

Codon

a

b

*Methylated base   **T** (Ribothymidine)   pU (Pseudouridine)   dU (Dihydrouridine)   **m⁷G** (7- methylguanidine)   **m²G** (2'-O-methylguanidine)

Fig. 18.2 RNA types and their secondary/tertiary structures. The three major types of RNA in eukaryotic cells are rRNA (80% of total), tRNA (15% of total), and mRNA (1 to 5% of total). All but mRNA are long-lived species. rRNA (e.g., 5S-rRNA) and tRNA (e.g., phenylalanyl-tRNA^Phe) exhibit extensive secondary structures, whereas mRNA is generally a linear molecule (although some mRNAs do contain stem-loop or hairpin structures in their untranslated regions). tRNA not only assumes a cloverleaf-like secondary structure but also contains a tertiary structure (not shown) that facilitates its function as an adapter in protein synthesis. tRNA is "charged" at its 3' end (red) when attached to its cognate amino acid. The anticodon loop (pink) contains a triplet nucleotide sequence that is complementary to the codon sequence on the mRNA. These complementary sequences form hydrogen bonds with each other on the assembled ribosome. tRNA also contains several unusual nucleotides, such as ribothymidine (T), dihydrouridine (dU), pseudouridine (pU), 7-methylguanosine (m⁷G), and 2'-0-methylguanosine (m²G).

mRNAs). The three major types of RNA present in animal cells are (▶ Fig. 18.2a, b):

1. **Ribosomal RNA (rRNA):** These represent 80% of total cellular RNA and are long-lived. rRNAs play a structural and functional role in ribosomes (the sites of protein synthesis) and have the following features:
   - They are GC rich and extensively folded into highly conserved configurations with numerous internal base pairs. rRNAs provide the scaffolding needed to assemble ribosomes. The addition of ribosomal proteins to rRNAs yields ribosomal subunits.
   - rRNAs also play a catalytic role in the formation of peptide bonds during protein synthesis.
   - There are four species of eukaryotic rRNAs: 28S (~ 5000 bases long), 18S (~ 2000 bases long), 5.8S (~ 150 bases long), and 5S (~ 120 bases long).

2. **Transfer RNA (tRNA):** These represent 15% of total cellular RNA and are also metabolically stable. tRNAs serve as "adapters" that carry an activated amino acid to ribosomes for incorporation into a growing polypeptide chain. Key features of tRNAs include the following:

- They are small, containing only 65 to 110 bases. Some of these bases are modified after transcription (becoming ribothymidine, pseudouridine, dihydrouridine, 7-methylguanosine, or 2'-O-methylguanosine). It is speculated that base modifications may provide increased stability to tRNAs and help in their interaction with the translational machinery.
- The 3' end of each tRNA is modified after initial synthesis to add three nucleotides, CCA, in a template-independent fashion. The 3' terminal A is the site of amino acid attachment.
- They have an extensive secondary structure that forms a "cloverleaf," and they fold into an *L*-shaped tertiary structure.
- Each tRNA contains an "anticodon" loop whose triplet sequence is complementary to the triplet codon sequence of the mRNA it associates with.
- When "charged," each tRNA contains an amino acid covalently attached to 3'-OH of the A of the CCA sequence at its 3' end. Each tRNA can accept only a single, specific amino acid, and each amino acid has at least one specific

Table 18.1 Types of RNA that exist in small amounts in eukaryotic cells

RNA type	Features/Function
snRNA (small nuclear RNA)	These are packaged with proteins to form small nuclear (or nucleolar) ribonucleoproteins (snRNPs or "snurps") that are part of "spliceosomes." They are involved in the splicing of precursor mRNA and export of mature mRNA. • Example: U1 snRNA
scRNA (small cytoplasmic RNA)	These are associated with small cytoplasmic ribonucleoproteins (scRNPs, "scryps") that are involved in protein processing and secretion. • Example: 7SL RNA or signal recognition particle RNA that is associated with the signal recognition particle needed for the translocation of nascent proteins containing a signal recognition sequence, from the cytoplasm to the endoplasmic reticulum
siRNA (short interfering RNA)	These are short (21–24 nucleotides) antisense transcripts derived from transposons and complementary to the coding regions of certain mRNAs. siRNAs inhibit the translation of target mRNAs and enhance their degradation in RNA-induced silencing complexes (RISCs).
miRNA (micro RNA)	Similar to siRNA, these short (~ 22 nucleotides) RNA are also involved in the posttranscriptional regulation of gene expression.
Mitochondrial RNA	Mitochondria contain their own protein-synthesizing machinery and therefore express unique RNA species, such as the 16S and 12S rRNAs, as well as 22 tRNAs and 13 mRNAs.

acceptor tRNA. There are 56 tRNAs, and different tRNAs that accept the same amino acid are called isoacceptors.

3. **Messenger RNAs (mRNA):** These represent only 1 to 5% of total cellular RNA but account for more than 50% of all new RNA synthesis. mRNAs tend to be very short-lived (typical of regulated biological messages) and have the following characteristics:
   • They encode proteins and thus serve as the direct carrier of genetic information from genes to ribosomes.
   • They are very heterogeneous in length and thus can be several thousands of bases long. The spectrum of mRNAs in each cell type is also variable.

4. **Other types of RNA:** Small amounts of other types of RNA are also present in eukaryotic cells. They include small nuclear RNA (snRNA), small cytoplasmic RNA (scRNA), ribonuclease P (RNase P), short interfering RNA (siRNA), micro RNA (miRNA), and mitochondrial RNA. Features and functions of each of the aforementioned types are summarized in ▸ Table 18.1.

Foundations
mRNA-processing bodies (P bodies)
Discrete cytoplasmic P bodies are sites where mRNAs that are not being translated accumulate. In addition to such mRNAs, P bodies contain hundreds of proteins and noncoding small RNAs that appear to be involved in mRNA degradation, translational repression, mRNA surveillance, and RNA-mediated gene silencing. Two such species of noncoding RNAs in P bodies are short interfering RNAs (siRNAs) and micro RNAs (miRNAs). Both of these classes of RNA associate with the conserved family of Argonaute proteins to form RNA-induced silencing complexes (RISCs). siRNAs are fully complementary to their target mRNAs and, through base pairing, guide the Argonaute proteins to degrade the target mRNAs in P bodies. Most miRNAs are only partially complementary and silence gene expression both by promoting mRNA degradation and by translational repression.

Therapeutics
Antipyrimidines
The methylation of uracil forms thymine. Addition of fluorine to carbon 5 of uracil produces 5-fluorouracil, an anticancer drug whose nucleotide derivative, 5-fluoro-dUMP, is a potent covalent (suicide) inhibitor of thymidylate synthase. 5-Fluorouracil also competes with orotic acid for condensation with 5-phospho-a-d-ribosyl 1-pyrophosphate (PRPP). Capecitabine is an orally administered fluoropyrimidine carbamate prodrug of 5-FU. Another antipyrimidine that is used as an anticancer drug is the nucleoside analogue cytosine arabinoside (Ara-C). Other clinically useful pyrimidine analogues are 5-azacytidine (used to treat myelodysplastic syndromes) and 2', 2'-difluoro-2'-deoxycytidine (Gemcitabine, used to treat advanced non-small cell lung, pancreatic and bladder cancers).

Foundations
Ribonucleotide reductase
Proliferating cells express the iron-dependent enzyme ribonucleotide reductase (RNR, also known as ribonucleoside diphosphate reductase), which converts the ribonucleotides CDP, UDP, ADP, and GDP into the deoxyribonucleotides dCDP, dUDP, dADP, and dGDP, respectively (see **Fig. 16.3**). The NADPH-dependent reduction reaction catalyzed by RNR substitutes an –H for the 2'-OH group on ribose.

18.2 Transcription

The purpose of transcription is to synthesize multiple types of RNA molecules that not only carry out the process of protein synthesis but also regulate it. Almost all RNA is synthesized (transcribed) from a DNA template; therefore, RNA is complementary to a portion of cellular DNA. Although a large fraction of the mammalian genome is transcribed into RNA (as high as

63% in the case of the mouse genome), only a small subset (~ 2%) of these transcripts, known as mRNAs, are actually translated into proteins.

18.2.1 RNA Polymerases

Transcription requires a DNA-dependent RNA polymerase that copies a template DNA by stringing together ribonucleoside monophosphates (derived from ATP, GTP, CTP, and UTP) in the 5' → 3' direction. Thus, the direction of growth of a new RNA chain is the same as that of a new DNA chain. The mechanism of RNA polymerization is also very similar to that of DNA but with two major differences:

1. Ribonucleotides are used in RNA synthesis (compared with deoxyribonucleotides in DNA synthesis).
2. RNA polymerase can carry out *de novo* chain assembly and thus does not require a primer (compared with DNA polymerases, which do).

RNA polymerases act catalytically to initiate, elongate, and terminate RNA chains. Although bacteria have a single RNA polymerase that is capable of synthesizing all types of RNA, eukaryotes express multiple RNA polymerases, each of which is specific for certain types of RNA and requires separate accessory proteins to initiate transcription. There are three different eukaryotic RNA polymerases (▶ Fig. 18.3):

1. **RNA polymerase I:** It is located in the nucleolus–a dense region within the nucleus composed of proteins and nucleic acids. It catalyzes the synthesis of a single large precursor rRNA (45S rRNA), which is cleaved after synthesis into three fragments to form the mature 28S, 18S, and 5.8S rRNAs.
2. **RNA polymerase II:** It is located in the nucleoplasm–the thick liquid component of the nucleus. It catalyzes the synthesis of precursor mRNA, also known as heterogeneous nuclear RNA (hnRNA), which is then processed into mature mRNA. It also synthesizes some snRNA and miRNA.

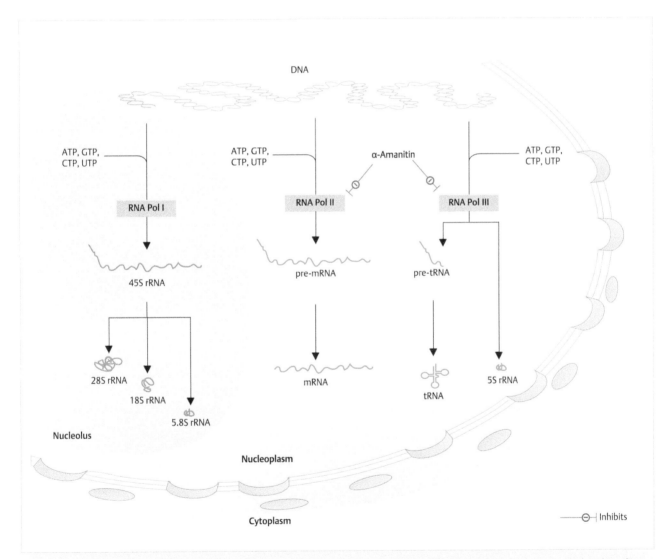

Fig. 18.3 RNA polymerases and the RNAs they transcribe. In the nucleolus, RNA polymerase I synthesizes a 45S precursor rRNA, which is cleaved into the 28S, 18S, and 5.8S rRNAs. In the nucleoplasm, RNA polymerase II synthesizes a precursor mRNA, which is then processed into mature mRNA. Also in the nucleoplasm, RNA polymerase III synthesizes small RNAs such as tRNAs and the 5S rRNA. α-Amanitin is a more potent inhibitor of RNA polymerase II than of RNA polymerase III.

3. **RNA polymerase III:** It is also present in the nucleoplasm and is responsible for the synthesis of small RNAs such as tRNA, 5S rRNA, and others such as U6 snRNA and scRNA.
   - α-Amanitin, a toxin produced by the *Amanita phalloides* mushroom, inhibits RNA polymerase II at low concentrations (1 µg/mL), and III at higher concentrations (10 µg/mL).

18.2.2 Functional Organization of a Gene

Before delving into the mechanism of transcription, one must understand the components of a gene that are necessary for transcription. For starters, DNA sequences are conventionally written 5′ to 3′ (from left to right), using the sequence of the top strand. For simplicity, the bottom strand is not usually shown, though it is understood that the DNA exists in a double-stranded form. The features of the functional organization of a gene that are necessary for transcription are as follows (▶ Fig. 18.4):

1. **The coding ("sense") strand:** This is the top, nontemplate strand, which is identical to the sequence the RNA would take, except that thymidine (T) is present in the coding strand where uridine (U) would be in the RNA transcript. As such, RNA polymerase "reads" the noncoding ("antisense") bottom template strand.

2. **Transcription start site:** The transcriptional start site is defined as the+ 1 position of a gene; some genes may contain more than one transcription start site. The initiating base at+ 1 is usually a purine (A or G), and the start site is defined by the assembly of an initiation complex formed by the binding of basal transcription factors and RNA polymerase.

3. **Transcription stop site:** One indicator of a stop site is the poly(A) addition signal (5′-AATAAA-3′). However, transcription does not terminate at this sequence but continues 500 to 2000 nucleotides beyond this site. During the processing of pre-mRNA, the RNA sequence 10 to 35 nucleotides downstream from the poly(A) signal site is cleaved and degraded, and a poly(A) tail is added in its place.

4. **Transcription unit:** This refers to the linear sequence of DNA from the transcription start site to the stop site. In contrast, a gene includes the transcription unit and the upstream elements such as the promoter and the proximal regulatory sequences. Upstream is toward the 5′ direction on the top strand, and downstream is toward the 3′ direction.

5. **The promoter:** This is a specific site located upstream of the transcription start site in each gene to which basal transcription factors (initiation factors) first bind and recruit the RNA polymerase. The promoter specifies both the start site and the polarity of transcription (i.e., which of the two DNA strands would serve as the template strand). There are two parts to the eukaryotic RNA polymerase II promoter–the core promoter and upstream regulatory sequences (URSs)–and each part employs two types of protein factors, as described here.
   - The core promoter of some eukaryotic genes contains the minimum sequence necessary for the initiation of transcription and may extend ~ 85 bp upstream of the start site. It includes the transcription start site and binding sites for basal transcription factors. The core promoter can consist of specific, conserved nucleotide sequences; a prominent example is a sequence called the TATA box (5′-TATAA(T)AA(T)A(G)-3′), which may be found 20 to 30 bp upstream of the transcription start site. Some TATA-less core promoters may contain a 6 bp downstream promoter element (DPE)+ 28 to+ 33 bp downstream of the transcription start site.
   - Additional elements such as a the "CAAT" box, may be present in the core promoter, where they are bound by general transcription factors or specific transcriptional regulatory proteins. Eukaryotic RNA polymerase II does not bind a specific sequence. Bacterial RNA polymerase holoenzyme does bind specific -10 and -35 sequences via the sigma subunit.
   - The sites of URS, to which additional transcription factors bind, may be found at position -250 or beyond. URSs include hormone response elements to which specific transcription factors bind to regulate the rate of

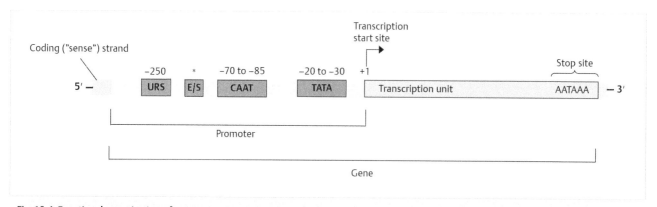

Fig. 18.4 Functional organization of genes. A transcription unit is the linear DNA sequence from the transcription start site (+ 1) to the polyadenylation (poly A) signal sequence (AATAAA). Eukaryotic RNA polymerases are recruited to the core promoter by basal (general) transcription factors that form a pre-initiation complex on the promoter. Formation of the initiation complex is complete when it includes RNA polymerase II. The TATA box is usually found 20 to 30 base pairs (bp) upstream of the transcription start site, and the CAAT box may be found 70 to 85 bp upstream of the start site. The upstream regulatory sequence (URS), to which specific transcription factors bind, may extend up to or beyond 250 bp upstream of the start site. Enhancer (E) and silencer (S) sequences can be anywhere (*) upstream, downstream, or within the transcription unit and on either the coding or the noncoding strand.

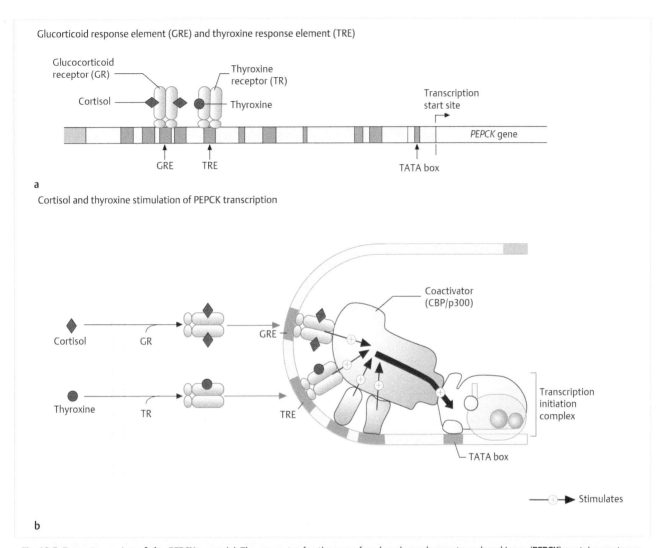

Glucorticoid response element (GRE) and thyroxine response element (TRE)

a

Cortisol and thyroxine stimulation of PEPCK transcription

b

Fig. 18.5 Promoter region of the *PEPCK* gene. (a) The promoter for the gene for phosphoenolpyruvate carboxykinase **(*PEPCK*)** contains upstream regulatory sequences such as the glucocorticoid response element (GRE) and thyroxine response element (TRE). **(b)** Transcription factors (hormone-receptor complexes) for cortisol and thyroxine bind to these sites. These transcription factors associate with the coactivator/mediator complex CBP/p300 to promote formation of the initiation complex and thus increase transcription *of PEPCK*. Cushing syndrome is a disorder marked by elevated cortisol levels.

transcription initiation. They can be located close to the core promoter (proximal sites) or farther away from the core promoter (distal sites). Their influence on the rate of formation of the initiation complex with basal transcription factors is mediated by other proteins, such as coactivators and co-repressors. This is the manner in which the hormones cortisol and thyroxine promote the transcription of the gene for phosphoenolpyruvate carboxykinase (PEPCK), a gluconeogenic enzyme (▶ Fig. 18.5).

6. **Enhancers and silencers:** These short (~ 8 bp) sequences can be located up to hundreds of thousands of base pairs away from the core promoter; upstream, downstream, or within the transcription unit; and on either the coding or the non-coding strand.

Enhancers and silencers are bound by specific transcription factors that act to increase or decrease the rate of transcription, respectively.

Foundations

cDNA

Double-stranded complementary DNA (cDNA) is created *in vitro* from a mature mRNA template via the action of reverse transcriptase (an RNA-dependent DNA polymerase) and DNA polymerase. Reverse transcriptase creates the first strand of DNA that is complementary to the mRNA template. After the mRNA template has been removed and the single-stranded DNA remains, the latter serves as the template for DNA polymerase to synthesize the second DNA strand, which is complementary to the first. This technique is used to create cDNA libraries (see **Fig. 21.9b**), which can be probed to identify the cDNAs of specific genes. Additionally, the technique is commonly coupled with real-time polymerase chain reaction (RT-PCR) (see **Fig. 21.8**) to measure the level of transcription of selected genes.

Foundations

Bacterial RNA polymerase and elements in prokaryotic promoter

The bacterial RNA polymerase core enzyme consists of five subunits ($\omega\alpha_2\beta\beta'$). A sixth dissociable subunit, σ (sigma factor), helps RNA polymerase to recognize the DNA sequence to be transcribed and to initiate transcription. RNA polymerase containing the sigma factor is the holoenzyme; without the sigma factor, it is called the apoenzyme. Bacterial RNA polymerase holoenzyme initially binds to a consensus sequence (called the -35 box) that reads 5′-TTGACA-3′ at position 30 to 40 bp upstream of the transcription start site (+ 1). Another consensus sequence, called the -10 box (or the Pribnow box), reads 5′-TATAAT-3′ and specifies a region ~ 7 bp upstream of the start site where the two DNA strands begin to unwind to initiate transcription.

Foundations

Alternative sequence to the TATA box

Some constitutively expressed eukaryotic housekeeping genes (especially those for β-actin, tubulin and RNA polymerase itself) do not contain a TATA box and may instead contain a nucleotide region that is rich in GC (5′-GGGCGG-3′, GC box). A second consensus sequence (CAAT box, 5′-GGC CAATCT-3′) may also be present ~ 80 bp upstream of the start site.

Foundations

Cis- and *trans*-acting elements

The expression of many genes is regulated by *cis*- and *trans*-acting elements. These elements are sequences in genomic DNA. The *cis*-acting elements are DNA sequences that modulate the transcription of genes on the same chromosome. They are not part of the coding sequence of the gene that is being regulated, but occur either upstream, near the promoter or the 5′-untranslated region of the gene. Sometimes, a *cis*-acting element may be located several kilobases downstream from the gene. The *trans*-acting elements code for transcription factors that regulate the expression of genes on many chromosomes. For example, the short 6 to 8 bp response element sequences found in the promoter regions of some genes are *cis*-acting elements, whereas the proteins that bind to such response elements are *trans*-acting factors.

Normal

Combinatorial control of gene expression

It should be emphasized that the control of gene expression by transcription factors is combinatorial in nature, meaning that the status of transcription of a regulated gene is the result of the integrated sum of positive and negative effects of all of the transcription factors associated with that gene. Combinatorial control allows multiple combinations of a small number (~ 2000) of transcription factors to regulate the expression of a large number (~ 21,000) of genes and to fine-tune such regulation in different cell types, tissues, and stages of development.

Normal

Transcription factors

Transcription factors are *trans*-acting proteins that regulate the transcription of genes across chromosomes. A general characteristic feature of transcription factors is that they have DNA-binding domains that enable them to bind to specific DNA sequences (response elements) in the upstream regulatory sequence (e.g., enhancer) regions of genes. Although the promoter regions of genes are located just upstream of the transcription start site, regulatory sequences may reside thousands of kb upstream or downstream from the transcribed gene. Transcription factors can either promote or repress the transcription of target genes. They bind to target sequences on DNA as homo- or heterodimers and once bound, recruit other proteins, including, in the case of activating factors, RNA polymerase. Proteins that bind to many lipophilic hormones (e.g., steroid and thyroid hormones, vitamin D) are transcription factors. Signals from hydrophilic molecules that act at the surface of a cell via G-protein-coupled receptors, receptor tyrosine kinases, or receptor-associated kinases modulate the activity of specific transcription factors to regulate gene expression. Such modulation of the activity of transcription factors usually involves regulated phosphorylation.

18.3 Mechanism of Transcription

The process of transcription in eukaryotic cells may be broadly classified into the following phases: assembly of the preinitiation complex, promoter clearance, elongation, and termination.

18.3.1 Assembly of Preinitiation Complex

RNA polymerases I, II, and III cannot bind by themselves to promoter sequences on a gene and initiate transcription. But rather, gene transcription in eukaryotes is regulated by basal or general transcription factors whose role is to form specific protein–DNA or protein–protein complexes on core promoters, upstream regulatory sequences, and enhancers. The respective RNA polymerases then bind to these complexes and initiate RNA synthesis.

Some of the roles of key members of preinitiation complexe are as follows:

1. **Recognition and binding to the TATA box:** Transcription factor TFIID, which contains TATA binding protein (TBP) and other protein factors, recognizes and binds to the TATA box (▶ Fig. 18.6a). TBP also binds to AT-rich regions in TATA-less promoters.
   - The binding of TBP/TFIID to the core promoter is sequentially followed by the recruitment of TFIIA, TFIIB, RNA polymerase II/TFIIF, TFIIE, and TFIIH. TFIIB helps in accurate positioning of RNA polymerase II at the transcription start site.

2. **Separation of DNA strands:** TFIIH, which has DNA helicase activity, uses the energy of hydrolysis of ATP to separate the

template and coding strands at the transcription start site by unwinding 11 to 15 base pairs of DNA. It also plays a role in DNA repair.

- Xeroderma pigmentosum, Cockayne syndrome, and trichothiodystrophy are disorders associated with mutations in the genes encoding two of the subunits of TFIIH.
- TFIIH also exhibits protein kinase activity which phosphorylates RNA poymerase II on its carboxy terminal domain (CTD) to activate it.

3. **Initiation of polymerization:** RNA polymerase II is capable of initiating the synthesis of a new RNA chain in the absence of a primer. It does so by catalyzing the formation of a dinucleotide starting from two ribonucleoside triphosphates in the presence of a DNA template. The driving force for this and subsequent polymerization reactions is provided by the hydrolysis of pyrophosphate (▶ Fig. 18.6c-2). It is important to note the following:

- Shortly after initiation, a capping enzyme adds a 7-methylguanosine (m^7G_{ppp}) cap to the 5′ terminal nucleotide of the pre-mRNA transcript in an unusual 5′-5′ triphosphate linkage (▶ Fig. 18.6c-3). This cap serves to protect the transcript from degradation by ribonucleases, enhances the efficiency of splicing, enhances the export of mature mRNAs into cytoplasm and later plays a role in binding mRNA to ribosomes for translation into protein.
- A cell's DNA exists as chromatin in which DNA is wrapped around histones in nucleosomes. Protein–DNA interactions are stabilized between the positively charged "tails" (due to lysine residues) in the N-terminal of histones and the negatively charged phosphate backbone of DNA. In order for transcription to occur, the chromatin must be remodeled so that the basal or general transcription factors can access the target DNA sequence. Such remodeling occurs via the action of histone acetyltransferases (HATs).
- HATs acetylate (add an acetyl group) the N-terminal lysine residues of histones. This removes their positive charge and reduces their interaction with DNA (▶ Fig. 18.6c-1).
- On the other hand, enzymes called histone deacetylases (HDACs) reverse the action of HATs by removing the acetyl group. This reestablishes the interactions between histones and DNA.

Transcription initiation by RNA polymerases I and III is analogous to that of RNA polymerase II except that they require their own polymerase-specific general transcription factors that recognize different DNA sequence elements.

18.3.2 Elongation and Termination

Subsequent elongation of the RNA chain by RNA polymerase II occurs by sequential addition of ribonucleotides in a 3′-5′ phosphodiester linkage (▶ Fig. 18.6b). Elongation factors join the transcription complex, and the RNA chain grows in the 5′ →3′ direction until RNA polymerase II encounters nonspecific ter-

mination signals 500 to 2000 nucleotides past the polyadenylation signal sequence (AAUAAA).

- Enzymes associated with the poly(A) polymerase complex cleave the mRNA transcript at sites located 10 to 35 nucleotides downstream of the polyadenylation signal and synthesize a poly(A) tail of 200 to 250 nucleotides in a template-independent fashion.
- The antibiotic actinomycin D and the organic compound acridine orange inhibit elongation in eukaryotes and bacteria. When they intercalate between the bases of the double helix, they bend the DNA and thus prevent RNA polymerase from moving along the DNA template.

Normal
TFIIH and DNA repair

TFIIH is one of the basal or general transcription factor proteins that make up the transcription initiation complex with RNA polymerase II. It contains seven subunits, two of which, XPB/ERCC-3 and XPD/ERCC-2, have DNA helicase activity. This activity contributes to the creation of the transcription bubble. Both *XPB* and *XPD* are members of the xeroderma pigmentosum (XP) complementation group genes and participate in nucleotide excision repair of DNA. Mutations in these genes are implicated in XP, Cockayne syndrome, and trichothiodystrophy. Thus, TFIIH plays a dual role in transcription and in DNA repair.

Therapeutics
Reversible acetylation of histones

Histones (H2A, H2B, H3, and H4) are at the core of the basic unit of chromatin, the nucleosome. They undergo multiple posttranslational modifications (e.g., acetylation, methylation, phosphorylation, ubiquitylation, sumoylation), and the combination of such modifications determines whether a gene is transcriptionally active or not. Histone acetyltransferases (HATs) are a diverse set of evolutionarily conserved enzymes that acetylate core histones to neutralize the positively charged lysines and facilitate chromatin decondensation, DNA repair, and gene transcription. HATs can also acetylate nonhistone substrates such as transcription factors. Inhibitors of HAT activity show promise in the treatment of several diseases (e.g., cancer, Alzheimer disease, rheumatoid arthritis). Garcinol, a natural product HAT inhibitor derived from *Garcinia indica*, inhibits osteoclast differentiation and acts as an antiarthritic agent. Curcumin and anacardic acid are other natural product HAT inhibitors. Isothiazolones and synthetic analogues of garcinol have been shown to exhibit antiproliferative activity in cultures of tumor cell lines.

Histone deacetylases (HDACs) are enzymes that remove acetyl groups from the lysines on core histones and nonhistone proteins. Cancer cells are very sensitive to inhibitors of such lysine deacetylases. Inhibitors of HDACs, such as valproic acid and vorinostat, are used as anticonvulsives and anticancer drugs.

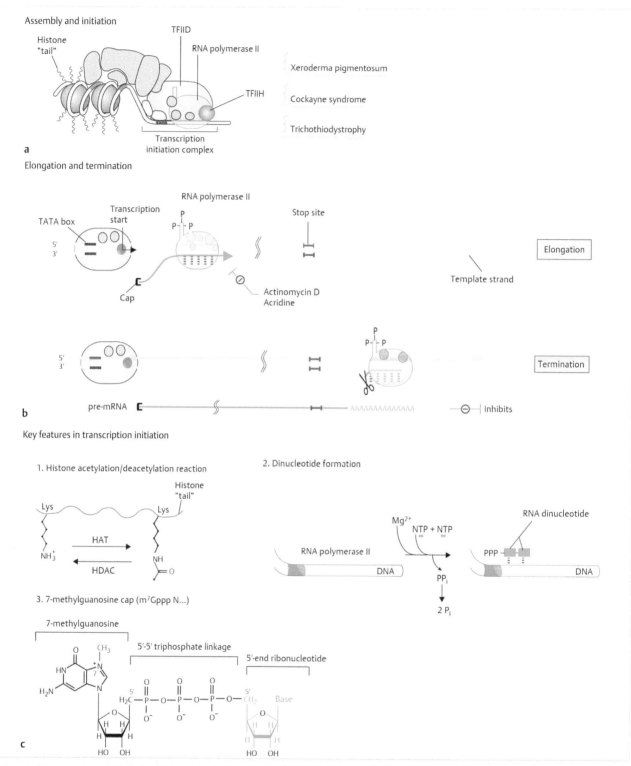

Fig. 18.6 Process of transcription. (a) Key components of the transcription initiation complex of eukaryotes are TFIID (which recognizes and binds to the TATA box), TFIIH (which separates the DNA strands), and RNA polymerase II (which catalyzes the polymerization of ribonucleotides into an RNA chain). **(b)** The elongation of mRNA chains proceeds in the 5' → 3'direction, 500 to 2000 nucleotides past the polyadenylation signal until RNA polymerase II encounters nonspecific termination signals. Poly(A) polymerase-associated enzymes then cleave the primary transcript at a site 10 to 35 nucleotides downstream from the polyadenylation signal. Actinomycin D and acridine inhibit elongation by intercalating between the bases of the DNA double helix. **(c-1)** DNA becomes accessible via the acetylation of lysine residues on histone tails. **(c-2)** RNA polymerase II initiates mRNA synthesis by catalyzing the formation of a dinucleotide from two ribonucleoside triphosphates. This (and subsequent) phosphodiester bond formation is driven by the hydrolysis of pyrophosphate (PP_i) into two inorganic phosphates (2 Pi). **(c-3)** Shortly after synthesis begins, a 7-methylguanosine cap is added to the 5'end of the mRNA transcript. HAT, histone acetyltransferase; HDAC, histone deacetylase.

Normal

Promoter-proximal pausing

The movement of RNA polymerase II between the 4th and 28th nucleotide of nascent pre-mRNA is considered to be the slow step of transcription. During this phase, the RNA-DNA hybrid is relatively strong. In some cases, initiation may be aborted during this slow phase, leaving abortive transcripts of 3 to 15 nucleotides in length. TFIIH and TFIIE appear to contribute to successful promoter escape of RNA polymerase II.

Due to the action of negative elongation factors, RNA polymerase II in the early elongation complex enters a paused state (promoter-proximal pausing) 20 to 50 nucleotides into elongation of some genes. The duration of pause is variable among different genes. The pausing may allow time for the capping enzyme and HATs to act. Phosphorylation of negative elongation factors by the kinase subunit of TFIIH allows the elongation complex to escape from the paused state.

Normal

Heterochromatin versus euchromatin

Eukaryotic cells contain highly condensed acidic DNA in a complex with basic histone proteins. In this state, the DNA is not available for transcription. This problem is overcome by modification of regions of chromatin to expose promoter regions to basal transcription factors. Actively transcribed chromatin (euchromatin) is more loosely packaged than transcriptionally inactive (dormant) regions of tightly packed chromatin (heterochromatin). Chromatin is rendered "open" by acetylation of histones using acetyl coenzyme A (CoA) as a substrate. Covalent modification of DNA, such as methylation, is associated with "silent" or transcriptionally inactive genes and with certain regions of chromosomal DNA (e.g., centromeres). Heterochromatin is characterized by extensive CpG DNA methylation that directs the deacetylation (and a specific type of methylation) of histones.

Therapeutics

Rifampicin inhibits bacterial RNA synthesis

Rifampicin is an antibiotic that inhibits RNA synthesis in bacterial cells by binding to the β subunit of RNA polymerase. In doing so, it prevents RNA polymerase from initiating translation. Human RNA polymerases are unaffected by this drug. Rifampicin is an effective drug for treating tuberculosis and is used as a prophylactic against some forms of bacterial meningitis. The drug needs to be taken for several months to eliminate *Mycobacterium tuberculosis*. Bacteria, however, tend to mutate their RNA polymerase to become rifampicin resistant. Therefore, rifampicin is not used in monotherapy but is co-administered with isoniazid, pyrazinamide, and streptomycin to substantially reduce the bacteria's chances of developing resistance to rifampicin. Side effects of rifampicin treatment include up-regulation of hepatic cytochrome P-450 enzymes (e.g., CYP-3A4, CYP-2C9) and thus an increase in the metabolism of other drugs (e.g., the anticoagulant warfarin) and hormones (e.g., contraceptive steroids) by this system.

Rifampicin transiently imparts red color to urine, sweat, and tears for a short time after administration.

Therapeutics

Actinomycin D

The antibiotic, actinomycin D, intercalates between successive G-C base pairs of the DNA double helix and prevents the movement of RNA polymerase, and thus inhibits the elongation phase of transcription. Due to its lack of specificity for prokaryotic transcription, actinomycin D is mostly used as a laboratory tool to study RNA synthesis. Actinomycin D is sometimes used to treat cancers such as Wilms tumor and neuroblastoma.

Therapeutics

α-Amanitin poisoning

Mammalian RNA polymerases that bind the mushroom toxin α-amanitin display differential sensitivity (RNA polymerase II > III > I) to it. Fifty percent inhibition of RNA polymerase II occurs at an α-amanitin concentration of 10 nM (9 ng/mL), while polymerases I and III are unaffected. Thus, amanitin is a useful agent with which to distinguish among these enzymes. α-Amanitin, a cyclopeptide of eight amino acids, is extremely hepatotoxic to humans and domestic pets that eat the wild mushroom *Amanita phalloides* or deathcap mushroom. It causes liver cells to lyse and release liver enzymes (e.g., alanine aminotransferase [ALT]) into circulation. The LD_{50} of α-amanitin is 0.1 mg/kg body weight. Symptoms of α-amanitin poisoning include cramps and diarrhea, followed by renal failure, liver failure, coma, and death. Treatment includes gastric lavage with activated charcoal and antibiotics. In cases of extreme poisoning, a liver transplant may be needed.

Therapeutics

Acridine orange

Acridine orange, a fluorochrome nucleic acid stain, fluoresces green when bound to double-stranded DNA and yellow-red when bound to single-stranded DNA or RNA. It provides a sensitive method for screening clinical specimens for the presence of bacteria. At a pH of 3.5, the dye-stained human cells appear green and bacteria appear bright orange, thus allowing easy and rapid detection. Acridine orange has been used to detect pathogenic bacteria such as *Trichomonas vaginalis* in vaginal specimens and parasites such as *Anaplasma marginale* and trypanosomes in blood samples.

18.4 RNA Processing

All mature RNAs found in eukaryotic cells are derived from primary transcripts that are processed in the nucleus before they are exported to the cytoplasm. Processing may be cotranscriptional or posttranscriptional and can involve capping, cleavage, addition of polyadenylate sequences, and base modifications.

V

The 40S and 60S ribosomal subunits

The formation of mature eukaryotic rRNAs is coupled to the assembly of the small 40S ribosomal subunit and the large 60S ribosomal subunit. Maturation of individual rRNA species and the small and large ribosomal subunits proceeds together in a tightly coupled manner. For instance, the 45S primary rRNA transcript is assembled into a 90S preribosomal complex. The 90S complex is initially cleaved to pre-40S and pre-60S ribosomal subunits. Incorporation of 5S rRNA from the nucleoplasm and additional cleavage and modifications follow to produce the mature ribosomal sub-units containing the 18S rRNA (40S subunit) and the 28S, 5.8S, and 5S rRNAs (60S subunit).

18.4.1 rRNA Processing

The primary transcript of eukaryotic RNA polymerase I is the 45S pre-rRNA, which contains the sequences for the 28S, 18S, and 5.8S rRNAs. Processing of the primary rRNA transcript in the nucleolus involves the following (▶ Fig. 18.7a):

1. Modifications of nucleosides (e.g., pseudouridine formation and methylation of 2'-OH groups of riboses)
2. Cleavage, which is performed by large preribosome complexes that contain small nucleolar ribonucleoproteins (snoRNPs), protein components of ribosomes, and a combination of endo- and exonucleases

The 5S rRNA, however, is made separately by RNA polymerase III in the nucleoplasm (▶ Fig. 18.7c-2).

18.4.2 mRNA Processing

The sequence of the nascent mRNA transcript known as heterogeneous nuclear RNA (hnRNA), or pre-mRNA, is complementary to the DNA template and identical (except for U's in place of T's) to the nontemplate strand. The pre-RNA is a faithful copy of the template DNA sequence and contains exons (expressed sequences that are present in mature mRNA and may be translated into protein) and introns (noncoding intervening sequences). Pre-mRNA processing, which occurs cotranscriptionally and continues in the nucleoplasm after the termination of transcription, includes the following (▶ Fig. 18.7b):

1. **Addition of 5' cap:** As mentioned earlier, the 5' end of pre-mRNA is capped by the addition of guanosine (G) in an unusual 5'-5' triphosphate linkage in which the 5'-terminal G is methylated at the 7 position using S-adenosyl methionine as the methyl donor to generate the m^7G_{ppp} cap (see ▶ Fig. 18.6c-3).
2. **Addition of poly(A) tail:** The 3' end of the premRNA transcript is cleaved 10 to 35 nucleotides downstream of the polyadenylation signal by an endonuclease. Poly(A) polymerase then adds 50 to 250 residues of adenylate to the new 3' end in a template-independent fashion.
3. **Splicing (removal of introns):** Splicing occurs in specialized nucleoprotein structures called spliceosomes whose

assembly is made possible by the energy obtained from the hydrolysis of ATP. Spliceosomes are composed of five small ribonucleoproteins (snRNPs) (U1, U2, U4, U5 and U6), and 50 to 100 other proteins. These snRNPs recognize the exon–intron junctions and initiate splicing of the primary transcript as it is being transcribed. When an intron is cleaved out, the two exons flanking it are joined together. After splicing, the introns are degraded in the nucleus. Notable features of the splicing mechanism include the following (▶ Fig. 18.8):

- The exon-intron junctions are recognized by snRNPs because intron sequences usually have GU at their 5' end and AG at their 3' end.
- Splicing involves first generating a "lariat" or lasso structure of the intron, then cleaving it out and joining the flanking two exons together.
- The autoimmune disease systemic lupus erythematosus is sometimes characterized by the body's production of antibodies against its own snRNPs.
- A hemoglobinopathy, β-thalassemia can develop in patients with point mutations (G → A) at the exon-intron junction of the pre-mRNA of β-globin chain.

4. After processing, the mature mRNA thus contains a central stretch of a protein-coding sequence called an open reading frame (ORF), untranslated regions (UTRs) of variable length on either side of the ORF (5'-UTR and 3'-UTR), as well as the 5'-7-methylguanosine cap and the 3' poly(A) tail.
    - In prokaryotes, mRNAs contain several consecutive ORFs that code for separate proteins (polycistronic). In eukaryotes, each mRNA usually contains a single ORF (monocistronic).
    - Each set of three bases in the ORF represents a "codon" that specifies a single amino acid or a stop signal.

18.4.3 tRNA Processing

The processing of tRNA in the nucleoplasm involves the following (▶ Fig. 18.7c-1):

1. **Cleavage of extra sequences at both 5' and 3' ends:** The 5' sequence of the primary transcript produced by RNA polymerase III is removed by ribonuclease P, a multisubunit ribonucleopreotein that functions as an endonuclease. The extra nucleotides at the 3' end are removed by an exonuclease, RRP6, which is a homologue of prokaryotic RNase D.
2. **Extensive modification of nucleotides:** These include methylations, deaminations, and reductions. Currently 93 such post-transcriptional modifications are known. On average, there are 13 modifications per each human tRNA molecule. Many of the modifications are location specific (see ▶ Fig. 18.2).
3. **Template-independent addition of nucleotides:** The trinucleotide sequence CCA is added to the 3' end by tRNA nucleotidyltransferase.
4. **Removal of an intron at the anticodon loop:** The intron is removed by an endonuclease and a ligase (similar to the DNA ligase) that reseals the tRNA chain.

V

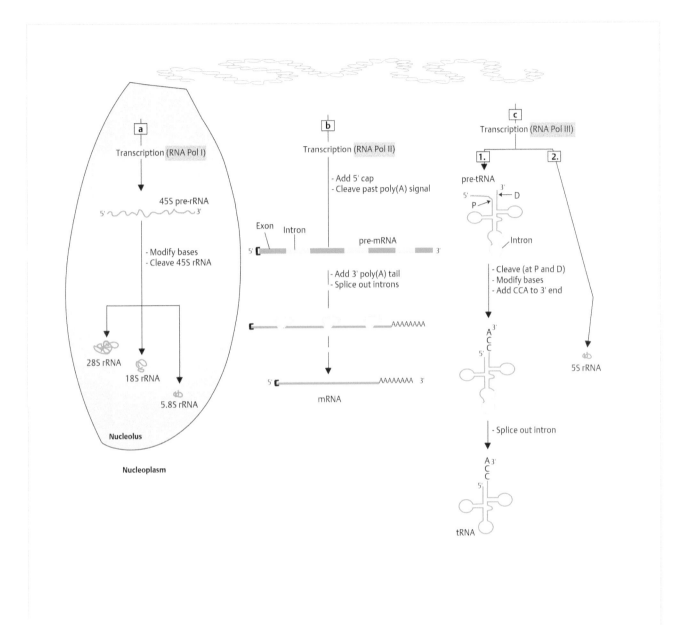

Fig. 18.7 Processing of eukaryotic rRNA. (a) Once the 45S pre-rRNA has been synthesized in the nucleolus by RNA polymerase I, modifications of nucleosides and cleavage results in the formation of the 28S, 18S, and 5.8S rRNAs. (b) In the nucleoplasm, the processing of the pre-mRNA (hnRNA) occurs co-transcriptionally and involves adding a guanosine cap to the 5'end, cleavage past the poly(A) stop signal, addition of a poly(A) tail, and splicing out of introns. (c-1) Processing of the pre-tRNA generated by RNA polymerase III in the nucleoplasm involves cleavage of the extra nucleotides at the 5' and 3'ends by RNase P (P) and RRP6 (D), splicing out of introns, modification of nucleotides, and the addition of a trinucleotide sequence (CCA) to the 3' end. and. (c-2) The 5S rRNA is synthesized in the nucleoplasm by RNA polymerase III.

Normal

Lupus

Lupus is an autoimmune disease in which the body generates antibodies against itself. In systemic lupus erythematosus (SLE), the antibodies target subunits of the U1 snRNP complex and the Ro/La antigenic complex comprising of small cytoplasmic ribonucleoproteins (scRNPs). Other chronic inflammatory rheumatic diseases such as mixed connective tissue disease and systemic sclerosis also exhibit similar antibodies. Antibodies may be directed against both protein and RNA components of the RNPs. Antigen-specific therapies are under investigation using a modified (e.g., phosphorylated) 21 amino acid U1 snRNP peptide (P140 peptide). When administered intravenously, P140 peptide prolonged the survival of mouse models of SLE.

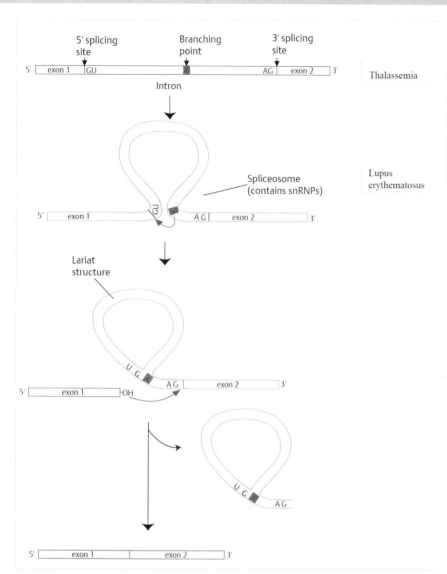

Fig. 18.8 Mechanism for splicing pre-mRNA. Intron sequences usually have GU at their 5' end and AG at their 3' end. An adenosine (A) is usually found at the branching point within the intron sequence. The snRNPs of the spliceosome recognize intron-exon junctions and splice out the intron as a "lariat" structure. One form of β-thalassemia is associated with a mutation (G to A) in the exon-intron junction. In systemic lupus erythematosus, the body produces antibodies against its own snRNPs (in particular U1 snRNP).

Therapeutics

Errors in splicing–thalassemia

Thalassemia is a disease resulting from the loss of synthesis of one of the two types of subunits (α or β) of hemoglobin, leading to an imbalance in the relative amounts of the two subunits. Although there are multiple mechanisms that cause such loss of gene expression, errors in mRNA splicing are an important cause. Patients with point mutations at the exon–intron junction (G →A) fail to correctly splice the β-globin mRNA. Under such conditions, the splicing machinery tries to find the next best splice site. Retaining all or parts of an intron severely interferes with the correct sequence of the ORF and thereby the primary sequence and activity of the translated protein product.

Normal

Alternative splicing: single gene, multiple mRNA products

Alternative mRNA splicing, in which different combinations of exons present in the nascent heterogeneous nuclear RNA (hnRNA) are spliced together, occurs for up to 80% of mRNAs. This leads to the generation of different protein isoforms that can have very different levels of activity or function. Thus, a single gene can produce more than one mRNA and more than one gene product in different tissues. In alternative splicing, special splicing-specificity factors operate as components of spliceosomes. It is conceivable that tissue-specific distribution of such factors could lead to alternative splicing patterns (e.g., tropomyosin in different types of muscle). Another mechanism is the presence of multiple polyadenylation signal sites in the primary transcript (e.g., diversity in the variable domains of immunoglobulin-heavy chains). In the case of the hormone calcitonin, utilization of both these mechanisms leads to the production of calcitonin in the thyroid gland and the production of calcitonin-gene-related peptide in the brain of rats (from the same hnRNA).

Normal

3'-UTR of mRNA

Translation of some mRNAs and/or mRNA stability may be inhibited by microRNAs (miRNAs), which are short (~ 22 nt) RNAs that hybridize to the 3'-UTR of mRNA. Unlike short interfering RNAs (siRNAs) whose sequences are totally complementary to open reading frame sequences in their target mRNAs, miRNAs are only partially complementary (as little as 7 out of 22 bases) to sequences in the 3'-UTR of their target mRNAs. Deadenylation of the poly(A) tail of mRNA followed by rapid degradation in RNA-induced silencing complexes (RISCs) seems to be the main mechanism by which miRNAs silence gene expression. It is estimated that the expression of up to 30% of all genes may be under miRNA control. The pattern of expression of specific mRNAs varies with tissue type and with development. It is, therefore, possible that by regulating the types of genes expressed, miRNAs play a role in cellular differentiation.

18.5 Regulation of Transcription

The efficiency of transcription of the ~21,000 protein-coding genes in the human genome is quite variable, and this highly complex process is regulated at many levels. Eukaryotic gene transcription regulation occurs at many levels such as remodeling of chromatin through histone acetylation; methylation of cytosines on DNA to silence transcription; formation of the pre-initiation complex near the transcription start site; and complex interactions between gene-specific transcription factors binding specifically to DNA at upstream regulatory sites and enhancer and silencer elements.

The formation of the preinitiation complex has been considered to be the rate-limiting step of transcription in prokaryotes. However, some studies point to promoter clearance (promoter-proximal pausing) as an alternative rate-limiting step in the process of RNA synthesis in eukaryotes.

Transcription factors do accelerate the rate of formation of initiation complex and help recruit enzymes that modify chromatin so that the core promoter region is accessible to RNA polymerase. Thus, regulation is achieved through the following:

- Interaction of multiple transcription factors that number more than 2000
- Interaction of coactivators and corepressors among themselves and with the basal transcription factors on one hand and the transcription-competent RNA polymerase on the other

Transcription of many genes for proteins in a single metabolic pathway or related pathways tends to be regulated in concert by the same set of hormones or end products. This result is achieved by the presence of response elements (e.g., steroid hormone response element) in the URS. Different genes would usually have different combinations of response elements to allow for fine-tuning of regulation in response to extracellular signals (e.g., hormones and neurotransmitters) or developmental cues.

- The transcription factors that interact with such elements share a common tripartite domain theme in their domain structure: a DNA-binding domain, a transcriptional activation domain, and a ligand-binding domain (in some). They bind to the palindromic response element sequence as homo- or heterodimers. Transcription factors are categorized by the presence of specific, conserved protein structures that bind DNA. Examples of common categories include the following:

1. **Homeodomain proteins:** First identified in the fruit fly *Drosophila*, they contain a conserved 60-residue DNA-binding motif called the homeodomain.
2. **Zinc-finger proteins:** These proteins have short (~ 25 amino acid) regions containing cysteine and histidine residues that interact with Zn^{2+} ions that produce multiple compact loops termed zinc fingers (e.g., the C2H2 and the C4 zinc fingers). These domains can insert into the major grooves of the DNA double helix. Zinc fingers are the most common DNA-binding factors in the human genome, with ~ 700 different proteins containing these structures (e.g., steroid hormone receptors).
3. **Leucine-zipper proteins:** These proteins contain dimerization domain sequences in which every seventh residue is leucine, a hydrophobic amino acid. The leucines help in dimerization of these factors and the formation of coiled coil structures. Other proteins with similar structure but containing hydrophobic amino acids other than leucine are known. All of these proteins are commonly referred to as basic zipper (bZIP) proteins.
4. **Basic helix-loop-helix (bHLH) proteins:** The DNA-binding domains of these proteins are similar to those of bZIP proteins except that the α-helical regions in these proteins are separated by a nonhelical loop sequence.

Although the assembly of the initiation complex on the promoter may be the rate-limiting step in overall transcription, the processes of elongation and termination are also regulated. For example, RNA chain elongation appears to be coupled to the recruitment of proteins that are involved in RNA processing such as capping, splicing, and polyadenylation. Many of these factors associate with the phosphorylated carboxy-terminal domain of RNA polymerase II.

Therapeutics

Transcription factors and cancer

Deregulation of transcription factors can lead to oncogenesis and cancer by inappropriate activation/inactivation of genes that control cell growth. Mutated genes for transcription factors represent a significant fraction of oncogenes. Misregulation can occur by an aberrant increase in the level of expression (e.g., an increase in gene copy number) or by mutations in the coding sequence that alter the activity of a transcription factor (e.g., loss of a phosphorylation site that is required for the regulated shutdown of its activity).

Therapeutics
Aberrant methylation of DNA

The fragile X mental retardation 1 (*FMR1*) gene encodes a protein involved in neurologic function. Its DNA sequence contains 30 repeats of the sequence CGG in exaon 1 in most people. In patients with fragile X mental retardation syndrome, this CGG repeat is expanded to >200 copies, and the *FMR1* gene becomes silent even though the triplet expansion occurs upstream of the protein-coding region. Expansion of CGG repeats leads to methylation of cytosine (via an unknown mechanism). As the methylated repeat region extends into the promoter area, transcription is turned off.

Foundations
Regulation of prokaryotic gene expression

In prokaryotic genomes, all the genes that encode proteins of a specific metabolic pathway are organized in clusters called operons. All the genes in an operon share a single promoter and are transcribed as a single transcript (polycistronic mRNA), thus allowing coordinated regulation of gene expression. The transcript is translated into proteins as it is being synthesized. In addition to containing a promoter, which is recognized by RNA polymerase, the operon contains a segment of DNA called an operator. Binding of a repressor protein to the operator prevents the RNA polymerase from transcribing the operon. The regulatory gene that constitutively produces the repressor is not a part of the operon. An inducer binds to the repressor protein and changes its conformation so that it cannot bind to the operator. Some operons are regulated by the binding of an activator protein to the operator. An inhibitor may bind to the activator to prevent its interaction with the operator.

Foundations
Homeobox and Hox genes

Some genes harbor a homeobox, an approximately 180-base pair sequence of DNA that encodes the DNA-binding domain (homeodomain) of the gene's protein product. Such domains are found in transcription factors encoded by Hox genes that regulate anatomic development (morphogenesis). Vertebrates express four banks of overlapping sets of Hox genes (*HoxA, HoxB, HoxC,* and *HoxD*) with each bank containing clusters of multiple (up to 13) genes. Spatial and temporal control of Hox gene expression regulates the patterning of the vertebrate body axis. Mutations in the 39 human Hox genes are known to cause congenital malformations (e.g., *HoxD13* in synpolydactyly and *HoxA13* in hand-foot-genital syndrome).

19 Translation and Posttranslational Modifications

19.1 Genetic Code and Mutations

Proteins are composed of linear chains of amino acids linked together by peptide bonds. There are 20 different amino acids commonly found in proteins, but there are only 4 different bases (A, T, G, C) that encode the genetic information in the DNA or mRNA. A grouping of 2 bases would yield a maximum of only 4^2, or 16 combinations. This is 4 short of the 20 combinations that would be needed to code for each amino acid. A grouping of 3 bases, however, yields a maximum of 4^3, or 64 combinations. Therefore,

• the minimum number of bases required to code for each of the 20 amino acids is 3, and
• there are 64 such 3-base combinations (codons) possible.

This is the basis for the genetic code–a set of rules that govern how cells translate the information in DNA and mRNA sequences into a protein chain. It takes into account the fact that genes are collinear with the proteins they encode. This means that the sequence of triplet deoxyribonucleotides in the coding (nontemplate) strand of DNA determines the corresponding sequence of ribonucleotide codons in mRNA (but U replaces T). This in turn determines the sequence of amino acids (▶ Fig. 19.1a). Initial experiments suggested the following general features about the genetic code:

1. **It is degenerate;** that is, some amino acids can be coded by more than one codon. Three codons (UAA, UGA, UAG), however, do not code for any amino acid, and they represent the stop or translation termination signal (▶ Fig. 19.1b).

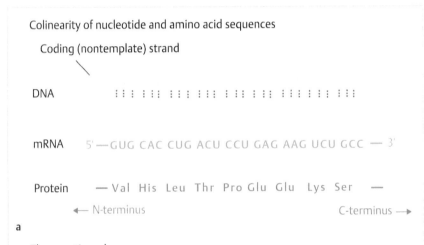

Colinearity of nucleotide and amino acid sequences

Coding (nontemplate) strand

DNA

mRNA   5'—GUG CAC CUG ACU CCU GAG AAG UCU GCC — 3'

Protein   — Val His Leu Thr Pro Glu Glu Lys Ser —

← N-terminus   C-terminus →

a

Fig. 19.1 Colinearity of nudeotide and amino acid sequences and the genetic code. (a) The sequence of triplet deoxyribonucleotides in the coding (sense or nontemplate) strand of DNA determines the corresponding sequence of ribonucleotide codons in mRNA (except that U replaces T), which in turn determines the sequence of amino acids in a protein. **(b)** A standard genetic code.

The genetic code

1st base in codon		2nd base in codon				3rd base in codon
		U	**C**	**A**	**G**	
U		Phe	Ser	Tyr	Cys	U
		Phe	Ser	Tyr	Cys	C
		Leu	Ser	STOP	STOP	A
		Leu	Ser	STOP	Trp	G
C		Leu	Pro	His	Arg	U
		Leu	Pro	His	Arg	C
		Leu	Pro	Gln	Arg	A
		Leu	Pro	Gln	Arg	G
A		Ile	Thr	Ans	Ser	U
		Ile	Thr	Ans	Ser	C
		Ile	Thr	Lys	Arg	A
		Met	Thr	Lys	Arg	G
G		Val	Ala	Asp	Gly	U
		Val	Ala	Asp	Gly	C
		Val	Ala	Glu	Gly	A
		Val	Ala	Glu	Gly	G

b

- A group of triplet nucleotides that code for the same amino acid is called a codon family. The first two bases of members of a codon family are the primary determinants of specificity, but the degeneracy appears to be concentrated in the third base (wobble position). For example:
  - Codons XYPy where Py is a pyrimidine (C or U) always code for the same amino acid.
  - Codons XYPu where Pu is a purine (A or G) usually code for the same amino acid.
2. **It is not punctuated and is without commas;** that is, no "extra" nucleotides are used between codons for punctuation or commas.
3. **It is nonoverlapping;** however, a few exceptions have been discovered (e.g., the transcripts for two of the subunits of mitochondrial ATP synthase [ATP-6 and ATP-8] are generated using different reading frames from overlapping segments of mitochondrial DNA).

Foundations
Genetic code: standard, not universal
The genetic code is standard but not quite universal. Exceptions to the genetic code are present, most notably in mitochondria, the subcellular organelle with its own genome and machinery for transcription and translation. The code also differs in mitochondrial genomes from different species. In human mitochondria, the codons AUA and AUU code for Met (instead of Ile), and AGA and AGG act as stop codons (instead of Arg). The standard stop codon, UGA, codes for Trp instead in mitochondria.

19.1.1 Mutations
Point mutations, those that affect a single base pair in the protein coding region or open reading frame (ORF) of a gene, may result in a different amino acid being incorporated into the protein. Such mutations may be classified into four categories:
1. A **silent mutation** is one that *does not change* the amino acid incorporated into the protein. This is due to the degeneracy of the genetic code. Typically, mutations in the wobble position are most likely to be silent.
2. A **missense mutation** is one that *does change* the amino acid inserted into the protein. Such amino acid substitutions can have little or no effect on protein function (a conservative substitution) or result in a protein with vastly different (or absent) function. Such a mutation would result in a polypeptide with altered function.
   - Sickle cell anemia is caused by a missense mutation in the β-globin gene in which a glutamate is changed to a valine.
3. A **nonsense mutation** results in a codon being changed to a stop signal, which causes premature chain termination. This most often prevents the production of a functional protein due to rapid degradation of both the altered message and its protein product. However, a nonsense mutation can sometimes result in a truncated protein with altered activity.
   - β⁰ thalassemias are marked by a lack of production of β-globin protein due to nonsense mutations giving rise to truncated transcripts that decay rapidly.
4. A **frameshift mutation** can occur when a number of nucleotides that are not multiples of 3 are deleted from or inserted into the ORF. Such insertions or deletions are commonly known as indels. If an indel is out of frame, it causes a change in the codon sequence downstream from the point of change. Such a mutation would alter the amino acid sequence of the protein product downstream of the indel often resulting in the introduction of a premature termination codon. Such transcripts and their truncated translation products (if any) are rapidly degraded.
   - Many cases of Duchenne muscular dystrophy are caused by out-of-frame internal deletions in the gene for the muscle protein dystrophin, resulting in internally truncated transcripts with translational frameshift. The resultant premature stop codons prevent such transcripts from producing a functional dystrophin protein.

Foundations
Nonsense mutations
Nonsense mutations that occur near the end of the coding sequence tend to generate nearly full-length transcripts that the translated into protein products. However, such defective proteins are often rapidly degraded. Nonsense mutations that occur near the beginning of the coding sequence produce transcripts that decay rapidly and are not not translated (nonsense-mediated decay).. Thus, a nonsense mutation is also called a null mutation.

Foundations
Selenocysteine and pyrrolysine
Selenocysteine (Sec) and pyrrolysine (Pyl) are considered by some as the 21st and 22nd proteinogenic amino acids. The former is present in both bacterial and eukaryotic proteins (most notably in the antioxidant enzyme glutathione peroxidase), whereas the latter is observed only among the proteins in methane-producing bacteria. Both of these nonstandard amino acids are encoded by the stop codons (UGA in case of Sec and UAG in case of Pyl). The UGA codon specifies Sec only when a *cis*-acting, hairpin structure known as the Sec insertion sequence (SECIS) is present in the 3'-UTR of selenoprotein mRNAs. The UGA stop codon is recognized by an activated Ser-tRNA on which the Ser is changed to Sec by a Sec synthase. Decoding of UAG as a Pyl codon requires both a downstream Pyl insertion sequence and unique Pyl tRNA.

Foundations
Conservative substitutions
During evolution across many species as well as among members of the same gene family, proteins that exhibit identical or similar function rarely have identical amino acid sequences. However, in regions critical for their function, the substituted residues tend to be conservative, meaning that they have similar chemical properties. Thus, a substitution of an Asp with a Glu, or a Lys with an Arg, is said to be a conservative substitution.

Therapeutics

Sickle cell anemia

The β-globin subunit in adult hemoglobin (HbA) is a polypeptide of 146 amino acids. A missense mutation that changes the codon for the 6th amino acid in both alleles of the gene for human β-globin (*HBB*) from GAG to GTG substitutes a Glu with a Val, giving rise to HbS. This nonconservative substitution, from a negatively charged amino acid to a hydrophobic branched-chain amino acid, alters the conformation of hemoglobin, particularly in its deoxy form. As a result, the mutated deoxyhemoglobin molecules aggregate, forming rigid rod-like structures, and cause the deformation of red blood cells into a sickle-like shape. The deformed erythrocytes tend to clog capillaries, thus restricting blood supply to various tissues. They also have a much shortened lifespan, leading to anemia. A variant form of sickle cell disease (HbSC) is caused in compound heterozygotes exhibiting a Glu to Lys mutation in one allele of *HBB* and the Glu to Val mutation in the other allele.

Therapeutics

Duchenne muscular dystrophy

Duchenne muscular dystrophy (DMD) is an X-linked, recessive disorder with an incidence of 1 in 3500 boys and leads to progressive muscle wasting. Affected males require confinement to wheel chairs by age 12 and die of respiratory failure within 10 years. A milder form of the disease with a later onset is called Becker muscular dystrophy (BMD). Both DMD and BMD are the result of mutations in the dystrophin gene that codes for the 427 kDa muscle protein dystrophin. Dystrophin is a rod-like protein that connects the cytoskeleton to basal lamina and stabilizes the membranes and participates in calcium handling. The dystrophin gene is the largest human gene known, spanning about 2.5 million base pairs of DNA on the P arm of the X chromosome. It contains 79 exons. Hundreds of mutations in the gene have been described, about two-thirds of which are due to large internal deletions. About half of such deletions are in-frame, and the other half are out-of-frame, causing a translational frame shift in the RNA transcript. The in-frame deletions observed in BMD patients give rise to a smaller dystrophin protein with partial function. The out-of-frame deletions seen in DMD patients lead to little or no expression of dystrophin due to the rapid turnover of both truncated transcripts and their products. The remaining third of the cases are due to very small deletions or point mutations that result in premature termination signals.

Therapeutics

β⁰ thalassemia

Thalassemias are disorders in the expression of globin subunits of hemoglobin (in contrast to hemoglobinopathies, such as sickle cell disease, which are disorders of hemoglobin structure and function). Homozygous β thalassemias are characterized by an absence (β^0) or much reduced expression (β^+) of the β-globin subunit. About 200 mutations have been identified in the β-globin gene, most of them being point mutations and only a handful of deletions. Homozygous mutations of splice sites (GU and AG dinucleotides) and nonsense mutations that introduce premature stop signals at codons 17 (exon 1) and 39 (exon 2) result in β^0 thalassemia. The transcripts produced due to nonsense mutations are rapidly degraded by a process known as nonsense-mediated decay (NMD). The function of NMD may be to prevent the expression of harmful truncated proteins in heterozygotes. Base insertions that result in a frameshift also cause β^0 thalassemia.

Therapeutics

Hemoglobin Constant Spring

Alpha (α) thalassemias occur when the production of the 141 residue α-globin protein is greatly reduced. The gene for α-globin is present in duplicate on chromosome 16. The majority of α thalassemias are the result of macrodeletions affecting either one or both alleles of both copies (four genes). On the other hand, a form of nondeletion α thalassemia prevalent in Southeast Asia and southern China, designated as hemoglobin Constant Spring (HbCS), is the result of a mutation that alters the stop codon of the α_2 copy (which is normally responsible for 75% of α-globin production). The terminal codon is mutated from UAA (stop) to CAA (Gln), and the chain is extended to 172 amino acids. The mutant α_2 mRNA, however, is unstable and fails to produce α-globin.

19.2 Protein Synthesis (Translation)

19.2.1 Key Components of the Translational Machinery

In eukaryotes, proteins are synthesized (translated) in the cytoplasm as linear polypeptides. This process is catalyzed by ribosomes. It requires mRNA as the template and various aminoacyl-tRNAs as the substrates. Key features of each of these components are as follows:

Ribosomes and mRNA

The translational machinery is assembled on ribosomes, which are large complexes of proteins and various rRNAs. The 80S eukaryotic ribosome consists of two subunits (▶ Fig. 19.2a):
1. **Large subunit (60S):** Made up of 49 proteins and 3 types of rRNA (28S, 5.8S, and 5S)
2. **Small subunit (40S):** Made up of 33 proteins and 1 type of rRNA (18S)

Prokaryotic ribosomes are also composed of a large subunit (50S; 31 proteins + 23S rRNA + 5S rRNA) and a small subunit (30S; 21 proteins + 16S rRNA). Aminoglycoside antibiotics such as streptomycin and gentamycin bind to the 16S rRNA of the 30S subunit and distort ribosome assembly (▶ Fig. 19.2b).

The large and small subunits are prompted to assemble into an active ribosomal complex by the presence of mRNA.

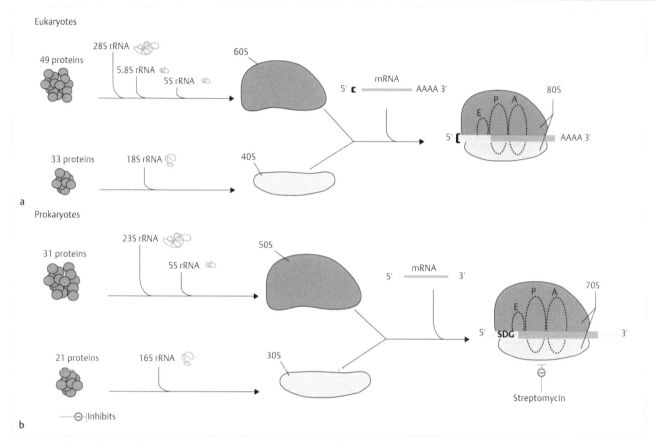

Fig. 19.2 **Ribosomal assembly and mRNA.** Ribosomes are large ribonucleoprotein complexes assembled from a large and a small ribosomal subunit and mRNA. Ribosomes catalyze the formation of peptide bonds between amino acids to produce a linear polypeptide according to the mRNA template. (**a**) The large eukaryotic 60S ribosomal subunit is composed of 49 proteins and 3 rRNA molecules. The smaller 40S ribosomal subunit is composed of 33 proteins and 1 rRNA molecule. Both subunits assemble with mRNA to form an 80S eukaryotic ribosome, which forms E, P, and A sites. Eukaryotic mRNA contains a 7-methylguanosinecap at the 5′end and a poly(A) tail at the 3′end. (**b**)The large prokaryotic 50S subunit is composed of 31 proteins and 2 rRNAs. The smaller 30S subunit is composed of 21 proteins and 1 rRNA. Both subunits assemble with mRNA to form a 70S prokaryotic ribosome (which also has E, P, and A sites). Assembly is distorted by streptomycin. Prokaryotic mRNA contains the Shine-Dalgarno (SDG) sequence.

There are three important sites of the ribosomal complex (► Fig. 19.2a):

1. **Acceptor (A) site,** the location where the mRNA codon is exposed and set to receive all aminoacyl-tRNAs (except the initiating methionine tRNA)
2. **Peptidyl (P) site,** the location where the aminoacyl-tRNA is attached to the growing polypeptide chain
3. **Empty (E) site,** the location that the empty tRNA (i.e., aminoacyl free) occupies just prior to exiting the ribosome

Aminoacyl tRNAs

These are the "activated" forms of amino acids that are esterified to the 3′-OH group of the 3′-terminal adenine in the acceptor stem of their cognate tRNA. When an amino acid is bound, the tRNA is said to be charged. The major fidelity/specificity of protein synthesis resides at the level of tRNA charging–a two-step energy-requiring activation process catalyzed by aminoacyl-tRNA synthetases, as follows (► Fig. 19.3a-c):

1. In the first step, which uses one adenosine triphosphate (ATP), an aminoacyl-tRNA synthetase catalyzes the activation of the amino acid by transferring adenosine monophosphate (AMP) to its α-carboxyl group. This reaction, which is driven by the hydrolysis of pyrophosphate, generates the enzyme-bound intermediate, aminoacyl-AMP.

2. In the second step, synthetase transfers the amino acid from aminoacyl-AMP to its cognate tRNA.
   - There is 1 aminoacyl-tRNA synthetase enzyme for each of the 20 different amino acids.
   - Charging is governed by "acceptor identity," which constitutes in essence a second genetic code. Specifically, the aminoacyl-tRNA synthetase enzymes recognize both the amino acid and its cognate tRNA by sensing a particular three-dimensional conformation. If the target amino acid does not match the tRNA, the amino acid is released before transfer to the tRNA.
   - There are two classes of aminoacyl-tRNA synthetases. One of the differences between them is in the mechanism of transfer of the aminoacyl group from aminoacyl-AMP to the 3′-OH of the A residue at the 3′ terminus. The class I enzymes transfer the aminoacyl group first to the 2′-OH of ribose and then to the 3′-OH by a transesterification reaction. Class II enzymes catalyze a direct transfer of the aminoacyl group to the 3′-OH of the 3′ terminal A residue on the cognate tRNA.

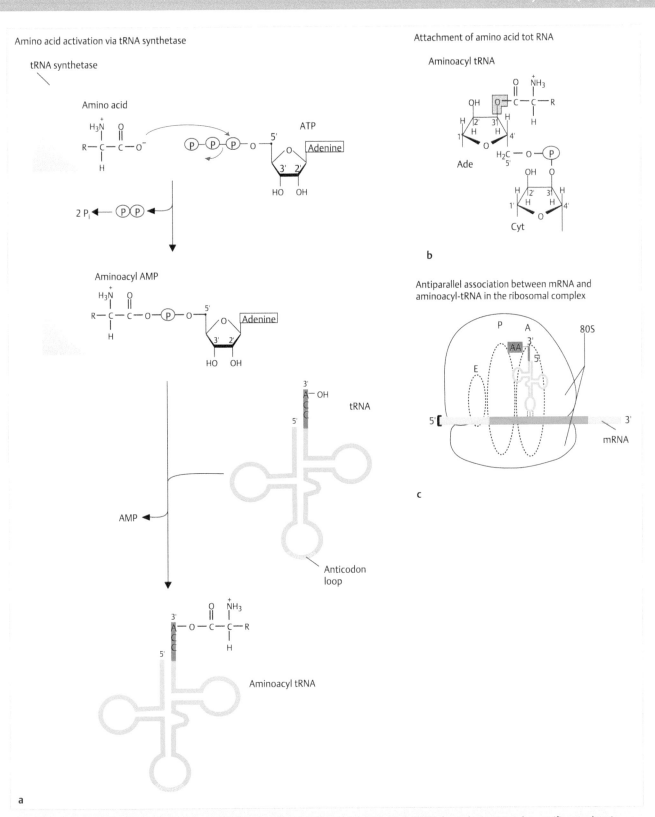

Fig. 19.3 Amino acid activation. (a) Amino acids are activated in an adenosine triphosphate (ATP)-dependent manner by specific cytoplasmic aminoacyl-tRNA synthetases that catalyze the transfer of an adenosine monophosphate (AMP) residue onto the carboxyl residue of the amino acid (forming aminoacyl-AMP). This reaction is driven by the energy obtained from the hydrolysis of pyrophosphate (PP_i) into two phosphates. tRNA synthetase then catalyzes the transfer of the amino acid from aminoacyl-AMP onto tRNA. This releases AMP and creates an aminoacyl-tRNA molecule, which brings the amino acid to the ribosome. (b) The ester bond formed between the carboxyl group of the amino acid and the ribose residue of the tRNA's terminal (3′) adenosine (Ade). (c) Aminoacyl-tRNAs associate in a manner that is antiparallel to the mRNA template. Cyt, cytosine.

19.2.2 Mechanism of Translation

Proteins are synthesized by ribosomes, which read mRNA sequences in the 5'→3' direction. In this section, we will focus on the steps in prokaryotic translation in order to point out the sites of action of specific antibiotics. The three major phases of translation are initiation, elongation, and termination.

1. **Initiation:** In this phase, a preinitiation complex (which lacks the large ribosomal subunit) is first assembled. Once the large ribosomal subunit is added, a complete initiation complex is formed. The preinitiation complex is made up of the following components (▶ Fig. 19.4a):
   - The small ribosomal subunit, to which initiation factors are bound. These initiation factors are abbreviated as IF in prokaryotes (▶ Fig. 19.4a) and eIF in eukaryotes (▶ Table 19.1).
   - The initiator tRNA, to which a guanosine triphosphate (GTP)–bound initiation factor is attached. The initiator tRNA in prokaryotes is N-formylmethionyl tRNA (fMet-tRNA$_i^{Met}$) (▶ Fig. 19.4), and in eukaryotes, it is methionyl tRNA (Met-tRNA$_i^{Met}$).
   - An mRNA strand whose start codon (AUG) always codes for methionine. Proper placement of the mRNA onto the small ribosomal subunit (30S) in bacteria is aided by the presence of the Shine-Dalgarno sequence (AGGAGG). It is found ~7 nucleotides upstream of the start codon and forms complementary base pairs with the 16S rRNA of the 30S subunit.
   - Proper placement of eukaryotic mRNA on the small ribosomal subunit (40S) is aided by the presence of the 5'-7-methylguanosine cap, the length of the 3' poly(A) tail, and an ATP-dependent scan in the 5'→3' direction to locate AUG.
   - Although eukaryotic mRNA does not have a Shine-Dalgarno sequence, it has the Kozak sequence, which is analogous. Whereas most of the time translation initiates at the first AUG after the methylguanosine cap, the Kozak sequence determines the "strength" of a given AUG.
   - The complete initiation complex is then formed by the binding of the large ribosomal subunit to the preinitiation complex and the release of initiation factors. This is driven by hydrolysis of the GTP (bound to the initiation factor associated with the initiator tRNA) into guanosine diphosphate (GDP) and inorganic phosphate (P$_i$). The initiating tRNA is positioned in the ribosome's P site with its anticodon base paired to the mRNA's codon.
   - Linezolid, which belongs to the oxazolidinone class of antibiotics, inhibits the initiation of protein synthesis in prokaryotes by preventing the formation of 70S ribosomal complex.

2. **Elongation:** In this phase, an activated amino acid is attached to the initiating methionine via a peptide bond. The polypeptide chain is extended via catalytic action of the ribosome and involves the following steps (▶ Fig. 19.4b):
   - Loading of an aminoacyl-tRNA onto the ribosome such that its anticodon base pairs with the codon positioned in the A site. Prior to loading, the aminoacyl-tRNA is attached to a GTP-bound elongation factor (▶ Table 19.1). Loading is marked by the hydrolysis of this GTP into GDP and P$_i$ and release of the GDP-bound elongation factor from the aminoacyl-tRNA.

Aminoglycoside antibiotics such as streptomycin and gentamycin distort prokaryotic ribosome assembly and cause misreading of mRNA codon in the A site.
- Tetracyclines are antibiotics that inhibit protein synthesis at the elongation phase by binding to the small 30S subunit of bacteria. In doing so, tetracyclines block entry of aminoacyl-tRNAs to the ribosome–mRNA complex (A site).
- Shiga toxin (produced by the bacterium *Shigella dysenteriae*) and ricin (a toxin produced by the castor oil plant *Ricinus communis*) both inhibit eukaryotic protein synthesis at the elongation phase by binding to the large 60S subunit. In doing so, they prevent aminoacyl-tRNAs from binding to ribosomes.
- Peptide bond formation (transpeptidation) between the amino acid residues in the A and P sites is catalyzed by peptidyl transferase, a ribozyme located in the large ribosomal subunit. In this reaction, the P site amino acid detaches from its cognate tRNA and, via its carboxyl group, attaches to the amino group of the A site amino acid.
- The energy for peptide bond formation comes from the high-energy bond between the amino acid and tRNA (which required ATP for formation during charging).
- Chloramphenicol is a broad-spectrum antibiotic that inhibits bacterial protein synthesis at the elongation phase by inhibiting peptidyl transferase.
- Similarly, cycloheximide, a toxin produced by the bacterium *Streptomyces griseus*, inhibits eukaryotic protein synthesis at the elongation phase through inhibition of peptidyl transferase.
- Once the peptide bond is formed, the ribosome moves (translocates) such that the next codon is positioned in the A site, the tRNA containing the growing peptide chain is transferred to the P site, and the deacylated tRNA (i.e., aminoacyl-free) is transferred to the E site. Hydrolysis of the GTP (bound to another elongation factor) into GDP and P$_i$ is used to power the ribosome's translocation along the mRNA strand. After translocation, the A site becomes vacant and ready for another aminoacyl-tRNA and another round of elongation. In this manner, the polypeptide chain grows from the N terminus to the C terminus.
- Macrolide-lincosamide-streptogramin B (MLS) class of antibiotics such as erythromycin and clindamycin inhibit prokaryotic protein synthesis at the elongation phase by binding to the nascent peptide exit tunnel in the 50S subunit. In doing so, they cause context-specific arrest of peptidyl transferase and early release of peptidyl-tRNAs. Thus, they block the synthesis of a subset of proteins rather than act as inhibitors of global protein synthesis.
- In addition to causing the misreading of mRNA codons, aminoglycoside antibiotics may also block the translocation of the 70S ribosome.
- Diphtheria toxin, released by the bacterium *Corynebacterium diphtheriae*, inhibits protein synthesis at the elongation phase by inactivating the GTP-bound elongation factor (eEF-2) that powers ribosomal translocation.

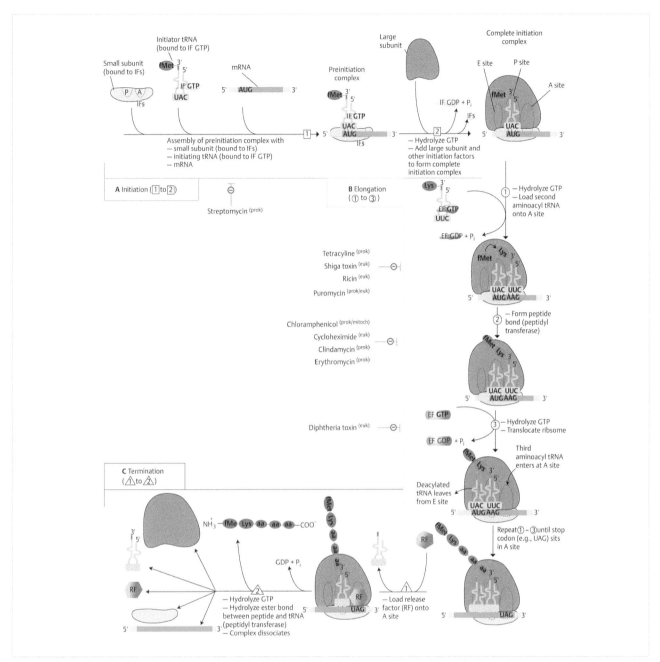

Fig. 19.4 General mechanism of translation (in prokaryotes). The mechanisms of translation for prokaryotes and eukaryotes are very similar. This figure summarizes prokaryotic translation, and ▶ Table 19.1 offers a comparison of the specific factors and sources of energy for translation in both systems. **(A)** Initiation of eukaryotic translation involves the assembly of the ribosomes of the complete initiation complex (70S in prokaryotes and 80S in eukaryotes) from small and large subunits, mRNA, and the initiator tRNA. This assembly is achieved with the help of proteins known as initiation factors (IFs in prokaryotes). **(B)** Elongation of the nascent polypeptide chain follows the initiation of translation. Amino acids are added sequentially to the initiating amino acid via multiple elongation cycles. Elongation consists of the binding of aminoacyl-tRNAs to guanosine triphosphate (GTP)-bound elongation factors (step 1). Binding of aminoacyl-tRNAs to the acceptor (A) site is driven forward by the energetically favorable hydrolysis of GTP (step 2). The formation of peptide bonds is catalyzed by peptidyl transferase, a ribozyme on the rRNA portion of the large ribosomal subunit (step 3). The C terminus of the amino acid occupying the P site is transferred onto the amino group of the residue in the A site. GTP hydrolysis of the GTP-bound elongation factor (EF) powers the translocation of the ribosome along the mRNA. This moves the peptidyl-tRNA to the P site and exposes a new mRNA codon in the A site. The next aminoacyl-tRNA can bind in the A site. **(C)** Termination of translation. A stop codon in the A site of the ribosome is recognized by release factors (RFs). Their binding to the A site causes cleavage of the peptide-tRNA linkage by peptidyl transferase and the release of the polypeptide chain. Following GTP hydrolysis, the ribosomal subunits dissociate.

Table 19.1 Components involved in prokaryotic and eukaryotic translation

Components	Prokaryotes	Eukaryotes	Key points to remember
Ribosome subunits	30S subunit 50S subunit	40S subunit 60S subunit	• Linezolid inhibits the assembly of 70S ribosome • Streptomycin binds to the 30S subunit to cause misreading of mRNA codons • Shiga toxin binds to the 60S subunit to disrupt elongation • Tetracyclines bind to the 30S subunit to disrupt elongation • Chloramphenicol inhibits peptidyl transferase of 50S ribosomal subunit • Erythromycin and clindamycin bind to the 50S ribosomal subunit to cause context-specific arrest of peptidyl transferase and early dissociation of peptidyl-tRNAs. • Cycloheximide inhibits eukaryotic peptidyl transferase • Diphtheria toxin inhibits eukaryotic protein synthesis by inactivating the GTP-bound elongation factor, eEF-2
Initiation: requires hydrolysis of one GTP (equivalent to one ATP)			
Initiation factor(s) bound to small ribosomal subunit	IF-1, IF-3	eIF1, eIF1A, eIF3, eIF5	• The initiation factors facilitate binding of the small ribosomal subunit to the initiator tRNA and base pairing between the anticodon and codon
Initiation factors bound to initiator tRNA (fMet-tRNA$_i^{Met}$/ Met-tRNA$_i^{Met}$)	IF-2-GTP	eIF2-GTP	• Hydrolysis of GTP to GDP + P$_i$ provides the energy for assembly of the initiation complex
Features of mRNA important for assembly of initiation complex	• AUG start codon • Shine-Dalgarno sequence	• AUG start codon • 5′ cap and poly(A) tail	• Additional initiation factors such as the eIF4 complex and eIF5B-GTP are required for the assembly of the final 80S initiation complex
Elongation: requires hydrolysis of two GTP per amino acid added (equivalent to two ATP)			
Elongation factors attached to aminoacyl tRNAs	Tu-GTP	EF1a-GTP	
Elongation factors that power the ribosome's translocation	EF-GTP	EF2-GTP	• Diphtheria toxin inactivates EF2-GTP and inhibits elongation
Termination: requires hydrolysis of one GTP (equivalent to one ATP)			
Release factor that recognizes the stop codon	RF-1 or RF-2	eRF-1	
Factor(s) that power dissociation of the ribosomal complex	EF-GTP	eRF-3-GTP	

Abbreviations: ATP, adenosine triphosphate; GDP, guanosine diphosphate; CTP, guanosine triphosphate; P$_i$ inorganic phosphate.
Note: The activation and charging of each amino acid to its cognate tRNA requires one ATP (▶ Fig. 19.3). Assembly of the complete 80S initiation complex in eukaryotes
requires the hydrolysis of two CTP molecules (one each associated with eIF2 and eIF5B).

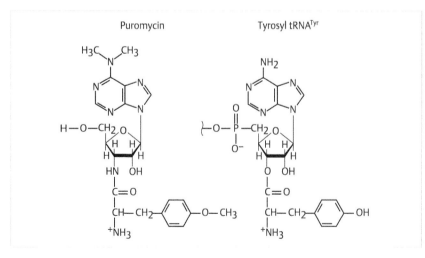

Puromycin   Tyrosyl tRNA^{Tyr}

Fig. 19.5 Structure of puromycin and tyrosyl-tRNA^{Tyr}. The structure of puromycin resembles the aminoacylated 3′end of tyrosyl-tRNA^{Tyr}.

- Puromycin is an antibiotic that inhibits both prokaryotic and eukaryotic protein synthesis at the elongation phase. Because its structure mimics that of the aminoacylated 3′ end of tyrosyl-tRNA^{Tyr} (▶ Fig. 19.5), puromycin can enter the A site and be incorporated into the growing peptide chain. However, because the peptidyl puromycin is not anchored to the ribosome, the growing polypeptide chain falls off the ribosome, and translation is prematurely terminated.

3. Termination: In this phase, the peptide chain is released from the ribosomal complex, and the latter dissociates into its component parts. Termination of protein synthesis is triggered when a stop codon (UAA, UAG, or UGA) resides in the A site of the ribosome. Subsequent general steps include the following (▶ Fig. 19.4c):
   - Recruitment of a release factor (RF) to the A site due to the presence of a stop codon. This triggers peptidyl transferase to cleave the ester bond between the peptide's C terminus and the tRNA in the P site.
   - The specificity of peptidyl transfer is altered such that the attacking moiety is water rather than the α-amino group of an amino acid bound to a tRNA at the A site. Water adds to the carbonyl carbon of the peptidyl tRNA in the P site, thereby releasing the polypeptide.
   - Following the hydrolysis of GTP, the ribosomal complex dissociates, setting the stage for another round of translation.

Polysomes

When clusters of 10 to 100 ribosomes are simultaneously attached to a single mRNA like beads on a string, they form a polysome. Each ribosome synthesizes one nascent polypeptide chain from the message, leading to efficient and rapid protein synthesis.

Normal
Mitochondrial protein synthesis

Mitochondria have their own translational machinery that includes mitochondrial ribosomes, mRNA, and a set of tRNAs. The genetic code of mitochondrial DNA differs from the standard genetic code. Interestingly, the process of translation in mitochondria bears several similarities to that in prokaryotes. This lends support to the hypothesis that mitochondria may be the descendants of a bacterial endosymbiont in the early stages of eukaryotic development. For instance:

- Mitochondrial mRNA does not contain the 7-methylguanosine cap seen in cytoplasmic mRNAs.
- The translation initiator tRNA in mitochondria is fMet-tRNA$_i^{Met}$, as in prokaryotes.
- The types and the number of protein factors necessary for the initiation, elongation, and termination of mitochondrial protein synthesis are similar to those observed in prokaryotes.
- Peptidyl transferase in mitochondria is sensitive to chloramphenicol, like that of the prokaryotic ribosome.

Foundations
Transcription and translation: spatial and temporal considerations

Because prokaryotic cells lack a nucleus, transcription is coupled to translation, and both take place in the cytoplasm. As such, translation of mRNA begins before its transcription is complete. In eukaryotes, however, transcription takes place in the nucleus, whereas translation occurs in the cytoplasm. Therefore, transcription and translation in eukaryotes are spatially and temporally separated.

Foundations
Eukaryotic mRNA and initiation

Along with the initiation factors that participate in the preinitiation complex, additional initiation factors are needed in eukaryotic protein synthesis to activate the mRNA. The multisubunit eIF4 complex contains factors that interact with both the 5′ cap structure and the poly(A) binding protein (PABP) that is bound to the 3′ poly(A) tail of the mRNA to be translated. The large eIF4G factor binds to PABP and interacts with the eIF4E attached to the cap structure to form a circular complex. Factors eIF4A and eIF4B then also bind to eIF4G. The activated mRNA then enters the preinitiation complex through an interaction between eIF4G and eIF3. Factor eIF4E is normally inactive due to the binding of an inhibitory protein (4EBP). Mitogenic agents (e.g., insulin, insulin-like growth factor 1 [IGF-1], platelet-derived growth factor [PDGF]) cause the phosphorylation of 4EBP via the AKT/PKB pathway to release active eIF4E.

19.3 Sites of Protein Synthesis

Protein biosynthesis begins on ribosomes in the cytoplasm and is terminated either in the cytoplasm or in the rough endoplasmic reticulum (RER). The site of termination depends on the final destination of the mature protein product. This may be an intracellular compartment, an extracellular location (for secreted proteins), or on membranes. There are two major pathways of protein sorting (▶ Fig. 19.6):

1. **Cytoplasmic pathway:** It is used for the synthesis of proteins destined for the cytoplasm, mitochondria, nucleus, and peroxisomes. In this pathway, protein synthesis begins and ends on free ribosomes in the cytoplasm. The absence or presence of specific targeting signals on the polypeptide plays a role in getting it to its final destination (▶ Fig. 19.6a).

2. **Secretory pathway:** It is used for the synthesis of proteins destined for the ER, lysosomes, secretion, or membranes. In this pathway, translation begins on free ribosomes in the cytoplasm but terminates on ribosomes sent to the ER. This sorting is facilitated by an ER-targeting translocation signal present in the first several amino acid residues of the polypeptide (▶ Fig. 19.6b).

V

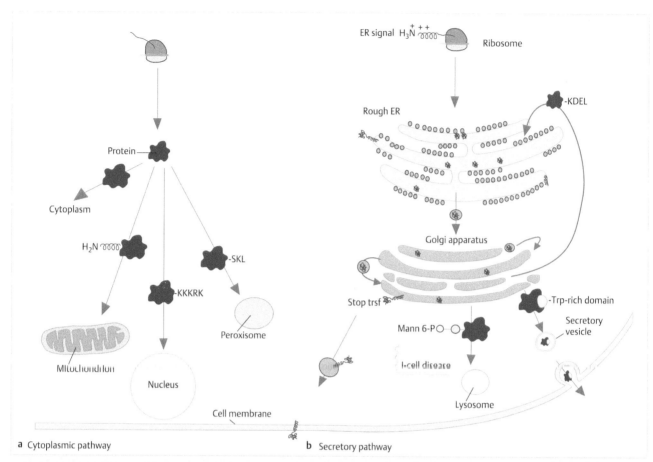

a Cytoplasmic pathway   b Secretory pathway

Fig. 19.6 Protein sorting. (a) Proteins destined for the cytoplasm, mitochondria, nucleus, and peroxisomes are synthesized via the cytoplasmic pathway. Their synthesis begins and ends on cytoplasmic ribosomes. Those proteins that lack a translocation signal remain in the cytoplasm. Others contain signal sequences that target them to specific organelles. (b) Proteins destined for membranes, lysosomes, and secretion are synthesized via the secretory pathway. Their translation begins on cytoplasmic ribosomes but ends on ribosomes directed to the rough endoplasmic reticulum (RER) by the presence of an ER-targeting translocation signal on the N terminus of the nascent peptide. The polypeptides are folded and processed into mature proteins in the ER lumen. Proteins are then transported in vesicles to the Golgi apparatus for further posttranslational modifications. (Note: Transport occurs through budding of vesicles from existing ER and Golgi membranes.) These proteins contain additional translocation signals that target them to their final destinations. When synthesized on the RER, future membrane proteins remain tethered in the RER membrane. These portions of the membrane then bud off and fuse with other membranes.

19.3.1 Protein Sorting via the Cytoplasmic Pathway

Proteins synthesized via the cytoplasmic pathway that lack any translocation signal will remain in the cytoplasm. Others destined for certain intracellular organelles contain specific translocation signals that aid in their import into structures such as mitochondria, the nucleus, and peroxisomes (▶ Fig. 19.6a, ▶ Table 19.2). Examples include the following:

- **N-terminal hydrophobic α-helix (for mitochondrial import):** Mitochondrial proteins synthesized in the cytoplasm must be imported across mitochondrial membranes. These proteins cannot cross the membranes in their folded (tertiary) form, and the linear form is susceptible to aggregation and degradation. The presence of the N-terminal hydrophobic α-helix, however, allows the protein to interact with specific auxiliary proteins (chaperones) from

the heat shock protein family (e.g., HSP70). These chaperones bind to and protect the protein's linear structure. Subsequent import of the target protein into mitochondria involves the following steps (▶ Fig. 19.7):

1. Recognition of the exposed signal peptide by two mitochondrial translocator complexes. These are pores in the outer and inner mitochondrial membranes known as the transporter outer membrane (TOM) and transporter inner membrane (TIM).
2. Movement of the linear peptide across the mitochondrial membrane with the aid of mitochondrial HSP70

- **Nuclear localization signals (for nuclear import):** Because proteins cannot be synthesized in the cell nucleus, they are imported via nuclear pores. Small proteins are able to pass through specific pores, but large proteins (> 40 kDa) require nuclear localization signals made up of four continuous basic residues (Arg and Lys) to enter the nucleus.

Table 19.2 Sorting of newly synthesized proteins

Cytoplasmic pathway		Secretory pathway (each protein contains the N-terminal hydrophobic a-helix ER signal peptide)	
Destination	**Translocation Signal**	**Destination**	**Translocation Signal**
Cytoplasm	None	ER lumen	C-terminal KDEL retention signal
Mitochondria	N-terminal hydrophobic α-helix signal peptide	Lysosomes	Mannose 6-phosphate signal group
			I-cell disease
Nucleus	KKKRK signal sequence	Secretion	Tryptophan-rich domain signal region, absence of retention motifs
Peroxisomes	C-terminal SKL signal sequence	Membranes	N-terminal apolar region (stop-transfer sequence)

Abbreviations: ER, endoplasmic reticulum; S, serine; K, lysine; L, leucine; R, arginine; D, aspartate; E, glutamate.
Note: Signal peptides are cleaved off after translation; signal sequences are not.

V

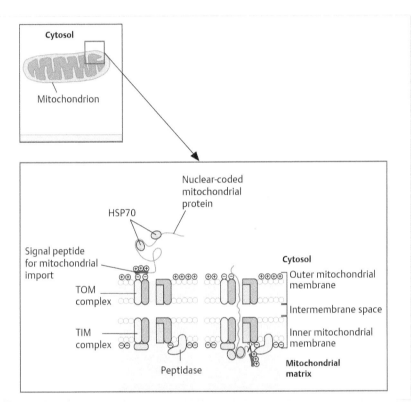

Fig. 19.7 Mitochondrial protein import.
Proteins are passed across the mitochondrial membranes via two translocator complexes: transporter outer membrane (TOM) in the outer membrane and transporter inner membrane (TIM) in the inner membrane. The unfolded proteins are protected by binding to chaperones, in particular heat shock proteins 70 (HSP70).

19.3.2 Protein Sorting via Secretory Pathway

Each protein synthesized via the secretory pathway contains an ER-targeting signal peptide of 15 to 60 amino acid residues at its N terminus. There are two key features of this signal peptide:

1. One to two extremely basic residues (e.g., Lys, Arg) near the N terminus
2. An extremely hydrophobic sequence (10 to 15 residues) on the C terminus side of the aforementioned basic residues

Once the signal peptide is exposed during translation, a ribonucleoprotein called the signal recognition particle (SRP) binds to both it and the ribosome (halting translation). SRP tethers the ribosome-mRNA-peptide complex to the ER membrane (▶ Fig. 19.8). Translation resumes in a manner that directs the newly synthesized polypeptide into the luminal space of the ER. Enzymes on the luminal side of the ER's membrane subsequently cleave the signal peptide to expose the proprotein.

The proprotein is converted to its mature form via posttranslational modifications in the ER and/or Golgi apparatus. The presence of additional signal sequences serves to guide each protein to its final destination (▶ Table 19.2). For instance, pro-

V

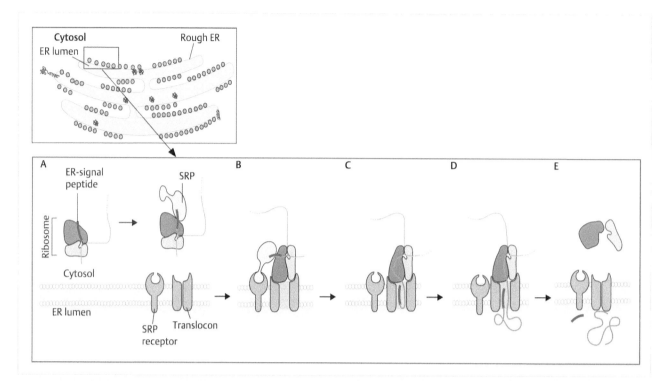

Fig. 19.8 Translation on the endoplasmic reticulum
Proteins that will be sent to some intracellular organelles or membranes or secreted require posttranslational modification in the endoplasmic reticulum (ER) or Golgi apparatus. The translation of these proteins is therefore directed to the rough ER (RER) via the presence of N-terminal signal peptides. (A) Once cytoplasmic translation has exposed the signal peptide (red), a signal recognition particle (SRP) binds to the peptide. (B) The SRP tethers the ribosome to the RER membrane. (C, D) Translation then resumes with the newly synthesized polypeptide being directed into the luminal space of the ER. (E) Enzymes on the luminal side of the ER's membrane cleave the signal peptide to expose the proprotein. The proprotein is then converted to its mature form via modification in the ER or Golgi apparatus.

teins destined for the ER lumen, secretion, or membranes contain the following signals (▶ Fig. 19.6b):
- **KDEL (for ER lumen proteins):** Proteins destined for the ER lumen are processed in the Golgi apparatus and redirected back to the ER lumen due to the presence of a C terminal KDEL retention signal (see **Fig. 4.2** for the identification of single letter codes of amino acids).
- **N-terminal apolar region (for membrane proteins):** Upon completion of translation, proteins destined for membranes remain embedded in the ER's membrane. This is aided by the presence of an apolar region in the N terminus of the polypeptide, which serves as a stop translation sequence. These ER membranes bud off as vesicles, which then fuse with other membranes (e.g., ER, Golgi, and cellular).
- **Mannose 6-phosphate (for lysosomal proteins):** Proteins destined for lysosomes are processed by the ER and Golgi such that they contain one or more phosphorylated mannose residues.
  - I-cell disease is a lysosomal storage disorder in which the tagging of lysosomal proteins with mannose 6-phosphate is defective. As such, these proteins are secreted from the cell rather than being sent to lysosomes.
- **Tryptophan domain (for secretory proteins):** Proteins destined for secretion may be processed via standard or signal-regulated pathways and secreted constitutively or in a regulated manner with the aid of a tryptophan-rich domain and the absence of retention motifs.

Normal
Smooth and rough endoplasmic reticulum
Endoplasmic reticulum (ER) in an animal or plant cell under an electron microscope can be distinguished into two types: rough ER and smooth ER. The rough ER (RER) is studded on the cytosolic face with ribosomes and predominates in cells involved in active protein synthesis. Cells involved primarily in the biosynthesis of lipids and steroid hormones will have more of the smooth ER (SER). Parts of the RER are contiguous with the nuclear envelope as well as with the SER. Proteins destined for the secretory pathway are synthesized in RER. In addition to lipogenic enzymes, SER is home for the cytochrome P-450 system.

Normal
Golgi apparatus
Golgi apparatus or Golgi complex is a subcellular organelle made up of stacked membranous sacks (cisternae). The Golgi complex may be functionally subdivided into four structural components: cis-Golgi, endo-Golgi, medial-Golgi and trans-Golgi. Each of the components contains a distinct set of enzymes that function in the maturation and sorting of proteins delivered from the endoplasmic reticulum through transport vesicles. Posttranslational modifications such as

glycosylation, phosphorylation, and sulfation involve passage of proteins through the Golgi complex. This organelle is also the site of synthesis of proteoglycans.

19.4 Posttranslational Protein Processing

Proteins destined for secretory pathway are synthesized on the RER. After translation, they are processed in the ER and/or Golgi apparatus. These processes include protein folding, proteolytic cleavage, and numerous covalent modifications.

19.4.1 Protein Folding

Although small proteins can fold into their native conformations spontaneously, large unfolded proteins cannot and are therefore subject to two major dangers:

1. **Aggregation:** Hydrophobic residues promote aggregation into insoluble, inactive protein clusters.
2. **Proteolysis:** Unfolded proteins are more susceptible to proteolysis by proteases.

Large proteins therefore require auxiliary proteins–known as chaperones (e.g., HSP70)–which protect the unfolded protein and help it fold into its proper tertiary structure. Other auxiliary proteins called chaperonins (e.g., HSP60) are barrel-shaped channels

Normal

Processing of preproinsulin to mature insulin

Preproinsulin produced in the β cells of the pancreas is a single polypeptide containing 104 amino acids. A 20-residue signal peptide is cleaved in the lumen of the endoplasmic reticulum to produce the proinsulin, which folds to allow the formation of two intramolecular disulfide bridges. Proinsulin passes through the Golgi apparatus into β granules, where it is cleaved twice to release the 33-residue C peptide, leaving behind mature insulin, which contains two peptides of 30 and 21 residues linked by two disulfide linkages. Mature insulin is stored in β granules as a Zn-bound hexamer until secretion. As mature insulin and C peptide are produced and released in equimolar amounts, an immunoassay for circulating C peptide is useful in the assessment of pancreatic β-cell function, particularly in patients in whom immunoassay for insulin is not possible due to circulating anti-insulin antibodies. Type 1 diabetic patients (and newborn infants of mothers treated with insulin) tend to express antibodies to injected bovine or porcine insulin. Assays for C peptide are also useful in distinguishing between hypoglycemic disorders due to islet cell tumors (overproduction of insulin) and the infusion of exogenous insulin (facetious hypoglycemia).

with two compartments that admit unfolded proteins and catalyze their folding in an ATP-dependent manner (▶ Fig. 19.9).

- α_1-Antitrypsin deficiency is a genetic disorder caused by mutations that prevent proper folding of the α_1-antitrypsin protein. As such, it aggregates and accumulates in the ER of liver cells.
- Cystic fibrosis is a genetic disorder caused by mutations that also prevent proper folding of the cystic fibrosis transmembrane conductance regulator (CFTR) protein. Consequently, CFTR is degraded by the action of proteases.
- Glucose 6-phosphate dehydrogenase (G6PD) deficiency is an X-linked genetic disease that is associated with mutations that cause misfolding and degradation of the enzyme.

Proteolytic Cleavage

Proteolytic cleavage is important for the conversion of inactive enzymes (zymogens) into active enzymes, as well as the post-translational processing of nascent precursor proteins into mature ones. For instance,

- during digestion, proteolytic cleavage converts trypsinogen and chymotrypsinogen into trypsin and chymotrypsin, respectively, and
- proteolytic cleavage converts preproinsulin into the two peptides of mature insulin.

Covalent Modifications

More than 200 covalent modifications of proteins have been described. Examples include glycosylation, phosphorylation, and disulfide bond formation. Several more are summarized in ▶ Table 19.3 and ▶ Fig. 19.9. Such modifications are often critical for appropriate expression of the activity and function of the protein.

Glycosylation. Extracellular proteins, including cell surface and plasma proteins (except albumin), are covalently linked to sugar residues. As the protein is being translated in the ER, sugar residues are added within the ER lumen. As the protein passes through the ER and Golgi apparatus, these residues are processed to a final mature glycoprotein (▶ Fig. 19.10).

- In *N*-linked glycosylation, the precursor oligosaccharide is cotranslationally transferred as a block of 14 sugars from a phosphorylated form of dolichol to a specific asparagine residue in the growing (nascent) polypeptide chain (▶ Fig. 19.11).
- Tunicamycin inhibits the transfer of phosphorylated *N*-acetyl-d-glucosamine (GlcNAc-P) from UDP-GlcNAc to dolichol diphosphate in the initial step of core oligosaccharide synthesis.
- *O*-linked glycoproteins are not synthesized via the dolichol phosphate cycle. Their synthesis is posttranslational, not sequence-dependent, occurs in the Golgi apparatus, and is catalyzed by specific glycosyl transferases.

Phosphorylation. This modification involves forming an ester bond between a phosphate group and the OH of an amino acid such as serine, threonine or tyrosine. The activity of many enzymes and signal transducers is acutely regulated by their phosphorylation status. This is particularly true in pathways that regulate metabolic homeostasis. Phosphorylation also plays a major role in cell growth, differentiation, and oncogenesis.

- For instance, in response to inputs from signaling pathways, serine/threonine kinases and tyrosine kinases can phosphorylate and alter the activity/function of a target protein. Protein phosphatases can remove such phosphates and similarly modulate protein function.

Table 19.3 Posttranslational protein modification

Modification		Functional group	Residue affected
Acylation	N-terminus bonded to acetyl or long-chain acyl residue	Amine (-NH)) Sulfhydryl (-SH)	N-terminus Cys
	Thioesterification with a long-chain acyl group		
Acetylation	Covalent linkage to amine	Amine (-NH))	Lys
Glycosylation	O-glycosylation	Hydroxyl (-OH)	Ser, Thr
	N-glycosylation	Acid-amide (-CONH2)	Asn
Phosphorylation	Phosphate linked via esterification	Hydroxyl (-OH)	Ser, Tyr, Thr; also Asp and His
γ-Carboxylation	Addition of -COOH group	γ-carbon	Glu
Ubiquitination	Covalent modification with ubiquitin	Amine (-NH$^+_3$)	Lys
Hydroxylation	Addition of -OH group	C-4	Pro and Lys
Disulfide bonds	Oxidation to achieve covalent linkage of cysteine residues	Sulfhydryl (-SH)	Cys
Prenylation	An isoprenoid group such as farnesyl or geranylgeranyl group added to cysteines in C-terminal CAAX or CC motifs		Cys

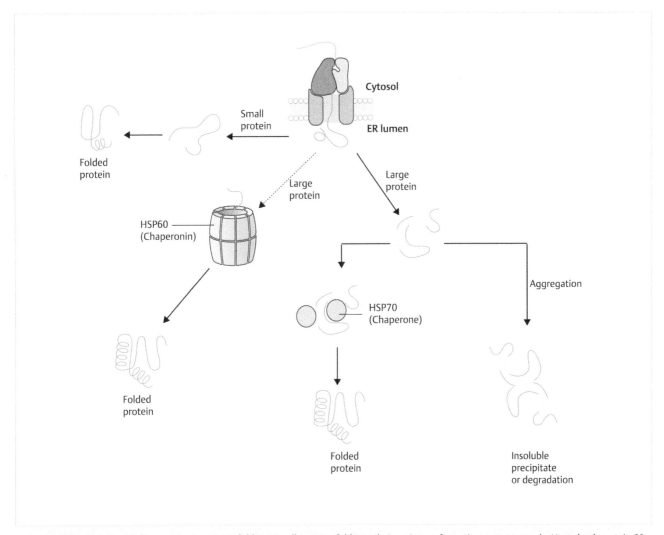

Fig. 19.9 Chaperones and chaperonins in protein folding. Small proteins fold into their native conformations spontaneously. Heat shock protein 60 (HSP60) is a large, barrel-shaped chaperonin pore. It contains two compartments that admit unfolded proteins and catalyze their folding in an adenosine triphosphate (ATP)-dependent manner. To protect large proteins from aggregation or degradation, chaperones such as HSP70 bind the polypeptide chain and aid in proper folding.

Disulfide bond formation. Both intra- and intermolecular disulfide bonds stabilize the structure of many proteins. These bonds form between the thiol (-SH) groups of two cysteine residues. The formation and rearrangement of such bonds are facilitated by protein disulfide isomerase in the ER lumen.

Foundations

Covalent modification of glutamate in vitamin K–dependent proteins

Posttranslational covalent modification of vitamin K–dependent proteins involved in blood coagulation such as prothrombin, factors VII, IX, and X, and proteins C, S, and Z, as well as the G1a protein involved in bone metabolism, is necessary for their function. In each case, certain glutamate residues of these proteins are carboxylated by the vitamin K–dependent γ-glutamyl carboxylase to generate γ-carboxyglutamate-rich domains (Gla).

Therapeutics

Posttranslational modification of collagen

The heterotrimeric type I collagen is the most abundant structural protein in vertebrates. Some of the lysines on procollagen are posttranslationally modified inside the cell to generate 5-hydroxylysines, some of which are further modified by glycosylation with the addition of galactose and glucose. Outside the cell, some of the lysines and hydroxylysines are oxidatively deaminated to aldehydic residues. Some of the prolines on procollagen are also hydroxylated to produce 4-hydroxy- and 3-hydroxyprolines. These modifications are essential to proper assembly and cross-linking of collagen helices. Mutations in lysyl hydroxylases result in skin, bone, and joint disorders (e.g., Ehlers-Danlos syndrome type VI, Nevo syndrome, Bruck syndrome type 2, epidermolysis bullosa simplex). Ascorbic acid (vitamin C) is essential for the activities of lysyl and prolyl hydroxylases.

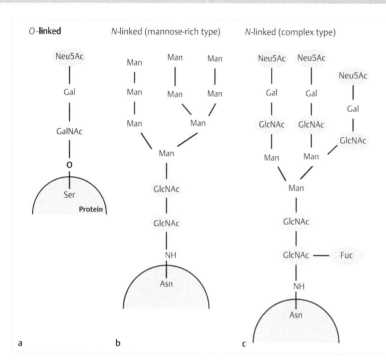

O-linked

Neu5Ac — Gal — GalNAc — O — Ser — Protein

N-linked (mannose-rich type)

Man, Man, Man — Man, Man, Man — Man, Man — Man — GlcNAc — GlcNAc — NH — Asn

N-linked (complex type)

Neu5Ac — Gal — GlcNAc — Man

Neu5Ac — Gal — GlcNAc — Man

Neu5Ac — Gal — GlcNAc — Man

Man — GlcNAc — GlcNAc — Fuc — NH — Asn

a   b   c

Fig. 19.10 Glycosylation forms. Glycoproteins display O-glycosidic and/or N-glycosidic linkage. (a) O-links are formed with the hydroxyl groups of Ser or Thr residues. N-links are always with the amino group of the Asn. There are two types of N-glycosidic linkages in glycoproteins: (b) mannose-rich and (c) complex types. NeuAc, N-acetylneuraminic acid; GalNAc, N-acetyl-D-galactosamine; Gal, galactose; GlcNAc, N-acetyl-D-glucosamine; Fuc, fucose.

Therapeutics
Congenital disorders of glycosylation

Congenital disorders of glycosylation (CDGs) arise from defects in the assembly of the 14-sugar core oligosaccharide on phosphorylated dolichol (Type I) or in their processing to complex types of glycoproteins in the Golgi apparatus (Type II). CDG1a is caused by a defect in phosphomannomutase which converts mannose 6-phosphate into mannose 1-phosphate. CDG1a accounts for 70% of CDG cases. CDG1b is caused by a defect in phosphomannose isomerase which converts fructose 6-phosphate into mannose 6-phosphate.

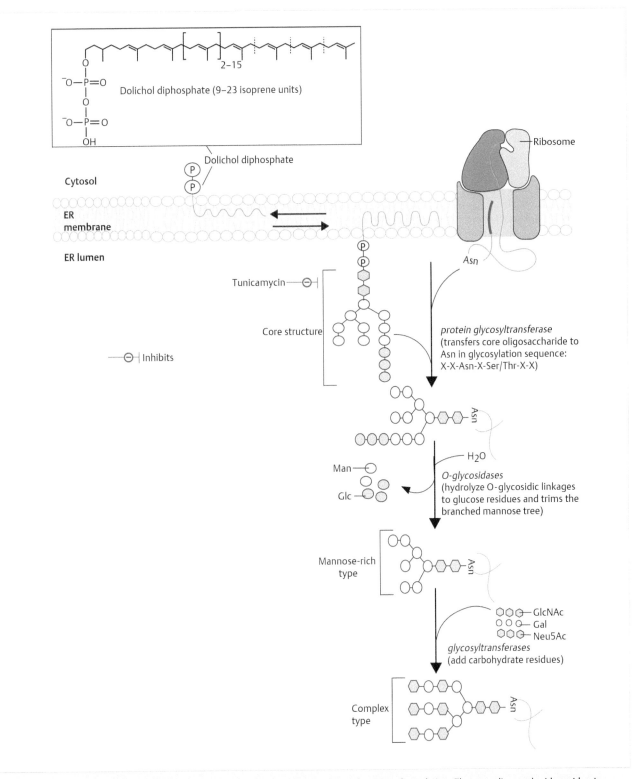

Fig. 19.11 Protein glycosylation. *N*-glycosidic linkage is the most common form of protein glycosylation. The core oligosaccharide residue is synthesized on a phosphorylated form of dolichol–an embedded endoplasmic reticulum (ER) membrane isoprenoid. The 14-residue-core oligosaccharide is transferred as a unit onto Asn residues within newly revealed glycosylation sequences (-Asn-X-Ser/Thr-) in a peptide. The core structure is then trimmed by ER *O*-glycosidases into the mannose-rich type of glycosylation. Subsequent monosaccharide transfers in the ER and Golgi apparatus produce the complex type of glycosylation. Tunicamycin inhibits the initial step in the formation of the core oligosaccharide attached to the phosphorylated form of dolichol. Neu5Ac, *N*-acetylneuraminic acid; Gal, galactose; Glc, glucose; GlcNAc, *N*-acetyl-D-glucosamine.

20 Cell Cycle, Apoptosis, and Cancer

20.1 Cell Cycle

The term *cell cycle* refers to the ordered process by which each living cell undergoes growth and cell division resulting in the formation of two daughter cells, each of which contains exactly the same genetic information as the parent. Eukaryotic cells divide on average once every 18 to 24 hours.

The molecular events of the cell cycle are very strictly controlled and monitored to ensure that no errors are introduced and passed on to the progeny. Homeostasis (maintenance of equilibrium by controlling internal physiological processes) also requires a balance between cell division and cell death.

- When the pathways of division and death become aberrant, the result is usually unchecked cell growth or cancer.

The cell cycle consists of three stages in which the cells are either growing, dividing, or resting. Each stage consists of various phases.

20.1.1 Cell Cycle Stages and Phases

Phases within the Growing Stage, Collectively Referred to as Interphase, are G_1, S, and G_2

- **G_1 (Gap 1):** RNA and protein synthesis occurs in response to exogenous growth factors (mitogens) to create the proteins that are needed to replicate DNA in the next phase.
- **S (synthesis):** DNA is replicated, and RNA and proteins are synthesized.
- **G_2 (Gap 2):** RNA and protein synthesis continues and the integrity (correctness, stability) of the DNA is checked as the cell prepares to split/divide into two.

Phase within the Dividing Stage Is M

- **M (mitosis):** Nuclear and cytoplasmic division occurs to create two identical daughter cells. This phase is further divided into prophase, metaphase, anaphase, telophase, and cytokinesis.

Phase within the Resting Stage Is G_0

- G_0 is a phase where cells have exited the cell cycle and are not growing or dividing; however, they synthesize just enough RNA and protein for general housekeeping or for specialized functions.
- Cells in G_0 are either quiescent, senescent, or terminally differentiated. Quiescent cells may reenter the cell cycle at G_1 after stimulation by molecules such as growth factors. Senescent cells are never able to reenter the cell cycle and are unable to proliferate even in the presence of growth factors. Terminally differentiated cells can be made to reenter the cell cycle by several means, such as the suppression of CKI expression (e.g., p21, p27), overexpression of cyclin D1, or introduction of viral oncogenes.

Foundations
DNA content
Resting mammalian cells in the G_1 phase have a DNA content of 2N (where N refers to the amount of DNA in a haploid genome). During the S phase, the content of DNA varies between 2N and 4N. The DNA content doubles to 4N in cells in the G_2 and M phases and returns to 2N after cytokinesis. By labeling cells with a DNA-binding fluorescent dye and sorting those in a fluorescence-activated cell sorter (FACS), cells in different phases of the cell cycle can be distinguished.

Foundations
Cell types
Cells in the human body are grouped into three broad classes: permanent, stable (quiescent), and labile. Permanent cells are those that remain in the G_0 phase and thus cannot be regenerated. These include cardiac muscle cells, neurons, and red blood cells. Stable cells are those that retain the ability to exit the G_0 phase to enter G_1 when stimulated by growth factors. This allows for the regeneration of damaged tissue. Examples of stable cell types include hepatocytes and epithelial cells of the kidney tubules. Labile cells never enter G_0 and are constantly dividing to replace cell populations that are continuously lost. Examples include cells in the gut epithelium, skin, hair follicles, and bone marrow.

Foundations
Chromosomes
Somatic cells, which are diploid, contain 46 chromosomes (i.e., 23 pairs inherited from mother and father). Germline cells (gametes), which are haploid, contain 23 unpaired chromosomes.

20.1.2 Cell Cycle Restriction Point and Checkpoints

Before the initiation of each major phase in the cell cycle, critical parameters are checked to make sure that errors are not introduced. If these "checks" fail, the cycle is arrested through a negative signal until repairs can be completed. The eukaryotic cell cycle includes one restriction point and three major checkpoints (▶ Fig. 20.1b):

Restriction Point

- When growth factors are limiting, the cell cycle is usually arrested in G_1 at a point approximately 2 hours before the initiation of the S phase. This is called the restriction point (R). When the cells pass the restriction point, they become growth factor independent and transit through the remaining phases.

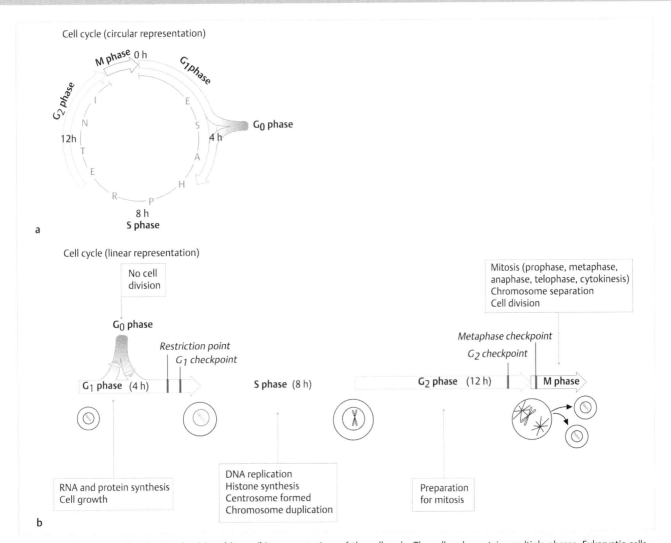

Fig. 20.1 Eukaryotic cell cycle. Circular (**a**) and linear (**b**) representations of the cell cycle. The cell cycle contains multiple phases. Eukaryotic cells divide during the mitotic phase (M). This phase is characterized by nuclear division (mitosis) at the beginning and by cell division (cytokinesis) at the end. The long growth period that follows the M phase is called interphase, which can be further divided into the Gap 1 (G_1) phase, DNA synthesis (S) phase, and Gap 2 (G_2) phase. When the nutrient or environmental conditions are not appropriate for division, cells usually arrest during the G_1 phase. This quiescent state is referred to as the G_0 phase. The restriction point and three checkpoints are marked in the phases in which they appear.

Checkpoints

1. **G_1 checkpoint:** This checkpoint verifies the integrity of DNA during the late G_1 phase, before proceeding to the S phase and DNA replication. Any damage to the DNA induces molecular mechanisms that arrest the cell cycle at this checkpoint. (It is very similar to the restriction point induced by mitogen deprivation but occurs instead in response to DNA damage.)
2. **G_2 checkpoint:** This checkpoint verifies the completeness and fidelity of genomic DNA replication before committing to mitosis.
3. **Metaphase checkpoint:** This checkpoint monitors the attachment of chromosomes to the mitotic spindle before proceeding into anaphase and chromosomal segregation during mitosis (cell division).

20.1.3 Cyclins and Cyclin-dependent Kinases

The transition of cells through the various phases of the cell cycle is dependent on the activity of a family of heterodimeric protein kinases, each of which contains
• a regulatory subunit called a cyclin and
• a catalytic subunit called a cyclin-dependent kinase (CDK).

Binding of cyclins to CDKs causes partial activation of their kinase activity. Cyclins not only help activate the CDKs but also direct them to specific proteins targeted for phosphorylation. The full activation of CDKs requires the action of the CDK-activating kinase (CAK).

There are multiple cyclins (e.g., cyclins A, B, D, E) and CDKs (CDK1, CDK2, CDK4, CDK6) in eukaryotic cells. Each cyclin can

Table 20.1 The four major classes of cyclins in vertebrate cells

Cyclin class	Function	Cyclin-CDK complex (es)
G$_1$ cyclin (D)	Helps the passage of cells through the restriction point in late G$_1$ phase	Cyclin D-CDK4 CyclinD-CDK6
G$_1$/S cyclin (E)	Helps the cells at the end of G$_1$ phase to commit to DNA replication and enter S phase	Cyclin E-CDK2
S phase cyclin (A)	Necessary for the initiation of DNA synthesis	Cyclin A-CDK2
M phase cyclins (A and B)	Necessary for the nuclear division during mitosis	Cyclin A-CDK1 Cyclin B-CDK1

complex with more than one CDK, and each CDK may interact with more than one cyclin. It is important to note the following:

- The levels of CDKs are constant throughout the cell cycle.
- The levels of individual cyclins vary considerably during the various phases of the cell cycle.

Cyclin–CDK Complex Activity during the Cell Cycle

The progression of the cell cycle through the aforementioned checkpoints is dependent on the action of various cyclin–CDK complexes. The activity of CDKs varies in different phases of the cell cycle due to the transient and cyclical availability of cyclins, of which there are four major classes (▶ Table 20.1).

The activities of different cyclin–CDK complexes oscillate through the cell cycle in the following manner (▶ Fig. 20.2b):

- At the beginning of G$_1$, cyclin D complexes with CDK 4 and 6. When the cells transit the restriction point (R) and enter the S phase, cyclin D is degraded rapidly.
- Cyclin E–CDK2 complex is active during the G$_1$ to S transition.
- Cyclin A–CDK2 is active during the S phase to induce the enzymes necessary for DNA synthesis.
- Cyclin A–CDK1 and cyclin B–CDK1 initiate mitosis.

Inhibitors of Cyclin–CDK Complex Activities

Phosphorylation of CDKs on specific residues by CAK (CDK-activating kinase) fully activates the cyclin–CDK complex. On the other hand, phosphorylation of CDK by another enzyme (WEE1 kinase) inhibits cyclin–CDK activity (▶ Fig. 20.2a).

- CDC25 is a phosphatase that can remove the phosphate group introduced by WEE1 to reactivate the cyclin–CDK complex.

Cyclin–CDK complex activities can be modulated by CDK inhibitor proteins (CKIs), which fall into two distinct families: CIP/KIP and INK4.

- The CIP/KIP family (e.g., p21, p27, and p57) inhibit G$_1$- and S-phase cyclin–CDK activities by binding to the cyclin–CDK complex and altering the conformation of the active site to render CDK inactive (▶ Fig. 20.2b).

- The INK4 family (e.g., p15, p16, p18, and p19) specifically inhibit the G$_1$ CDKs (4 and 6) by binding to them, which prevents CDK4 and CDK6 from associating with cyclin D (▶ Fig. 20.2b).

Foundations

Proteolysis of cyclins

A major mechanism to terminate the activity of cyclin–CDK complexes is to degrade the transiently expressed cyclin proteins through regulated proteolysis. Targeting of cyclins for proteolysis is accomplished by polyubiquitination (see **Table 4.2, Fig. 4.7**) catalyzed by ubiquitin ligases (e.g., APC/CDC20). Specific ubiquitin ligases (e.g., SCF) can also ubiquitinate CKIs and target them for degradation, thereby releasing the inhibition of S phase cyclin–CDK complexes.

Foundations

Meiosis for the division of germline cells

Mitosis describes a process by which a diploid (2N) somatic cell divides to produce two identical daughter cells, each of which also contains 2N amount of DNA. Meiosis, on the other hand, is a process by which a diploid (2N) germline cell divides into haploid (1N) gametes. Meiotic cell division occurs in two stages:

In Meiosis I, following an interphase, the chromosomes divide as in mitosis, and during prophase, the duplicated homologous chromosomes pair up to form a structure called a bivalent. Thus, in a bivalent, there are four chromatids corresponding to each chromosome.

This pairing allows homologous recombination in which fragments of maternal and paternal chromatids are exchanged, leading to genetic diversity. Following the recombination, cell division proceeds to generate two daughter cells, each of which contains one unmodified parental chromosome and one recombinant chromosome.

Meiosis II then follows without any further DNA synthesis. The sister chromatids in each cell separate to produce a total of four gametes, each with 1N amount of DNA.

Cyclin–CDK Complexes Phosphorylate Retinoblastoma Protein

The retinoblastoma (RB) protein is a substrate of G$_1$ and G$_1$/S cyclin-CDK complexes. RB is known as a tumor-suppressor protein because it can arrest the cell cycle at the G$_1$ checkpoint (▶ Fig. 20.3).

- The hypophosphorylated form of RB binds to E2F transcription factors. This action sequesters E2Fs and prevents them from triggering the transcription of cyclin E (a G$_1$/S phase cyclin) and cyclin A (an S phase cyclin), as well as proteins involved in DNA replication.
- Hyperphosphorylation of RB, however, by the G$_1$ and G$_1$/S CDKs releases E2Fs and allows for the transcription of cyclin E

V

Activation and inhibition of cyclin–CDK complexes

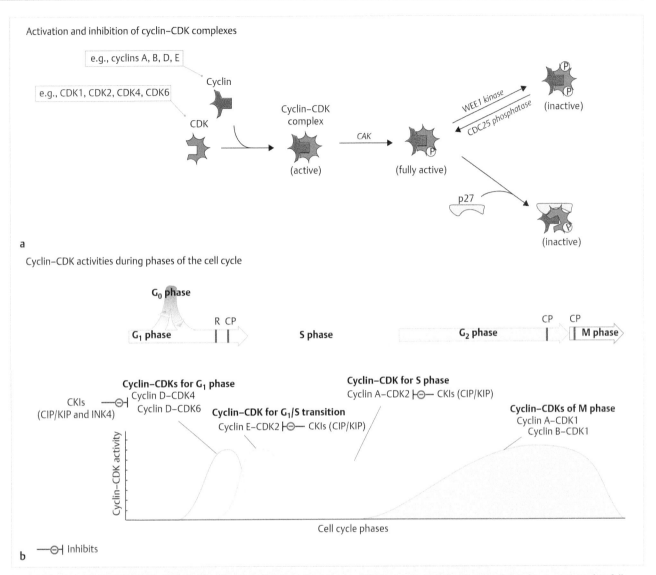

a

Cyclin–CDK activities during phases of the cell cycle

b —⊖| Inhibits

Fig. 20.2 Cyclin-CDK activity. (a) Binding of cyclins to cyclin-dependent kinases (CDKs) causes partial activation of their kinase activity, but full activation requires the action of the CDK-activating kinase (CAK). The CIP/KIP family of CDK inhibitors (CKIs), such as p27, binds to the cyclin-CDK complex to inactivate the kinase activity of CDK. (b) The periods of the cell cycle during which the cyclin-CDK complexes are active are shown as colored curves. Curve height indicates the amount of appropriate cyclin and the kinase activity of the heterodimer. At the beginning of G_1, cyclin D complexes with CDKs 4 and 6. When the cells transit the restriction point (R) and enter the S phase, cyclin D is rapidly degraded. The cyclin E-CDK2 complex is active during the G_1–S phase transition. Cyclin A-CDK2 is active during the S phase to induce the enzymes necessary for DNA synthesis. Cyclin A-CDK1 and cyclin B-CDK1 initiate mitosis. The CIP/KIP family of CKIs bind to G_1 and S phase cyclin-CDK complexes to inactivate the kinase activity of CDK. The INK4 family of CKIs bind specifically to G_1 CDKs, which prevents them from associating with cyclin D. CP, checkpoint.

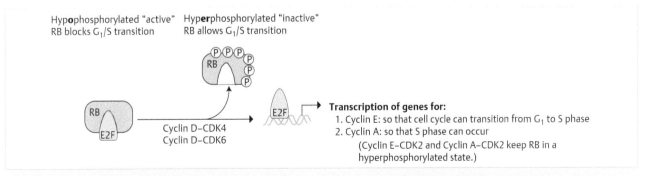

Fig. 20.3 Hypo- and hyperphosphorylated RB modulates the passage of cells from the G_1 to the S phase. Initiation of S phase protein synthesis requires the E2F transcription factors. These factors are sequestered by the hypophosphorylated form of the retinoblastoma (RB) tumor suppressor protein. Hyperphosphorylation of RB by successive cyclin–CDK complexes releases the E2F factors to allow transition of cells past the G_1 checkpoint.

to occur so that cells can transit the late G_1 checkpoint and enter the S phase.

- S phase and M phase cyclin–CDK complexes keep RB in the phosphorylated state. Degradation of these cyclins during the later stages of mitosis allows for the dephosphorylation of RB for the next round of the cell cycle.

p53 Arrests Cell Cycle at Interphase Checkpoints

When DNA is damaged by physical or chemical agents, replication of such DNA prior to repair and segregation of damaged chromosomes could invoke the possibility of transmitting the damage to the daughter cells. The DNA damage checkpoints in interphase are designed to prevent the entry of cells into the S phase as well as into mitosis when the DNA fails an integrity check. In mammalian cells, DNA damage appears to stabilize another tumor suppressor protein known as p53 (▶ Fig. 20.4).

- In the absence of DNA damage, p53 is rapidly degraded by the action of murine double minute 2 (MDM2), a ubiquitin ligase.
- However, when DNA damage is detected, p53 is phosphorylated and stabilized. Consequently, it can stimulate the transcription of many genes, including p21, a member of the CIP/ KIP family of CKI. Inhibition of cyclin–CDKs by p21 can lead to arrest of cells in G_1, S, and G_2 phases.
- For example, expression of p21 in G_1 would prevent the inactivation of RB protein via hyperphosphorylation.
- If the damage is not repaired, then the cell undergoes a process of programmed cell death (apoptosis).

Therapeutics
Retinoblastoma and the RB protein
Retinoblastoma is a childhood disease of retinal development with an incidence rate of one in 20,000. Tumors develop due to unchecked division of precursor cells in the immature retina. The hereditary form of retinoblastoma affects both eyes; in the nonhereditary form, only one eye is affected. Through examination of the microdeletions in chromosome 13 in affected individuals, the *RB1* gene was identified. In the

hereditary form of the disease, one copy of the *RB1* gene is mutated or lost in every cell, and the cells become predisposed to becoming cancerous. When the good second copy of the gene is damaged due to a somatic mutation, the cells lose control of the G_1 checkpoint. In the nonhereditary form of the disease, cancerous cells contain different somatic mutations in the two copies of the *RB1* gene.

Therapeutics
p53 and cancer
More than 50% of all human cancers exhibit mutations in the *TP53* gene. Examples of cancers in which p53 fails to activate include Li-Fraumeni syndrome and ataxia telangiectasia. Metabolic activation of benzo(a)pyrene, which is present in cigarette smoke, produces a potent mutagen. Activated benzopyrene causes mutations in genes such as *TP53* by G → T transversions. Afatoxin, a fungal metabolite that is present as a contaminant in moldy grain and peanuts, also induces G→T transversions in the *TP53* gene. Both benzopyrene and aflatoxin are called carcinogens because the mutations they cause lead to cancer.

Foundations
Replicative cell senescence
Primary human skin fibroblasts in cell culture stop dividing after 30 to 50 population doublings, even when abundant growth factors are present in the culture medium. This type of aging of somatic cell cultures is termed replicative cell senescence and appears to be due to a progressive shortening of the telomeres of chromosomes with each cell division (see Chapter 17). Many somatic cells lack the enzyme telomerase, which is necessary to maintain the telomeres by preserving their length as well as protecting them from damage by promoting end cap structures. DNA damage leads to p53-mediated cell cycle arrest at the G_1 checkpoint. It is thought that aging-induced DNA damage could be mediated by an accumulation of reactive oxygen species.

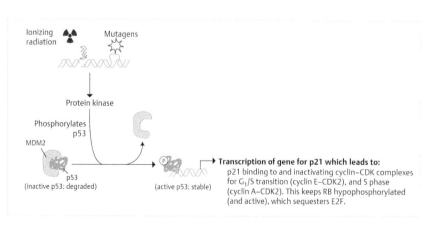

Fig. 20.4 p53 and the cell cycle. DNA damage, induced by chemical agents or by physical agents such as X-rays, activates protein kinases, which phosphorylate and stabilize the p53 protein. Activation of p53 leads to increased transcription of p21, a CDK inhibitory protein (CKI). Binding and inactivation of cyclin-CDK complexes by p21 causes cell cycle arrest. MDM2, murine double minute 2.

20.2 Apoptosis

When eukaryotic cells accumulate DNA damage that is beyond their repair capacity, they activate a process of programmed cell death called apoptosis (from the Greek word for "falling off").

- Apoptosis is also the mechanism by which unneeded cells are eliminated during development (e.g., formation of fingers and toes).
- Apoptosis differs from necrosis, which occurs after acute injury. In necrosis, cells swell and burst; in apoptosis, they shrink and condense.
- Lysis of a cell's membrane in necrosis tends to damage neighboring cells due to the release of degradative enzymes

and the resultant inflammatory response. In contrast, in apoptosis, the integrity of the cell is maintained, and no inflammatory or immunological response is invoked.

Apoptosis is performed by a cascade of intracellular proteases called caspases. They are synthesized as inactive zymogens (procaspases) that are activated by cleavage by other caspases at aspartic acid residues. The two major pathways for the induction of apoptosis differ mainly in their mode of initiation (e.g., the extrinsic pathway initiates outside the cell, whereas the intrinsic pathway is triggered within the cell). Both pathways culminate in mitochondrial damage triggering a caspase cascade (▶ Fig. 20.5).

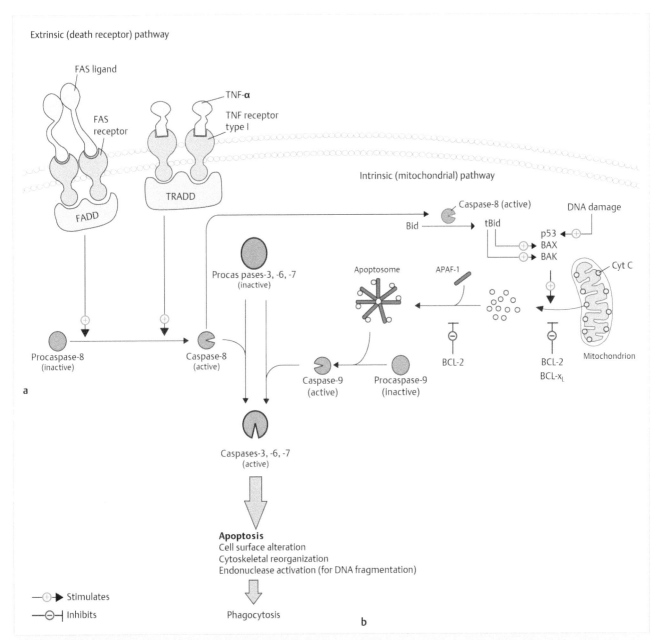

Fig. 20.5 Extrinsic and intrinsic pathways of apoptosis. (a, b) Both intrinsic and extrinsic pathways act through adaptor proteins that activate initiator caspases, which in turn triggers a caspase cascade. The cascade modifies the cell surface to cause blebbing, causes collapse of the cytoskeleton and dissolution of the nuclear envelope, and activates endonucleases that cleave chromatin between nucleosomes. The cell surface changes are detected by phagocytic cells such as macrophages. BAX and BAK are proapoptotic proteins, whereas BCL2 and BCLx_L are antiapoptotic. APAF-1, apoptotic peptidase activating factor 1; FADD, Fas-associated death domain protein; TNF, tumor necrosis factor; TRADD, tumor necrosis factor receptor type 1-associated death domain protein. tBID, truncated BID.

1. **Extrinsic pathway:** This is also known as the death receptor pathway and is triggered by the binding and activation of an external death ligand (e.g., tumor necrosis factor α, Fas ligand) to its receptor on the plasma membrane.
   - Adaptor proteins containing death domains (e.g., Fas-associated death domain protein [FADD]) bind to the intracellular regions of the activated receptor and recruit procaspase-8.
   - Autocatalysis of procaspase-8 generates caspase-8, which then initiates a caspase cascade involving other caspases (e.g., -3, -6, and -7).

2. **Intrinsic pathway:** This is also known as the mitochondrial pathway and is triggered by events such as growth factor withdrawal, DNA damage (which increases p53), and cell cycle defects. Cytochrome-c released by stressed mitochondria binds to an adaptor protein known as apoptotic peptidase activating factor 1 (APAF-1), which recruits and activates procaspase-9. (Cytochrome-c release is facilitated by proapoptotic proteins BAX and BAK, which reside in the mitochondrial outer membrane.)
   - Activated caspase-9 then triggers a caspase cascade involving caspases -3, -6, and -7.
   - This pathway is regulated by the relative amounts of anti-apoptotic (e.g., BCL2, BCLx_L) and proapoptotic (e.g., BAX, BAK) proteins.
   - Caspase-8 cleaves the cytosolic proapoptotic protein BID. Truncated BID (tBID) acts on mitochondrial BAK and BAX to initiate cytochrome-c release and to cause nuclear condensation and cell shrinkage.
   - Activation of MAP kinase and PK-B (AKT) signaling pathways (see Chapter 7) by mitogenic growth factors causes phosphorylation and inactivation of BAD, which prevents BAK and BAX from facilitating cytochrome-c release from the mitochondria. As a result, the caspase cascade is halted.
   - Cell cycle arrest by p53 can lead to the activation of the intrinsic pathway of apoptosis.

20.3 Cancer

Cancer is defined as the uncontrolled growth and proliferation of somatic cells. It occurs due to the failure of the normal regulatory mechanisms that control the cell cycle and apoptosis. Cancer is a genetic disease in the sense that it involves an abnormal increase or decrease in the expression of a set of critical genes. Such abnormal gene expression is the result of genetic damage caused by chemical or physical agents, hormones, and, in some cases, viruses.

Mutations in two types of genes have been observed to make normal cells susceptible to oncogenesis or carcinogenesis.

1. **Proto-oncogenes:** These encode proteins that promote cell growth and division. They tend to be members of cell-signaling pathways, such as growth factors, growth factor and hormone receptors, signal transducers, and transcription factors.
   - Mutations in proto-oncogenes that change the structure of their protein products or increase their level of expression may convert proto-oncogenes into oncogenes, which leads to the production of oncoproteins (▶ Fig. 20.6a, b). Such

"gain of function" mutations often appear to be inherited in an autosomal dominant fashion.

Proto-oncogenes may be converted to oncogenes via the following three mechanisms (▶ Table 20.2):

1. A point mutation or a deletion in the coding sequence would lead to the formation of a protein with an abnormally high activity (e.g., *KRAS, ERBB2, EGFR*).
2. Gene amplification, caused by abnormal DNA replication, leads to multiple copies of a proto-oncogene. This could result in an overproduction of the encoded protein. In this case, even though the protein is normal (i.e., not an oncoprotein), its increased amount can lead to growth stimulation (e.g., *ERBB2, N-MYC*).
3. Chromosomal translocation—a type of genetic rearrangement—may either bring a proto-oncogene under the control of a different and strong promoter or generate a fusion protein that is hyperactive (e.g., *c-MYC, BCR-ABL*).

2. **Tumor suppressor genes:** These typically encode proteins involved in the control of cell proliferation, especially those that normally regulate the cell cycle checkpoints.
   - Even one good copy of a tumor suppressor gene is usually sufficient to provide normal regulation. Therefore, mutations in tumor suppressor genes appear to be autosomal recessive mutations, and both copies of such genes have to be damaged to make the cells prone to the onset of cancer. Such mutations are known as "loss of function" mutations (▶ Table 20.3). Thus, oncogenesis results when somatic mutations in such genes occur in combination with the inheritance of recessive mutations and so both alleles become dysfunctional. There are five types of such proteins:
   1. Proteins that regulate a particular phase of the cell cycle (e.g., RB1 protein in G_1)
   2. Proteins that monitor checkpoints to arrest the cell cycle (e.g., p53)
   3. Proteins that are components of growth-inhibitory signaling pathways (e.g., TGFβ receptor, APC protein)
   4. Proteins that promote apoptosis (e.g., FAS, BAX)
   5. Proteins that participate in DNA damage repair (e.g., NER proteins implicated in xeroderma pigmentosum, see Chapter 17)

Foundations

Loss of Heterozygosity (LOH)

Mutations in tumor suppressor genes lead to a loss of function and are, therefore, normallt inherited in a recessive manner. Thus, heterozygous individuals who inherit one mutant copy of a tumor suppressor gene would be expected to have the same phenotype as homozygous nrmal individuals. However, it is observed that in the case of several tumor suppressor genes (e.g., *RB1, TP53, BRCA1/2*), heterozygotes are at an increased risk of developing cancers, suggesting a dominant pattern of inheritance. This paradox is explained by the concept of loss of heterozygosity (LOH). LOH states that in certain tissues of heterozygotes, the normal copy of a tumor suppressor gene may be at a higher propensity of becoming defective through somatic mutation or deletion making such tissue homozygous for the defective gene. Such tissue then becomes cancerous while the surrounding heterozygous cells remain normal.

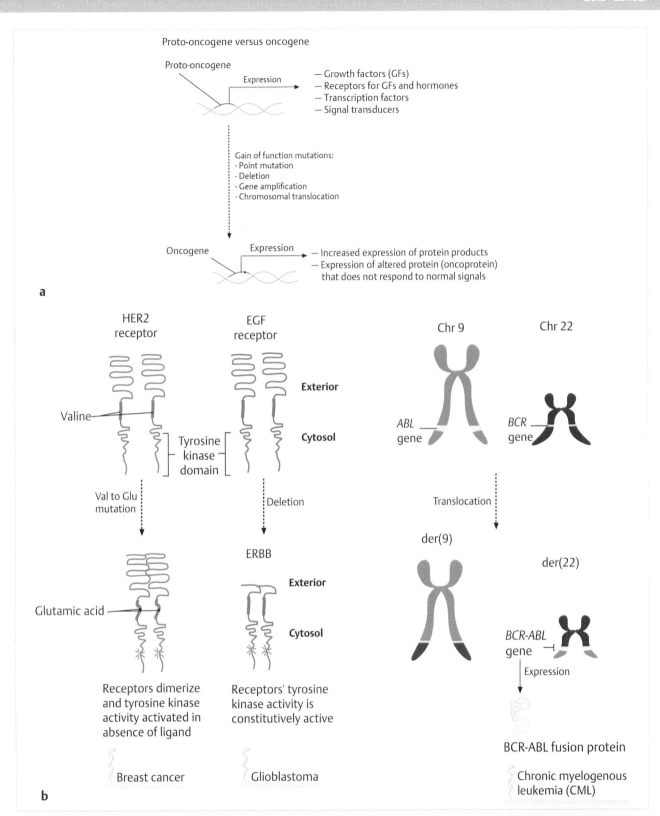

Fig. 20.6 Oncogenic transformation by point mutation or deletion. (a) Proto-oncogenes, which encode proteins that promote cell growth and division, are converted to oncogenes via gain of function mutations. **(b)** The HER2 and epidermal growth factor (EGF) receptors are products of proto-oncogenes *ERBB2* and *EGFR*, respectively. A point mutation that changes valine (Val) to glutamic acid (Glu) in the transmembrane domain of HER2 activates its tyrosine kinase activity. HER2 can heterodimerize with other EGFRs and exhibit tyrosine kinase activity even in the absence of a ligand. **(b, bottom)** A deletion of the extracellular ligand-binding domain in the EGF receptor changes it into the constitutively active EGFRvIII oncoprotein. In chronic myelogenous leukemia (CML), a translocation between chromosomes 9 and 22 results in the formation of der(22) Philadelphia chromosome and leads to the production of the fused protein kinase BCR-ABL.

Cell Cycle, Apoptosis, and Cancer

Table 20.2 Gain of function mutations in proto-oncogenes

Proto-oncogene	Genetic change	Oncoprotein characteristics and associated disease
Point mutations/deletions		
RAS	Point mutation changes glycine to valine (at codon 12)	The resulting RAS oncoprotein is perpetually active Occurs in ~ 25% of all cancers
ERBB2 (a member of the family of EGF receptors)	Point mutation changes a valine to glutamine	The resulting oncoprotein is called HER2/NEU Observed in some breast cancers
EGF receptor	Deletion in part of gene	The resulting oncoprotein (called EGFRvIII) lacks the extracellular ligand-binding domain and constitutively signals in the absence of ligand Observed in glioblastoma
Gene amplification		
ERBB2 (a member of the family of EGF receptors)	–	Results in overexpression of HER2 Observed in many breast cancers
N-MYC	-	Results in elevated levels of the N-MYC transcription factor Observed in neuroblastoma
Chromosomal translocation		
c-MYC	Reciprocal translocation between chromosomes 8 and 14	Causes the MYC transcription factor to be overexpressed because the translocation puts c-MYC under the influence of the immunoglobulin heavy-chain gene enhancer Observed in Burkitt lymphoma
BCR-ABL	Translocation occurs between chromosomes 9 and 22, which generates a derivative of chromosome 22 (der(22)) known as the Philadelphia chromosome	Generates the BCR-ABL fusion oncoprotein (an unregulated protein tyrosine kinase) because the translocation creates a BCR-ABL fusion gene Causes chronic myelogenous leukemia (CML)

Abbreviation: EGF, epidermal growth factor.

Table 20.3 Loss of function mutations in tumor suppressor genes

Gene	Chromosome (Chr) location and normal function	Characteristics of mutated protein product
TP53	Chr 17 Monitors checkpoints of cell cycle	Observed in > 50% of all human tumors
RB1	Chr 13 Regulates G_1 phase of cell cycle	Observed in retinoblastoma
APC	Chr 5 Regulates cell proliferation	Observed in familial adenomatous polyposis; is an early event that occurs in the progression toward colon cancer
DCC	Chr 18 Plays a role in cell proliferation, migration, and apoptosis	Observed in colon cancer
BRCA1/BRCA2	Chr 17 Plays a role in DNA repair and apoptosis	Observed in breast cancer; inheritance of a mutated BRCA1 gene increases the chance of developing breast cancer by the age of 50 by 30-fold
NF-1	Chr 17 Encodes a GTPase-activating protein (GAP), called p120GAP, which normally turns of activated RAS protein	Mutations in the NF-1 gene lead to neurofibromatosis

Abbreviations: APC, adenomatous polyposis coli; BRCA1/BRCA2, breast cancer type 1/2; DCC, deleted in colorectal carcinoma; NF-1, neurofibromatosis type 1; RB1, retinoblastoma.

20.3.1 Multistep Progression of Cancer

Although mutations in proto-oncogenes or tumor suppressor genes may be oncogenic, mutation in a single gene is usually not sufficient to result in cancer. According to the "multihit" model of cancer, it takes mutations in multiple genes over a period of time for the development of full-blown cancer. Each successive mutation increases the genetic instability and facilitates the subsequent mutation. In the model shown here, the development of metastatic colon carcinoma over many years appears to involve the following events:

1. An early loss of the anaphase-promoting complex (*APC*) tumor suppressor gene from the long arm of chromosome 5
2. Activation of the *KRAS* oncogene (with a Val$_{12}$ mutation) on the short arm of chromosome 12
3. Loss of the deleted in colorectal carcinoma (*DCC*) tumor suppressor gene from the long arm of chromosome 18
4. Loss of the *TP53* tumor suppressor gene from the short arm of chromosome 17
5. Other events (e.g., stimulated angiogenesis)

20.3.2 Hallmarks of Cancer

There are some acquired traits that appear to be common to most tumor cells. Hanahan and Weinberg[1] initially identified the first six such hallmarks of cancer cells, followed by an additional four (▶ Table 20.4).

Therapeutics

Mutations and cancers

Mutations of several tumor suppressor genes have been observed in human cancers. For instance, von Hippel-Lindau (VHL) disease, which predisposes individuals to multisystem tumors, is caused by mutations in the *VHL* tumor suppressor gene found on chromosome 3. VHL is a protein that plays a role in the ubiquitination and degradation of the transcription factor hypoxia-inducible factor (HIF), which is involved in regulating gene expression in response to oxygen levels. Familial melanoma is associated with mutations in the *CDKN2A*

gene (located on chromosome 9), which encodes the tumor suppressor protein p16 (a CDK inhibitor from the INK family). Wilms tumor is associated with mutations in the *WT1* gene (located on chromosome 11). WT1 is a transcription factor that plays a role in cell differentiation and development of organs, such as the kidneys and gonads. Ataxia telangiectasia (a childhood disease that affects the nervous system) is associated with mutations in the gene for ataxia telangiectasia mutated (*ATM*) located on chromosome 11. ATM is a serine/threonine protein kinase that, in response to DNA double-strand breaks, causes phosphorylation of p53 and CDC25 phosphatase to promote cell cycle arrest and apoptosis.

20.3.3 Viral Oncogenesis

A small number of benign as well as malignant human tumors are known to be caused by viruses. Both DNA and RNA viruses have been implicated in certain cancers (▶ Table 20.5). The generation of oncogenic retroviruses is thought to involve the following steps (▶ Fig. 20.7):
1. A nontransforming retrovirus infects its host.
2. As a part of its life cycle, its RNA genome is reverse transcribed into DNA and integrated into the host genome.
3. When the virus replicates, it accidentally incorporates an adjacent host proto-oncogene into its genome.
4. At some subsequent point, a mutation converts the proto-oncogene into an oncogene.

Table 20.4 Hallmarks of cancer cells (Hanahan and Weinberg)

Of the first six traits listed, five appear to be shared by both benign and malignant tumors. Only the characteristic of invasion and metastasis is unique to malignant tumors.

Trait	Description
1. Self-sufficiency in growth signals	Tumor cells show a lack of necessity of external growth factors because many oncogene products mimic growth signaling
2. Evading growth suppressors	Tumor cells resist growth inhibitory signals from neighboring cells (e.g., contact inhibition of growth)
3. Activating invasion and metastasis	Primary tumor masses spawn pioneer cells that move out and invade adjacent and distal sites, forming new colonies where nutrients and space are not limiting Metastases are the cause of 90% of cancer deaths
4. Enabling replicative immortality	Normal cells exhibit replicative cell senescence due to the loss of telomeres
	Cancer cells continue to express telomerase activity, which prevents telomere shortening
5. Inducible angiogenesis	All cells in a tissue must reside within 100 μm of a capillary blood vessel to ensure an adequate supply of nutrients
	To progress to a larger size, cancers demonstrate an ability to induce the development of new blood vessels
6. Resisting cell death	Cancer cells appear to be defective in both intrinsic and extrinsic pathways of apoptosis and also exhibit higher levels of cell survival pathways
In 2011, Hanahan and Weinberg revised their list of hallmarks to add four additional characteristics:	
7. Deregulating cellular energetics	Cancer cells exhibit "aerobic glycolysis," or the ability to express high rates of glycolysis by upregulating their GLUT1 glucose transporters
8. Avoiding immune destruction	Cancer cells appear to be invisible to the body's immune surveillance by the T and B lymphocytes
9. Tumor-promoting inflammation	Immune cells are often present in neoplastic lesions, leading to an inflammatory response Reactive oxygen species released during such responses may accelerate mutagenesis of cancer cells
10. Genome instability and mutation	It appears that in cancer cells each mutation may enhance the frequency of a subsequent mutation by epigenetic mechanisms, thus facilitating the multistep tumor progression

[1] Cell, 100:57, 2000 and 144:646, 2011.

Table 20.5 DNA and RNA viruses implicated in certain cancers

DNA viruses	Associated human tumors
Epstein-Barr virus (EBV)	Burkitt lymphoma, Nasopharyngeal carcinoma
Hepatitis B virus	Liver cancer (hepatocellular carcinoma)
Human papillomavirus (HPV)	There are several strains of HPV; specific ones are associated with benign warts, cervical and uterine cancers
RNA viruses	
Human T cell leukemia virus type 1 (HTLV-1)	Adult T cell leukemia/lymphoma
Kaposi sarcoma–associated herpesvirus (KSHV)	Kaposi sarcoma • Observed in those infected with human immunodeficiency virus (HIV) because the latter alters immune defenses, allowing endothelial cells to be transformed by KSHV and flourish as a tumor instead of being destroyed by the immune system

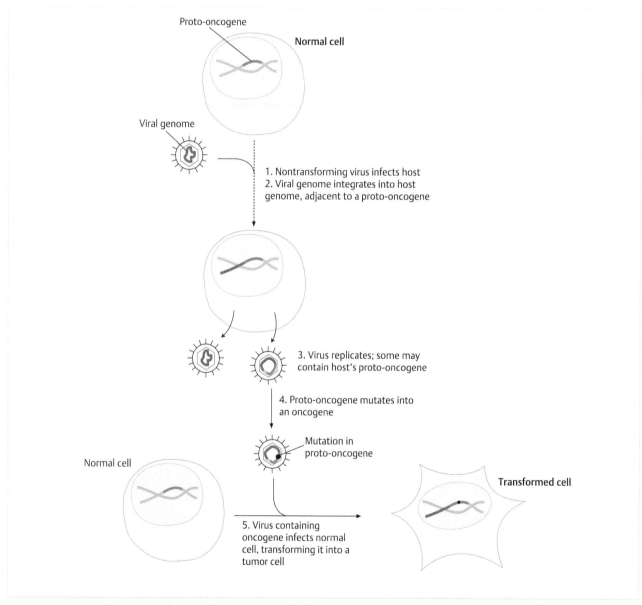

Fig. 20.7 Generation of transforming retroviruses. A transducing retrovirus infects a host cell and integrates into the host genome. During replication, the virus may accidentally integrate a part of the host DNA containing a proto-oncogene into its genome. The proto-oncogene may be converted into an oncogene by a subsequent mutation, thus generating a species of retrovirus capable of transforming its host cells.

5. The virus containing the oncogene can now transform normal cells and cause tumors.

Foundations
Fibrosarcomas in chickens
Pioneering work by Peter Rous in the early 20th century recognized that the Rous sarcoma retrovirus (RSV) could cause fibrosarcomas in chickens. The transforming factor introduced by the RSV was identified as v-src, a tyrosine kinase. The v-*src* gene is the oncogenic form of the normal host proto-oncogene c-*SRC*.

20.3.4 Cancer Chemotherapeutics

The use of ionizing radiation and of cytostatic or cytotoxic drugs in the treatment of tumors is based on the rationale that because such treatments mainly affect rapidly dividing cells, they would tend to preferentially target cancer cells. However, the many side effects of such treatments, such as nausea, gastrointestinal disturbances, fatigue and hair loss, are the result of collateral damage to healthy tissue. Nevertheless, such treatment options still represent an effective and less expensive first line of defense. These agents may be classified into six types of drugs, as summarized in ▶ Fig. 20.8.

Targeted Inhibition of Oncoproteins

A more recent approach is to target particular oncoproteins with monoclonal antibodies or specific inhibitors. Examples of such agents include

- Herceptin (Roche-Genentech, San Francisco, CA) (trastuzumab), for breast cancer, is a monoclonal antibody (mAb) directed against HER2/NEU epidermal growth factor (EGF) receptors whose gene copy number is amplified in ~20% of breast cancers (▶ Fig. 20.9a). This drug has proven to be of use in some late-stage cancers. Even though the mAb was generated in mice, it was later developed to be humanized by a process in which the antigenic portions of the protein are replaced by sequences of human origin, thereby reducing the chances of an adverse immune reaction to treatment.
- Lapatinib (Novartis Pharmaceuticals, East Hanover, NJ) and neratinib (Puma Biotechnology, Los Angeles, CA) are small molecule inhibitors of the tyrosine kinase activity of EGFR

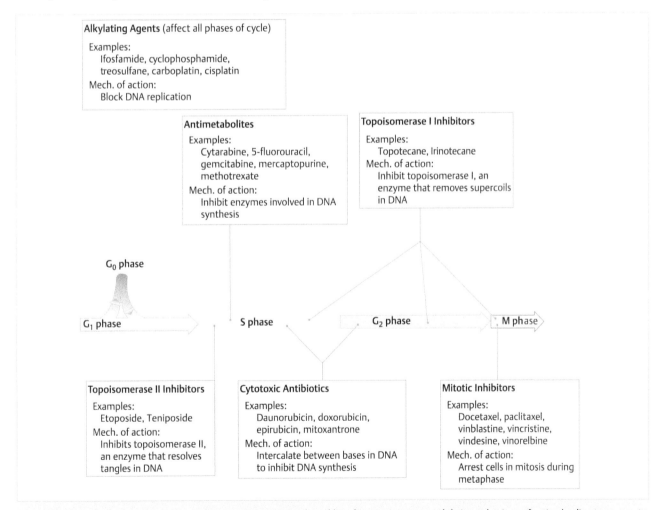

Fig. 20.8 Sites of action of cancer chemotherapeutic agents. A selected list of cytotoxic agents and their mechanisms of action leading to an arrest of the cell cycle at specific phases.

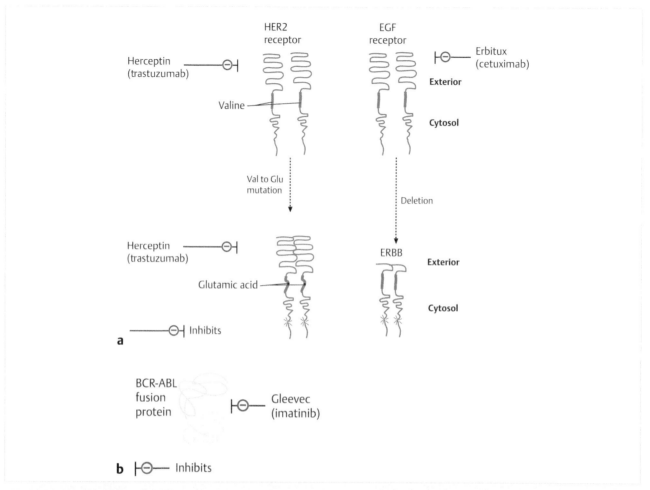

Fig. 20.9 Targeted inhibition of oncoproteins. (a) Herceptin (Genentech) is a monoclonal antibody directed against HER2, a member of a family of epidermal growth factor (EGF) receptors, which forms heterodimers with other members (HER1-HER4). The gene copy number of *ERBB2* is greatly amplified in ~20% of breast cancers. Herceptin also targets non-amplified HER2 molecules containing activating point mutations (e.g., Val → Glu). Erbitux (ImClone) is another monoclonal antibody directed against the EGF receptor overexpressed in the colon. Herceptin is an effective treatment in HER2-positive breast cancers, and Erbitux has successfully been used to treat colorectal cancers. **(b)** Gleevec (imatinib, Novartis) is an inhibitor that kills chronic myelogenous leukemia (CML) cells by inhibiting the BCR-ABL tyrosine kinase. Gleevec binds to the active site of the enzyme and prevents the binding of substrate proteins. In the absence of phosphorylation of critical target proteins, the tumor cells cannot proliferate.

family and may be effective in some trastuzumab-resistant breast cancers.

- Erbitux (ImClone, New York, NY) (cetuximab), for colorectal cancer, is a mAb directed against the EGF receptor that is over-expressed in colorectal cancer.
- Gleevec (Novartis Pharmaceuticals, East Hanover, NJ) (imatinib), for chronic myelogenous leukemia (CML), is an

inhibitor that binds to the active site of the BCR-ABL tyrosine kinase and inhibits its activity (▶ Fig. 20.9b). In laboratory studies, it appeared to be remarkably specific for CML cells, having little effect on normal white cells in the blood. It was approved by the US Food and Drug Administration in 2001 as a drug that targets an oncoprotein (BCR-ABL) that is unique to cancer cells.

21 Molecular Biotechniques

21.1 Techniques for the Study of Biomolecules

As our understanding of the role of genes and gene products in disease processes has developed, so has the need for techniques to study these biomolecules in detail. Many different techniques have been developed over the past few decades to study DNA, RNA, and proteins. This chapter provides a brief overview of just a few of these techniques. These tools may be classified into the following categories:

21.1.1 Methods

1. Cloning methods, which involve the use of restriction endonucleases (see 21.2.1 and recombinant DNA tools, such as the following:
   - Cell-based cloning and cell-free or polymerase chain reaction (PCR)-mediated cloning (see 21.6.3); real-time/quantitative PCR (see 21.6.4); multiplex PCR (see 21.6.4)
   - Genomic and cDNA libraries (see 21.6.5)
2. Electrophoretic methods to separate mixtures of macromolecules (see 21.3).
3. Hybridization methods to identify specific macromolecules. These techniques include
   - Southern blot and its derivatives: membrane hybridization, fluorescence in situ hybridization (FISH), and DNA microarray (see 21.4.1)
   - Northern blot (see 21.4.2)
4. Methods to characterize the sequence and the structure of DNA:
   - The Sanger and automated methods of DNA sequencing (21.5)
5. Methods to amplify and express macromolecules:
   - PCR amplification of DNA (see 21.6.3), production of recombinant proteins and antibodies (see 21.8)

21.1.2 Applications

- Detecting infectious agents (see 21.7.1), variations in sequence [restriction fragment length polymorphism (RFLP)] and variable number of tandem repeats (VNTR) (see 21.7.2), or diagnosis of disease-causing mutations (see 21.7.3)
- DNA microarrays to detect changes in gene copy number or gene expression (see 21.4.1)
- Gene therapy (see 21.8.4)
- Creating transgenic and knockout animals (see 21.8.3)
- Enzyme-linked immunosorbent assay (ELISA) and Western blot are used for protein analysis (see 21.9.1).

21.2 Restriction Endonucleases and DNA Ligase

21.2.1 Restriction Endonucleases

Restriction endonucleases are bacterial enzymes that recognize a specific palindromic restriction sequence (i.e., the sequence is the same on both DNA strands when read in the $5' \rightarrow 3'$ direction) and cleave both strands at the same point (▶ Fig. 21.1a).
- Some restriction enzymes cleave the double-stranded DNA in a staggered fashion to yield cohesive (sticky) ends with either 5'or 3' overhangs.
- Others cut DNA at the same position on both strands to yield flush or blunt ends.
- Most recognition sites for type II restriction enzymes (which usually cut DNA within the recognition sequence), commonly used in biotechnology, are four to six base pairs in length.

21.2.2 DNA Ligase

DNA ligase from bacteriophage T_4 is the most commonly used enzyme to join DNA fragments with either sticky or blunt ends (▶ Fig. 21.1b). This enzyme, which is dependent on adenosine triphosphate (ATP), catalyzes the formation of a phosphodiester linkage between the 5'-phosphate group at the end of one strand of DNA and the 3'-OH group at the end of the other strand.
- An adenosine monophosphate (AMP) molecule derived from ATP is covalently linked to the ε-amino group of a lysine residue of the enzyme and serves as an intermediate in the ligase reaction.

Foundations
Bacterial DNA ligases

Bacteriophage T4 ligase and eukaryotic DNA ligases use ATP as their source of AMP, whereas bacterial DNA ligases use nicotinamide adenine dinucleotide (NAD^+).

Foundations
Lysine ε-amino group modifications

Lysine is an essential, ketogenic amino acid that plays a significant role in the structure and catalytic function of proteins. The positively charged ε-amino group of lysine can undergo many different covalent modifications, such as acetylation (e.g., histones), biotinylation (e.g., acetyl coenzyme A [acetyl CoA] carboxylase and pyruvate carboxylase), mono-, di-, or trimethylation (e.g., histones and calmodulin), hydroxylation (e.g., collagen), adenylylation (e.g., DNA ligase), and ubiquitination and sumoylation (to mark proteins targeted for proteasomal degradation).

V

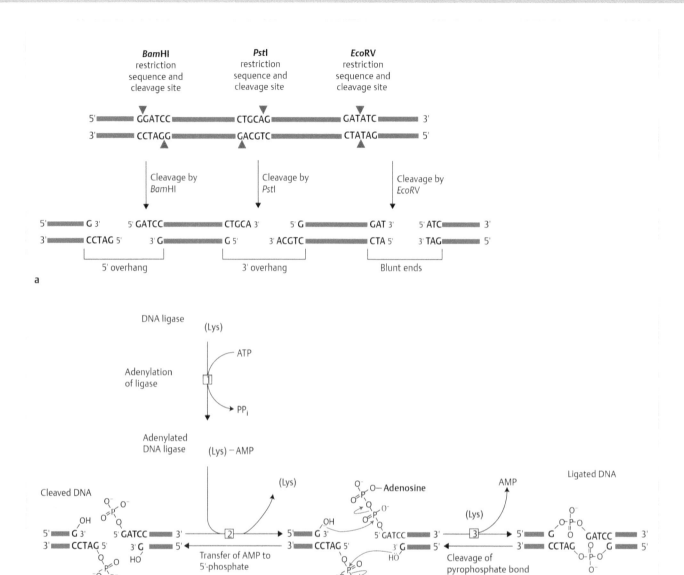

Fig. 21.1 Restriction endonucleases and ligase. (a) The palindromic restriction sequences and the cleavage sites (red triangles) for the restriction endonucleases *Bam*HI, *Pst*I, and *Eco*RV are depicted. Cleavage of DNA on both strands produces cohesive (sticky) ends that have 5′ or 3′ overhangs and blunt ends that lack overhangs. **(b)** Mechanism of DNA ligase reaction. The DNA ligase reaction involves three steps. In step 1, a covalent linkage is formed between the ε-amino group of a lysine (lys) residue on DNA ligase and the phosphate group of adenosine monophosphate (AMP), which was derived from an adenosine triphosphate (ATP) molecule. In step 2, AMP is transferred to the 5′-phosphate group at the nick that is to be sealed. The pyrophosphate bond is cleaved to release AMP (step 3) and allow the formation of a 5′→3′ phosphodiester bond.

21.3 Electrophoretic Separation of Macromolecules

DNA, RNA, and proteins may be separated from other members of their respective macromolecule group based on differences in their movement in a gel matrix (made of agarose, acrylamide, starch, or cellulose acetate) under the influence of an electrical current, due to their size, shape, and the electrical charge.

- Nucleic acids, which possess an essentially constant charge-to-mass ratio, can be separated based entirely on their size on nondenaturing gel matrices. The separation medium of choice is the polysaccharide agarose (▶ Fig. 21.2a).
  - After the electrophoretic run, the gel is briefly placed in a solution of ethidium bromide. Ethidium bromide is an intercalator that fluoresces strongly under ultraviolet (UV) light when complexed to DNA (▶ Fig. 21.2b).
- RNA mixtures can be similarly separated on agarose gels except that formaldehyde is incorporated into the gel as

Agarose gel electrophoresis: separates
population of DNA or RNA molecules based on size

Agarose gel electrophoresis result (photograph)

SDS-polyacrylamide gel electrophoresis:
separates population of proteins based on size

SDS-polyacrylamide gel electrophoresis result (silver stain)

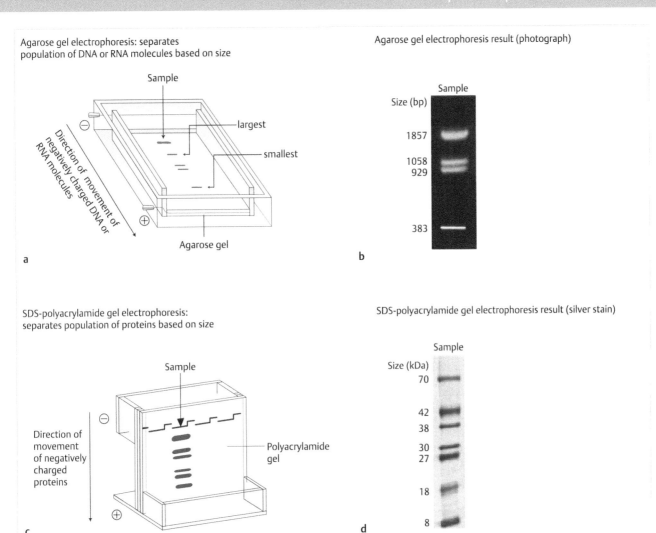

Fig. 21.2 Agarose and SDS-polyacrylamide gel electrophoresis. (a) Separation of DNA or RNA by agarose gel electrophoresis involves applying the DNA or RNA sample to preformed wells in a horizontal agarose gel. When RNA is to be separated, formaldehyde is added to provide a denaturing environment. The agarose gel is then submerged in the separation buffer and separated according to mass by applying an electrical current. (b) After electrophoresis, the ethidium bromide–stained gel is photographed under ultraviolet (UV) light. The smaller DNA or RNA molecules move faster than the larger ones. Size of separated bands is measured as the number of base pairs (bp) of DNA by comparison to DNA bands of known sizes. (c) Separation of proteins by sodium dodecyl sulfate (SDS)–polyacrylamide gel electrophoresis (SDS-PAGE) involves mixing the protein mixture with SDS in the presence of b-mercaptoethanol or dithiothreitol and loading it into wells. When an electrical current is applied, the rate of migration of each protein in the mixture is proportional to its molecular mass. (d) The separated protein bands are visualized by silver staining (or Coomassie Blue staining). The smaller proteins move faster than the larger ones. Size is measured in molecular mass, kilodaltons (kDa) by comparison to known size markers.

a denaturing agent to prevent the secondary structures of RNA from influencing their migration through the gel.
- Large genomic DNA fragments (up to 2×10^6 base pairs) can be separated by pulsed field gel electrophoresis in which the voltage applied is varied among three directions.
- Proteins can be separated based mainly on their size on polyacrylamide gels, which have smaller pore sizes than

agarose gels, in the presence of a denaturant such as sodium dodecyl sulfate (SDS). In such denaturing gels, the influences of shape and individual charge are eliminated (▶ Fig. 21.2c).
◦ Separated protein bands are visualized by staining with Coomassie Blue dye or with metallic silver (▶ Fig. 21.2d).

V

Foundations

Denaturing versus nondenaturing conditions

Polyacrylamide gel electrophoresis (PAGE) at concentrations of acrylamide ranging from 4 to 15% is routinely used for high-resolution separation of nucleic acids and proteins. PAGE can be run under either nondenaturing (native) or denaturing conditions. Sodium dodecyl sulfate (SDS) is a commonly used denaturant for proteins and while urea, formamide, and formaldehyde are used for nucleic acids. Under denaturing conditions, the separation of polypeptides depends entirely on their hydrodynamic size. Under native conditions, the separation depends on the size as well as the conformation and the intrinsic charge of the proteins. Nondenaturing gels are used for the separation of double-stranded DNA molecules in their native conformation, whereas denaturing conditions (which prevent base pairing) are used for the separation of single-stranded nucleic acids. Nondenaturing PAGE is preferred when studying alterations in charge and/or shape of proteins due to covalent modifications and also when recovery of separated species in their native state is desired. SDS-PAGE is used for the determination of size and purity of polypeptides. Polyacrylamide sequencing gels containing urea are capable of resolving DNA fragments that differ in length by a single nucleotide and are used to sequence DNA.

21.4 Hybridization

Hybridization is a fundamental property of double-stranded DNA molecules in which two complementary nucleotide strands base pair with each other to form a DNA–DNA or a DNA–RNA hybrid heteroduplex (▶ Fig. 21.3a, b). This property is advantageous for detecting the presence of a specific species of DNA (or RNA) in a mixture and in estimating the quantity of such DNA.

- In hybridization techniques, the single-stranded DNA that is used to detect the unknown DNA (or RNA) is called a probe. A DNA probe may be an oligonucleotide that is just a few nucleotides (nt) in length (~ 15 to 20), or it could be several kilobases long.

When the target nucleic acid is immobilized on a solid support such as nylon or nitrocellulose membrane, the hybridization technique is referred to as blotting. There are two types of techniques to detect nucleic acids:

1. Southern blot, in which both the probe and target nucleic acids are DNA
2. Northern blot, in which the probe is single-stranded DNA, whereas the target is usually mRNA

21.4.1 Southern Blots

Southern blots are useful to verify the presence of specific target DNA in a genomic DNA sample. In this technique, the genomic DNA sample is usually immobilized on a solid support (e.g., nylon, or nitrocellulose membrane) and denatured with alkali to convert DNA into single-stranded structures. The single-stranded probe DNA is either radiolabeled or fluorescently labeled prior to hybridization.

The following are a few techniques derived from Southern blotting:

- **Membrane (filter) hybridization:** Used for the identification of bacterial colonies containing the target gene (▶ Fig. 21.4a). A nitrocellulose filter is briefly overlaid on an agar plate containing multiple bacterial colonies. Some of the bacteria in

DNA–DNA hybridization (feature of Southern blots)

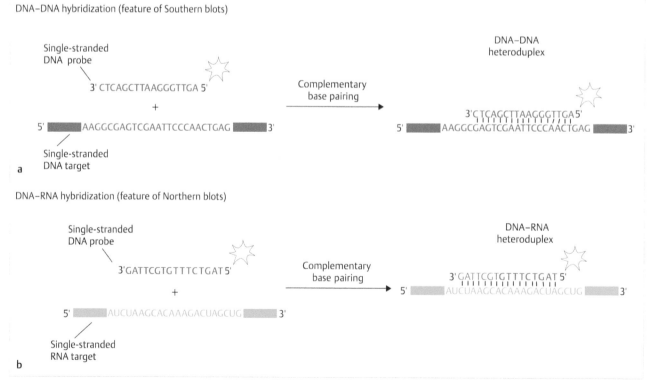

DNA–RNA hybridization (feature of Northern blots)

Fig. 21.3 Hybridization. Hybridization observed between (**a**) a DNA probe and a DNA target and (**b**) a DNA probe and an RNA target.

Filter hybridization: to identify the bacterial colonies that harbor the DNA of interest

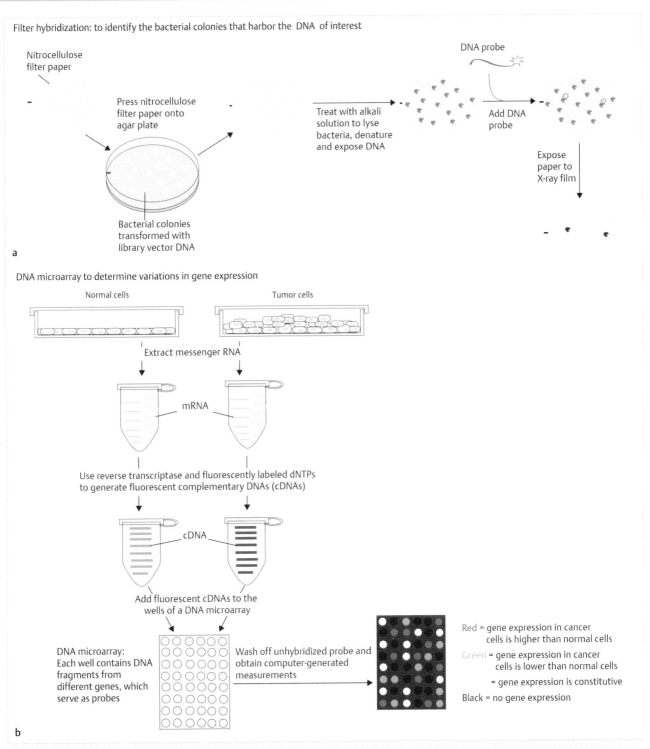

a

b

Fig. 21.4 Membrane hybridization and DNA microarray techniques. (a) In membrane hybridization for colony screening, a nitrocellulose membrane is overlaid on an agar plate containing multiple bacterial colonies. Some of the bacteria in each colony adhere to the membrane. Alkali treatment followed by heat disrupts the bacteria and fixes the released denatured DNA to the membrane. It can then be probed with a labeled DNA probe to identify the colonies containing target DNA. **(b)** (*See page 414*) In DNA micro-array, thousands of unique oligonucleotides (expressed sequence tags, ESTs), immobilized on glass slides, are probed with fluorescently labeled cDNAs synthesized from total mRNA isolated from tissues or from specific cell populations. By this technique, variation in gene expression between two types of cells (e.g., normal and cancerous cells) can be compared by using different fluorescent tags for the two cDNA pools (e.g., green versus red).

V

each colony transfer to the paper in a process called replica plating. The filter is then treated with alkali to lyse the bacteria and to denature the DNA, then baked to fix the denatured DNA. The filter containing a DNA replica of the original colonies is probed to identify the specific colonies that contain the desired DNA.

- **Fluorescence in situ hybridization (FISH):** In this technique, fluorescently labeled DNA probes are used to screen the interphase or metaphase spread of chromosomes on a glass slide. The technique is useful in determining the specific chromosomal localization of genes and other markers.
- **DNA microarrays:** These are a collection of thousands of tiny amounts of known single-stranded gene fragments immobilized on a solid support (e.g., glass). Each DNA fragment serves as a probe. These gene chips are hybridized to pools of fluorescently labeled genomic DNA or complementary DNA (cDNA), which is obtained from reverse transcription of mRNA populations of different sources (▶ Fig. 21.4b). DNA microarrays aid in determining variations in gene copy number (when probed with genomic DNA) or in gene expression (when probed with cDNA).

21.4.2 Northern Blots

Northern blots are also used to measure gene expression. In this technique, poly(A)-containing RNA (i.e., mRNA) is isolated from cells or tissues and separated on a denaturing agarose gel, as already described. The term *Northern blotting* refers to the process by which the RNA is transferred to a nylon or nitrocellulose membrane and immobilized using UV light or heat. A probe corresponding to an exon sequence of a specific gene is then labeled and hybridized to the blot.

Therapeutics

Karyotyping

Karyotyping is a technique that allows determination of the number, size, and gross structure of metaphase chromosomes. Although karyotyping is the cytogenetic method used in identifying several chromosomal abnormalities associated with genetic disorders, it does not provide information at the molecular level.

Therapeutics

FISH and aneuploidy screening

Rapid aneuploidy screening of chromosomes 21, 18, 13, X, and Y using FISH is an alternative method for the detection of disorders such as Down syndrome and other common aneuploidies (abnormal chromosome number).

21.5 DNA Sequencing

21.5.1 Sanger Method

The genetic information carried in a DNA molecule resides in the sequence of its bases. Therefore, it is vital to know the sequence of genes to identify the mutations that change the normal sequence. Rapid determination of DNA sequences up to a few hundred bases became possible by the discovery of an enzymatic method of sequencing known as the Sanger dideoxy chain termination method in the 1970s.

- In this technique, a target DNA strand is replicated in vitro using a primer, DNA polymerase, and a mixture of deoxyribonucleoside triphosphates for adenosine, guanosine, cytidine, and thymidine (dNTPs - dATP, dGTP, dCTP, and dTP) in four separate reaction tubes (▶ Fig. 21.5a, b).
  - Each reaction also contains a small amount of one of the four radiolabeled dideoxyribonucleoside triphosphates (ddNTPs - ddATP, ddGTP, ddCTP, and ddTTP) lacking the 3′-hydroxyl group, which is necessary for the extension of the DNA chain through phosphodiester linkages. Thus, whenever a dideoxy analog is introduced into the growing complementary strand, the chain terminates at that point.

- When the reaction is complete, each tube contains a mixture of radiolabeled DNA fragments of various lengths, each terminating in a particular dideoxynucleotide. These fragments are separated on a denaturing urea-polyacrylamide gel that is capable of resolving sequences that vary in length by a single nucleotide (▶ Fig. 21.5b, d).

21.5.2 Automated Method

In later years, the Sanger method was automated with the use of nonradioactive, fluorescently labeled ddNTPs, and subtle modifications were introduced to allow rapid sequencing of several thousands of bases at a time. Starting in the 1990s, these techniques allowed the sequencing of thousands of whole genomes, ranging from bacteria to humans.

- In the automated Sanger method, each of the four dideoxyribonucleoside triphosphates is labeled with a tag that fluoresces a different wavelength (color), and the polymerization reaction is performed in a single tube (▶ Fig. 21.5c).
- The fluorescent DNA products are separated by capillary gel electrophoresis where separation occurs in narrow-bore capillary columns filled with a matrix such as non-cross-linked linear polyacrylamide gel. A laser detector is used to monitor the elution of fluorescent peaks, and the sequence is read by measuring the specific fluorescence of each peak (▶ Fig. 21.5c, d).

21.6 Recombinant DNA Techniques

The term *recombinant DNA* refers to an artificial construct that is composed of DNA sequences from two or more sources (species). Because most inherited diseases result from the dysfunction of one or more proteins, it is clear that the structure and function of any protein are primarily determined by the sequence of nucleotides in the DNA that encodes it. Therefore, knowledge of the molecular techniques used in isolating, amplifying, analyzing, and manipulating the macromolecules of life—DNA, RNA, and proteins—is essential to the understanding of both normal and disease states.

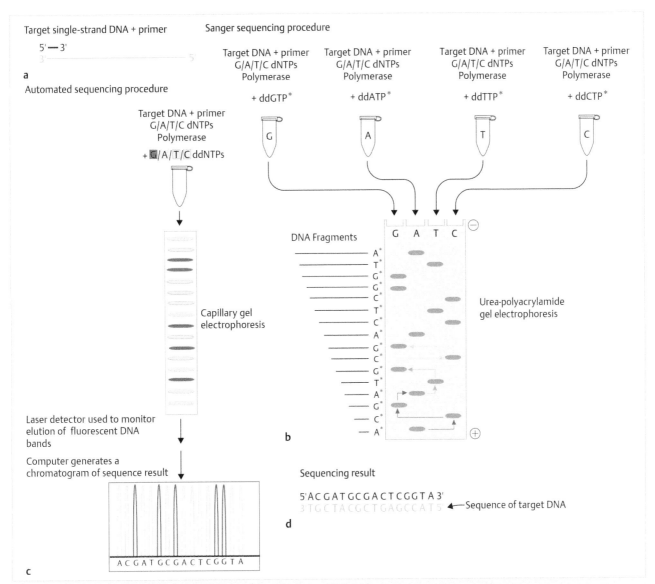

Fig. 21.5 The original and automated versions of the Sanger method of DNA sequencing. (a) The target DNA (whose sequence is unknown) is in blue; the synthetic sequencing primer is in black. **(b)** Each of the four reaction tubes used in the original Sanger method of sequencing contains the target DNA, primer, all four deoxyribonucleoside triphosphates, DNA polymerase, and a specific radiolabeled (*) dideoxyribonucleoside triphosphate. Each polymerase reaction generates a mixture of DNA fragments complementary to the target sequence, and they are separated on a denaturing urea-polyacrylamide gel. Each lane contains fragments terminating in a specific radiolabeled dideoxyribonucleotide analogue. The bands on the image of the gel can be read from bottom to top (shorter to longer fragments) to provide the sequence of the complementary strand and thereby that of the target strand. **(c)** In the automated sequencing method, a single reaction tube is used, containing the target DNA, primer, all four deoxyribonucleoside triphosphates, and all four dideoxyribonucleoside triphosphates (each labeled with a different fluorescent color label). The polymerase reaction generates DNA fragments that are separated by capillary gel electrophoresis. The fluorescence emission of each peak is monitored by a laser detector and presented as a computer-generated chromatogram. The sequence is read from left to right. **(d)** Sequencing result for **(b)** and **(c)**.

Recombinant DNA technology allows DNA to be amplified many-fold, especially because

- the amount of total DNA available for examination, particularly from sources such as human tissue, is very small and insufficient for proper laboratory studies, and
- availability of sufficient quantities of genomic DNA facilitates its study at the molecular level

21.6.1 DNA Cloning

The term *cloning* refers to the process by which either a part (e.g., specific genes) or all of genomic DNA can be copied multiple times yet remain identical to the original. Cloning is desirable, for example,

- to study the identification and organization of various elements of a gene,

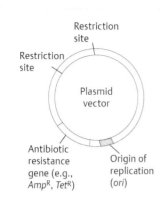

Fig. 21.6 A typical plasmid cloning vector. A typical plasmid vector has three basic features: an origin of replication that is recognized by the host enzymes to initiate replication, one or more selectable markers such as antibiotic resistance genes, and several restriction sites that can be cut by specific restriction enzymes. In other engineered vectors, the restriction sites are usually clustered together in a polylinker site.

• to study the regulation of gene expression, or
• to produce a recombinant gene product.

The two basic approaches through which cloning can be accomplished are cell-based cloning and cell-free cloning, also known as polymerase chain reaction (PCR).

21.6.2 Cell-based Cloning

In this approach, the desired DNA sequence is first inserted into a "vector," which is a stretch of DNA capable of replicating in host cells (e.g., bacteria) in a manner that is usually independent of the host genome (▶ Fig. 21.6). By this process, a foreign DNA insert can be copied and amplified many-fold in a fairly short time.

• The choice of a vector is determined by the length of the DNA fragment to be cloned, as well as by the choice of the host cell. Many bacterial cells have the ability to host extrachromosomal circular DNA vectors known as plasmids.
• These plasmids possess origins of replication that allow them to replicate independently from the bacterial genome.
• Plasmids multiply faster than the host bacteria.

▶ Table 21.1 provides an outline of the five steps of cell-based cloning in bacteria.

Foundations

Limitations of plasmid vectors
The efficiency of transformation of bacterial cells with recombinant plasmid vectors decreases drastically with increasing size of the insert. Thus, plasmid vectors are limited to cloning of DNA fragments that are less than 10,000 base pairs in size. Larger genomic DNA fragments can be cloned using bacterial artificial chromosomes (BACs), which can accept 1 to 3×10^5 base pairs inserts, and yeast artificial chromosomes (YACs), which can accept inserts up to 2×10^6 base pairs long.

21.6.3 Cell-free Cloning (also known as Polymerase Chain Reaction [PCR])

In this approach, the copying of the DNA sequence is performed in vitro by the addition of appropriate nucleotide substrates and a special heat stable DNA polymerase in a process known as polymerase chain reaction. PCR is a remarkably simple and rapid technique to amplify a sequence of target DNA up to 10^9-fold in just a few hours. It is a valuable tool in medicine because it allows for the amplification of even trace amounts of DNA for the following purposes:

• **Diagnosing infections:** PCR can be used to determine whether an individual has been infected by microorganisms (e.g., bacteria, fungi, viruses) much earlier than is possible by other techniques. For instance, human immunodeficiency virus (HIV), which has a long latency of infection, is detected by PCR, which amplifies a target sequence of the proviral DNA that has been incorporated into the host DNA. Other infections caused by bacterial and fungal strains (e.g., Lyme disease and meningitis) are also detected using PCR.
• **Genetic testing:** Mutations of specific genes can be detected via PCR. For instance, it allows for the detection of mutations in certain genes associated with cystic fibrosis, thalassemia, and hereditary hemochromatosis. PCR is also used to detect mutations of genes due to expansion of short tandem repeats (STRs) in inherited disorders, such as Huntington disease and fragile X syndrome.

PCR Procedure

The following materials are essential for PCR reactions (▶ Fig. 21.7):

1. **DNA template:** A sample of double-stranded DNA (dsDNA) containing the target sequence to be amplified is needed to serve as the template from which copies are made. dsDNA is obtained from fluid or tissue samples from an individual. When subjected to high temperatures (94 to 95 °C), dsDNA denatures (separates) into single-stranded DNA.
2. **Primers:** Two primers—each a single-stranded piece of synthetic DNA made up of 20 to 35 nucleotides—are needed. They are designed to be complementary to the $3'\rightarrow5'$ sequences that flank either end of the DNA sequence that is targeted for amplification. At temperatures 3 to 5 °C below the melting points of the oligonucleotide primers, the primers anneal (hybridize) to their complement on the separated DNA template strands. Annealing temperatures are usually in the range of 55 to 60 °C.
3. **Deoxyribonucleoside triphosphates (dNTPs):** All four dNTPs (dATP, dCTP, dGTP, and dCTP) are necessary for the synthesis of DNA copies.
4. **Taq DNA polymerase:** This enzyme from the bacterium, *Thermus aquaticus,* synthesizes DNA copies by adding deoxyribonucleotides to the primer in the $5'\rightarrow3'$ direction, generating copies that are complementary to the template DNA. Taq DNA polymerase functions at high temperatures (72 to 78 °C) and requires Mg^{2+} and proper ionic and pH environments for optimal activity. It has a half-life of 40 min at 95 °C, and thus can withstand multiple cycles of PCR.
5. **PCR thermocycler and micro test tubes:** The reaction components listed in 1 through 4 are combined in a thin-walled microtube and placed in a machine with

V

Table 21.1 Steps in cell-based cloning

1. Isolate DNA fragment to be cloned

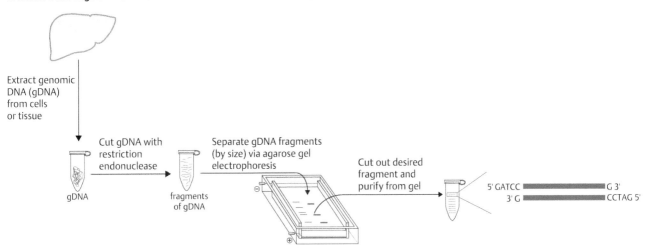

Extract genomic DNA (gDNA) from cells or tissue

gDNA

Cut gDNA with restriction endonuclease

fragments of gDNA

Separate gDNA fragments (by size) via agarose gel electrophoresis

Cut out desired fragment and purify from gel

5' GATCC　　　　　G 3'
3' G　　　　　CCTAG 5'

V

2. Prepare plasmid for cloning

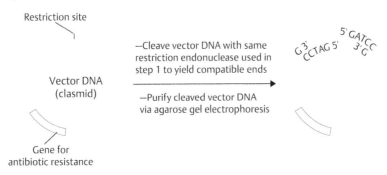

Restriction site

Vector DNA (clasmid)

Gene for antibiotic resistance

—Cleave vector DNA with same restriction endonuclease used in step 1 to yield compatible ends

—Purify cleaved vector DNA via agarose gel electrophoresis

G 3'　5' GATCC
CCTAG 5'　3' G

3. Generate recombinant DNA molecule

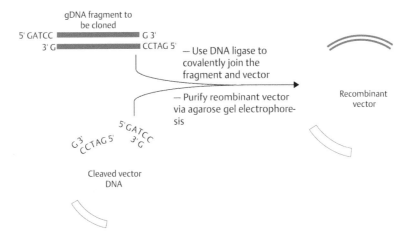

gDNA fragment to be cloned

5' GATCC　　　　　G 3'
3' G　　　　　CCTAG 5'

— Use DNA ligase to covalently join the fragment and vector

— Purify recombinant vector via agarose gel electrophoresis

Recombinant vector

G 3'　5' GATCC
CCTAG 5'　3' G

Cleaved vector DNA

V

4. Introduce recombinant DNA molecule into host cell

A useful trick in distinguishing between the colonies that contain recombinant plasmid and those that contain an empty vector is to engineer the vector in such a way as to place the cloning site in the middle of a reporter gene, such as bacterial β-galactosidase. The transformed bacteria are grown on a medium containing a colorless substrate, X-gal (5-bromo-4-chloro-3-indolyl-β-d-galactopyranoside).

- A functional β-galactosidase activity converts X-gal to a colored product such that the colony would appear blue to the naked eye.
- In the recombinant vector, however, the β-galactosidase gene is disrupted, and the colonies containing an insert DNA appear white.

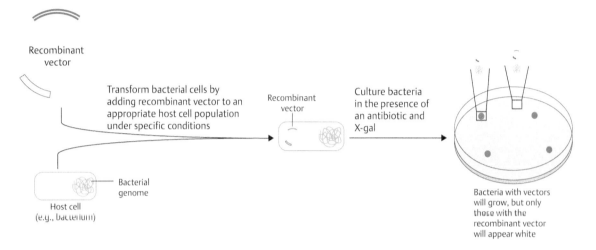

5. Isolate and purify cloned DNA fragment

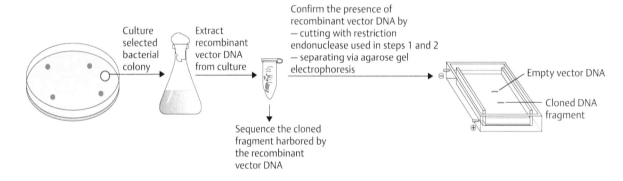

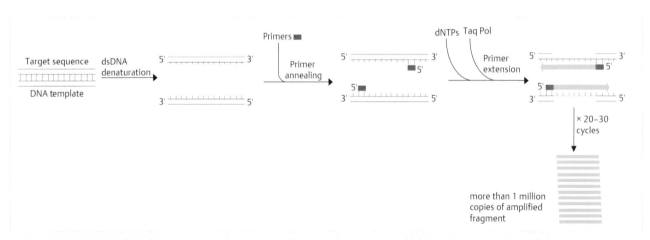

Fig. 21.7 Polymerase chain reaction procedure. The procedure of polymerase chain reaction (PCR) greatly amplifies the target DNA sequence whose flanking sequences are known. In this procedure, short (20 to 35 base pairs) primers complementary to the 3′ends of each strand of the target sequence are extended by a heat-stable DNA polymerase in a series of 20 to 30 cycles, each consisting of a double-stranded DNA (dsDNA) denaturation phase, a primer annealing phase, and a primer extension phase. dNTPs, deoxyribonucleoside triphosphates.

programmable temperature settings and number of reaction cycles. The amount of DNA is doubled during each cycle; therefore, after 20 cycles, there is a 2^{20} ($\sim 10^6$)-fold increase in DNA molecules and a 10^9-fold increase after 30 cycles. In each cycle, the alternating temperatures serve to

- denature (separate) the double-stranded template DNA (e.g., 95 °C for 30 sec),
- allow the primer to anneal to the template (e.g., 55 °C for 30 sec), and
- extend the primers by $5'\rightarrow3'$ polymerization (e.g., 72 °C for 1 min).

Advantages of the PCR procedure

- Rapid amplification of the target DNA sequence. As already described, a 10^9-fold amplification of DNA can be achieved in just a few hours.
- Because of the magnitude of amplification possible, only minute amounts of template DNA are needed.

Limitations of the PCR procedure

- The flanking sequence of target DNA must be known for proper primer design.
- The polymerization is somewhat error prone because of the fact that Taq polymerase does not have $3'\rightarrow5'$ exonuclease activity required for proofreading ability. (However, nowadays, optimized versions of high-fidelity polymerases with proofreading ability, such as the heat-stable *Pfu* polymerase from *Pyrococcus furiosus*, are commercially available.)
- The procedure reliably amplifies only short (200 to 5000 base pairs) stretches of target sequence (although "long" PCR methods have been developed to amplify sequences up to 20+ kb).
- Unwanted amplification of even a very minor amount of contaminating DNA that contains the primer sequences or the primers' target sequence is possible.

21.6.4 Other Types of PCR

Real-time PCR

The increase in the amount of PCR product depends on the amount (copy number) of the target sequence being amplified in the sample. This fact can be utilized to compare the copy numbers of a specific gene in two populations of cells (e.g., normal vs cancer cells) using the technique of real-time PCR (RT-PCR), also known as quantitative PCR (qPCR).

- In this technique, a probe that fluoresces only in the presence of PCR product is included in the reaction. This allows real-time detection of the PCR product at the end of each cycle. A probe may be a fluorescent dye that intercalates into double-stranded DNA or, more specifically, a complementary oligonucleotide with a fluorescent tag.
  - The cycle number (C_t) at which the amount of PCR product crosses a threshold and starts to increase exponentially is determined for each sample (▶ Fig. 21.8). The sample with the higher amount of target sequence will have a smaller C_t. The relative amounts of target sequence in the two samples may be calculated from the difference in C_t numbers.
  - RT-PCR can be used to measure the levels of an infectious agent within a human body.
  - RT-PCR is often coupled to cDNA production from isolated mRNA samples using reverse transcriptase to determine the levels of gene expression.

Multiplex PCR

In this technique, multiple primer sets are used to amplify either different loci in a single large gene or loci on multiple genes in a single PCR reaction.

- Multiplex PCR is useful in detecting deletions in a large gene, such as in the dystrophin gene, which cause Duchenne muscular dystrophy, or in the hypoxanthine phosphoribosyltransferase gene, which cause Lesch-Nyhan syndrome.

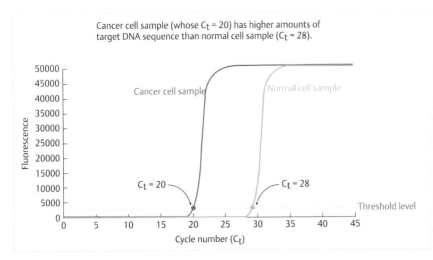

Cancer cell sample (whose $C_t = 20$) has higher amounts of target DNA sequence than normal cell sample ($C_t = 28$).

Fig. 21.8 Real-time polymerase chain reaction quantitation of target DNA copy numbers. In real-time polymerase chain reaction (RT-PCR), the amount of fluorescent signal emitted by the probe in the presence of PCR product is determined at the end of each cycle and plotted against the cycle number. A threshold level of fluorescence can be determined above which the signal increases exponentially. A sample that has a greater copy number (i.e., higher amount) of target DNA sequence would reach the threshold at an earlier cycle number (C_t) than the sample with a smaller copy number. In the example provided, the cancer cell sample has a C_t that is smaller than the normal cell sample by 8. Thus, the relative difference in the target DNA copy number is $2^8 = 256$.

• Multiplex PCR is also useful in DNA typing in paternity testing, forensic identification, and population genetics.
• An important use of multiplex PCR is in rapid screening for multiple pathogens in a single reaction. For instance, amplification of multiple regions (*gag*, *env*, and *pol*) of the HIV retroviral genome is desirable for accurate identification due to high rates of mutation. Multiplex PCR also simultaneously screens for both HIV-1 and HIV-2.

21.6.5 DNA Libraries

A library is a collection of cloned recombinant DNA molecules each containing the same vector but different DNA inserts. There are two types of genetic libraries:

1. **Genomic libraries:** The entire genome of an organism is cleaved using appropriate restriction enzymes into many thousands of fragments, and each fragment is cloned into an appropriate vector (▶ Fig. 21.9a). A genomic library therefore contains a combination of expressed and nonexpressed sequences.
   • Genomic libraries are useful for large-scale sequencing projects and also for studying the organization of a gene, such as its promoter and enhancer sequences and its exon-intron makeup.

2. **cDNA libraries:** A cDNA library represents only the expressed sequences (those that are transcribed into mature mRNA) of a genome. The total mRNA (eukaryotic messenger RNA containing poly (A) tails) is first isolated from a single organ or a cell population.
   • The mRNA is then converted into complementary DNA (cDNA) using a reverse transcriptase enzyme obtained from a retrovirus (▶ Fig. 21.9b). Short, double-stranded

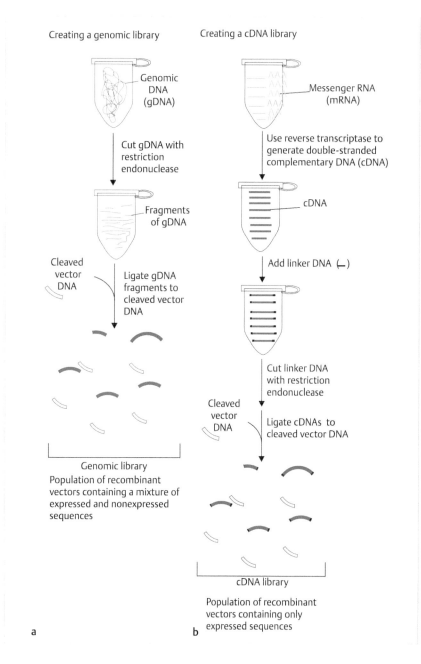

Fig. 21.9 Genomic and cDNA libraries. (a) Total genomic DNA isolated from an organism is fragmented by physical (e.g., shearing) or enzymatic methods to yield appropriately sized fragments, which are then inserted into the appropriate vector to produce a genomic library. (b) Poly (A)-containing mRNA, isolated from a eukaryotic cell population, is first converted into double-stranded complementary DNA (cDNA) using retroviral reverse transcriptase. Short DNA linkers containing a restriction site are ligated to each cDNA prior to digestion with a restriction enzyme. The resulting cDNAs are cloned into an appropriate vector to generate cDNA libraries.

Creating a genomic library

Genomic DNA (gDNA)

Cut gDNA with restriction endonuclease

Fragments of gDNA

Cleaved vector DNA

Ligate gDNA fragments to cleaved vector DNA

Genomic library
Population of recombinant vectors containing a mixture of expressed and nonexpressed sequences

Creating a cDNA library

Messenger RNA (mRNA)

Use reverse transcriptase to generate double-stranded complementary DNA (cDNA)

cDNA

Add linker DNA (⌐)

Cut linker DNA with restriction endonuclease

Cleaved vector DNA

Ligate cDNAs to cleaved vector DNA

cDNA library
Population of recombinant vectors containing only expressed sequences

a

b

linkers containing a restriction site are ligated to the fragments prior to digestion and cloning into an appropriate vector.

- The resulting cDNA library is representative of the distinctive expression pattern of the source cell population. Such libraries are useful in identifying a specific gene and characterizing its tissue-specific expression.
- cDNA clones of a specific gene in an expression vector are also used for the production of the recombinant protein expressed by that gene. Expression vectors are plasmids that contain promoter and enhancer sequences to allow for the expression of the cDNA insert in a suitable host (e.g., bacteria).

21.7 Applications of Molecular Biotechniques

Nucleic acid–based detection techniques have been widely used in diagnosing infectious diseases, genetic diseases, and cancer. They have also been a valuable part of forensic procedures.

21.7.1 Detection of Infectious Agents

In recent years, complete genomes of over 5000 pathogens have been sequenced. This information has led to state-of-the-art molecular biological tools for the rapid detection and identification of many disease-causing organisms in biological samples.

1. **Hybridization:** Short, single-stranded oligonucleotides are designed and synthesized to hybridize to complementary sequences of microbial genomes.
2. **PCR and qPCR:** These techniques eliminate the need for culturing microbes that are difficult to culture under laboratory conditions (e.g., *Chlamydia*).

A list of Food and Drug Administration (FDA)–approved nucleic acid–based assays for the detection of microbial pathogens is provided in ▶ Table 21.2. ▶ Table 21.3 contains a list of inher-

ited disorders for which PCR has been successfully used in detecting associated mutations.

21.7.2 Detection of Variations in DNA Sequence

Restriction Fragment Length Polymorphism

Polymorphisms refer to sequence changes in genomic DNA that occur in at least 1% or more of the population. A vast majority of such changes occur as single nucleotide polymorphisms (SNP). Individual human genomes vary by as much as 1 in every 1000 base pairs. Most of such variations are benign or silent in the sense that they do not affect either the expression or the function of any gene. Some of these variations occur in the recognition sequences for restriction enzymes such that when the genomes from two different individuals are cleaved with a set of restriction enzymes and the fragments are resolved on an agarose gel, the size distribution of the fragments from each sample forms a "fingerprint" that is different for each individual.

- Such variation is referred to as restriction fragment length polymorphism (RFLP). It is a component of DNA typing or DNA fingerprinting. Applications of RFLP include forensic analysis (▶ Fig. 21.10a) and paternity testing.
- Of noteworthy mention is sickle cell disease, a condition caused by a single A → T mutation in the β-globin gene, which causes a valine residue to replace the normal glutamic acid residue in position 6. Interestingly, this change results in a loss of a *Dde*I (as well as a *Mst*II) restriction site in the DNA (▶ Fig. 21.10b). *Dde*I recognizes the site 5′-CTNAG-3′ while *Mst*II recognizes 5′-CCTNAGG-3′, where N is any nucleotide. This RFLP may be detected by probing a Southern blot of genomic DNA fragments with a probe derived from the N-terminus of the β-globin gene.

Variable Number of Tandem Repeats

Another common variant in DNA sequence is the copy number of short tandem repeats (STRs) that occur throughout the human genome.

- Such variable number of tandem repeat (VNTR) regions may be obtained from each genomic sample either by using either

Table 21.2 Pathogens and nucleic acid–based assays approved for their detection

Pathogen	Detection method
Chlamydia	PCR
Cytomegalovirus (CMV)	PCR
Hepatitis C	PCR
Mycobacterium tuberculosis	PCR
Neisseria gonorrhoeae	PCR
Streptococcus	qPCR
HIV	qPCR
Trichomonas vaginalis	Hybridization
Cardnerella vaginalis	Hybridization

Abbreviations: HIV, human immunodeficiency virus; PCR, polymerase chain reaction; qPCR, quantitative PCR.

Table 21.3 Inherited disorders diagnosed via polymerase chain reaction

Adenosine deaminase deficiency	Maple syrup urine disease
α₁-Antitrypsin deficiency	Ornithine transcarbamoylase deficiency
Cystic fibrosis	Phenylketonuria
Duchenne muscular dystrophy	Retinoblastoma
Fabry disease	Sickle cell anemia
Familial hypercholesterolemia	Tay-Sachs disease
Glucose 6-phosphate dehydrogenase deficiency	β- and δ-Thalassemia
Gaucher disease	von Willebrand disease
Hemophilia A and B	
Lesch-Nyhan syndrome	

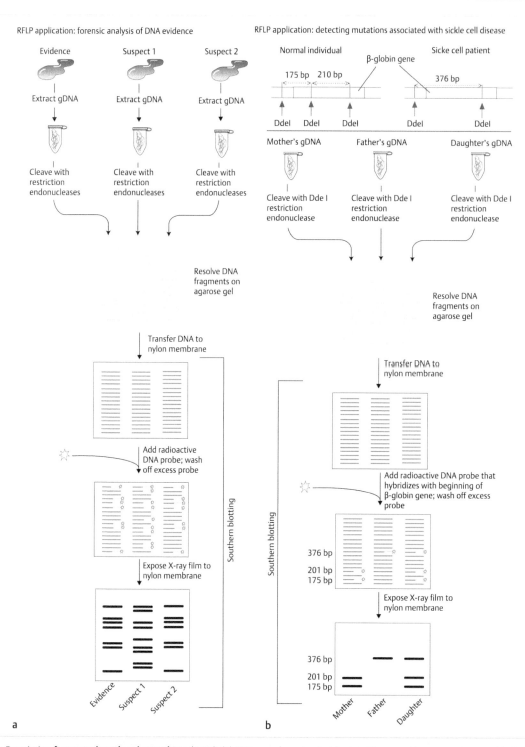

Fig. 21.10 Restriction fragment length polymorphism (RFLP). (a) DNA samples extracted from evidence and two suspects are subjected to cleavage by restriction enzymes, resolved on an agarose gel, then analyzed by Southern blotting. Hybridization of the blot to a specific radiolabeled DNA probe followed by autoradiography reveals the specific pattern of complementary fragments in each sample of DNA. The pattern generated by suspect 2 matches that of the evidence. **(b)** The normal allele for the b-globin gene contains three *Dde*I sites, whereas the mutated allele (seen in patients with sickle cell disease) contains only two. Cleavage of genomic DNA by the restriction enzyme *Dde*I, followed by agarose gel electrophoresis and Southern blotting (in which a DNA probe for the beginning of the b-globin gene is used), reveals two fragments of 175 and 201 base pairs (bp) from the normal b-globin gene (as seen in the sample from the Mother), whereas the homozygous mutant b-globin gene yields a single fragment of 376 bp (as seen in the sample from the Father). In the heterozygote (sample from the Daughter), who carries both normal and mutant alleles, all three fragments are seen.

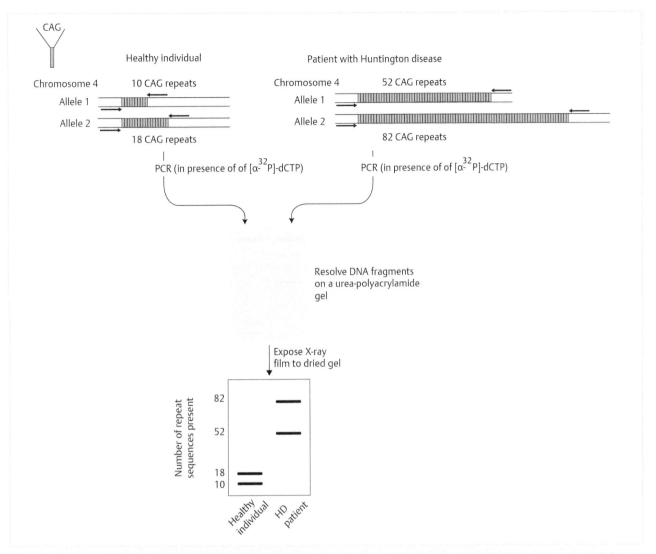

Fig. 21.11 Variable number of tandem repeats DNA in fingerprinting. The variable number of tandem repeat (VNTR) region in exon 1 of the huntingtin gene on chromosome 4 of genomic DNA samples is amplified by polymerase chain reaction (PCR) in the presence of [α-^{32}P]-dCTP. The products, along with a DNA size ladder, are separated by denaturing urea-polyacrylamide sequencing gel electrophoresis, and the dried gel is subjected to autoradiography to determine the number of CAG repeats: ≥ 40 CAG repeats are associated with Huntington disease (HD), whereas 10 to 26 CAG repeats are considered normal. Primers flanking the CAG repeat sequences in each allele are indicated by the arrows.

flanking restriction sites or through PCR. Southern blotting once again reveals the differences in the DNA fingerprint. VNTR analysis is also helpful in determining the probability and severity of inherited diseases associated with expansion of unstable trinucleotide repeats, such as Huntington disease (▶ Fig. 21.11), fragile X syndrome, myotonic dystrophy, and Friedreich ataxia.

- In each case, a particular repeat sequence is expressed only as a small number of tandem repeats in normal individuals but is greatly expanded in patients with the disease (▶ Table 21-4).
- The number of repeats tend to increase with each successive generation of affected individuals in a phenomenon termed "anticipation."
- Trinucleotide repeats are present in individuals without clinical disease; progressive increase in the number of repeats leads to the onset of clinical symptoms, although a pre-mutant phase has been described in some disorders, such as in fragile X site A (FRAXA) or in the gene for Huntingtin, where expansions larger

than normal are found but with minimal or no clinical features. These pre-mutant states give rise to carriers—parents who can subsequently pass on an expanded triplet repeat to their offspring, which may result in the disease.

21.7.3 Diagnosis of Disease-causing Mutations

In addition to diagnosing disease-causing VNTRs, as already described, molecular techniques can be used to detect subtler changes in genes that lead to inherited diseases. Genetic screening is useful in the following cases:

1. **Prenatal diagnosis:** Amniocentesis or chorionic villus sampling is used to detect the occurrence of a disorder in the fetus when both parents are carriers of a disease trait. Genetic testing may also be employed prior to implantation of embryos generated through in vitro fertilization.

2. **Newborn screening:** Blood from newborns can be used in diagnosing over 60 inherited disorders, such as phenylketonuria, sickle cell anemia, and cystic fibrosis. Such screening is mandatory in all the states in the US, although the list of diseases screened may vary from state to state.

3. **Carriers of disease:** Heterozygotes that are asymptomatic for diseases such as Duchenne muscular dystrophy, cystic fibrosis, and Tay-Sachs disease may be detected by screening blood samples.

21.8 Production of Clinically Relevant Proteins

21.8.1 Recombinant Proteins

The cDNAs of therapeutic proteins can be inserted into expression vectors engineered to allow high levels of replication, transcription, and translation in specific hosts.

Table 21.4 Disorders associated with trinucleotide repeats

Disorder	Repeat sequence	Number of repeats in normal (N) versus individuals with disorders (D)
Dentatopallidoluysian atrophy (DRPLA)	CAC	N: 7–34 D: 49–88
Fragile X site A (FRAXA)	CCC	N: 6–60 D: >200
Fragile X site E (FRAXE)	CCC	N: 4–39 D: 200–900
Fragile X site F (FRAXF)	CCC	N: 6–29 D: >500
Fragile 16 site A (FRA16A)	CCC	N: 16–49 D: 1000–2000
Friedereich ataxia	GAA	N: 6–32 D: 200–1700
Huntington disease	CAG	N: 10–26 D: ≥40
Kennedy disease	CAG	N: 17–24 D: 40–55
Machado–Joseph disease (SCA III)	CAG	N: 12–36 D: 69–79 +
Myotonic dystrophy	CTG	N: 5–35 D: 50–4000
Spinocerebellar ataxia	CAG	N: 6–39

- This allows large-scale production and rapid purification of proteins such as human insulin, growth hormone, erythropoietin, clotting factors (e.g., factor VIII, which is deficient in hemophilia), and vaccines against diseases such as influenza and malaria, as well as viral infections.

21.8.2 Antibodies

Another application of recombinant DNA technology is in the production of humanized monoclonal antibodies used as anti-cancer drugs. Monoclonal antibodies (mAbs) that are specific for a single epitope on an antigen can be generated by single clones of immortalized B lymphocytes. Immortalization is achieved by fusing the B cells with a tumor cell such as a mouse myeloma to generate a hybridoma cell.

- The purpose of humanization is to minimize the immunogenicity of mAbs and to prolong their lifespan in the human patient. ▶ Table 21.5 contains a list of some of the chimeric mAbs currently in use.

Therapeutics

Improving on insulin

With recombinant DNA technology, it is possible to generate modified forms of a protein that exhibit greater biological activity than the native form. For example, normal human insulin has a proline at position 28 and a lysine at position 29 at the C-terminus of the B chain. Lispro (Humalog, Eli Lilly, Indianapolis, IN) is an insulin analogue engineered to reverse the positions of these two residues. Lispro is faster acting and is more readily absorbed than normal insulin. Together with normal insulin, Lispro provides a tighter glycemic control. Insulin aspart (NovoLog, Novo Nordisk, Princeton, NJ), in which the proline at position 28 of the B chain is replaced by aspartic acid, behaves similarly to lispro. Insulin glargine (Lantus, Sanofi-Aventis, Bridgewater, NJ) is a longer-acting analogue of insulin in which an asparagine at position 21 of the A chain is replaced by glycine, and two arginines are added to the C-terminus of the B chain.

Table 21.5 Chimeric monoclonal antibodies, their targets and uses

Chimeric mAb (trade name)	Target antigen	Clinical use
Abciximab (ReoPro Eli Lilly, Indianapolis, IN)	Glycoprotein IIb/IIIa receptor	Inhibits platelet aggregation
Baciliximab (Simulect, Novartis, New York, NY)	α Chain of interleukin (IL)-2 receptor	Prevents rejection of transplanted kidney
Cetuximab (Erbitux, ImClone, New York, NY)	Epidermal growth factor receptor	Treats metastatic colorectal cancer
Infiximab (Remicade, Janssen Biotech, Hor-sham, PA)	Tumor necrosis factor α	Treats autoimmune diseases
Retuximab (MabThera, Roche, Indianapolis, IN)	CD-20 on B cells	Treats lymphomas, leukemias
Bevacizumab (Avastin, Roche-Genentech, San Francisco, CA)	Vascular endothelial growth factor (VEGF)	Treats colorectal cancer, non-squamous cell lung cancer, glioblasoma and renal cell carcinoma
Trastuzumab (Herceptin, Roche-Genentech, San Francisco, CA)	HER-2 growth receptor	Treats HER2-positive breast cancer

21.8.3 Transgenic and Knockout Animals

Transgenic Animals

Although bacteria such as *Escherichia coli* remain a valuable host for the production of recombinant proteins such as human insulin (Humulin, Eli Lilly, Indianapolis, IN), large farm animals such as goats, sheep, pigs, and cows offer some advantages in serving as the hosts for transgenes, as follows:

1. **Large-scale and renewable production:** The gene of interest (GOI) is engineered to be under the direction of a tissue-specific promoter such as the lactoglobulin promoter. Thus, the gene product is only produced in the mammary glands and is secreted into milk in large quantities, making it easy to obtain and purify.
2. **Posttranslational processing:** Synthesis in a mammalian system allows for proper folding of the gene product and for posttranslational modifications such as glycosylation, phosphorylation, or proteolytic maturation that may not take place in a prokaryotic system.
3. **As models for human diseases:** Transgenic animal models, particularly mice, are available for more than 100 inherited human diseases. Such animals are generated by mutating the same gen responsible for the disease condition in humans.

Knockout Animals

Knockout animals are transgenics in which one or more specific genes have been rendered inoperative (knocked out) by replacing a part of the gene with an artificial construct. Scientists use such knockout animals to understand the role of particular genes in disease process. Genes involved in obesity, heart disease, diabetes, arthritis, and aging have been studied by this technique. Mice are the animal of choice to generate a gene knockout because of the following characteristics:

- their similarity to human metabolism
- ease of handling large numbers
- short generation times

21.8.4 Gene Therapy

Gene therapy is a process by which inherited single-gene disorders may be corrected by the introduction of a functional transgene. Two types of gene therapy are possible.

1. **Somatic cell therapy:** Nonreproductive cells of the patient are altered to correct the gene defect. The correction may be short term, and the defective gene may still be passed on to the offspring.
   - The cells of choice for somatic cell therapy vary from one disorder to the next but are usually bloodborne cells or skin fibroblasts that may be removed and reintroduced easily. However, there are several problems associated with such therapy:
   - Transformation is inefficient, although the use of viral vectors has somewhat alleviated this problem. On the other hand, the use of such vectors can lead to production of harmful or immunogenic viral gene products.

- Integration of the transgene into host chromosomes is often random. In some cases a vital normal gene may be disrupted.
- The choice of vectors includes naked DNA, liposomes, and modified adeno- and retroviruses. Integration of the transgene into host chromosomes is more efficient with the retroviral vectors. The choice of a particular vector is often determined by the size of the transgene and the target tissue.

2. **Germline and stem cell therapy:** In this case, reproductive cells or multipotent stem cells are altered with the transgene. For ethical reasons, germline cell therapy is not used in humans.

   Two well-publicized cases where gene therapy has been successful to some extent in humans involve the diseases severe combined immune deficiency (SCID) and sickle cell anemia.
   - In ADA-SCID, the defective gene is adenosine deaminase (ADA), which is involved in purine catabolism. The resultant accumulation of dATP is toxic to both T- and B-lymphocytes of the immune system, due to its inhibition of ribonucleotide reductase. The standard treatment for ADA-SCID is with enzyme replacement therapy using bovine ADA modified with polyethylene glycol (PEG-ADA). If available, transplantation of bone marrow hematopoietic stem cells (HSC) from a normal, human leukocyte antigen (HLA)–matched sibling provides a more permanent cure.
   - Many patients, mostly in Europe, have been successfully treated with autologous HSC transformed with cDNA for normal human ADA in a retroviral vector. Most of such patients no longer require enzyme replacement therapy.
   - In sickle cell anemia, the defect is in the β-globin gene in erythrocyte precursor cells. Gene therapy in some cases of sickle cell anemia patients has involved replacing the defective bone marrow cells with HSC from umbilical cord blood.

3. **Gene editing:** A recent development in gene therapy is the ability to precisely edit specific target genes in order to either disable or correct a mutant gene. An example of such targeted editing is the use of a Zn-finger nuclease which is a fusion protein consisting of a Zn-finger domain which is capable of recognizing a specific hexamer DNA sequence and a nuclease (e.g., FOK1) domain capable of cutting the DNA at or near such a sequence. Another example is the use of CRISPR-Cas9 system which is derived from a bacterial defense mechanism against viral infections (▶ Fig. 21.12). CRISPR stands for clustered regularly interspaced short palindromic repeat sequences in DNA and Cas9 is a CRIPR-associated bacterial nuclease. The CRISPR tool is constructed using a guide RNA that complements the defective sequence of a target gene attached to the Cas9 nuclease. When the guide RNA hybridizes to the complementary DNA sequence, Cas9 cuts both strands of target gene. The cell tries to repair the double-strand break by the preferred but error-prone mechanism of nonhomologous end joining (NHEJ, see 17.4). However, NHEJ results in nonspecific insertions or deletions (Indel) of bases at the cut ends leading to the generation of a premature stop codon and the disabling of gene expression. If, on the other hand, the goal is to correct the mutated sequence in the target gene, a donor DNA with the correct

V

V

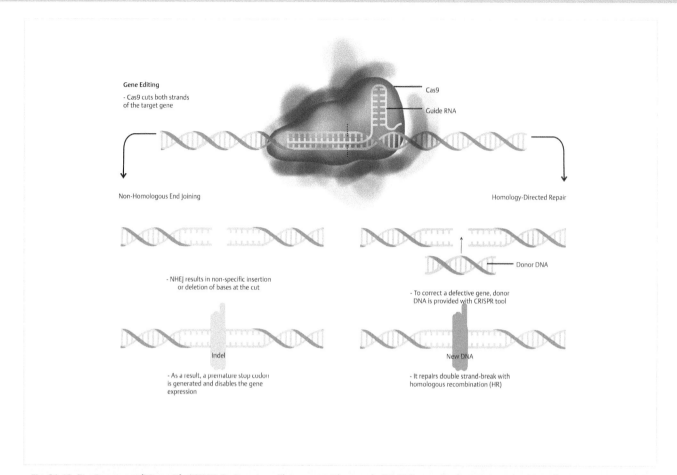

Gene Editing
- Cas9 cuts both strands
of the target gene

Cas9

Guide RNA

Non-Homologous End Joining

Homology-Directed Repair

- NHEJ results in non-specific insertion
or deletion of bases at the cut

Donor DNA

- To correct a defective gene, donor
DNA is provided with CRISPR tool

Indel

New DNA

- As a result, a premature stop codon
is generated and disables the gene
expression

- It repairs double strand-break with
homologous recombination (HR)

Fig. 21.12 Precise gene editing with CRISPR-Cas9 system. The green guide strand of RNA directs the Cas9 enzyme to a complementary sequence in the mutant target gene, adjacent to a protospacer adjacent motif (PAM) sequence (NGG) specific to Cas9 from a given bacterial species. Cas9 cuts both strands of genomic DNA. The double-strand break is usually repaired by nonhomologous end joining (NHEJ) process which is error-prone. As a result, the mutant gene is disabled due to an insertion or deletion (Indel) leading to a premature termination codon. On the other hand, if a donor DNA with correct base sequence is provided, the double-strand break is repaired using homologous recombination (HR) mechanism and the mutation in the target gene is corrected.

base sequence is provided along with the CRISPR tool. The cell then repairs the double-strand break using homologous recombination mechanism (see 17.4) and the defective gene is corrected. The safety and the lack of adverse off-target modifications of the genome for this technique are yet to be established.

Therapeutics
Adverse effects of gene therapy

Serious adverse events following gene therapy due to random integration of retroviral vectors into a patient's genome are rare but have been reported. For example, a patient with X-linked SCID, treated with HSC transformed with a retroviral vector containing cDNA for γc cytokine receptor subunit, responded well initially but developed leukemia after 2½ years. The leukemia was the result of an oncogenic transformation of T lymphocytes due to the insertion of the retroviral vector in the first intron of the *LMO-2* gene on chromosome 11 and the resulting overexpression of the gene product. Lentiviral vectors appear to preferentially integrate into transcriptionally active genes. Additional adverse effects of gene therapy may result

from unregulated, prolonged expression of the transgene, persistence of the viral vector, and altered expression of other host genes.

Therapeutics
Embryonic Stem cells (ES cells) & Induced pluripotent stem cells (iPS cells)

After fertilization the zygote undergoes equal divisions to create two, four, eight cells, and so on. These cells are considered *totipotent* (i.e., each cell has the ability to form an entire new organism). Approximately 4 days after fertilization and several mitotic divisions the totipotent cells begin to specialize, forming a hollow sphere of cells, called a *blastocyst*. An outer layer develops, which will eventually become the placenta and other supporting tissues. An inner cell mass (ICM) develops, which will eventually form every type of cell found in the human body. These ICM cells are considered *pluripotent* because they can give rise to many types of cells but not all types necessary for fetal development. ICM cells have been grown in culture and used to derive embryonic stem cell lines (ES cells) which hold great therapeutic potential because research suggests that they may be used to treat such conditions as spinal cord injuries, heart failure, Parkinson disease, type 1 diabetes, arthritis, osteoporosis, and liver failure. However, the isolation of ES cells involves an ethical controversy because it involves the destruction of human embryos. Therefore, recombinant DNA technology approaches are being utilized to develop pluripotent stem cells starting from differentiated adult cells. In recent years it has been shown that the introduction of active genes for four transcription factors (e.g., Oct4, Sox2, Nanog, and Lin28) can induce adult human cells to exhibit many of the properties of ES cells. Further research is needed to establish the promise of iPS cells. An exciting prospect of this approach is the prospect of generating patient-specific induced pluripotent stem (iPS) cells that may have the potential to correct many currently incurable conditions.

21.9 Molecular Techniques for Protein Analysis

Biomolecular techniques that analyze proteins are useful to study functional aspects of gene expression. Pathogens can be detected by the presence of unique proteins produced by them. Many disorders result not from mutant forms of gene products but from altered levels of expression of one or more normal proteins. Detection and quantitation of proteins often make use of their immunological properties.

21.9.1 Enzyme-linked Immunosorbent Assays

Solid phase enzyme-linked immunosorbent assay (ELISA) measures the levels of specific antigen or antibody concentrations in biological samples using a corresponding immobilized antibody or antigen (▶ Fig. 21.13a-c).
- In a sandwich ELISA, the target protein bound to a specific immobilized antibody is then reacted with a second specific antibody linked to an enzyme, for example, horseradish peroxidase (HRP), followed by the addition of a chromogenic substrate. The intensity of the resulting color reflects the levels of target protein.
- Medical uses of sandwich ELISA are exemplified by the applications listed hereafter.

ELISA Application: Measurement of Cardiac-specific Troponin Isoforms

Troponin is the contractile regulating protein of striated muscle and contains three subunits—troponin I, troponin C, and troponin T. The cardiac isoforms of troponin T and I increase in serum after acute myocardial infarction (▶ Fig. 21.13b) and serve as useful diagnostic markers of acute ischemia along with myoglobin and creatine kinase.

1. Polystyrene microtiter plates coated with specific antibodies to human troponin T are incubated with serum samples.
2. After washing to remove nonspecifically bound antigens, another antitroponin antibody conjugated to HRP is added.
3. The microtiter wells are washed again to remove any excess secondary antibody and incubated with a chromogenic substrate for HRP.
4. After development, the color is read in a spectrophotometer.

ELISA Application: Diagnosis of HIV Infection

Humans produce specific antibodies to surface proteins of human immunodeficiency virus (HIV) that are detectable 4 to 6 weeks after infection. ELISAs are the most commonly used screening assays for such detection due to their rapidity, sensitivity, and low cost. However, they occasionally produce both false-negative and false-positive results and require confirmation by a second approach, such as Western blotting.
- In this application of ELISA, an immobilized HIV antigen is used to capture the antibodies in a biological sample. The captured antibodies are then reacted with an enzyme-linked antihuman immunoglobulin G (IgG) followed by incubation with a chromogenic substrate (▶ Fig. 21.13c).

ELISA Application: Hormone Immunoassays

ELISAs are widely used for the quantitation of several hormone levels in biological fluids. The sandwich assays usually employ monoclonal antibodies that recognize different epitopes on the same human hormone.

21.9.2 Western Blots

In Western blots (immunoblots), a specific monoclonal (usually from mouse) or polyclonal (usually from rabbit) antibody is used to detect the target protein in a mixture after electrophoretic separation and transfer to nitrocellulose or polyvinylidene fluoride (PVDF) membranes (▶ Fig. 21.14).
- After blocking (e.g., with bovine serum albumin or casein) to minimize nonspecific binding, the membrane (blot) is incubated with the primary antibody that binds to the immobilized target protein. Then the blot is washed and incubated with a secondary antibody directed against the primary antibody.
- The secondary antibody is raised in a different animal species. For example, if the primary antibody is of rabbit origin, the secondary antibody could be the goat antirabbit IgG. The secondary antibody is also tagged with either a radioactive, chromogenic, chemiluminescent, or fluorescent label to allow visualization.
- The use of a secondary antibody amplifies the signal and makes detection of target protein easier. The intensity of the visualized bands on the blot is used as a measure of the amount of target protein present in the sample.

V

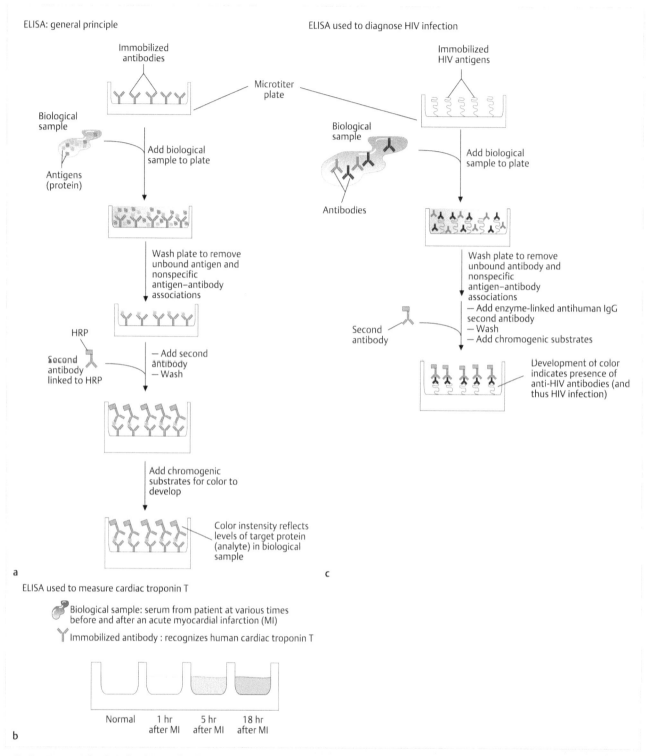

ELISA: general principle

Immobilized antibodies

Microtiter plate

Biological sample

Antigens (protein)

Add biological sample to plate

Wash plate to remove unbound antigen and nonspecific antigen–antibody associations

HRP

Second antibody linked to HRP

— Add second antibody
— Wash

Add chromogenic substrates for color to develop

Color instensity reflects levels of target protein (analyte) in biological sample

a

ELISA used to measure cardiac troponin T

Biological sample: serum from patient at various times before and after an acute myocardial infarction (MI)

Immobilized antibody : recognizes human cardiac troponin T

Normal | 1 hr after MI | 5 hr after MI | 18 hr after MI

b

ELISA used to diagnose HIV infection

Immobilized HIV antigens

Biological sample

Antibodies

Add biological sample to plate

Wash plate to remove unbound antibody and nonspecific antigen–antibody associations
— Add enzyme-linked antihuman IgG second antibody
— Wash
— Add chromogenic substrates

Second antibody

Development of color indicates presence of anti-HIV antibodies (and thus HIV infection)

c

Fig. 21.13 Principle of sandwich ELISA for the measurement of an antigen or detection of antibodies. (a) A microplate is precoated with a capture antibody, which is immobilized to the plate's surface. Any analyte (e.g., target protein) from standard or biological samples will be captured (bound) to the antibody when added to the well. Unbound/nonspecifically bound molecules are washed away. A second antibody conjugated with horseradish peroxidase (HRP) is added and binds to the captured analyte. After the unbound second antibody is washed away, the HRP substrate, tetramethylbenzidine (TMB), is added to the wells. Blue color is developed proportional to the amount of analyte in the sample. (b) Application of enzyme-linked immunosorbent assay (ELISA) in measuring serum levels of cardiac troponin T in serum from normal patients and after an acute myocardial infarction. (c) Application of ELISA in diagnosing human immunodeficiency virus (HIV) infection. The immobilized molecule is an HIV antigen, which will only be bound by HIV-specific antibodies. IgG, immunoglobulin G.

Western Blot Application: Early Detection/ Confirmation of HIV Infection

Even prior to the appearance of anti-HIV antibodies in infected patients there is an increase in the circulating levels of HIV p24 surface antigen, which can be detected by Western blot analysis. Western blot is considered the gold standard for validation of HIV infection and is used to confirm the results of ELISA. In addition to p24, several other HIV proteins such as gp160, gp120, p66, p55, p51, gp41, p31, p17, and p15 can be detected by Western blot technique.

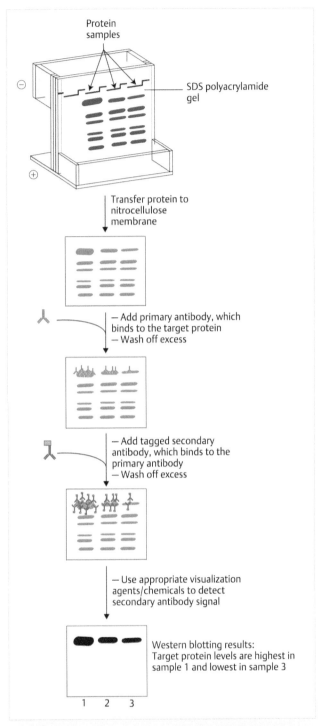

Protein samples

SDS polyacrylamide gel

Transfer protein to nitrocellulose membrane

— Add primary antibody, which binds to the target protein
— Wash off excess

— Add tagged secondary antibody, which binds to the primary antibody
— Wash off excess

— Use appropriate visualization agents/chemicals to detect secondary antibody signal

Western blotting results: Target protein levels are highest in sample 1 and lowest in sample 3

1 2 3

Fig. 21.14 Western blot. A mixture of proteins is separated by sodium dodecyl sulfate polyacrylamide gel electrophoresis (SDS–PAGE) and then transferred to a nitrocellulose membrane. The membrane is incubated with the first (primary) antibody directed against the target protein followed by a second (tagged) antibody directed against the first.

V

Questions and Answers: Genetics and Cell Cycle

V

1. A nucleotide sequence, 5′-TCCGAT-3′, within human genomic DNA underwent a spontaneous mutation resulting in a nucleotide substitution, producing the sequence 5′-TTCGAT-3′. Which one of the following chemical reactions could account for such a mutation?
   A) Conversion of a deoxyribosyl group to a ribosyl group
   B) Deamination of a pyrimidine
   C) Hydrolysis of the *N*-glycosidic bond in a purine
   D) Hydrolysis of a phosphodiester bond
   E) Methylation of a cytosine

2. Which of the following characteristics of nucleosomes is important for their ability to package genomic DNA into chromatin?
   A) The histone constituents of nucleosomes contain a relatively high proportion of lysine and arginine amino acids.
   B) Multiple posttranslational modifications can be present on multiple amino acids in the N-terminal regions of histones within nucleosomes.
   C) Nucleosomes consist of two copies each of histone H2A, H2B, H3, and H4
   D) The wrapping of DNA around nucleosome particles induces negative supercoils in the DNA molecule.
   E) The histones form ionic bonds with positively charged DNA and have no sequence specificity.

3. Which of the following observations is evidence for semiconservative DNA replication?
   A) One double-helix is completely original, and one is newly synthesized.
   B) DNA synthesis occurs on both lagging and leading strands in the replication fork.
   C) After DNA synthesis, each daughter molecule contains one parental strand and one new strand.
   D) During DNA synthesis, replication proceeds in both directions from the origin of replication.
   E) DNA synthesis in eukaryotes requires the activity of more than one DNA polymerase enzyme.

4. The following DNA sequence is the template for the synthesis of newly transcribed RNA:
   5′-TAGACCAC-3′
   Which of the following sequences represents the RNA synthesized from the template?
   A) 5′-GUGGUCUA-3′
   B) 5′-UAGACCAC-3′
   C) 5′-CACCAGAU-3′
   D) 5′-AUCUGGUG-3′
   E) 5′-CACCAGAT-3′

5. The anticancer drug cytarabine can be metabolically activated into the compound shown below. Which of the following enzymes is inhibited by this compound?

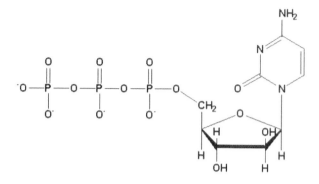

   A) DNA polymerase δ
   B) DNA primase
   C) Ribosome
   D) RNA polymerase II
   E) Helicase

6. One mechanism of potential mutations is the insertion of an incorrect nucleotide into the newly synthesized DNA molecule. Which of the following enzymes, present at the replication fork, repairs nucleotide misincorporation during DNA synthesis?
   A) DNA ligase
   B) DNA helicase
   C) DNA topoisomerase
   D) DNA polymerase δ
   E) DNA polymerase α

7. The PEPCK-C gene is transcribed in the liver under normal conditions, and its transcription is induced significantly by glucocorticoids. It was reported in the literature that a nucleotide substitution, at a position outside the protein coding region of the PEPCK-C gene, resulted in consistently elevated levels of PEPCK-C transcription that were only increased slightly by glucocorticoid treatment. Which of the following regulatory elements is most likely the site of this mutation?
   A) Core promoter
   B) Enhancer element
   C) Silencer element
   D) Transcriptional start site
   E) Polyadenylation site

8. p16 is a member of the INK family of CDK inhibitor proteins (CIP). What effect does the action of p16 have on the cell cycle?
   A) p16 promotes the associations between CDK4/6 and cyclin D.
   B) p16 triggers the release of E2F from RB.
   C) p16 blocks passage of cell cycle through restriction point in late G_1.
   D) p16 promotes the hyperphosphorylation of RB.
   E) p16 inhibits S phase cyclin CDK activities.

9. A strain of bacteria resistant to a specific antibiotic was isolated in a hospital laboratory. Biochemical analysis demonstrated that treatment of the sensitive strain with the antibiotic resulted in a block in bacterial RNA synthesis, whereas in the resistant strain, RNA synthesis was unaffected. The antibiotic in the question is:
   A) Chloramphenicol
   B) Tetracycline
   C) Rifampicin
   D) Acyclovir
   E) Amoxicillin

10. Ciprofloxacin, a fluoroquinolone, exerts its antimicrobial effect by inhibiting which of the following enzymes?
    A) DNA polymerase III
    B) DNA gyrase
    C) Helicase
    D) Reverse transcriptase
    E) Primase

11. Which of the following is an essential characteristic of the intrinsic pathway of apoptosis?
    A) Activation of caspase 8
    B) Cleavage of the proapoptotic factor, BID by caspase 8
    C) Involvement of Fas-associated death domain protein (FADD)
    D) Release of cytochrome c from mitochondria
    E) Death receptor pathway

12. Genetic mutations in proto-oncogenes contribute to cancer by
    A) altering the amount or the structure of the gene's protein product.
    B) disrupting the protein product's ability to repair damaged DNA.
    C) disrupting the protein product's ability to arrest the cell cycle.
    D) causing a reduction in the amount of the gene's protein product.
    E) disrupting the protein product's ability to promote apoptosis.

13. Which of the following DNA sequences (only one strand of the double-stranded sequence is shown) would have the highest thermal stability?
    A) GGAATCCG
    B) TTATTCCG
    C) AGGATTTC
    D) GGCTTTTT
    E) CCCCGGGA

14. A drug, used clinically to treat seizures, is an inhibitor of histone deacetylase. The drug in question is:
    A) Streptomycin
    B) Doxorubicin
    C) Didanosine
    D) Rifampicin
    E) Valproic acid

15. Cells from a patient that cannot produce the enzyme GlcNAc phosphotransferase would be unable to transport newly synthesized glycoproteins to which of the following locations?

A) Extracellular space
B) Lysosomes
C) Plasma membrane
D) Mitochondria
E) Nucleus

16. The DNA translocation generating the Philadelphia chromosome involves which of the following proto-oncogenes?
    A) *RAS*
    B) *ERBB2*
    C) *c-MYC*
    D) *ABL*
    E) *N-MYC*

17. During the elongation phase of prokaryotic translation, for each amino acid added to the growing peptide chain, two GTP molecules are hydrolyzed to GDP. One GTP molecule is hydrolyzed when an amino acyl tRNA is inserted into the A site and a second is expended during the
    A) peptide bond formation
    B) translocation process
    C) binding of CAP-binding complex to the 7-methyl-guanosine cap of mRNA
    D) assembly of the small and large ribosomal subunits

18. The mRNA sequence 5′-GCG ACG UCC-3′, is being translated by a ribosome. Which of the following sequences represent the anticodons of the aminoacyl-tRNAs that were used (in order) during translation?
    A) 5′-UCC-3′ 5′-ACG-3′ 5′-GCG-3′
    B) 5′-GGA-3′ 5′-CGU-3′ 5′-GCG-3′
    C) 5′-GCG-3′ 5′-ACG-3′ 5′-UCC-3′
    D) 5′-CGC-3′ 5′-CGU-3′ 5′-GGA-3′
    E) 5′-CGC-3′ 5′-GCA-3′ 5′-UCC-3′

19. Which one of the following antibiotics blocks the synthesis of a subset of proteins by an ealy release of peptidyl-tRNA in prokaryotic organisms?
    A) Erythromycin
    B) Tetracycline
    C) Streptomycin
    D) Chloramphenicol
    E) Puromycin

20. You are cloning BamHI-cut genomic DNA into the plasmid vector pBR322, which has both an ampicillin resistance gene and a tetracycline resistance gene. If the inserts are ligated into the BamHI site in the tetracycline resistance gene of the vector, the entire population of transformed bacteria should first be grown on
    A) media containing no antibiotic
    B) media containing ampicillin
    C) media containing tetracycline
    D) media containing both ampicillin and tetracycline

21. When the ribosome reaches a stop codon on mRNA, release factors act to change the specificity of peptidyl transferase so that the growing peptide chain is transferred to:
    A) Water
    B) eIF4F
    C) Formyl-methionine
    D) UDP-GlcNAc
    E) The E site

V

V

22. Recombinant human granulocyte-macrophage growth factor (GMCSF), a hematopoietic factor used to treat neutropenia, can be produced in a human cell line engineered to synthesize the protein. Analysis of the glycosylation of recombinant GMCSF (rGMCSF) was performed with PNGase F, an enzyme that catalyzes the complete removal of N-linked oligosaccharides from proteins at the site of attachment. Treatment of rGMCSF released an oligosaccharide containing eight residues. Which of the following is true regarding the glycosylated rGMCSF?
A) The oligosaccharide is attached to rGMSCF at an amino acid that can also serve as a site of phosphorylation.
B) The oligosaccharide is attached to rGMSCF via a mechanism that is insensitive to tunicamycin treatment.
C) The oligosaccharide is attached to rGMCSF via a hydroxyl functional group.
D) The oligosaccharide is attached to rGMCSF via an acid amide functional group.
E) The oligosaccharide is attached to rGMCSF via a mechanism that does not require dolichol phosphate.

23. The genome of a bacterial species is found to be composed of 23% deoxycitidine. What would the predicted percentage of deoxyadenosine be?
A) 23%
B) 27%
C) 29%
D) 32%
E) 77%

24. During the interphase of the cell cycle, euchromatin is
A) condensed chromatin conformation.
B) associated with histone deacetylation activity.
C) transcriptionally active region of genome.
D) usually localized near nuclear periphery during interphase.
E) intense dark stained region with Giemsa.

25. Mutations in the BRCA1 gene lead to a predisposition to breast and ovarian cancers caused by a defect in which of the following DNA repair pathways?
A) Base excision repair
B) Nucleotide excision repair
C) Homologous recombination repair
D) Mismatch repair
E) Nonhomologous End Joining repair

26. A 31-year-old man who emigrated from Vietnam and recently returned from a visit to his home country presents in your office with a chief complaint of sore throat, fever, and malaise. Upon physical examination, you observe a gray membrane that covers his tonsils and pharynx. Upon questioning, you find that he has never been vaccinated for diphtheria. In cells exposed to the toxin, which of the following proteins related to gene expression is affected as a direct result of the action of the diphtheria toxin?
A) Initiation factor
B) Sigma factor
C) Release factor
D) Rho factor
E) Elongation factor (EF-2)

27. The public health department in your state recently reported the isolation of a tetracycline-resistant strain of *Treponema pallidum* in your area. Biochemical analysis has determined that the resistance is associated with a change in ribosome structure, which alters the ribosome's function. Which of the following events in protein synthesis is most likely to be altered in the tetracycline-resistant strain of *T. pallidum*?
A) Assembly of the 30S preinitiation complex
B) Entry of the 50S ribosomal subunit to create the initiation complex
C) Binding of aminoacyl-tRNAs to the A site
D) Peptidyl transferase activity of the 70S ribosome
E) Translocation of the 70S ribosome

28. You must evaluate the genetic status of a family with a history of Huntington disease and wish to determine the number of triplet repeats in each individual. The best way to estimate the number of triplet repeats is by variable number of tandem repeat (VNTR) analysis and will test for repeats of which of the following nucleotide sequences?
A) CGG
B) CTG
C) CAG
D) GAA
E) CCTG

29. A couple expecting their second child requests for prenatal genetic testing for cystic fibrosis (CF). They already have a 4 year old son who suffers from CF. You administer a PCR amplification test for the ΔF508 mutation responsible for 70% of all cases of CF and obtain the data diagrammed below. It can be concluded that:

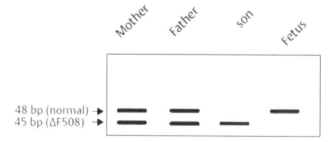

48 bp (normal) →
45 bp (ΔF508) →

A) The fetus does not carry the *ΔF508* mutant allele for the CF gene.
B) The mother is homozygous for the *ΔF508* CF mutation.
C) The fetus is heterozygous for the *ΔF508* CF mutation.
D) The fetus is homozygous for the *ΔF508* CF mutation.
E) The son does not carry the *ΔF508* mutant allele for the CF gene.

30. The following table lists the GC content of the genomes of several pathogenic bacteria:

Organism	% GC content of genome
Mycobacterium tuberculosis	65.5
Clostridium botulinum	28.2
Francisella philomiragia	32.6
Burkholderia mallei	68.5
Escherichia coli O157H7	50.3

Based on the difference in thermal stability of the organisms' genomes, which of the following pairs of organisms would be suitable candidates for developing a PCR-based clinical laboratory assay that would allow the amplification of DNA from one pathogen but not the other?
A) M. tuberculosis and B. mallei
B) E. coli and M. tuberculosis
C) B. mallei and E. coli
D) F. philomiragia and B. mallei
E) C. botulinum and F. philomiragia

31. A 44-year-old woman who emigrated from Poland three years earlier comes to your office with a chief complaint of fatigue of six months' duration. A previous doctor told her she was anemic and had prescribed oral iron supplements, which she stopped taking because of the taste. Physical examination was unremarkable. During your conversation, she remarks that her mother had died from colon cancer at age 51, as did her maternal grandfather at age 55. Laboratory tests indicate she was indeed anemic, and a fecal occult blood test was positive. On a follow-up visit, colonoscopy and following pathologic examination of biopsied lesions resulted in the diagnosis of colon adenoma with villous features. Genetic testing indicated that the woman has a mutation resulting in a defect of a DNA repair pathway. Which of the following pathways is most likely dysfunctional in this patient?
A) Homologous recombination repair
B) Mismatch excision repair
C) Nonhomologous end-joining repair
D) Nucleotide excision repair
E) Transcription coupled repair

32. Bloom syndrome is characterized by skin sensitivity and risk of cancer due to a defect in the BLM gene that encodes for:
A) Topoisomerase
B) DNA ligase
C) Excision endonuclease
D) DNA glycosylase
E) DNA Helicase

33. A 2-year-old male patient was brought to the physician by his mother, who stated that her son's left eye had a glow similar to that of a cat's eye caught in headlights. She also noticed that his eyes appeared crossed, and he appears to have diminished vision in his left eye. The physician sends the child to an ophthalmologist, who confirms that the child has tumors in his retina due to:
A) A "loss of function" mutation in the *TP53* gene
B) A chromosomal translocation involving the *BCR* and *ABL* genes
C) A "gain of function" mutation in the *RAS* gene
D) A "loss of function" mutation in the *RB1* gene
E) A point mutation in the *N-MYC* gene

34. A novel pharmaceutical agent in development is claimed to inhibit the activity of CDK2. The effect of this agent on the cell cycle should include
A) inhibition of the G_1/S transition
B) maintenance of RB in a hyperphosphorylated state

C) inhibition of the CDK inhibitor proteins p21 and p27
D) promotion of the transcription of genes for cyclin E and cyclin A
E) rapid degradation of cyclin D

35. You carry out an experiment in which the expression of a human protein is analyzed via hybridization to an antibody. Which of the following best describes the hybridization technique used in this experiment?
A) Western blotting
B) Southern blotting
C) Northern blotting
D) DNA microarray
E) SDS-PAGE

36. A mother brings his 6-year-old son to the clinic with the primary complaint of altered learning behavior in school. She informs the physician about personality changes in the son. Physical examination reveals a long face with large ears; prominent jaw and forehead. Further examination of the son reveals delayed development of speech and language and intellectual disability. The mother gives a family history of death of her young cousin due to Fragile X syndrome. Knowing that Fragile X syndrome is marked by > 230 CCG repeats in the X-linked gene that encodes for Fragile X mental retardation (FMR1) protein, which of the following modifications of cytosines in the promoter sequence silences transcription from the gene leading to the loss of normal function of FMR1 protein?
A) Acetylation
B) Phosphorylation
C) Methylation
D) Deamination
E) Dephosphorylation

37. While working in a medical mission in a small village in Honduras, a 7-year-old male child is brought to you by his parents. The parents tell you that the child has always had "very bad skin and been very sick," and whenever they can afford it, they take the boy to a hospital in the nearest city for treatment of his skin lesions. While the child was still an infant, the doctors told the parents that he cannot ever be exposed to sunlight, a restriction that is difficult to impose as both parents work in the fields all day. Upon examination of the boy, you find significant patches of discolored skin with areas of severe blistering on his face, arms, and neck that are oozing and raw, indicative of xeroderma pigmentosum. Molecular analysis of the DNA from the boy's skin keratinocytes would reveal an abundance of which of the following types of lesions?
A) Double-stranded breaks
B) Pyrimidine dimers
C) Chromosomal translocations
D) Nucleotide deletions
E) Nucleotide substitutions

38. A recent report identified a G → C transversion in the gene encoding the hematopoietic transcription factor GATA1 in the genome of a patient with the congenital syndrome Diamond-Blackfan anemia. The mutation caused a loss of exon 2 in the transcribed mRNA. Biochemical analysis of cells homozygous for this mutation indicated that no

V

functional GATA1 protein was produced. What is the likely location of the nucleotide substitution in the *GATA1* genes of this patient?[1]
A) 5'-UTR
B) 3'-UTR
C) Splice donor site
D) Promoter
E) Enhancer

39. A child born from consanguineous parents has a congenital defect in pituitary development. Genetic analysis revealed a five-nucleotide deletion associated with the child's *PIT1* genes that was associated with significantly diminished levels of PIT1 mRNA. Biochemical analysis of cells biopsied from the child determined that the acetylation of chromatin associated with the *PIT1* core promoter was significantly lower than in matched cells from a healthy donor. The five nucleotide deletion is likely in which of the following elements associated with the *PIT1* gene?
A) Enhancer
B) Polyadenylation signal sequence
C) Silencer
D) Splice donor site
E) Transcriptional start site

40. A 26-year-old woman in generally good health comes to your clinic for a check-up, as she and her husband have decided to start a family. She is currently using a skin patch for transdermal delivery of low-dose synthetic estrogen and progesterone and will discontinue its use immediately. Both of these drugs activate gene transcription through mechanisms similar to another steroid family member, glucocorticoids. At genes that are activated by estrogen, what changes in histone protein will likely occur in the short term (hours to days) once the woman discontinues her use of the contraceptive patch?
A) Decreased acetylation
B) Increased acetylation
C) No change in acetylation
D) Variable changes in acetylation, depending on the gene
E) Loss of positive charge

41. Following the treatment of cells with a low dose of the mushroom toxin α-amanitin, polyadenylated RNA in these cells was found to be decreased, whereas ribosome number and transfer RNAs (tRNAs) were unchanged. The activity of which of the following proteins is inhibited by low-dose α-amanitin?
A) Transcription factor II D (TFIID)
B) RNA polymerase II
C) RNA polymerase III
D) Histone acetyl transferase (HAT)
E) Capping enzyme

42. A nitrogenous base and the deoxy sugar in a deoxyribonucleotide of a double-stranded DNA molecule are connected by which of the following types of chemical bonds?
A) Electrostatic
B) Glycosidic
C) Hydrogen
D) Phosphodiester
E) Van der Waals

43. The compound palbociclib, or PD 0332991 (Pfizer Inc., New York, NY), is a selective potent inhibitor of CDK4 and CDK6 in retinoblastoma protein (RB) positive cancer cell lines. Which of the following effects would be a consequence of treatment with PD 0332991?[2]
A) Progression of tumor cell cycle through the G_1-S phase
B) Stimulation of RB phosphorylation
C) Reduction in the transcription of genes under the control of E2F
D) Arrests cells in the G_2 phase
E) Promotion of E2F release

44. Fabry disease is an X-linked recessive disorder caused by defects in the activity of the lysosomal enzyme α-galactosidase. This results in the accumulation of glycolipids in the plasma and cellular lysosomes of the brain, heart, and kidneys. Patients affected by Fabry disease present with rashes, peripheral neuropathy, cardiac disease, and kidney failure. The pedigree below shows inheritance of the X-linked recessive Fabry disease. Which statement is a correct interpretation of this family's pedigree?

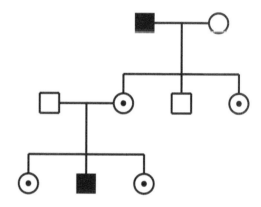

A) Both males and females of all generations are affected.
B) All female children of an affected male are also affected.
C) Sons of heterozygous mothers have a 50% chance of being affected.
D) The genetic mutation cannot be passed on to great-grandchildren (third generation).
E) All male descendants of the affected male are carriers.

45. Li-Fraumeni syndrome (LFS) is an autosomal dominant inherited cancer syndrome characterized by mutations in the *TP53* gene that prevent activation of the p53 protein in response to DNA damage. Consequently, patients with LFS develop tumors early (before age 45), develop multiple types of tumors (in an individual), and have several relatives who have been diagnosed with some type of cancer before the age of 45. What is a possible consequence of a defective p53 in response to DNA damage?
A) Sequestration of E2F
B) Decreased transcription of p21
C) Hypophosphorylation of RB
D) Decreased transcription of cyclin A
E) Cell cycle arrest

46. Which of the following mutations is an example of a "gain of function" mutation that converts a normal gene (proto-oncogene) into an oncogene that leads to the production of oncoproteins?
A) A mutation in *BRCA1* that disrupts homologous recombination
B) A mutation in *TP53* that prevents phosphorylation of p53 in response to DNA damage
C) A mutation in *NF-1* that prevents activated RAS protein from being turned off
D) A point mutation in *ERBB2* that allows the protein product to signal in absence of ligand
E) A microdeletion in *RB1* that results in loss of control of the G_1 checkpoint

47. A mutation in a gene coding for a specific type of RNA molecule from which class of eukaryotic RNAs could potentially cause amino acid misincorporations in a wide variety of proteins?
A) Small interfering RNA (siRNA)
B) mRNA
C) Micro RNA (miRNA)
D) snRNA
E) tRNA

48. During protein synthesis, the energy for peptide bond formation comes from which of the following chemical bond reaction?
A) The ester bond joining the amino acid and the terminal ribose of tRNA
B) The phosphoanhydride bond of adenosine triphosphate (ATP), hydrolyzed by the catalytic rRNA.
C) The phosphoanhydride bond of guanosine triphosphate (GTP), hydrolyzed by an elongation factor
D) The phosphoanhydride bond of GTP, hydrolyzed by an initiation factor
E) The phosphoanhydride bond of GTP, hydrolyzed by a release factor

49. A mutation resulting in a nucleotide substitution was observed within the open reading frame of a gene. When the protein produced from this gene was analyzed, it was found that no changes in amino acid sequence were present. Which of the following characteristics of the genetic code accounts for these observations?
A) Nonoverlapping
B) Not punctuated
C) Degenerate
D) Triplet code
E) Universal

50. Cycloheximide causes a significant disruption of which of the following processes of eukaryotic protein synthesis?
A) Blocks the initiation of protein synthesis.
B) Causes premature chain termination.
C) Inhibits peptidyl transferase activity of 60S ribosome.
D) Inhibits release of polypeptide.
E) Inhibits binding of aminoacyl transfer RNA.

51. A 65-year-old woman presents to her physician complaining of fatigue, lack of energy, and weight loss. Physical exam reveals splenomegaly, and laboratory tests indicate an elevation in white blood cell count. Bone marrow analysis reveals the presence of a shortened version of chromosome 22 caused by a reciprocal translocation of DNA between chromosomes 9 and 22. Which of the listed drugs is a suitable first-line therapeutic agent to treat this patient's condition?
A) Trastuzumab (Herceptin)
B) Imatinib (Gleevec)
C) Cetuximab (Erbitux)
D) Infliximab (Remicade)
E) Basiliximab (Simulect)

52. Six weeks after possible exposure to the human immunodeficiency virus (HIV), a 28-year-old man visits his doctor to request an HIV test. Blood was drawn, and an enzyme-linked immunosorbent assay (ELISA) for specific HIV antigens was positive. What additional antigen-antibody test must be performed to rule out the possibility that the ELISA result was a false-positive?
A) Southern blot
B) Western blot
C) DNA microarray
D) Fluorescence in situ hybridization (FISH)
E) Northern blot

53. The antineoplastic drug 5-fluorouracil (5-FU) can be metabolized in cells to 5-fluorouridine triphosphate (5-FUTP), whose structure is shown below. Which of the following enzymes would use 5-FUTP as a substrate?

A) DNA polymerase
B) Protein kinase
C) Ribosome (peptidyl transferase activity)
D) RNA polymerase
E) Telomerase

54. Which among the following is correct regarding the process of DNA synthesis?
A) DNA synthesis is bidirectional.
B) DNA primase is required only for the initiation of new DNA synthesis at origins of replication but not for ongoing DNA synthesis.
C) Single-stranded DNA-binding (SSB) proteins are helix stabilizing proteins.
D) DNA synthesis requires strand separation by topoisomerase.
E) The parental DNA molecule is conserved in one of the daughter cells.

55. The monoclonal antibody cetuximab has shown activity against colorectal cancers. A 2010 study showed that administration of cetuximab to patients with advanced colorectal cancer resulted in a significant improvement in overall survival and in progression-free survival. For this study, the clinical scientist specifically chose patients who may benefit from cetuximab treatment based on detectable amounts of a specific protein that shows up on immunohistochemical analysis of a patient's cancer.[3] This protein is:
A) Retinoblastoma (RB)
B) BCR-ABL
C) Epidermal growth factor (EGF) receptor
D) p53
E) Neurofibromatosis type 1 (NF-1)

56. Following a day spent at the beach, which of the following types of DNA damage would most commonly be found in melanocytes within the basal layer of the epidermis?
A) Apurinic sites caused by depurination
B) Intrastrand cross-links
C) Double-strand breaks
D) Pyrimidine dimers
E) Nucleotide alkylation

57. A psuedouridine loop is found in the product of which of the following enzymes?
A) RNA polymerase I
B) RNA polymerase II
C) RNA polymerase III
D) DNA polymerase α
E) DNA polymerase δ

58. The overexpression of BCL-2 observed in certain types of B cell lymphoma serves as one of the first and strongest forms of evidence that failure of cell death contributes to cancer. Tumors expressing high levels of BCL-2 (and other antiapoptotic family members) are frequently found to be resistant to radiation therapy and chemotherapeutic agents. Early advances in BCL-2 targeted therapy involved the use of antisense technology that aimed at inhibiting BCL-2 expression. One promising antisense oligonucleotide was G3139 (oblimersen). Which experimental result would provide evidence that G3139 is effective at overcoming the antiapoptotic effects of elevated BCL-2 in B cell lymphoma?
A) Organization of the cytoskeleton remains unchanged
B) decrease in the cleaved form of caspase-3
C) An increase in the cleaved form of caspase-9
D) An increase in BCL-2 mRNA
E) An increase in the number of cells that swell and burst

59. Lentiviral particles such as the human immunodeficiency virus (HIV) contain an RNA genome. Upon infection, the RNA is converted into double-stranded DNA, which integrates into the host cell's genome. Which of the following enzymes is responsible for the conversion of the RNA genome into DNA?
A) DNA polymerase δ
B) Poly(A) polymerase
C) Reverse transcriptase
D) RNA polymerase II
E) Telomerase

60. An investigator is comparing the properties of the eukaryotic 80S and prokaryotic 70S ribosomes. However, during the preparation of ribosomal samples, he neglects to label the tubes. He suspects the tube labeled A contains the 80S ribosomes. Which antibiotic would inhibit protein synthesis in tube A and thus unambiguously identify it as the tube containing 80S ribosomes?
A) Chloramphenicol
B) Cycloheximide
C) Erythromycin
D) Puromycin
E) Tetracycline

61. Which type of mutation in a codon would lead to recruitment of release factor to the ribosome when the codon is present in the A site?
A) Transversion
B) Transition
C) Missense
D) Nonsense
E) Thymidine dimer

62. One treatment modality for the treatment of tularemia is the antibiotic chloramphenicol in combination with one other antibiotic that inhibits a different phase of protein translation. Which of the following drugs would be the appropriate choice to pair with chloramphenicol?
A) Erythromycin
B) Puromycin
C) Tetracycline
D) Streptomycin
E) Cycloheximide

63. Actinomycin D, a chemotherapy medication used to treat a number of types of cancer including Wilms tumor, acts by inhibiting:
A) DNA polymerase alpha
B) RNA polymerase I
C) Type I Topoisomerase
D) Peptidyl transferase
E) Reverse transcriptase

64. A 29-year-old woman presents at the clinic with a chief complaint of joint pain of 8 weeks' duration. She also reports loss of appetite, fatigue, and general malaise of similar duration. More recently, she noted her hair was thinning in places, which spurred her to visit the doctor. Upon physical examination, you observe several red, scaly, disc-shaped lesions on her scalp and face, indicative of systemic lupus erythematosus (SLE). You order blood work and suspect the test may find autoantibodies directed against components of the cellular machinery responsible for:
A) DNA synthesis
B) RNA splicing
C) Protein synthesis
D) RNA synthesis
E) DNA recombination

65. Poly ADP-ribose polymerase (PARP-1) is a nuclear enzyme found in eukaryotes. It has a high affinity for single stranded DNA breaks. Upon binding to DNA strand breaks PARP-1

builds a branched polymer of ADP-ribose on itself which recruits:
A) DNA glycosylase
B) AP endonuclaease
C) DNA polymerase β
D) DNA polymersase I
E) DNA polymerase ξ

66. A recent development in gene therapy is the ability to precisely edit specific target genes in order to either disable or correct a mutant gene. One such tool is CRISPR (clustered regularly interspaced short palindromic repeat sequences), which is constructed using a guide RNA attached to the:
A) Telomerase
B) Cas 9 nuclease
C) Zn finger nuclease
D) Reverse transcriptase
E) RNA polymerase I

Answers and Explanations: Genetics and Cell Cycle

1. B Deamination of cytosine converts the base to a uracil. Uracil will be replaced by thymidine either by repair mechanisms or during the next round of DNA replication.

A Spontaneous conversion of deoxribose to ribose is not a common reaction and could not, in any case, account for the mutation listed in the question.

C Hydrolysis of the *N*-glycosidic bond of a purine/pyrimidine does occur in cells, resulting in abasic sites in the DNA that must be repaired by the base excision repair pathway. However, this process cannot explain the C to T mutation.

D Hydrolysis of a phosphodiester bond would result in a single-stranded break in the DNA backbone. It is highly unlikely that this would produce a nucleotide base change.

E Methylation of cytosine does not alter its base pairing and is not mutagenic.

2. A The relatively high percentage of positively charged lysine and arginine residues in histones facilitates wrapping of the negatively charged DNA molecule around the surface of the nucleosome.

B Posttranslational modification of N-terminal tails in histones influences the structure of chromatin and the accessibility of DNA. However, these modifications are not necessary for chromatin to form.

C Although nucleosomes do consist of two copies each of histone H2A, H2B, H3, and H4. However, this fact contributes only to the content of DNA per nucleosome (147 bp) and not to chromatin formation itself.

D It is true that the wrapping of DNA around nucleosome particles induces negative supercoils in the DNA molecule. However, this is an effect and not the cause.

E While it is true that the histones form ionic bonds with DNA and have no sequence specificity, histones are basic proteins with positively charged tails which interact with negatively charged sugar-phosphate backbone of DNA.

3. C (A) During semiconservative replication, the parental DNA molecule is unwound (by the helicase enzyme), and the two single strands serve as templates for synthesis of new DNA. After synthesis is complete, each of the two resulting DNA molecules contain one parental strand and one newly synthesized strand; that is, the parental strand is "semiconserved" in the product.

B DNA synthesis on leading and lagging strands is evidence of simultaneous replication of both parental strands.

D DNA synthesis is bidirectonal, proceeding in both directions from the origin of replication. However, this does not account for the semiconservative nature of DNA synthesis.

E DNA synthesis in eukaryotes requires the activity of more than one DNA polymerase enzyme. However, this does not account for the semiconservative nature of DNA synthesis.

4. A RNA synthesis proceeds in the $5' \rightarrow 3'$ direction. Therefore, the template strand is "read" by the RNA polymerase enzyme in the $3' \rightarrow 5'$ direction, with the resulting RNA complementary to the DNA template.

B This sequence is identical (except for the substitution of uracil for thymidine) to the template strand. RNA synthesized from the DNA template strand will be complementary; that is, the nucleotides in the RNA will base pair with the DNA template and have the opposite $5' \rightarrow 3'$ orientation

C This sequence is reversed but not complementary to the DNA (and has a substitution of uracil for thymidine). RNA synthesized from the DNA template strand will be complementary; that is, the nucleotides in the RNA will base pair with the DNA template and have the opposite $5' \rightarrow 3'$ orientation

D This sequence is not complementary to the template strand; its $5' \rightarrow 3'$ orientation will not allow it to base pair with the template strand.

E This sequence is reversed but not complementary to the template DNA (and has no substitution of uracil for thymidine). RNA synthesized from the DNA template strand will be complementary; that is, the nucleotides in the RNA will base pair with the DNA template and have the opposite $5' \rightarrow 3'$ orientation

5. A The activated form of cytarabine competes with the normal, cellular substrate deoxycytidine 5'-triphosphate (dCTP), inhibiting the activity of DNA polymerases, including DNA polymerase δ. Inhibition of DNA synthesis is lethal to actively dividing cells.

B DNA primase, part of the DNA polymerase α -DNA primase complex, synthesizes short RNA primers to initiate DNA replication. Primase uses ribonucleoside triphosphates as substrate. The metabolite of cytarabine shown in the question has a hydrogen at the 2' position, making this an isomer of a deoxyribonucleoside triphosphate, a substrate for DNA polymerases.

C Ribosomes polymerize amino acids, synthesizing proteins from an mRNA template. Aminoacyl-tRNAs are the substrate for protein synthesis by ribosomes. Aminoacyl-tRNAs do not resemble the metabolite of cytarabine shown in the question.

V

D RNA polymerase II polymerizes ribonucleotide triphosphates to make mRNAs. The metabolite of cytarabine shown in the question has a hydrogen at the 2′ position, making this an isomer of a ribonucleoside triphosphate, a substrate for DNA polymerases but not RNA polymerases.

E Helicase unwinds the DNA double helix to provide access to single-stranded DNA template by the DNA polymerases. Helicase consumes adenosine triphosphate (ATP) as a source of energy during the DNA unwinding. The metabolite of cytarabine shown in the question contains arabinose rather than ribose and has a hydrogen at the 2′ position, and the base is cytosine, which are major structural differences with ATP.

6. D DNA polymerase δ has 3′ → 5′ exonuclease (proofreading) activity that allows the enzyme to backtrack and remove a misincorporated nucleotide and insert the correct nucleotide.

A DNA ligase is important for several DNA repair pathways that operate to remove mutations that arise via multiple mechanisms. However, the vast majority of nucleotide misincorporations are repaired during the DNA synthesis process by the proofreading activity of DNA polymerases δ and ε.

B DNA helicase unwinds the DNA double helix during DNA replication. It is also involved in several DNA repair pathways that operate to remove mutations that arise via multiple mechanisms. However, the vast majority of nucleotide misincorporations are repaired during the DNA synthesis process by the proofreading activity of DNA polymerases δ and ε.

C DNA topoisomerase removes supercoils generated ahead of the replication fork, the result of the unwinding of the DNA double helix during DNA replication. It is not specifically involved in the repair of nucleotide misincorporation during DNA synthesis.

E DNA polymerase α, along with the primase enzymes, synthesizes short primers that are elongated by DNA polymerases δ and ε during DNA synthesis. It is not specifically involved in the repair of nucleotides misincorporated during DNA synthesis.

7. C A silencer element reduces or completely suppresses transcription of associated genes when it is bound by specific, repressive transcription factors. A mutation in a silencer element that prevents its interaction with a repressive factor would result in higher than normal transcription of the associated gene. Because many enhancers and transcriptional activator proteins oppose the actions of silencers, the observation that PEPCK-C transcription was only increased slightly by glucocorticoids is consistent with a mutation in a silencer element.

A Because the mutation did not reduce transcription of the PEPCK-C gene, the core promoter elements must be functioning normally. As such, the mutation cannot be in the core promoter sequences.

B Activation of transcription by glucocorticoids is mediated by binding of the hormone-glucocorticoid receptor (GR) complex to a specific nucleotide sequence (the glucocorticoid response element; GRE) that is present in enhancers associated with genes regulated by these hormones. A mutation in the GRE sequence would result in loss of inducibility by glucocorticoids but would not result in consistently elevated levels of PEPCK-C transcription.

D The transcriptional start site is the nucleotide position of a gene where the RNA polymerase initiates polymerization of mRNA. The transcriptional start site is not a specific, conserved nucleotide sequence. Rather, it is determined primarily by the location of core promoter elements (e.g., the TATA box). A nucleotide substitution at the transcriptional start site would likely have no stimulatory effect on the efficiency of transcription.

E Transcription is terminated when is an essential step in at sites located downstream of the polyadenylation signal sequence (AAUAAA). Following cleavage, 80 to 250 adenylate residues are added in a tepmplate-independent fashion to the end of the mRNA by Poly(A) polymerase. A mutation in this sequence would likely decrease the stability of the transcript but would not affect the rate of transcription.

8. C Binding of p16 to CDK4 and CDK6 prevents them from associating with cyclin D. Without active cyclin D-CDK4/6 complexes, cells cannot pass the restriction point in late G_1.

A. Binding of p16 to CDK4 and CDK6 prevents (not promotes) the associations between CDK4/6 and cyclin D.

B Binding of p16 to CDK4 and CDK6 (which prevents associations between CDK4/6 and cyclin D) blocks the hyperphosphorylation of RB (by cyclin D-CDK4/6) and thus prevents the release of E2F from RB.

D Binding of p16 to CDK4 and CDK6 (which prevents associations between CDK4/6 and cyclin D) blocks the hyperphosphorylation of RB (by cyclin D-CDK4/6).

E p16 specifically inhibits the G1 CDKs (4 and 6) and does not affect S phase cyclin CDK activities.

9. C Rifampicin inhibits the initiation of RNA synthesis by RNA polymerase holoenzyme in bacteria.

A Chloramphenicol is a broad-spectrum antibiotic that inhibits protein synthesis at the elongation phase by inhibiting peptidyl transferase activity of the bacterial ribosome.

B Tetracyclines bind to the small 30S subunit of bacterial ribosomes and inhibit translational elongation.

D Acyclovir is an inhibitor of viral DNA replication; it is not active against bacteria.

E Amoxicillin is a β-lactam antibiotic that inhibits bacterial cell wall synthesis by blocking the cross-linking of peptidoglycan polymers.

10. B (A, C, D, E) Type II Topoisomerase breaks the phosphodiester bonds between nucleotides (creates nicks) on both strands. It allows another part of the dsDNA to pass through the break and then reseals the break. Ciprofloxacin is an inhibitor of bacterial Type II topoisomerase (DNA gyrase). It has no direct effect on other enzymes of prokaryotic DNA replication.

11. D Release of cytochrome c from mitochondria is is an essential step in the intrinsic pathway of apoptosis.

A Activation of caspase 8 is characteristic of the extrinsic pathway of apoptosis.

B Cleavage of BID to tBID is catalyzed by caspase 8 (extrinsic pathway) .

C Recruitment of procaspase 8 by FADD is characteristic of the extrinsic pathway of apoptosis.

E Extrinsic pathway is also known as the death receptor pathway and is triggered by binding and activation of an external ligand to its receptor on plasma membrane.

12. A Mutations in proto-oncogenes, that change the structure of the gene's protein product, or increase the level of the normal protein product contribute to the development of cancer.

B Mutations in the genes for tumor suppressors (not proto-oncogenes) may disrupt the encoded protein's ability to repair damaged DNA.

C Mutations in genes for tumor suppressors (not oncogenes) may disrupt the encoded protein's ability to regulate the cell cycle.

D Mutations in proto-oncogenes are associated with an increase (not a reduction) in the amount and/or activity of the gene's protein product.

E Mutations in genes for tumor suppressors (not oncogenes) may disrupt the protein product's ability to promote apoptosis.

13. E This sequence has the greatest number of G:C base pairs (seven total). G:C base pairs are held together by three hydrogen bonds, compared with two hydrogen bonds for A:T base pairs, and therefore require more energy (heat) to denature. The higher the GC content, the higher the T_m, the temperature at which ½ of the helical structure is lost.

A Of the sequences listed, this sequence does not have the greatest number of G:C base pairs and therefore does not have the greatest thermal stability. G:C base pairs are held together by three hydrogen bonds, compared with two hydrogen bonds for A:T base pairs, and therefore require more energy (heat) to denature.

B Of the sequences listed, this sequence does not have the greatest number of G:C base pairs and therefore does not have the greatest thermal stability. G:C base pairs are held together by three hydrogen bonds, compared with two hydrogen bonds for A:T base pairs, and therefore require more energy (heat) to denature.

C Of the sequences listed, this sequence does not have the greatest number of G:C base pairs and therefore does not have the greatest thermal stability. G:C base pairs are held together by three hydrogen bonds, compared with two hydrogen bonds for A:T base pairs, and therefore require more energy (heat) to denature.

D Of the sequences listed, this sequence does not have the greatest number of G:C base pairs and therefore does not have the greatest thermal stability. G:C base pairs are held together by three hydrogen bonds, compared with two hydrogen bonds for A:T base pairs, and therefore require more energy (heat) to denature.

14. E Histones are rich in the basic amino acids arginine and lysine. Acetylation occurs only on the positively charged ε-amino groups of lysine residues. This neutralizes the basic charge and reduces the affinity of DNA for nucleosomes, making it more accessible to the transcriptional machinery. Arginine has a positive charge and is an important constituent of histones. However, it is not subject to acetylation. Treating cells with Vlaproic acid will likely alter the charge of lysine in histones.

A Streptomycin is an antibiotic and acts by inhibiting translation in bacteria.

B Doxorubicin is a chemotherapeutic drug and is an inhibitor of topoisomerase.

C Didanosine (2′,3′-dideoxyinosine) used in antiretroviral therapy for HIV infections is an inhibitor of reverse transcriptase.

D Rifampicin, an antibiotic commonly used to treat infections by Mycobacterium tuberculosis, is an inhibitor of RNA polymerase.

15. B The enzyme GlcNAc phosphotransferase phosphorylates terminal mannoses on asparagine-linked oligosaccharide chains. Cells from a patient that cannot produce the enzyme GlcNAc phosphotransferase would be unable to transport newly synthesized glycoproteins to lysosomes. Proteins destined for lysosomes are processed by the endoplasmic reticulum (ER) and Golgi such that they contain one or more phosphorylated mannose residues. Defects in GlcNAc phosphotransferase cause I cell disease.

A The presence of phosphorylated mannose residues on proteins does not play a role in directing them for secretion. Instead, proteins destined for secretion may be processed via standard or signal-regulated pathways and secreted constitutively or in a regulated manner with the aid of a tryptophan-rich domain and the absence of retention motifs.

C The presence of phosphorylated mannose residues on proteins does not play a role in directing them to plasma membranes. Instead, proteins destined for plasma membranes remain embedded in the outer layer of the ER. This is aided by the presence of an apolar region in the N-terminus of the polypeptide that serves as a stop translation sequence.

D The presence of phosphorylated mannose residues on proteins does not play a role in directing them to mitochondria. Instead, proteins destined for mitochondria contain an *N*-terminal hydrophobic α-helix that interacts with specific auxiliary proteins (chaperones) from the heat shock protein family (e.g., HSP70).

E Proteins destined for the nucleus contain a KKKRK signal sequence and are typically not glycosylated.

16. D The Philadelphia chromosome (der (22)) results from the reciprocal translocation of the abl proto-oncogene from chromosome 9 to chromosome 22 and the BCR region of chromosome 22 to 9. This translocation creates a BCR-ABL fusion gene (and an unregulated tyrosine kinase protein product) and is associated with chronic myelogenous leukemia (CML).

A The Philadelphia chromosome does not involve the RAS G protein. Mutations in the RAS G protein involve point mutations (not translocations).

B The Philadelphia chromosome does not involve HER2. HER2 is overexpressed in many breast cancers.

C The Philadelphia chromosome does not involve c-MYC. c-MYC is overexpressed in Burkitt's lymphoma due to a translocation between chromosomes 8 and 14.

E The Philadelphia chromosome does not involve n-MYC. Elevated levels of N-MYC transcription factor are observed in neuroblastoma.

17. B One GTP molecule is hydrolyzed by the G protein elongation factor-1 (EF-1 in eukaryotes) when an amino acyl tRNA is inserted into the A site. A second is expended during the translocation of ribosome to the next codon.

A The energy for peptide bond formation comes from an ATP consumed during charging of the tRNA by aminoacyl tRNA synthetases. The energy from that ATP is stored in the bond between the amino acid and the tRNA.

V

C The binding of the eIF4F (CAP binding complex) to the 7-methyl-guanosine cap of mRNA occurs at the initiation of mRNA translation and does not consume GTP.

D The assembly of the small and large ribosomal subunits on the mRNA occurs during the initiation of translation.

18. D Codons and anticodons pair in an antiparallel manner. If the mRNA has the sequence 5'-GCG ACG UCC-3', the first aminoacyl-tRNA anticodon would have the sequence 5'-CGC-3', to base pair with the mRNA. The second aminoacyl-tRNA anticodon would be 5'-CGU-3'; the third anti-codon would be 5'-GGA-3'.

A Codons and anticodons pair in an antiparallel manner. This sequence is not complementary to the mRNA; that is, it cannot base pair in an anti-parallel fashion with the mRNA.

B Codons and anticodons pair in an antiparallel manner. This sequence is not complementary to the mRNA; that is, it cannot base pair in an anti-parallel fashion with the mRNA.

C Codons and anticodons pair in an antiparallel manner. This sequence is not complementary to the mRNA; that is, it cannot base pair in an anti-parallel fashion with the mRNA.

E Codons and anticodons pair in an antiparallel manner. This sequence is not complementary to the mRNA; that is, it cannot base pair in an anti-parallel fashion with the mRNA.

19. A Erythromycin and clindamycin inhibit prokaryotic protein synthesis at the elongation phase by binding to the nascent peptide exit tunnel in the 50S subunit. In doing so, they cause context-specific arrest of peptidyl transferase and early release of peptidyl-tRNAs. Thus they block the synthesis of a subset of proteins rather than act as inhibitors of global protein synthesis.

B Tetracyline is a broad-spectrum antibiotic that binds the 30S ribosomal subunit in bacteria and impedes access to the acceptor (A) site by amino acyl-tRNAs.

C Aminoglycoside antibiotics such as streptomycin and gentamycin distort prokaryotic ribosome assembly and cause misreading of mRNA codon in the A site. In addition to causing the misreading of mRNA codons, aminoglycoside antibiotics may also block the translocation of the 70S ribosome.

D Chloramphenicol binds the bacterial 50S ribosomal subunit and inhibits peptidyl transferase activity. It does not inhibit eukaryotic ribosomes. However, at high (toxic) doses, it can inhibit mitochondrial protein synthesis. This can lead to severe toxicity in individuals who lack the ability to metabolize chloramphenicol (e.g., neonates).

E Puromycin acts upon both eukaryotic and prokaryotic peptidyl transferases, releasing small peptides ending in puromycin at their C-terminal ends.

20. B Because a genomic DNA insert will inactivate the tetracycline resistance gene, the transformants must be grown on ampicillin. This will select against any bacterial cells that were not transformed by a plasmid.

A The absence of any antibiotic in the growth media would allow transformed (contains plasmid) and untransformed (lacks plasmid) to grow.

C Ligation of the inserts into the tetracycline resistance gene inactivates its ability to confer tetracycline resistance to transformed bacteria. Therefore, only bacteria transformed with an empty plasmid (no insert) will grow in media containing tetracycline.

D Ligation of inserts into the tetracycline resistance gene inactivates its ability to confer tetracycline resistance to transformed bacteria. Although the transformed bacteria are resistant to ampicillin, they (and the untransformed bacteria) will not grow on a plate containing tetracycline.

21. A Release factors interact with peptidyl transferase, allowing it to transfer the nascent polypeptide chain to water instead of to the α amino group of an incoming aminoacyl tRNA.

B eIF4F is the complex that binds the 7-methyl guanosine cap of mRNA to seed the formation of the preinitiation complex in eukaryotes.

C Formyl-methionine is charged to the initiator tRNA in prokaryotes. It is the first amino acid of all proteins made in prokaryotes, but it does not participate in any way with termination.

D UDP-GlcNAc is the substrate for the initial step of N-linked glycosylation of proteins following their synthesis. It does not participate in translational termination.

E The E (or exit) site is the position on the ribosome where the spent tRNA in the P site is transferred to during ribosomal translocation.

22. D N-linked glycosylation of asparagine residues is via an acid amide ($CONH_2$) functional group.

A N-linked glycosylation occurs on asparagine residues. Phosphorylation is limited to serine, threonine, and tyrosine residues.

B Tunicamycin inhibits N-linked glycosylation at the first step of core oligosaccharide synthesis (the transfer of phosphorylated N-acetyl-D-glucosamine [GlcNAc-P] from UDP-GlcNAc to dolichol phosphate).

C O-linked glycosylation is via a hydroxyl functional group, on either serine or threonine amino acids.

E Dolichol phosphate is required for the initial N-linked glycosylation of asparagine on the target protein.

23. **B** (A, C, D, E) Erwin Chargaff's rule of base composition aided in elucidation of the DNA structure. %A = %T and %G = %C; A + T + C + G = 100% or (%A + %G) = (%T + %C); total purines=total pyrimidines. If we know the percentage of even one of the nucleotides, we can determine that of all the others. In the above case %C = 23%; %G = 23%; (A + T) + (G + C) = 100; (A + T) + (23 + 23) = 100; (A + T) + 46 + 100; A + T = 54; %A = 27.

24. C Euchromatin is a relatively open chromatin conformation present during the interphase; appear as light stained areas after Giemsa staining; transcriptionally active (genes are expressed); associated with histone acetylation activity.

A, B, D, E Heterochromatin is condensed chromatin conformation present during interphase; appear as intensely dark stained areas after Giemsa staining; transcriptionally inactive (genes are silent); associated with histone deacetylation activity; during interphase usually localized near nuclear periphery.

25. C (A, E) Homologous recombination repair DNA repair pathway is impaired when mutations render BRCA1 dysfunctional. *BRCA1* codes for a protein involved in the homologous recombination repair pathway. This pathway is particularly important in repairing double-stranded breaks in the DNA without errors. Ionizing radiation, such as X-rays, are capable of producing double-stranded breaks (among other types of damage).

B Xeroderma pigmentosum is associated with defects in nucleotide excision DNA repair mechanism.

D Hereditary Nonpolyposis Colon Cancer (HNPCC) is associated with defect in mismatch DNA repair mechanism.

26. E Diphtheria toxin catalyzes the covalent attachment of ADP to the catalytic unit of eEF-2, irreversibly inactivating it. Translocation, and therefore elongation, is blocked in eukaryotic cells.

A Diphtheria toxin does not affect initiation factor.

B Diphtheria toxin does not affect sigma factor.

C Diphtheria toxin does not affect release factor.

D Diphtheria toxin does not affect Rho factor

27. C Tetracyclclines bind to the small 30S subunit of bacteria, blocking access of aminoacyl-tRNAs to the A site. An alteration in ribosome structure, perhaps affecting the A site, could potentially disrupt the binding of tetracycline to the ribosome, generating a resistant phenotype.

A The 30S preinitiation complex consists of initiation factors, the 30S ribosomal subunit, and fMet-tRNA$_i^{Met}$ and the mRNA. Tetracycline does not affect the formation of this complex and therefore is unlikely to be altered in a tetracycline-resistant strain of bacteria.

B Once the preinitiation complex is formed, the 50S ribosomal subunit joins to create the initiation complex. Tetracycline does not affect the formation of this complex and therefore is unlikely to be altered in a tetracycline-resistant strain of bacteria. Linezolid, which belongs to the oxazolidinone class of antibiotics, inhibits the initiation of protein synthesis in prokaryotes by preventing the formation of 70S ribosomal complex.

D Formation of a peptide bond between the aminoacyl-tRNA in the A site and the peptidyl-tRNA in the P site is catalyzed by a ribozyme that has peptidyl transferase activity and is located in the large ribosomal subunit. Tetracycline does not affect this activity and therefore is unlikely to be altered in a tetracycline-resistant strain of bacteria. Chloramphenicol, however, is an antibiotic that inhibits peptidyl transferase.

E Once a peptide bond is formed, the hydrolysis of one GTP by an elongation factor is associated with translocation of the ribosome, one codon down the mRNA. Tetracycline does not affect this activity and therefore is unlikely to be altered in a tetracycline-resistant strain of bacteria. Aminoglycoside antibiotics (e.g., streptomycin, gentamycin), which cause misreading of mRNA codons in the A site, may also block the translocation of the 70S ribosome

28. C Huntington disease is associated with the presence of a variable number of tandem repeats (VNTR) regions in which the sequence CAG is found repeated between 36 and 100 times. Huntington diesease is marked by CAG repeats in the coding sequence of the gene that encodes huntingtin protein. As CAG codes for Gln (Q), this disease is characterized as a PolyQ disease.

A Fragile X syndrome is marked by CGG repeat in the X linked gene that encodes for fragile X mental retardation protein (FMR1).

B Myotonic dystrophy (DM1) is marked by CTG repeats in the gene that encodes for dystrophia myotonica protein kinase (DMPK).

D Friedreich ataxia is marked by GAA repeats in the gene for the mitochondrial protein, frataxin.

E Myotonic dystrophy 2 (DM2) is associated with tetranucleotide repeat expansion of CCTG.

29. A The fetus does not carry the *ΔF508* mutant allele for CF.

B The fetus does not carry the *ΔF508* mutant allele for CF. Its mother is heterozygous.

C The fetus is not heterozygous for the *ΔF508* mutant allele. Its father is heterozygous.

D The fetus is not homozygous for the *ΔF508* mutant allele. It is homozygous for the normal allele.

E The fetus does not carry the *ΔF508* mutant allele for CF. Its brother is homozygous for the *ΔF508* mutant allele.

30. D The difference in genomic GC content between *F. philomiragia* and *B. mallei* is the largest of the pairings provided. The temperature at which the strands of the DNA double helix of the *F. philomiragia* genome separates would be much lower than the temperature at which the genomic DNA of *B. mallei* denatures.

A The GC-content and hence the thermal stability of these two organisms are very close, which would make exploiting the small difference difficult if not impossible.

B Although there is a modest difference in GC content in the genomes of these two organisms, it is not the most significant of the pairings provided. The relative similarity in GC content and hence thermal stability of these two organisms would make exploiting differences in thermal stability difficult.

C Although there is a modest difference in GC content in the genomes of these two organisms, it is not the most significant of the pairings provided. The relative similarity in GC content and hence thermal stability of these two organisms would make exploiting differences in thermal stability difficult.

E The GC content and hence the thermal stability of these two organisms are very close, which would make exploiting the small difference difficult if not impossible.

31. B The woman has a mutation in one of the genes necessary for mismatch excision repair (MER), resulting in hereditary nonpolyposis colorectal cancer. The familial history of colon cancer and the early onset of her disease are consistent with her diagnosis. The absence of MER results in the inability to repair nucleotide misincorporations that are not fixed during replication by the proofreading activity of DNA polymerase δ.

A Genetic defects in homologous recombination repair (BRCA1/2 mutations, Fanconi's anemia) are typically not associated with hereditary colon cancer. Given the patient's family history, it is unlikely that this pathway would be affected.

C Genetic defects in nonhomologous end-joining repair are associated with severe, early-onset phenotypes (e.g., severe combined immunodeficiencies) and are typically not associated with hereditary colon cancer. Given the patient's medical history and her family history, it is unlikely that this pathway would be affected.

D Genetic defects in NER pathways are associated with severe, early-onset phenotypes (e.g., xeroderma pigmentosum) and are typically not associated with hereditary colon cancer.

V

Given the patient's medical history and her family history, it is unlikely that this pathway would be affected.

E Genetic defects in transcription coupled repair pathways are associated with severe, early-onset phenotypes (e.g., tricothiodystrophy) and are typically not associated with hereditary colon cancer. Given the patient's medical history and her family history, it is unlikely that this pathway would be affected.

32. E (A, B, C, D) The BLM gene encodes a protein which is a member of the helicase family. The RecQ family of helicases are enzymes that unwind DNA so that replication, transcription, and DNA repair can occur. They are required for DNA replication, recombination, repair and important for genomic maintenance. Blooms Syndrome is due to the mutations in the BLM gene.

33. D This patient has retinoblastoma marked by tumors in the retina. Retinoblastoma is linked to "loss of function" mutations and deletions in the *RB1* gene.

A A "loss of function" mutation in the *TP53* gene is not linked to retinoblastoma (marked by tumors in the retina) but to Li-Fraumeni syndrome.

B A chromosomal translocation involving the *BCR* and *ABL* genes is linked to chronic myelogenous leukemia (CML), not retinoblastoma.

C A "gain of function" mutation in the *RAS* gene is not linked to retinoblastoma.

E A point mutation in the *N-MYC* gene is linked to neuroblastoma (not retinoblastoma).

34. A Inhibition of the activity of CDK2 would prevent cells from exiting the G_1 phase and entering the S phase.

B Because cyclin E/A-CDK2 complexes keep RB in the hyperphosphorylated state, this CDK2 inhibitory agent would do the opposite.

C p21 and p27 are natural inhibitors of CDK2 and are not noted as targets of the novel CDK2 inhibitor.

D This CDK2 inhibitor would promote the hypophosphorylated state of RB and thus decrease the transcription of cyclin E and cyclin A.

E The rate of degradation of cyclin D is not affected by the status of CDK2.

35. A Western blotting refers to a process by which proteins (immobilized on a membrane) are probed with antibodies.

B Southern blotting refers to a process by which DNA (immobilized on a membrane) is probed with a complementary DNA molecule.

C Northern blotting refers to a process by which RNA (immobilized on a membrane) is probed with a complementary DNA molecule.

D DNA microarray refers to a process by which DNA (immobilized on a solid support) is probed with genomic or complementary DNA (cDNA) molecules.

E SDS-PAGE (sodium dodecyl sulfate-polyacrylamide gel electrophoresis) separates the proteins on the basis of their molecular weights. The separated proteins are subsequently blotted on to a membrane and probed by hybridization with an antibody.

36. C (A, B, D, E) Fragile X syndrome is an X-linked disorder marked by CGG repeat in the 5′-UTR of the FMR1 gene. The mutation in the disease allows for the expansion of CGG repeats

(> 230) in the 5′-terminus of the FMR1 gene in subsequent generations. The consequence of the very large number of CGG repeats in the DNA is extensive methylation of the entire promoter region of the FMR1 gene. The CGG expansion creates a CpG island that is hypermethylated. This leads to silencing of the FMR1 gene.

37. B The boy has the genetic condition xeroderma pigmentosum due to a defect in nucleotide excision repair. The most common form of DNA damage resulting from sunlight exposure is the production of thymidine dimers. Nucleotide excision repair recognizes and removes bulky adducts that alter or distort the normal shape of DNA, which includes thymidine dimers.

A The boy has the genetic condition xeroderma pigmentosum due to a defect in nucleotide excision repair. Double strand breaks are often caused by ionizing radiation (e.g., X-rays) and involve repair mechanisms (nonhomologous end-joining and homologous recombination repair) distinct from nucleotide excision repair.

C The boy has the genetic condition xeroderma pigmentosum due to a defect in nucleotide excision repair. Chromosomal translocations are swapping of large DNA fragments between chromosomes, usually the result of significant double strand breaks that are repaired by nonhomologous end joining. Nucleotide excision repair does not influence this pathway.

D The boy has the genetic condition xeroderma pigmentosum due to a defect in nucleotide excision repair. Nucleotide deletions are primarily the result of errors in replication and are not repaired by nucleotide excision repair pathways.

E The boy has the genetic condition xeroderma pigmentosum due to a defect in nucleotide excision repair. Nucleotide substitutions are primarily the result of errors in replication and are not repaired by nucleotide excision repair pathways.

38. C Mutations in intron-exon boundaries that affect splicing tend to cause loss of exons in the transcribed mRNA. In this case, the loss of exon 2 leads to the production of GATA1 that lacks the transactivation domain.

A The 5′-UTR can contain sequences that influence translation efficiency. However, such a mutation is extremely unlikely to result in loss of an exon, as was observed in this case.

B The 3′-UTR can contain sequences that influence translation efficiency and mRNA stability, as well as the signal for termination and polyadenylation. However, it is essentially impossible that a mutation in this region would result in the loss of an exon.

D The promoter is required for gene transcription. Because the transcript was detected, the promoter is operating normally.

E Enhancers influence the activity of associated promoters to increase the transcription of genes. Because the transcript was detected, any enhancers must be operating normally.

39. A PIT1 gene activity is required for normal pituitary development. Enhancers are bound by transcription factors that activate transcription of an associated core promoter. One mechanism for achieving this is the recruitment of histone acetyltransferase (HAT) enzymes, which act as coactivator, by the enhancer-bound transcription factor. Because the histone acetylation levels were diminished in the patient, it is likely that the deletion was in an enhancer that resulted in the absence of HAT enzyme recruitment.

B Transcription is terminated when the mRNA transcript is cleaved at sites located downstream of the polyadenylation signal sequence (AATAAA). Following cleavage, 80 to 250 adenine nucleotides are added to the end of the mRNA by enzymes associated with the RNA polymerase II complex. A mutation in this sequence would not alter the acetylation of histones in the chromatin.

C Silencer elements are bound by transcription factors that repress transcription of an associated genes. One mechanism for achieving this is the recruitment of histone deacetylase (HDAC) enzymes by the silencer-bound transcription factor. The observation of diminished histone acetylation levels in the patient is the exact opposite of what would be predicted if the silencer element was mutated.

D A splice donor site is the sequence at exon-intron boundary. As such, these sequences have no influence on histone acetylation at the promoter of the gene.

E The transcriptional start site is the nucleotide position of a gene where the RNA polymerase initiates polymerization of mRNA. The transcriptional start site is not a specific, conserved nucleotide sequence, although most transcripts do initiate with a purine. Rather, it is determined primarily by the location of core promoter elements (e.g., the TATA box). A nucleotide substitution at the transcriptional start site would likely have no effect on histone acetylation.

40. A The estrogen receptor functions in a manner similar to the glucocorticoid receptor. It is a ligand-activated nuclear transcription factor that binds DNA. The estrogen receptor recruits coactivators with histone acetyltransferase (HAT) activity to the genes it activates. The HAT enzymes acetylate histones on chromatin, leading to a decompacted structure and subsequent transcription. The loss of estrogen delivery once she discontinues the patch will result in the loss of estrogen receptor binding and activity at these genes. Histone deacetylase enzymes will then remove the acetyl groups on modified histones at these genes, resulting in reduced transcription.

B Increased acetylation is associated with transcriptional activation by the ligand-bound estrogen receptor. Discontinuing the contraceptive estrogen patch will have the opposite effect, resulting in loss of histone acetylation.

C The estrogen receptor (ER) is a ligand-activated nuclear transcription factor that binds DNA, leading to histone acetylation at genes that it activates. Discontinuing the delivery of estrogen will lead to loss of ER binding at target genes and a reduction in histone acetylation.

D Histones within nucleosomes associated with genes activated by estrogen will always have elevated acetylation. As such, discontinuing the delivery of estrogen will lead to a reduction in histone acetylation.

E Discontinuing the contraceptive estrogen patch will result in loss of histone acetylation and a gain of positive charge.

41. B RNA polymerase II, which synthesizes precursor messenger RNA (mRNA), is inhibited by low-dose α-amanitin.

A TFIID binds to core promoter DNA sequences (e.g., TATA box) and promotes the formation of the transcriptional preinitiation complex. The activity of TFIID is not influenced by α-amanitin.

C RNA polymerase III synthesizes precursor tRNA, 5S RNA, and some small nuclear RNA (snRNA) genes. It is inhibited by high doses of α-amanitin, which is why the tRNA levels did not decrease in cells treated with low doses of this toxin.

D HATs are enzymes that acetylate specific lysine residues on nucleosomal histones. Their action "loosens" the structure of chromatin so that it is easily accessible by the transcriptional machinery structure to a protranscriptional state. HAT enzymes are not influenced by α-amanitin.

E Capping enzyme adds a 7-methylguanosine residue to the 5′ end of mRNAs. The activity of capping enzyme is not influenced by α-amanitin.

42. B A glycosidic bond forms the link between a base and the deoxyribose moiety in linking a deoxyribonucleotide.

A Electrostatic forces contribute to the final structure of the DNA double helix, but they are not involved in a base and the sugar.

C Hydrogen bonds that form between nucleotide bases on the two opposing strands of a double-stranded DNA hold the double helix together.

D Phosphodiester bonds link adjacent nucleotides in DNA and RNA.

E Van der Waals forces occur among nucleotide bases stacked within the double helical DNA molecule and contribute to the final structure of the helix.

43. C Cyclin dependent kinases (CDK4/6) are key targets for cancer chemotherapy. Studies show that oral administration of PD 0332991 to mice harboring human tumor xenografts resulted in a broad spectrum of anticancer activity and caused the regression of certain tumors. Inhibition of CDK4/6 by PD 0332991 inhibits the phosphorylation of RB in tumor cells. Consequently, E2F remains sequestered by RB and unable to promote the transcription of target genes.

A Treatment of tumor cells with PD 0332991 inhibits CDK4/6 and thus prevents the transcription of E2F target genes such as cyclin E and cyclin A. Without the aforementioned cyclins, the transition from the G_1 to the S phase will not occur.

B Inhibition of CDK4/6 by PD 0332991 would inhibit (not stimulate) the phosphorylation of RB.

D Inhibition of CDK4/6 by PD 0332991 would arrest the cells in G_1, not G_2.

E Because inhibition of CDK4/6 by PD 0332991 inhibits the phosphorylation of RB, hypophosphorylated RB would sequester (not release) E2F.

44. C For X-linked disorders, sons of heterozygous mothers (i.e., carriers) have a 50% chance of having the disorder.

A Only male children of female carriers are affected.

B All female children of an affected male are carriers.

D The genetic mutation can be passed on to a third generation because a second-generation female is a carrier, and her male offspring could be affected.

E X-linked traits are not passed from father to son.

45. B The transcription of p21 will be decreased when p53 is defective. When p53 retains its ability to become activated in response to DNA damage, it triggers the transcription of p21, which binds to and inactivates cyclin-CDK complexes (e.g., cyclin D-CDK2, cyclin E-CDK2). Inactivation of these complexes prevents the phosphorylation and inactivation of RB, thus allowing the hyperphosphorylated RB to sequester E2F. Sequestration of E2F prevents it from promoting the transcription of cyclins (cyclin A and cyclin E) that allow the cell cycle to transition through its various phases.

(p53 → p21 ⊣Cyclin D/E-CDK2 → RB (hyperphosphorylated) → E2F (release) → Cyclin A/E transcription → Cell cycle transition)

A Defective p53 would allow E2F to be released (not sequestered) by RB.

C Defective p53 would allow the cyclin A/E-CDK2 complexes to keep RB in a hyperphosphorylated (not hypophosphorylated) state

D Defective p53 would allow the transcription of cyclins A and E to increase, due to the release of E2F from RB.

E Defective p53 would allow the cells to transition through the cell cycle instead of cell cycle arrest.

46. D *ERBB2* is a proto-oncogene that encodes *HER2* (a member of the family of epidermal growth factor receptors). A point mutation in *ERBB2* that changes a valine to glutamine converts it into an oncogene whose oncoprotein product is Neu. The dimerization of tyrosine kinase activity of Neu is triggered in the absence of ligand.

A *BRCA1/BRCA2* are tumor suppressor genes, not proto-oncogenes.

B *p53* is a tumor suppressor gene, not a proto-oncogene.

C *NF-1* is a tumor suppressor gene, not a proto-oncogene.

E *RB1* is a tumor suppressor gene, not a proto-oncogene.

47. E tRNA "charging" is governed by "acceptor identity," which constitutes in essence a second genetic code. Specifically, the tRNA synthetase enzymes recognize both the amino acid and its cognate tRNA by sensing a particular three-dimensional conformation. As such, a mutation in a tRNA could potentially alter its structure such that the mutant tRNA is recognized by an incorrect tRNA synthetase that "charges" the mutant tRNA with the wrong amino acid.

A Small interfering RNA (siRNA) would bind to its target mRNA to inhibit its translation and increase its degradation. A mutation in a specific siRNA would not lead to amino acid misincorporations in a wide variety of proteins.

B A mutation in a specific mRNA coding for a specific protein would not lead to amino acid misincorporations in a wide variety of proteins.

C miRNAs influence the stability and translation efficiency of mRNAs. A mutation in a specific miRNA would not lead to amino acid misincorporations in a wide variety of proteins.

D snRNAs are a structural component of small nuclear ribonucleoproteins (snRNPs) that are involved in pre-mRNA splicing. A mutation in a specific snRNA would not lead to amino acid misincorporations in a wide variety of proteins.

48. A During the charging of tRNAs by aminoacyl tRNA synthetases, ATP is consumed to form an ester bond between the amino acid and the 3'-OH of the terminal adenosine of tRNA. The energy stored in this bond is then consumed to form a peptide bond during protein synthesis.

B The catalytic rRNA of the ribosome does not consume ATP directly. Rather, ATP is consumed to form an ester bond between the amino acid and the 3'-OH of the terminal adenosine of tRNA during tRNA charging. The energy stored in this bond is then consumed to form a peptide bond during protein synthesis.

C As is true for all G proteins, GTP hydrolyzed by elongation factors alters the conformation/function of the protein during ribosome translocation. It does not provide energy for peptide bond formation.

D As is true for all G proteins, GTP hydrolyzed by initiation factors alters the conformation/function of the protein during the formation of the initiation complex. It does not provide energy for peptide bond formation.

E As is true for all G proteins, GTP hydrolyzed by release factors alters the conformation/function of the protein during the termination of protein synthesis. It does not provide energy for peptide bond formation.

49. C The degenerate nature of the genetic code means that some amino acids are represented by multiple codons. For example, phenylalanine is coded for by TTT and TTC. If a mutation alters the third T in the codon to C, then no amino acid change would be observed. This is known as a silent mutation.

A The genetic code is nonoverlapping in the vast majority of genes, although there are a few exceptions, typically in viruses and prokaryotes. However, this would not explain why a nucleotide change in the gene could be silent with respect to the amino acid that is inserted into a protein.

B The genetic code is not punctuated, which means that there are no "extra" nucleotides between codons; they are read contiguously by the ribosome. However, this would not explain why a nucleotide change in the gene could be silent with respect to the amino acid that is inserted into a protein.

D The genetic code is a triplet code; each three nucleotides making up a codon represent a single amino acid. However, this would not explain why a nucleotide change in the gene could be silent with respect to the amino acid that is inserted into a protein.

E The genetic code is universal among species, with very few exceptions. However, this would not explain why a nucleotide change in the gene could be silent with respect to the amino acid that is inserted into a protein.

50. C Cycloheximide inhibits eukaryotic protein synthesis at the elongation phase through inhibition of peptidyl transferase.

A. Linezolid, which belongs to the oxazolidinone class of antibiotics, inhibits the initiation of protein synthesis in prokaryotes by preventing the formation of 70S ribosomal complex.

B. Puromycin structurally mimics an aminoacyl-tRNA and inhibits peptidyl transferase activity; it becomes incorporated into peptides being synthesized and serves as a chain terminator of the elongating peptide in both prokaryotes and eukaryotes. Although not used frequently in the clinic, it is effective against gram-negative bacteria.

C Amoxicillin is a β-lactam antibiotic that inhibits bacterial cell wall synthesis by blocking the cross-linking of peptidoglycan polymers.

D There are not many inhibitors of polypeptide release from the ribosome. Blasticidin S blocks such release in both prokaryotes and eukaryotes by interfering with the P-site tRNA.

E Tetracycline is a broad-spectrum antibiotic that binds the 30S ribosomal subunit and impedes access to the acceptor (A) site by aminoacyl-tRNAs. Tetracycline acts after the formation of the initiation complex.

51. B The patient has chronic myelogenous leukemia (CML), which is driven by the unregulated tyrosine kinase activity of the BCR-ABL protein product of the Philadelphia chromosome (der 22). Imatinib binds to the active site of the BCR-ABL tyrosine kinase and inhibits its activity.

A Trastuzumab targets the HER2 receptors, which are amplified in some breast cancers.

C Cetuximab targets the epidermal growth factor (EGF) receptor, which is overexpressed in colorectal cancer.

D Infliximab targets tumor necrosis factor-α (TNF-α) for the treatment of autoimmune diseases.

E Basiliximab targets the α chain of the interleukin-2 (IL-2) receptor and is administered to prevent the rejection of a transplanted kidney.

52. B The Western blot (immunoblot) is the gold standard for validation of HIV infection and is used to confirm the results of an ELISA. It allows for the detection of some circulating HIV proteins whose levels increase prior to the appearance of anti-HIV antibodies (which are detected in HIV ELISAs).

A Southern blot is a hybridization technique in which both the probe and target molecule are DNA.

C DNA microarray is a DNA/complementary DNA (cDNA)-based technique derived from Southern blotting. It is performed on gene chips that allow for variations in gene expression to be determined.

D FISH is a DNA/DNA-based technique derived from Southern blotting. It is used to determine the specific chromosomal location of particular genes.

E Northern blot is a hybridization technique in which the probe is single-stranded DNA, and the target molecule is mRNA.

53. D 5-FUTP is a ribonucleoside triphosphate and therefore can be incorporated into RNA by RNA polymerases.

A DNA polymerase enzymes use deoxyribonucleoside triphosphates as substrates to synthesize DNA in a template-directed manner. Although 5-FUTP cannot be used as a substrate by DNA polymerase, 5-FUDP can be further metabolized in the cell by ribonucleotide reductase to 5-fluorodeoxyuridine di-phospate (5-FdUDP), which, after conversion to 5-FdUTP, can be incorporated into DNA by DNA polymerase.

B Protein kinases catalyze the addition of phosphate onto serine, threonine, or tyrosine residues of target proteins. Adenosine triphosphate (ATP) (or guanosine triphosphate [GTP] for a few kinases) is the substrate for phosphate addition; these enzymes cannot use 5-FUTP.

C The energy for peptide bond formation comes from the ATP consumed by aminoacyl-transfer RNA (tRNA) synthetases during tRNA charging. 5-FUTP cannot be used in this reaction.

E Telomerase has DNA polymerase activity and uses deoxyribonucleoside triphosphates as substrates to synthesize DNA.

54. A DNA synthesis is bidirectional and is preceded by unwinding and separation of the two strands that form a replication bubble. As DNA strands replicate, the bubbles expand in both directions simultaneously, giving rise to the bidirectional nature of DNA replication.

B DNA polymerase can synthesize DNA only in a 5′ →' 3′ direction. On one strand of the DNA molecule (the lagging strand), the polymerase synthesizes a series of short DNA poly-

mers (Okazaki fragments) that each require a primer. Therefore, new primers synthesized by primase are required for ongoing DNA synthesis, not just when DNA synthesis initiates at origins of replication.

C Single-stranded DNA-binding (SSB) proteins are helix destabilizing proteins. They bind to single-stranded DNA and keep the 2 strands of DNA separated in the area of the replication origin preventing reformation of the double helix

D DNA synthesis does require strand separation by helicase enzymes.

E DNA synthesis is semiconservative; that is, the two daughter strands produced by DNA replication each contain one parental strand that served as the template for synthesis.

55. C Cetuximab is a monoclonal antibody that targets the EGF receptor. It is used in the treatment of colorectal cancer.

A The RB protein is not a target of cetuximab, and its mutated form is associated with retinoblastoma, not colorectal cancer.

B The oncoprotein BCR-ABL is associated with chronic myelogenous leukemia (CML), not colorectal cancer. Imatinib (Gleevec) not cetuximab, is the therapeutic agent used to target BCR-ABL.

D More than 50% of all human cancers harbor mutant p53. However, cetuximab does not specifically target p53.

E NF-1 is not a target of cetuximab, and its mutated form is associated with neurofibromatosis (not colorectal cancer).

56. D Ultraviolet (UV) radiation in sunlight most commonly causes the formation of pyrimidine dimers.

A Depurination is typically a spontaneous type of mutation, but it can also be caused by free-radical damage. Although UV light can generate free radicals, the primary damage caused by UV light is the formation of pyrimidine dimers.

B Intrastrand cross-links are generated by the reaction of DNA with specific chemical agents known as cross-linking agents (e.g., nitrogen mustard, cisplatin, mitomycin C, and carmustine). Although they are mutagenic themselves, many cross-linking agents are used as antineoplastic drugs.

C Double-strand breaks are typically caused by high-energy ionizing radiation. Although a person at the beach will be exposed to some ionizing radiation from cosmic rays, the DNA damage produced is negligible compared with the generation of pyrimidine dimers from UV light exposure.

E The addition of alkyl groups to DNA requires exposure to alkylating agents such as dimethyl sulfate (DMS) and methylmethane sulfonate (MMS). The primary damage caused by UV light is the formation of pyrimidine dimers.

57. C A CCA sequence is added to the 3′ end of tRNAs following their synthesis. Post-transcriptional modification of tRNA includes the isomerization of uridine into the atypical base psuedouridine. Psudeouridine is most commonly located within the T-psi-C loop of the tRNA. RNA polymerase III synthesizes small RNAs such as tRNA, 5S rRNA, and others, including U6 small nuclear RNA (snRNA) and small cytoplasmic RNA (scRNA).

A RNA polymerase I synthesizes a single large precursor 45S ribosomal RNA (rRNA), which is cleaved into three fragments to form the mature 28S, 18S, and 5.8S rRNAs.

B RNA polymerase II synthesizes mRNA in eukaryotic cells.

D DNA polymerase α extends RNA primers to ~25 nucleotides.

E DNA polymerase δ is responsible for DNA synthesis during replication of the genome.

58. C Overexpression of BCL-2 would prevent the cleavage of caspase-9 into its active form. Thus, G3139 may be deemed effective if its use results in an increase in the cleaved form of caspase-9.

A If treatment of cells with G3139 was successful at inhibiting BCL-2 expression, then apoptosis would occur, and one would observe reorganization of the cytoskeleton.

B. Decreased expression of BCL-2 would increase the cleavage of caspase-3, -6, and -7.

D Because G3139 is an antisense oligonucleotide aimed at inhibiting BCL-2 expression, one would expect BCL-2 mRNA levels to decrease (not increase). However, a decrease in BCL-2 RNA expression is not solid proof that the antiapoptotic effects of elevated BCL-2 have been overcome.

E Cells that undergo apoptosis shrink and condense. Those that undergo necrosis swell and burst. Therefore, if G3139 were to overcome the antiapoptotic effects of elevated BCL-2, then there would be an increase in the number of cells that shrink and condense.

59. C Reverse transcriptase is an RNA-dependent DNA polymerase that copies the retrovirus's RNA genome into complementary DNA (cDNA). This enzyme action is inhibited by the chain terminator, azidothymidine (AZT).

A DNA polymerase δ is a DNA-dependent DNA polymerase that copies the host genome. It does not participate in the conversion of the RNA genome of HIV into DNA.

B Poly(A) polymerase adds 50 to 250 adenosine residues to the 3′ end of mRNA in eukaryotic cells. It does not participate in the conversion of the RNA genome of HIV into DNA.

D RNA polymerase II is a DNA-dependent RNA polymerase that synthesizes mRNA, some snRNAs, and micro RNAs (miRNAs) in eukaryotes. It does not participate in the conversion of the RNA genome of HIV into DNA.

E Telomerase is required for synthesizing DNA at the ends of linear chromosomes in eukaryotes. It is an RNA-dependent DNA polymerase, but it does not participate in the conversion of the RNA genome of HIV into DNA.

60. B Eukaryotic (80S) ribosomes are inhibited by cycloheximide, whereas prokaryotic (70S) ribosomes are not.

A Chloramphenicol inhibits prokaryotic (70S) but not eukaryotic (80S) ribosomes. It would not inhibit the protein synthesis activity in tube A.

C Erythromycin inhibits prokaryotic (70S) but not eukaryotic (80S) ribosomes. It would not inhibit the protein synthesis activity in tube A.

D Puromycin inhibits both prokaryotic (70S) and eukaryotic (80S) ribosomes. Therefore, it would not unambiguously identify the contents of tube A.

E Tetracycline inhibits prokaryotic (70S) but not eukaryotic (80S) ribosomes. It would not inhibit the protein synthesis activity in tube A.

61. D Nonsense mutations are those that result in the generation of a stop codon in place of an amino acid codon. When a stop codon is present in the A site of a ribosome, it leads to recruitment of release factor, which triggers peptidyl transfer-

ase to hydrolyze the ester bond between the peptide's C terminus and the tRNA in the P site.

A A transversion is the substitution of a purine for a pyrimidine, or vice versa. (e.g., C substituted by G; A substituted by T). However, without knowing the exact nucleotide substitution, it is impossible to determine what the effect on translation will be.

B A transition is the substitution of one pyrimidine for another or one purine for another. However, without knowing the exact nucleotide substitution, it is impossible to determine what the effect on translation will be.

C A missense mutation is when the codon is changed such that a different amino acid will be incorporated into the protein encoded by the mutated gene.

E Thymidine dimers can lead to nucleotide substitutions in DNA. However, without knowing the exact nucleotide substitution, it is impossible to determine what the effect on translation will be.

62. D Meningitis is a rare and very serious complication of tularemia, which is caused by *Francisella tularensis* infection. Antibiotic drugs inhibit protein translation in prokaryotes by interfering with the initiation, elongation, or translocation. Streptomycin binds to the 16S rRNA of the 30S subunit and distorts ribosome assembly to cause misreading of mRNA codons. Because chloramphenicol inhibits the elongation phase (by blocking peptidyl transferase activity), the two drugs inhibit different aspects of translation and are synergistic.

A Erythromycin inhibits protein synthesis at the elongation phase by binding to the 50S subunit and blocking translocation of the ribosome. Chloramphenicol also inhibits the elongation phase of translation.

B Puromycin inhibits the elongation phase of translation in both prokaryotes and eukaryotes. Puromycin's structure mimics the aminoacylated 3′ end of tyrosyl-tRNA^{Tyr} and can enter the A site and be incorporated into the growing peptide chain, serving as a chain terminator. Chloramphenicol also inhibits the elongation phase of translation.

C Tetracycline inhibits protein synthesis at the elongation phase by binding the 30S ribosomal subunit in bacteria and impedes access to the acceptor (A) site by amino acyl-tRNAs. Chloramphenicol also inhibits the elongation phase of translation.

E Cycloheximide is a potent inhibitor of eukaryotic translation and does so by inhibiting the elongation phase. Chloramphenicol also inhibits the elongation phase of translation.

63. B (A, C, D, E) Actinomycin D intercalates between successive G:C base pairs of the DNA double helix and prevents movement of RNA polymerase I and thus inhibits the elongation phase of transcription. Treatment of cells with actinomycin D results in the dissolution of nucleoli, the site of rRNA synthesis. RNA polymerase I is inhibited by doses of actinomycin D that are 50 to 100-fold lower than those needed to inhibit RNA polymerase II or III. RNA polymerase II transcribes mRNA and is inhibited only by high doses of actinomycin D. RNA polymerase III transcribes tRNA, 5S rRNA, and a few snRNA genes and is only inhibited by high doses of actinomycin D.

64. B Antibodies against small nuclear ribonucleoproteins (snRNPs)—the components of the RNA spliceosome, which splices out introns from pre-mRNA molecules and ligates the exons together to form functional mRNAs—are frequently found in the serum of patients with SLE.

A Although anti-DNA antibodies are commonly present in the serum of patients with SLE, antibodies directed against the proteins involved in DNA synthesis are not present.

C Antibodies against factors involved in protein synthesis (e.g., ribosomal proteins; initiation, elongation, and termination factors; aminoacyl-tRNA synthetases) have not been observed in patients with SLE.

D Antibodies against factors directly involved in RNA synthesis (e.g., RNA polymerase, transcription factors) have not been observed in patients with SLE.

E Antibodies against factors involved in DNA recombination have not been observed in patients with SLE.

65. C (A, B) Spontaneous deaminations and small, nondistorting alterations are repaired by base excision repair. Once an altered base is detected, the enzyme DNA glycosylase then hydrolyzes the N-glycosidic linkage to remove the altered base, leaving an abasic site. This AP site is recognized by an AP endonuclease, which cuts the phosphodiester linkage. The deoxyribose phosphate is removed by an AP lyase. The single strand break (SSB) is recognized by Poly ADP-ribose polymerase (PARP-1) which is activated by binding to the break site. PARP-1 builds a branched polymer of ADP-ribose on itself which recruits DNA polymerase β, X-ray cross-complementing protein-1 (XRCC1) and the associated DNA ligase III. PARP-1 dissociates and DNA polymerase β and DNA ligase then replace the excised base and seal the nick, respectively, to complete the repair.

D, E DNA polymerase ξ (polymerase I in the case of E. coli) functions in translesion synthesis of DNA during DNA repair.

66. B (C) A recent development in gene therapy is the ability to precisely edit specific target genes in order to either disable or correct a mutant gene. An example of such targeted editing is the use of CRISPR-Cas9 system which is derived from a bacterial defense mechanism against viral infections. CRISPR stands for clustered regularly interspaced short palindromic repeat sequences in DNA and Cas9 is a CRIPR-associated bacterial nuclease. The CRISPR tool is constructed using a guide RNA that complements the defective sequence of a target gene attached to the Cas9 nuclease. When the guide RNA hybridizes to the complementary DNA sequence, Cas9 cuts both strands of target gene. The cell tries to repair the double-strand break by the preferred but error-prone mechanism of nonhomologous end joining. However, NHEJ results in nonspecific insertions or deletions (Indel) of bases at the cut ends leading to the generation of a premature stop codon and the disabling of gene expression. If, on the other hand, the goal is to correct the mutated sequence in the target gene, a donor DNA with the correct base sequence is provided along with the CRISPR tool. The cell then repairs the double-strand break using homologous recombination mechanism and the defective gene is corrected. The safety and the lack of adverse off-target modifications of the genome for this technique are yet to be established.

A Telomerases use their built-in RNA template to fill in these hexameric repeat sequences at the shortened 5′ end of chromosomal DNA.

D Double-stranded complementary DNA (cDNA) is created in vitro from a mature mRNA template via the action of reverse transcriptase (an RNA-dependent DNA polymerase) and DNA polymerase.

E RNA polymerase I catalyzes the synthesis of a single large precursor rRNA (45S rRNA), which is cleaved after synthesis into three fragments to form the mature 28S, 18S, and 5.8S rRNAs.

References

[1] Sankaran VG, Ghazvinian R, Do R, et al. Exome sequencing identifies GATA1 mutations in Diamond-Blackfan anemia. J Clin Invest. 2012; 122(7):2439–2443

[2] Fry DW, Harvey PJ, Keller PR, et al. Specific inhibition of cyclin-dependent kinase 4/6 by PD 0332991 and associated antitumor activity in human tumor xenografts. Mol Cancer Ther. 2004; 3(11):1427–1438

[3] Tol J, Punt CJ. Monoclonal antibodies in the treatment of metastatic colorectal cancer: a review. Clin Ther. 2010; 32(3):437–453

Appendix: Normal Laboratory and Physical Exam Values

Test	Reference Ranges	
	Conventional Units	SI Conversions
Blood, Plasma, Serum		
Alanine aminotransferase (ALT), serum	8–20 U/L	8–20 U/L
Amylase, serum	25–125 U/L	25–125 U/L
Aspartate aminotransferase (AST), serum	8–20 U/L	8–20 U/L
Bilirubin, serum (adult) Total Direct	0.1–1.0 mg/dL 0.0–0.3 mg/dL	2–17 µmol/L 0–5 µmol/L
Calcium, serum (Ca^{2+})	8.4–10.2 mg/dL	2.1–2.8 mmol/L
Cholesterol, serum	Rec: < 200 mg/dL	<5.2 mmol/L
Cortisol, serum	8:00 AM: 5–23 µg/dL 4:00 PM: 3–15 µg/dL 8:00 PM: ≤ 50% of 8:00 AM	8:00 AM: 138–635 nmol/L 4:00 PM: 82–413 nmol/L 8:00 PM: Fraction of 8:00 AM is ≤ 0.50
Creatine kinase, serum	Male: 25–90 U/L Female: 10–70 U/L	Male: 25–90 U/L Female: 10–70 U/L
Creatinine, serum	0.6–1.2 mg/dL	53–106 µmol/L
Electrolytes, serum Bicarbonate (HCO_3) Chloride (Cl^-) Magnesium (Mg^{2+}) Potassium (K^+) Sodium (Na^+)	22–28 mEq/L 95–105 mEq/L 1.5–2.0 mEq/L 3.5–5.0 mEq/L 136–145 mEq/L	22–28 mmol/L 95–105 mmol/L 3.5–5.0 mmol/L 0.75–1.0 mmol/L 136–145 mmol/L
Estriol, total, serum (in pregnancy) 24–28 wks 32–36 wks 28–32 wks 36–40 wks	30–170 ng/mL 60–280 ng/mL 40–220 ng/mL 80–350 ng/mL	104–590 nmol/L 208–970 nmol/L 140–760 nmol/L 280–1210 nmol/L
Ferritin, serum	Male: 15–200 ng/mL Female: 12–150 ng/mL	Male: 15–200 µg/L Female:12–150 µg/L
Follicle-stimulating hormone, serum/plasma	Male: 4–25 mIU/mL Female: premenopause: 4–30 mIU/mL midcycle peak: 10–90 mIU/mL postmenopause: 40–250 mIU/mL	Male: 4–25 U/L Female: premenopause: 4–30 U/L midcycle peak: 10–90 U/L postmenopause: 40–250 U/L
Gases, arterial blood (room air) pH PCO_2 PO_2	7.35–7.45 33–45 mm Hg 75–105 mm Hg	[H^+] 36–44 nmol/L 4.4–5.9 kPa 10.0–14.0 kPa
Glucose, serum	Fasting: 70–110 mg/dL 2 hour postprandial: <120 mg/dL	Fasting: 3.8–6.1 mmol/L 2 hour postprandial: < 6.6 mmol/L
Growth hormone - arginine stimulation	Fasting: < 5 ng/mL Provocative stimuli: >7 ng/mL	Fasting: < 5 µg/L Provocative stimuli: > 7 µg/L
Immunoglobulins, serum IgA IgE IgG IgM	76–390 mg/dL 0–380 IU/mL 650–1500 mg/dL 40–345 mg/dL	0.76–3.90 g/L 0–380 kIU/L 6.5–15 g/L 0.4–3.45 g/L
Iron	50–170 µg/dL	9–30 µmol/L
Lactate dehydrogenase, serum	45–90 U/L	45–90 U/L

V

Table A.1 ▶ Normal Laboratory and Physical Exam Values (*continued*)

Test	Reference Ranges Conventional Units	SI Conversions
Luteinizing hormone, serum/plasma	Male: 6–23 mIU/mL Female: follicular phase: 5–30 mIU/mL midcycle: 75–150 mIU/mL postmenopause: 30–200 mIU/mL	Male: 6–23 U/L Female: follicular phase: 5–30 U/L midcycle: 75–150 U/L postmenopause: 30–200 U/L
Osmolality, serum	275–295 mOsmol/kg H_2O	275–295 mOsmol/kg H_2O
Parathyroid hormone, serum, N-terminal	230–630 pg/mL	230–630 ng/L
Phosphatase (alkaline), serum (p-NPP at 30°C)	20–70 U/L	20–70 U/L
Phosphorus (inorganic), serum	3.0–4.5 mg/dL	1.0–1.5 mmol/L
Prolactin, serum (hPRL)	<20 ng/mL	<20 µg/L
Proteins, serum Total (recumbent) Albumin Globulin	 6.0–7.8 g/dL 3.5–5.5 g/dL 2.3–3.5 g/dL	 60–78 g/L 35–55 g/L 23–35 g/L
Thyroid-stimulating hormone, serum or plasma	0.5–5.0 µU/mL	0.5–5.0 mU/L
Thyroidal iodine (123I) uptake	8–30% of administered dose/24 hour	0.08–0.30/24 hour
Thyroxine (T4), serum	5–12 µg/dL	64–155 nmol/L
Triglycerides, serum	35–160 mg/dL	0.4–1.81 mmol/L
Triiodothyronine (T3), serum (RIA)	115–190 ng/dL	1.8–2.9 nmol/L
Triiodothyronine (T3) resin uptake	25–35%	0.25–0.35
Urea nitrogen, serum (BUN)	7–18 mg/dL	1.2–3.0 mmol urea/L
Uric acid, serum	3.0–8.2 mg/dL	0.18–0.48 mmol/L
Cerebrospinal Fluid		
Cell count	0–5 cells/mm^3	0–5 × 106 cells/L
Chloride	118–132 mEq/L	118–132 mmol/L
Gamma globulin	3–12% total proteins	0.03–0.12
Glucose	40–70 mg/dL	2.2–3.9 mmol/L
Pressure	70–180 mm H_2O	70–180 mm H_2O
Proteins, total	<40 mg/dL	<0.40 g/L
Hematology		
Bleeding time (template)	2–7 minute	2–7 minute
Erythrocyte count	Male: 4.3–5.9 million cells/mm^3 Female: 3.5–5.5 million cells/mm^3	Male: 4.3–5.9 × 1012/L Female: 3.5–5.5 × 1012/L
Erythrocyte sedimentation rate (Westergren)	Male: 0–15 mm/hr Female: 0–20 mm/hr	0–15 mm/hr 0–20 mm/hr
Hematocrit	Male: 41–53% Female: 36–46%	0.41–0.53 0.36–0.46
Hemoglobin A1c	≤6%	≤0.06
Hemoglobin, blood (Hb)	Male: 13.5–17.5 g/dL Female: 12.0–16.0 g/dL	2.09–2.71 mmol/L 1.86–2.48 mmol/L
Hemoglobin, plasma	1–4 mg/dL	0.16–0.62 mmol/L
Leukocyte count and differential Leukocyte count Segmented neutrophils Bands Eosinophils Basophils Lymphocytes Monocytes	 4,500–11,000 cells/mm^3 54–62% 3–5% 1–3% 0–0.75% 25–33% 3–7%	 4.5–11.0 × 109 cells/L 0.54–0.62 0.03–0.05 0.01–0.03 0–0.0075 0.25–0.33 0.03–0.07

Table A.1 ▶ Normal Laboratory and Physical Exam Values (*continued*)

	Reference Ranges	
Test	**Conventional Units**	**SI Conversions**
Mean corpuscular hemoglobin (MCH)	25.4–34.6 pg/cell	0.39–0.54 fmol/cell
Mean corpuscular hemoglobin concentration (MCHC)	31–36% Hb/cell	4.81–5.58 mmol Hb/L
Mean corpuscular volume	80–100 μm^3	80–100 fL
Partial thromboplastin time (activated) (aPTT)	25–40 second	25–40 seconds
Platelet count	150,000–400,000 cells/mm^3	150–400 × 10^9 cells/L
Prothrombin time	11–15 second	11–15 seconds
Reticulocyte count	0.5–1.5% of red cells	0.005–0.015
Thrombin time	<2 second deviation from control	<2 second deviation from control
Volume Plasma	Male: 25–43 mL/kg Female: 28–45 mL/kg	Male: 0.025–0.043 L/kg Female: 0.028–0.045 L/kg
Red cells	Male: 20–36 mL/kg Female: 19–31 mL/kg	Male: 0.020–0.036 L/kg Female: 0.019–0.031 L/kg
Physical Exam		
Body mass index (BMI)	Adult: 19–25 kg/m^2	
Sweat		
Chloride	0–35 mmol/L	0–35 mmol/L
Urine		
Calcium	100–300 mg/24 hour	2.5–7.5 mmol/24 hour
Creatinine clearance	Male: 97–137 mL/min Female: 88–128 mL/min	
Estriol, total (in pregnancy) 30 wks 35 wks 40 wks	6–18 mg/24 hour 9–28 mg/24 hour 13–42 mg/24 hour	21–62 μmol/24 hour 31–97 μmol/24 hour 45–146 μmol/24 hour
17-Hydroxycorticosteroids	Male: 3.0–10.0 mg/24 hour Female: 2.0–8.0 mg/24 hour	8.2–27.6 μmol/24 hour 5.5–22.0 μmol/24 hour
17-Ketosteroids, total	Male: 8–20 mg/24 hour Female: 6–15 mg/24 hour	28–70 μmol/24 hour 21–52 μmol/24 hour
Osmolality	50–1400 mOsmol/kg H_2O	
Oxalate	8–40 μg/mL	90–445 μmol/L
Proteins, total	<150 mg/24 hour	<0.15 g/24 hour

Index

Note: Page numbers in **bold** refer to boxes and *italics* refer to figures.